A history of surgery

DANIEL DE MOULIN
Institute for the History of Medicine,
Catholic University, Nijmegen, The Netherlands

A history of surgery

with emphasis on the Netherlands

1988 **MARTINUS NIJHOFF PUBLISHERS**
a member of the KLUWER ACADEMIC PUBLISHERS GROUP
DORDRECHT / BOSTON / LANCASTER

Distributors

for the United States and Canada: Kluwer Academic Publishers, P.O. Box 358, Accord Station, Hingham, MA 02018-0358, USA
for the UK and Ireland: Kluwer Academic Publishers, MTP Press Limited, Falcon House, Queen Square, Lancaster LA1 1RN, UK
for all other countries: Kluwer Academic Publishers Group, Distribution Center, P.O. Box 322, 3300 AH Dordrecht, The Netherlands

Library of Congress Cataloging in Publication Data

Moulin, Daniel de.
A history of surgery.

Bibliography: p.
1. Surgery--History. 2. Surgery--Netherlands--Surgery. I. Title. [DNLM: 1. Surgery--history--Netherlands. WO 11 GN4 M9h]
RD19.M67 1988 617'.09 87-22133

ISBN-13: 978-94-010-8008-8 e-ISBN-13: 978-94-009-3357-6
DOI: 10.1007/978-94-009-3357-6

Dedicated to the Association of Surgeons of the Netherlands on the occasion of its 85th anniversary

Table of Contents

CHAPTER 2: THE WESTERN MIDDLE AGES

CHAPTER 3: THE RENAISSANCE

CHAPTER 4: THE GOLDEN AGE

CHAPTER 5: THE AGE OF ENLIGHTENMENT

CHAPTER 6: PRACTICAL SURGERY IN THE 17TH AND 18TH CENTURIES

CHAPTER 7: THE BEGINNING OF MODERN SURGERY

CHAPTER 8: ANTISEPSIS: A TURNING POINT IN SURGERY

CHAPTER 9: THE GERMAN PERIOD IN DUTCH SURGERY

CHAPTER 10: SURGERY IN THE PAST 75 YEARS

Introduction

Surgery as a medical discipline has from its beginnings appealed to the imagination of many. It is therefore not surprising to find that its colourful past has induced quite a few authors to take up their pens.

The truth of this in the Netherlands is witnessed by a number of dissertations and monographs and especially by the numerous articles related to the history of surgery which have appeared in the medical weekly *Nederlands Tijdschrift voor Geneeskunde*, particularly during the two decades preceding the Second World War.

The memorial volume, published in 1977 by the 'Nederlandse Vereniging voor Heelkunde' (Association of Surgeons of the Netherlands) has thoroughly covered the history of Dutch surgery since the turn of the century, but a chronological survey of the earlier events which led to these modern achievements is still wanting.

This book has been written with a view to meeting this need. In it, Dutch surgery has by no means been taken as an isolated phenomenon, but considered in its context with European surgery as a whole. Foreign influences on the Netherlands and, conversely, Dutch influences on surgery abroad are discussed whilst contemporary medical thinking is set against a cultural and political background. It is hoped that this approach will allow the book to exceed the narrow boundaries of 'campanilismo' and make it of interest to non-Dutch readers as well.

It is aimed primarily at practising surgeons and physicians in Holland and elsewhere, although it is hoped that it will be of some interest to medical historians and also to the public at large.

The history of surgery in the Low Countries begins in the fourteenth century with the appearance of surgical treatises in a Flemish dialect, together with Middle Dutch translations of texts of the Italian school and the manuals of the great French surgeons of the time.

Since the medical and surgical literature of the Western Middle Ages is founded on the writings of Greek and Roman Antiquity, some knowledge of the classical sources is indispensable for a proper understanding of surgery as it first made its appearance in our medical heritage. It was therefore necessary, by way of introduction, to summarize in the first chapter the major works of classical surgical literature and to describe the routes and byways via which they became available to Northwest Europe.

The arrangement of the subject matter is largely chronological. Instead of attempting the impossible task of a fully comprehensive description of the evolution of all practical surgery, we will restrict our attention mainly to a representative selection of developing surgical techniques. In the course of Chapters 1 to 7, these will include the treatment of wounds, fractures and joint injuries, head injuries, tumours and herniae, with amputations and lithotomy as examples of major surgery.

In order not to burden still further the already heavily laden lists of annotations, we have abstained from documenting such well-known facts and biographical details as may be found in general histories, of which a number have been included in our bibliography. This also applies to cultural and political information of a general nature.

This book could not possibly have been written without the support of others. First of all I have to mention the help of my good-humoured secretary Ms Marian Poulissen, who not only took upon herself the tedious task of styling the text but also showed herself to be a capable research assistant. Professor Ria Jansen-Sieben of Brussels supplied me with important details on the Middle Ages for which I am sincerely grateful. My thanks are also due to my translators Drs. V. Piket and Drs. C. van Heertum (chapters 1, 2 and 5) and Mrs. J. Abma-Hill (chapters 3, 4, 7, 8) at Nijmegen and Drs. J. Klerkx (chapters 9 and 10) at Maastricht: a text like the one before us is none too easy to turn into a foreign language.

I am under a special debt to my good friend Dr. John Cule, emeritus professor of medical history at the University of Wales College of Medicine for his careful revision of the semi-finished text: I feel sure that the final product benefitted greatly from his many thoughtful remarks and suggestions. Any remaining linguistic singularities are entirely my own responsibility since I could not always resist the urge to make last-minute amendments.

There are numerous libraries and museums in this country and abroad from which I derived my source material. I thank them all sincerely, in particular the Library of the Royal Dutch Medical Association, incorporated in the University Library of Amsterdam, where Mr. W. K. Gnirrep spared no efforts to help me out, and the library of the Medical Faculty at Nijmegen. In Nijmegen I have also to thank the very cooperative staff of the Photographic Service of the Faculty of Medicine and Dentistry.

I gratefully acknowledge the financial support from the Association of Surgeons in the Netherlands, 'the Stichting Prof. Michaël-van Vloten Fonds' at The Hague and the St. Cosmas and Damian Foundation at Nijmegen.

Last but not least I wish to express my feelings of gratitude to my wife for her continuous encouragement and support in many ways.

Professor of Medical History
Institute for the History of Medicine
Catholic University Nijmegen

D. DE MOULIN

List of Illustrations

CHAPTER 1

The Roots of Western Surgery

1.1. ANTIQUITY

1.1.1. *Greece*

1.1.1.1. Cultural Setting

The tourist who today climbs the Acropolis in Athens and walks over the sacred road through the Propylaea, finds himself confronted with the Parthenon which, with its unmatched proportions, forms the peak of Hellenic architecture. The Parthenon was once a temple dedicated to the virgin Athena, patroness of all the arts, sciences and crafts and goddess not only of the art of war but also of wisdom. This temple and the adjoining Erechtheion were built in the fifth century B.C., the century of the astonishing Golden Age of Greek cultural history. It produced such minds as the statesman Pericles, the philosophers Socrates, Plato, Xenophon and Protagoras, the tragedians Sophocles, Euripides and Aeschylos, the comedy dramatist Aristophanes, the sculptors Phidias, Praxiteles and Polyclitus, and the historians Herodotus and Thucydides. It was, moreover, the age of the physician Hippocrates (Fig. 1). Hippocrates is often called the Father of Medicine, but considering the high level of maturity of the medicine which he represents, Hippocrates cannot possibly have stood at the beginning of that discipline.

1.1.1.2. Hippocrates

Hippocrates (c. 460—c. 377 B.C.) was born on the isle of Cos facing the coast of Asia Minor. Little else is known about his life save that he seems to have travelled extensively and emerges as the important representative of the famous medical school of his native island. Today the tourist is still directed to the plane tree, in the shade of which Hippocrates is said to have taught his pupils. Both Plato and Aristotle testify to his great reputation as a clinician. His fame for posterity is due to the collection of medical writings, exceeding sixty, attributed to him. This *Corpus Hippocraticum* forms the basis of Western medical literature. In it are discussed numerous aspects of theoretical and clinical medicine. That not all of these treatises can possibly have been written by Hippocrates, is no matter of concern here. Whoever wrote them, they reflect the state of medicine in the fifth century B.C.

An important aspect of these works is that they are free from theurgic beliefs.

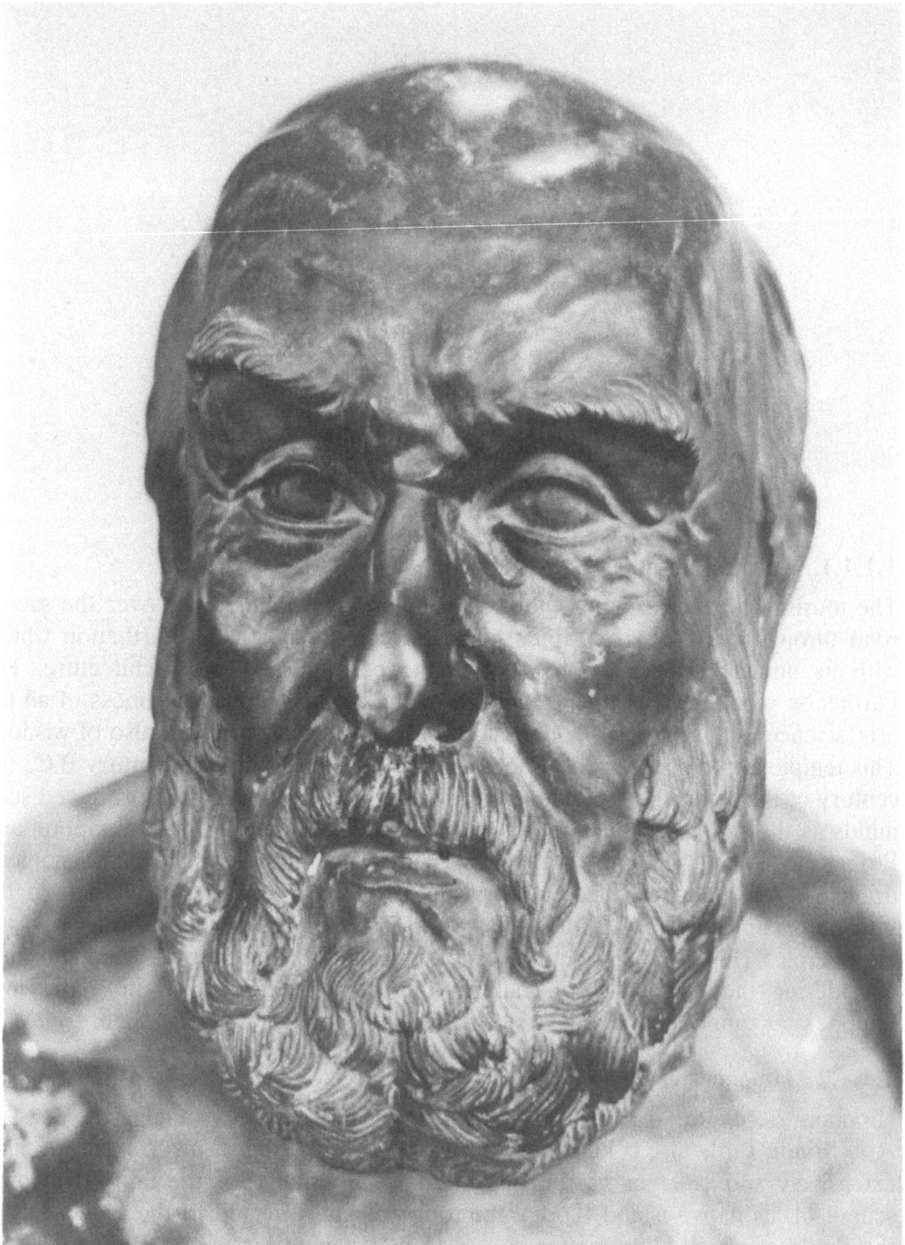

Fig. 1. Hippocrates. Bronze bust by the Dutch sculptor Oswald Wenckebach, in the possession of the Royal Dutch Medical Association.

The theoretical foundation of classical medicine consisted of the humoral pathology, which will be considered briefly when we come to Galen. It is in the Galenic adaptation the Hippocratic humoral pathology had such an overriding influence on Western medicine.

Hippocrates' medical practice was characterized by a careful bed side observation. His therapy was expectant and cautious. Because of this, and because of the high ethical notions which are reflected again and again in his works, Hippocrates has become the epitome of the ideal physician through the centuries.

1.1.1.3. Surgery in the Corpus Hippocraticum

The surgical sections are undoubtedly amongst the best work of the Hippocratic corpus. They must be the product of a long process of endeavour. Much material relating to surgery is also to be found in the non-surgical texts, indicating that internal medicine and surgery were not yet separate disciplines. Indeed, the Hippocratic physician was both physician and surgeon. On account of his using his hands in his work he was classed with the craftsmen.

Wound treatment is mainly discussed in the book *De ulceribus.*[1] The description is not always uniformly clear, which is partly due to the fact that the Greek word 'helkos', here translated as 'ulcus', can mean 'wound' as well as 'ulcer'. Since the formation of a small amount of pus in fresh wounds was apparently regarded as unavoidable, it was of prime importance to bring about such suppuration as quickly as possible and to see to it that the matter could escape freely. One should be careful, however, not to generate more pus than was necessary and the use of irritating medicaments was therefore to be avoided. The wound should in fact not be wetted at all except with wine: 'for the dry is nearer to the sound and the wet to the unsound, since a wound is wet, but a sound part is dry', was the guiding principle of the Hippocratic surgeons. Moderate suppuration should be looked upon as a normal stage in the healing process and not as a sign of inflammation, with which Hippocrates' translator Francis Adams in 1849 still agreed.[2] Hippocrates was well aware of inflammation as a pathological condition, but he did not state precisely what he understood by it. He confined himself to the remark that the wounded part becomes inflamed when rigor and throbbing supervene at the moment suppuration is about to take place.[3] Pus was evidently thought to play a part in cleansing the wound. Its generation therefore should be particularly promoted in contused wounds: the bruised and tattered flesh would melt away by becoming putrid and being converted into pus. Hippocrates assumed that pus was nothing else but vitiated blood — 'a wound suppurates when the blood is changed and becomes heated' — a view which was held until well into the nineteenth century and considered too evident to require much argument. On various occasions he wrote that the most favourable pus was white and smooth, uniform and not offensive to the smell, while pus of the opposite character was the worst.[4] For further treatment it was recommended that fresh wounds be covered with a dry rather than a wet sponge and that plenty of leaves be bandaged over it. Overhanging skin edges should be cut away. Emollients and oily substances should not be applied until healing was well on its way.

Slowly healing and putrid ulcers should be treated by cataplasms prepared according to prescriptions offered by our author.[5] For the healing, giving rest to the wounded part, a sparse diet with water as the only beverage and gentle purging were considered essential, but no reference was made to venesection. Suturing was only mentioned in passing without providing any technical details: Hippocrates either preferred healing by second intention or he thought the procedure too well known to describe in detail.

Although Hippocrates did not specify the difference between arterial and venous haemorrhage, he would undoubtedly have known the one from the other. It was probably first put into words by the Cnidian physician Euryphon, his older contemporary.[6] Vascular ligature was as yet unknown in the days of Hippocrates. Hippocratic surgeons tried to effect haemostasis by the elevation of the limb, by cold applications or compresses wetted in wine. They also used a choice of styptic medicines and, for exceptional cases, the red-hot iron. However, one should make no great haste in staunching the bleeding, for an abundant flow of blood would prevent inflammation by leaving the wound in a drier state. This advice, too, was well adhered to until the middle of the last century.

The wound treatment recommended by Hippocrates is somewhat ambiguous: the wound should be kept dry, yet the formation of moderate suppuration encouraged. This explains why in later centuries an appeal could be made to Hippocrates by both the proponents of wound treatment aimed at primary union and those in favour of healing by suppuration. Wound complications like erysipelas and tetanus were well-known at the time. Later in this book we will have occasion to observe that from Albucasis onwards, undesirable developments in wound healing were attributed to a nefarious influence of the air. Hippocrates does not appear to have subscribed to this view. Yet, in his treatise *Nature of Man*, he attributes the outbreak of epidemics to such an influence.[7] It is said that during the so-called plague of Athens, described by Thucydides, he ordered big fires to be lit in the streets to purify the atmosphere (Fig. 2).[8]

The survey below of the surgery of Hippocrates is compiled from a number of different books in the collection. The order 'from head to toe' is followed here, because it was the sequence common to the mediaeval and later surgical textbooks.

Traumatology of the head is given a great deal of attention, and even forms the subject of a separate book, *De capitis vulneribus*.[9] This remained an authoritative text until well into the eighteenth century, while in the seventeenth century a separate Dutch translation went through several editions. The author distinguishes five different kinds of injuries involving the skull: the simple fracture or fissure, the contusion without fracture, the depressed fracture, the indentation by a weapon, the counter fissure.[10] Hippocrates was aware of the fact that skull injuries could lead to contralateral convulsions. Neither was he unfamiliar with the clinical manifestations of concussion of the brain. He elaborately describes the way in which the wounded head ought to be examined, directing attention to the danger of mistaking the sutures for fissures. The use of the probe should be avoided if possible. When the skin wound does not afford a sufficient view of the cranium, one must not hesitate to enlarge it. If there exists any doubt about the presence or the depth of a fracture, one can pour a black liquid into the wound, wash it out the next day, after which a fracture will show as a black line. By means of the raspatory it is possible, while chafing, to determine how deep the fracture is. When a fracture cannot be made to disappear by scraping, the injury is a case for trepanation.

In the case of fractures and contusions early operative treatment is indicated.

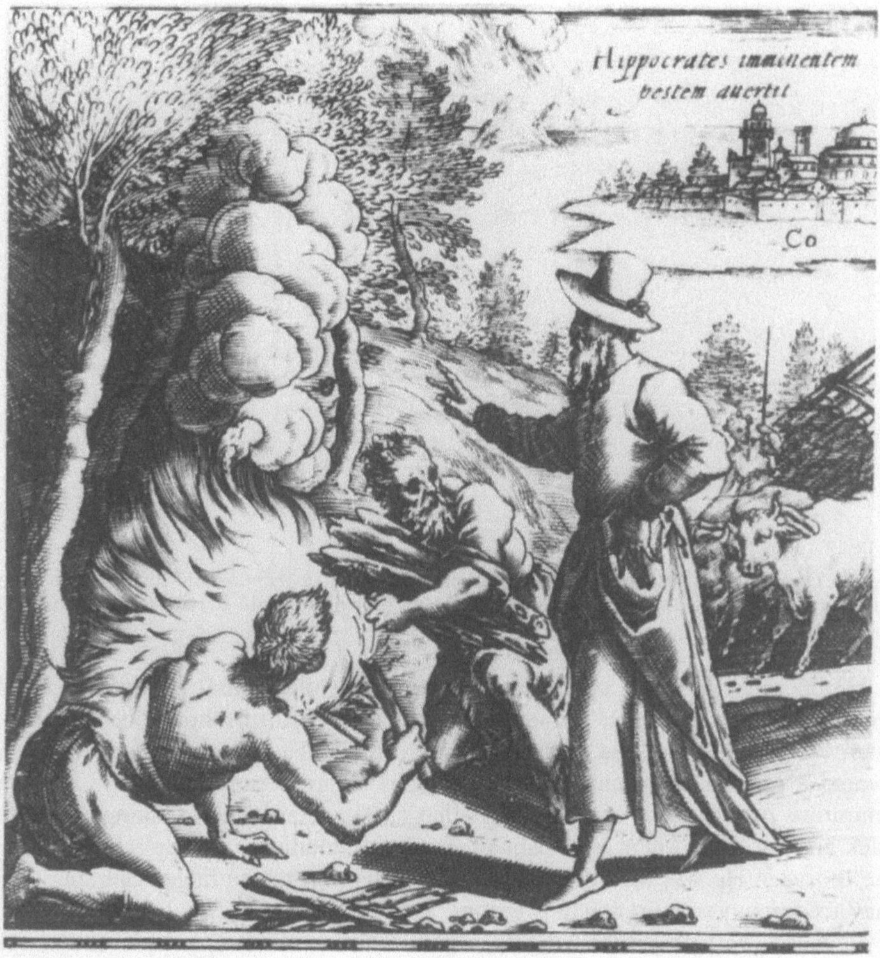

Fig. 2. Hippocrates purifies the infective air by burning fires during the plague of Athens.

The idea was to afford an issue to extravasated blood collected within the cranium.[11] Hippocrates provides careful, practical instructions for the technique of trepanation (Fig. 3). In cases of depressed fractures one should never proceed with this operation, but remove the loose fragments after a few days, when granulations have appeared. The lesion will granulate the faster as one succeeds in bringing about suppuration at an early stage, and so cause the cranial wound to cleanse itself.

As far as prognosis is concerned, he notes it will be less favourable when fever develops, the wound loses its colour and the bone becomes necrotic. If trepanation has not been performed by this stage, it is then urgently required. When treating head injuries the use of liquid substances is proscribed, even wine is not recommended. The best course to take is to fill the wound with lint and to apply a dry dressing.

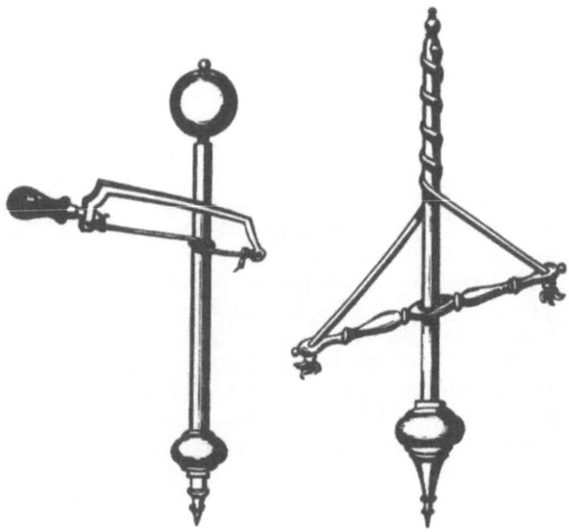

A B

Fig. 3. Trepanation instruments as they may have appeared in Hippocratic times. *A*: the *auger*, which is wound by means of a bow. *B*: the *terebra*, which is wound by means of a thong on a crossbeam.

Hippocrates does not shrink from removing swollen nasal polyps and cutting ulcerated tonsils.[12] In cases of pleural empyema he performs thoracocentesis via an intercostal incision or via trepanation of a rib.[13] He has apparently seen and treated a great many such cases: he provides a fine description of the signs and symptoms including the several noises that can be heard when shaking the patient back and forth, or when, by means of direct auscultation, one applies one's ear to the thorax.[14] He was also the first to draw attention to the finger clubbing which may accompany suppurating lung lesions.[15]

In dealing with abdominal surgery, Hippocrates mentions opening liver abscesses with the red-hot iron. Injuries of the gastrointestinal tract were invariably fatal in those days, Hippocrates does not seem to have performed intestinal suture. He is very familiar with the syndrome of ileus, which he treats with enemas or blowing in air via the rectum.[16] His description of the facies of patients whose acute diseases have taken a turn for the worse is well known: 'nose sharp, eyes hollow, temples' sunken, ears cold and contracted with their lobes turned outwards, the skin about the face hard, tense and parched, the colour of the face as a whole being yellow or very dark'.[17]

The signs and symptoms of several urological disorders are described in detail. He devotes particular attention to the bladder stone, a condition which he ascribes to the quality of the drinking water.[18] The treatment must be operative, although he himself would not undertake it: neither does he discuss any details of its technique. In the famous *Oath*, which still today is the basis of medical ethics, he declares: 'I will not use the knife on sufferers from stone, but I will leave it to such as are craftsmen therein'.[19] This sentence points to the existence of specialized lithotomists in ancient Greece, but nothing further is known about them.

Hippocrates treats perianal fistulae and haemorrhoids by means of ligature and cautery. That they were common in his day can be judged by the fact that each complaint is represented by a separate text in the Hippocratic collection.

Hippocrates' comments on herniae are strikingly few. He contents himself with the statement that they usually occur in the groin, but can also be found slightly above the navel. The latter may cause pain, nausea, and faecal vomiting. Herniae are caused either by a blow or by distention.[20] As he does not give any information on their treatment, it may have been left to specialized empirics as well. Ascitic fluid is tapped via a stab incision. Purulent inflammation of the hip joint is drained.

The treatment of fractures and dislocations reached a high level.[21] Reduction is carried out skilfully and thoughtfully, preferably on the same day. The rule is that 'in treating fractures and dislocations the physician must make the extension as straight as possible, for this is the most natural direction'. This admonition was heeded until the eighteenth century. Immobilization of the set fractures is accomplished by artfully applied bandages in several layers with compresses placed in between. Only after a week, when the oedema and the haematoma have subsided, are the splints applied, if necessary after repeated reduction. During tbe entire period of treatment the occurrence of any passive congestion, gangrene and pressure sores ought to be carefully watched. Fractures of the upper leg are very difficult to reduce, 'for the fleshy part is thick and powerful'. Yet one should try and prevent permanent shortening by all means, 'for the disgrace and harm are great if the result is a shortened leg'. Hippocrates uses long splints for their immobilization. Some surgeons tie the patient's foot to the end of the bed in case of fractures of the leg, probably in an attempt to exert continuous extension. Hippocrates does not consider this method to be of any use, because the body slides down 'and thus extension will not be maintained'.

It is advisable when dealing with compound fractures, to aim firstly at healing the wound, and to perform the reduction only when repair is well on its way. Sometimes it is necessary to make use of iron elevators when reducing open fractures. If subsequently convulsions develop, however, the patient is doomed.

Hippocrates also describes in detail the dislocation of large and small joints, and the ways in which they ought to be treated. Reduction of a shoulder luxation for instance, can be effected in several ways: by pulling on the affected arm while counter-pressure is being applied either by the surgeon's heel (Fig. 4), the surgeon's shoulder, a pole or the rung of a ladder placed in the axilla, or, particularly in old chronic cases, with the aid of a lever. This consisted of a narrow plank to which the arm was secured in extension. One end of the plank was put in the armpit under the head of the humerus. Then the arm was levered over a crossbar placed in the axilla (Fig. 49). Hippocrates treats recurrent dislocation of the shoulder joint with the cautery, the intention being to reduce flexibility in the skin of the armpit by means of the cicatrization which occurs after a burn.

He mistakes the fracture of the carpal extremity of the radius for a luxation. The ankle fracture was also wrongly regarded as a dislocation in Antiquity.

Curvature of the spine may be either spontaneous or result from trauma. Patients suffering from the first variety often cough and are short-winded, they may have hard tubercles in their lungs. This condition is incurable. The observa-

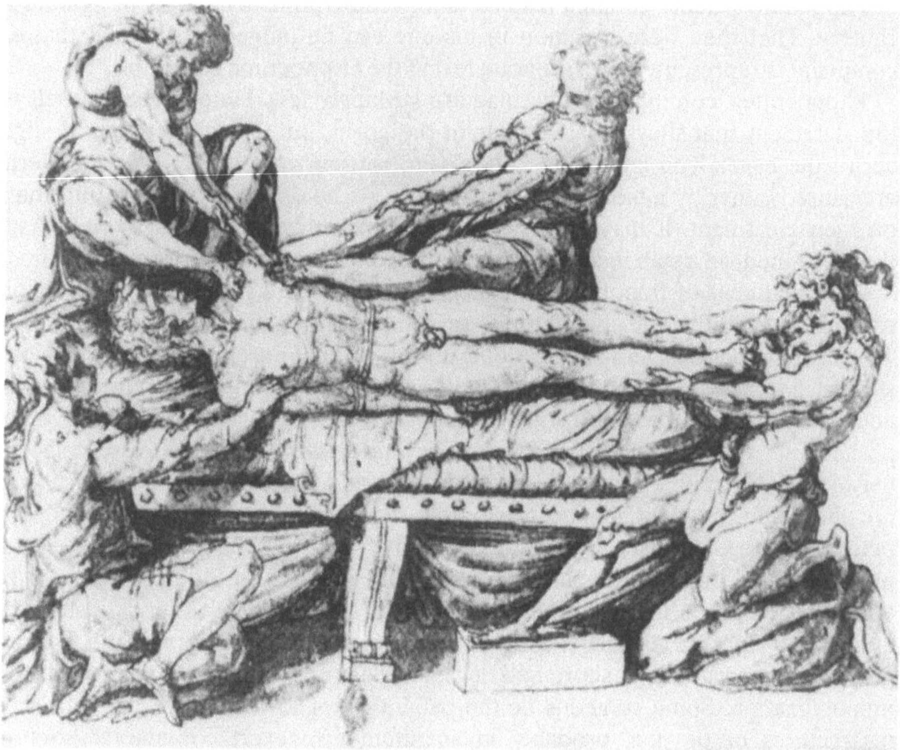

Fig. 4. Renaissance representation of the reduction of a dislocated shoulder joint, according to Hippocrates.

tion on an intrapulmonary lesion would seem to suggest that autopsies were carried out on the bodies of the deceased, although there is no further evidence of this in the writings ascribed to Hippocrates. If the kyphosis has been sustained by a fall, attempts at reduction may be made. The patient has to be placed face downward on a extension table thus mechanically enabling the surgeon to exert traction and countertraction in the longitudinal axis of the body, whilst at the same time exerting manual pressure on the prominent vertebrae. The neurological complaints which may accompany vertebral fractures were well-known at the time.

The extension equipment just mentioned, known ever since Galen as the scamnum of Hippocrates or the Hippocratic bench,[22] can also be used to advantage in the reduction of dislocations of the hip joint, four kinds of which are known and described by him. Particular attention is also paid to the clubfoot, which deformity he considers a congenital dislocation and of which he distinguishes several types.[23]

Amputations are only performed in cases of gangrene. In order to avoid bleeding, the division is made in the gangrenous area, preferably in a joint. For when one cuts in the living flesh, it will cause the patient such pain that he may lose consciousness. Collapses of this kind have brought sudden death to many.

Hippocrates prefers to adopt an expectant attitude, especially in the case of a compound fracture, and await a spontaneous shedding of the necrotic part. He does not mention the use of the saw in this connection, nor does he make any references to prostheses for the amputation patient.

The art of bandaging has reached a very advanced level in Hippocrates and is the main subject of the book *In the surgery*.[24]

As far as tumours are concerned, Hippocrates adopts a conservative attitude. The hidden, that is the not yet ulcerated carcinoma, is not treated by him at all, because an operation would shorten rather than lengthen the patient's lease of life.[25] Operative surgery was indeed considerably restricted in those days by the lack of reliable haemostatic means. Another obstacle was provided by the poor knowledge of anatomy — apart from osteology — which was based on information obtained by animal dissections; the opening of human bodies was not yet practised.

Hippocrates also supplies directions for the physician's consulting room, which must be spacious, airy and well-lit, as well as his armamentarium which must be simple and easy to clean. The physician must observe personal cleanliness and above all have clean nails. His diagnostic and technical skills must conform to certain standards. According to Hippocrates one is not a good doctor 'when one does not recognize pus in a wound or an abscess; when one is not able to insert the catheter into the bladder; when one fails to establish the presence of a stone in the bladder; when one fails to diagnose by concussion the presence of a pleural empyema; when one does not reach the required depth when cutting or burning, or when one cuts or burns where it is not necessary'.[26]

The best known book out of the entire Hippocratic corpus, however, is perhaps *Aphorisms*, a collection of pithy sayings relating to medical practice. They were probably meant to be learnt by rote by the pupils in an age when books were still too expensive to be purchased generally. Among these maxims there are quite a few relating to surgery. The best known aphorism is the last: 'Those diseases that medicines do not cure are cured by the knife. Those that the knife does not cure are cured by fire. Those that fire does not cure must be considered incurable'. In later ages the aphorisms repeatedly appeared in separate editions, in the Netherlands for instance they were printed several times in Latin and Greek in the seventeenth century.[27]

The Hippocratic collection of medical writings has exerted an enormous influence on medical thought for more than twenty centuries. Some of its books belong to the most widely read works of world literature. As late as 1790 the Amsterdam surgeon David van Gesscher published an annotated Dutch edition of the surgical books of Hippocrates which also appeared in German.[28] François Zacharias Ermerins, professor of medicine at Groningen, brought out an annotated Greek—Latin edition of the collected works in 1859—65, which was commissioned by the Royal Dutch Academy of Sciences. Even today medical terminology includes numerous terms and expressions which go back to the learned physician of Cos.

In conclusion we may state that the school of Hippocrates led conservative surgery to a height which was not always reached in later centuries. This applies in particular to traumatology, especially to injuries of the head and to fractures and dislocations. As far as bloody operations are concerned, Hippocratic surgery did not rise above the most elementary application of the knife.

1.1.2. *Hellenism*

1.1.2.1. Cultural Setting

The battle of Chaeronea in 338 B.C. put an end to the political independence of the Greek city-states which were now brought under the hegemony of Macedonia. The campaigns of conquest which the Macedonian king Alexander the Great (356—323 B.C.) undertook in Asia Minor, North Africa and the Near East, as a result of which entire realms, including those of Egypt and Persia, fell into his hands, strongly contributed to the dissemination of Greek language and culture. After Alexander's death his empire was divided amongst his military commanders or diadochi. Egypt came under the rule of a Greek-Macedonian dynasty, which descended from Alexander's general Ptolemy who had assumed the royal title. The Ptolemies spared no trouble or expense to turn their capital Alexandria into a centre of Hellenistic science and culture. For one they founded the famous academy of sciences, the so-called Museion, where scholars could devote themselves entirely to science at the expense of the state. The museum and the temple of the god Serapis held the richest libraries ever to have been collected in Antiquity, and at a one stage they together contained more than 700 000 book scrolls. It was allegedly in this city that the texts ascribed to Hippocrates were assembled in a *Corpus Hippocraticum.* Apart from libraries, there were in Alexandria laboratories, an observatory, and a botanical and zoological garden. The lighthouse was considered one of the Seven Wonders of the World. Amongst the scholars who were active in Alexandria were the mathematician Euclid, the mathematician and inventor Archimedes, and the geographer, astronomer and mathematician Ptolemy. From all over the then known world students travelled to Alexandria to attend the lectures which were given on a great number of subjects.

Medicine was an important branch of study. This ensued to no small extent from the fact that in Alexandria for the first time systematic anatomical research was conducted on human bodies, at least from the third century B.C. (Fig. 5). The blossoming of surgery in Alexandria may also be related to this. Religious strife was an important factor in determining the end of this period of cultural and scientific prosperity in the third century. In 642 the city was conquered by the Arabs.

We are familiar with the names of a great number of surgeons from the Alexandrian school, quoted by Celsus and Galen and other authors from the first centuries A.D. Unfortunately their writings have largely perished through the ensuing centuries, helped by the repeated fires in Alexandrian libraries which were the result of war and civilian strife. Only fragments of their works have been preserved in the large anthologies of the Byzantine encyclopaedists Oribasius (fourth century A.D.) and Aëtius (sixth century A.D.).[29] On the other hand one may wonder with Daremberg, to what degree the appearance of such compilatory works may have contributed to the loss of original texts.[30]

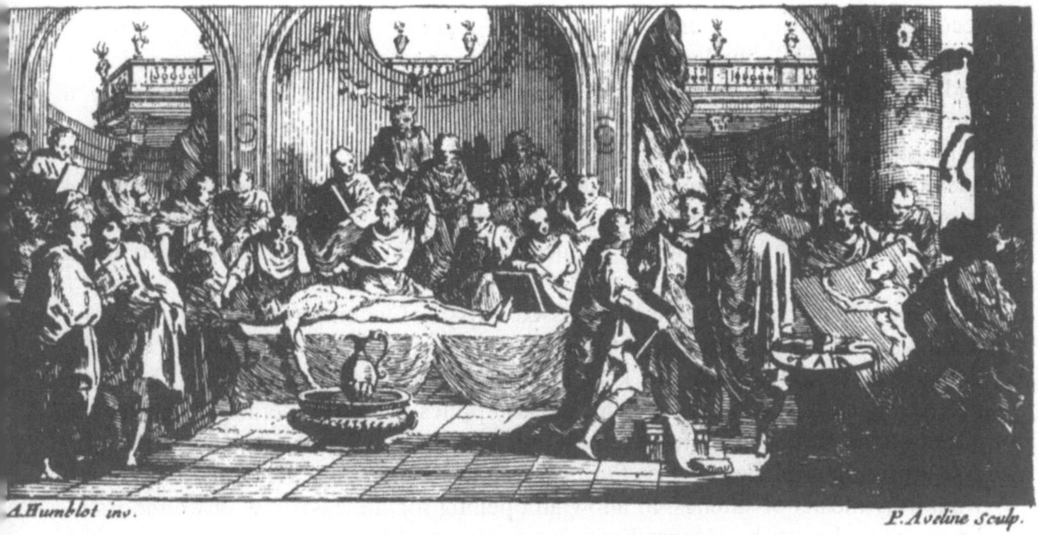

Fig. 5. Anatomical dissection at Alexandria in Hellenistic times.

1.1.2.2. Celsus

The state of Hellenistic surgery at the beginning of our era can be gathered from the work *De medicina* of the Roman encyclopaedist Aulus Cornelius Celsus, about whom nothing is known other than that he must have lived in the first century A.D. Considering the fact that he quotes more than 90 authors in his work, he must have been widely read. The book is not written in Greek, the scholarly language of Antiquity, but in Latin and as such may have been intended for a larger audience. It is, for that matter, written in superb Latin which is in no sense inferior to that of the best Roman literary authors. Its clear arrangement and its careful explanations make this book the best didactic work which classical medicine, which was largely a Greek affair, has to offer.

The work consists of eight books. The first book offers an historical introduction, a survey of contemporary medical schools and a discussion of the usefulness of a knowledge of anatomy for the physician. The anatomical knowledge of Celsus is still limited in our modern judgement, but nevertheless constitutes a notable advance over Hippocrates: the abdominal and thoracic organs appear to have become rather well-known by his time.

For our purpose book five and book seven are of particular importance.[31] The fifth book includes traumatology.[32] After having considered the effects of age, and constitution — which concept played no part in Hippocrates' thinking — the way of life and the time of the year on the healing of wounds, Celsus discusses in detail the symptoms which indicate injuries of the several thoracic and abdominal organs. He also elaborates on the various sorts of pus which may develop in a wound, together with their prognostic significance.[33] The linen vascular ligature is mentioned in the paragraph on haemostasis, together with tamponade, compression, the application of a vinegar bandage and the use of caustics. Celsus recommends leaving the ends of the thread uncut and hanging out of the wound, so that after a while the ligature, when it is loosened as a result of inflammation — and no longer of any use because the vessel has already been plugged by a thrombus — can be removed easily.[34] If the application of a vascular ligature is impossible, the red hot iron is the only remedy left. In the case of severe haemorrhages it may be useful to derivate the course of the blood by means of a cupping glass applied elsewhere on the body. Celsus believed with Hippocrates that the risk of inflammation is reduced by allowing the wound to bleed for a while.

Unlike Hippocrates, suture is discussed as part of wound treatment. This can be done with needle and thread, but also by means of a 'fibula': a pin passed through both edges of the wound and kept in place by a thread twisted round both the protruding ends in a figure of eight. Celsus applies the latter method whenever the edges of the wound cannot be closely approximated, in order to narrow the gap. As suture material Celsus uses thin wool. One should take care, when closing the wound by means of stitches, to allow an opening for the easy flow of wound issue. Every wound must be cleansed with a sponge wetted in vinegar or wine or, when these are not available, in cold water. It is certainly possible to heal a wound without the use of medicaments. Celsus does not in principle aim at the generation of pus but in his description of the further treatment he does give the impression that suppuration was the rule rather than the exception. Dressings must be applied in such a way that the wound edges approximate each other closely, although they must not be too tight. Like Hippocrates Celsus recommends rest for the afflicted part, and a meagre or even liquid diet. Celsus is familiar with wound complications such as inflammation, gangrene, erysipelas and tetanus. An old wound should be converted into a fresh one by excision of the edges, after which the same treatment is to be adopted as is indicated for recent wounds.

The seventh book is entirely devoted to surgical subjects. It opens with the following description:

> The third part of the Art of Medicine — next to dietetics[35] and the use of drugs — is that which cures by the hand . . . . The effects of this treatment are more obvious than any other kind; inasmuch that in diseases good fortune is of great help and it may be doubted whether recovery was due to medicine or a sound body or pure luck. . . . But in that part of medicine which cures by hand, it is obvious that all improvement chiefly comes from this, even if it is to be assisted somewhat in other ways.[36]

A little further on Celsus enumerates the requirements which a good surgeon must meet in the well-known passage:

> Now a surgeon should be youthful or at any rate nearer youth than old age; with a strong and steady hand which never trembles, and ready to use the left hand as well as the right; with vision sharp and clear, and spirit undaunted; filled with pity, so that he wishes to cure his patient, yet is not moved by his cries to go too fast, or cut less than is necessary; but he does everything just as if the cries of pain cause him no emotion.[37]

Of all that is dealt with in the seventh book, an anthology will be provided only of those subjects which are either not discussed at all by Hippocrates, or else very perfunctorily.[38] In this book one may find for example, the rib resection for thoracic fistula, the couching of cataracts, which Celsus was the first to describe in detail, as well as the treatment of numerous other eye diseases, and the sliding skin flap for covering certain superficial defects. The book also contains information on tonsillectomy and the treatment of goitre; Celsus regards the latter tumour entirely as a neoplasm, to which he gives the Greek name 'bronchocele'.[39] One treatment consists in the application of caustic agents to the skin which gradually attack the growth by eating away the skin and the subcutaneous parts. Celsus himself prefers the knife. The incision is made down to the tumour. The 'morbid pouch' is turned out with the finger and removed. Should this prove impossible, it is dusted with a caustic agent.

Unlike Hippocrates Celsus gives a great deal of attention to herniology. The umbilical hernia is treated surgically by reduction of the contents, then seizing the emptied protrusion at the base between two rods until it mortifies and drops off. It is also possible to encircle and close the base with a stitch ligature. Prior to discussing the aetiology and the therapy of the inguinal herniae, he provides an anatomical description of the contents of the scrotum. It consists of the testicles, each of which are suspended from the groin by means of a cord — Celsus speaks of 'nervus' — which the Greeks call 'cremaster' (suspender). He believes the testicles themselves to be insensible: that what hurts in cases of inflammation and trauma are the surrounding coverings. Veins and arteries run through the cremasters. They are ensheathed in a thin, white, bloodless tunic which the Greeks call 'elytroides' (tunica vaginalis), which is covered by a second, thicker tunic which the Greeks name 'dartos'.

A hernia is brought about by a rupture in these membranes, either as the result of an illness, or else a trauma. As these membranes also serve to separate the abdominal cavity from the scrotal pouch, their rupture will cause an intestinal loop or a tag of omentum to slip down into the scrotum under their own weight. The first eventuality is referred to as an enterocele, the second as an epiplocele. Celsus elaborately describes the signs whereby a hernia can be recognized, and how to differentiate between both types.[40] He also provides a fine description of the hydrocele, including the sign of translucency. This disorder is not caused by a rupture in the membranes.

In the case of ruptures in young children one can apply a bandage before resorting to the knife in the hope that the tunics become agglutinated together. A strangulated hernia — which he does not call by that name although he does describe the clinical symptoms — is inoperable. Treatment should consist of bloodletting, fasting, and immersion in a warm bath. In those cases of hernia which are suitable for operation — for which Celsus fails to give the precise criteria — an incision should be made in the groin down to the middle tunic (the elytroides?). This has to be split open. If the patient is a stout man, the surgeon puts the left index finger in the split, forces the testicle up into the wound and separates the blood vessels and nerve from the surrounding membranes. The middle tunic is cut away and the testicle replaced. Finally a strip has to be pared from the wound edges in the groin so that the wound, which apparently has to heal by second intention, will form a broader scar. In the case of an epiplocele featuring a sizeable mass of omentum, it will be exposed in the manner described above, and left to hang out of the wound until it mortifies and drops off.

It cannot be accurately gathered from these descriptions what exactly takes place. The operation would appear to consist of the removal of the hernial sac. There is no reference to closing its neck by means of a ligature, as one might expect the surgeon to do. But it is evident, however, that the testis and the blood vessels are spared, and in this respect the method described by Celsus compares favourably with the operative treatment of Paul and of the Middle Ages, which involved a hemicastration.

In the case of penetrating abdominal injuries a perforation of the large intestine may be closed by suture. Although the result of the intestinal suture is dubious, it must nevertheless be attempted, 'quod dubia spes certa desperatione sit potior'.[41] This should be done as soon as possible, because the intestines are unaccustomed to exposure to outside air. There is no need to take much trouble over the small intestine, since its suture always proves to be unsuccessful. Unfortunately Celsus does not provide any details about the way in which the enterorrhaphy ought to be carried out. The protruding intestines are returned, after which the patient is gently shaken to assure that they will fall back into their proper place. Abdominal wounds are closed using a running suture in two layers. For this Celsus uses a thread provided with a needle at each end. One needle is pushed from within outwards through each of the 'inner membranes' of both wound margins. When each margin has been traversed once, the needles cross to pass the thread through the inner membrane further down at the opposite side, once again from within outward and so on until the wound is closed. Using the same thread and needles, the skin is then closed by a similar procedure going back to the beginning.

That surgeons 2000 years ago were also confronted with the problem of varicose veins appears from a short but fine chapter. One can apply two principles in their treatment, either that of sclerotherapy — by means of the red-hot iron — or by excision.[42]

One of the most interesting parts of book seven is the clear description of lithotomy. Cutting for the stone had apparently been admitted to regular sugery in the course of the four hundred years which lapsed after Hippocrates had dissociated himself so emphatically from this procedure. The operation consists of the surgeon inserting his left index and middle fingers into the rectum of the patient, who lies on his back with his legs drawn up high, held down by a few strong men. While the right hand is placed on the hypogastrium to prevent the stone from slipping back to the fundus, the fingers of the left hand bring the stone down to the neck of the bladder, where it is fixed. Subsequently a semilunar incision is made to the left of the anus, the horns of which must point to the hip. Via a second incision, made at right angles to the first one, the soft parts underneath the skin are separated and the neck of the bladder is opened. A small stone can be expelled with the fingers which are still in the rectum, larger stones must be removed with a spoon specially constructed for the purpose. The wound is allowed to bleed for a while in order to prevent inflammation. In order to stop the bleeding the patient is seated in a hip bath filled with strong vinegar to which a little salt has been added. It may take as long as three months to a year before the urinary fistula, which perforce results from such an incision, has closed. The operation must preferably be performed when the patients — usually boys — are between nine and fourteen years old, and springtime is considered the most favourable season.

Book seven concludes with a chapter on amputation, which is indicated in cases of gangrene. Performed on a large extremity, it involves great risk because patients often die under the operation, either from loss of blood or syncope, a condition about which the author does not provide any details. It is of no use debating whether the remedy is safe enough, for unfortunately it is the only option open to the patients and their surgeons. Unlike Hippocrates, Celsus does not recommend performing the amputation through a joint; he makes the incision through healthy flesh. When the bone is reached, the muscles are detached from it over some distance and retracted by an assistant. After the bone is sawn through and the cutting-plane smoothed down, the soft parts are folded over the stump of the bone and arranged to cover it as far as possible. What cannot be covered with skin, is filled up with lint wetted in vinegar. The use of vascular ligature and skin sutures are not mentioned by Celsus in this context. The use of the saw and the amputation through healthy tissue is, however, an advance on the technique current in the days of Hippocrates.

The eighth and last book deals with fractures and dislocations, and is clearly inspired by the Hippocratic texts on these subjects. Unlike Hippocrates, Celsus recommends the refracturing of bones healed in an unsatisfactory position.

This small sample from the work of Celsus may suffice to demonstrate the considerable height reached by Hellenistic surgery in the first century A.D., making clear the advances made since Hippocrates. Oddly enough this excellent book, which must be included among the 'classics' of surgical literature, for centuries remained virtually unknown. Galen completely ignores it, and Oribasius is the only Byzantine encyclopaedist to quote him occasionally, and then usually without identifying his source. There are indications that the work of Celsus was available in the early Middle Ages, at least in Italy and in France where it was known in. Chartres and Rheims. But it had no effect whatsoever on the contemporary practice of surgery which, as will be seen, had in those days fallen to a very low level. The surgical writers of the late Middle Ages, including Jan Yperman and Thomas Scellinck, do not refer to him. But after the book's appearance in print in 1478, as one of the very first medical works ever to go to the press, its success was virtually unlimited. There were at least 60 Latin editions, of which a considerable number were produced in the Netherlands from the end of the fifteenth century onwards. It also appeared in a great many translations. The Leyden surgeon Trioen quoted Celsus with great appreciation as late as 1743, and even in 1832 the Amsterdam physician Pool published an anthology of the work of the ancient Roman author; an edition which was not intended as a historical monument!

1.1.2.3. Galen

Classical medicine reached a second peak in the person of Galen. Born in Pergamum around 130 A.D., this Greek studied philosophy and medicine in his native town and in several other Hellenistic centres of learning: Smyrna, Corinth and Alexandria. He lived and practised in Rome, where he acquired a considerable reputation. He was a prolific writer. Although a great number of his works are lost, the written legacy of Galen is more voluminous than that of any other author in the entire history of medicine. His publications are very versatile.

For his physiological and anatomical studies, he made use of live and dead experimental animals. Galen is even regarded as the founder of experimental physiology. The discoveries which he made in the two fields of these basic disciplines are numerous. Galen's anatomical and physiological concepts found universal acceptance until the sixteenth and seventeenth centuries. Unfortunately they contain not a few errors because the anatomical findings in animals were simply transposed to humans. His view on the movement of the blood in the body was only superseded by William Harvey's theory of the circulation of the blood after fierce academic debate.

Galenism

Galen's aim was to develop medicine into an exact science based on general theoretical foundations, in which anatomy and physiology, pathology, therapy and prophylaxis were each clearly defined. Although he was only partly successful in this impressive attempt, his synthesis nevertheless made such a marked impression on later generations, that for centuries Galenism as the theoretical foundation of medicine held a position of almost unquestioned authority.[43] This holds particularly true for the humoral pathology as further elaborated and refined by Galen.

Humoral Pathology

The four cosmic elements (earth, water, fire and air) out of which the universe is made up, are also to be found in the microcosm, i.e. the living creature, in the form of 'humours': blood, phlegm, yellow bile and black bile. These humours, which arise from different organs, namely the heart, the brain, the liver and the spleen, have the same features which characterize each of the cosmic elements. Two main qualities are attributed to each of the four humours. The qualities are linked to each other in pairs as in the four cosmic elements. The properties of the elements correspond with those of the humours. Both the air in the world around us, and the blood in our bodies have the qualities of being warm and moist; fire, the element, and yellow bile, the humour, have the properties of being warm and dry. As in the earth, the qualities coldness and dryness are found in black bile; as in water, the qualities coldness and moistness occur in phlegm.

These Aristotelian 'qualities' do not only represent actual physical concepts, but also have potential properties. Warmness not only refers to the physical heat of fire, but also includes the potential heat stored in peppercorns, and which can readily be experienced if one bites through one. Health, according to this theory, is a balanced condition of the qualities which are active in the body. Such a balance depends on a proper blending ('krasis' or 'temperament') of the humours. The physiological processes are activated and controlled by the intangible vital spirits or 'pneuma'. Generalized or local dominance of one of the cardinal humours would involve a general or localized preponderance of the associated qualities, and would lead to illnesses characterized by these qualities. But disease might also result from a decomposition or decay of any of the humours. No desire was apparently felt to express such humoral maladjustments in measure and number.

Therapy should in principle consist in expulsion of that humour, which in its excessive or decayed condition is responsible for the existing disorder. Apart from emetics, laxatives, and sudorifics, expulsion could be brought about by bleeding — to be discussed in greater detail below — cupping or the application of a setaceum or a vesicatory.[44] A second principle of treatment is that diseases are cured by their contraries — contraria contrariis —: cold by warmth for instance, or repletion by evacuation.

Such humoral pathological concepts — although with different emphases and several modifications — dominated medical thought far into the eighteenth century and even beyond: most enduring was the belief that 'fevers' were caused by decomposition of vital humours. For surgical pathology, which until the second half of the nineteenth century was largely confined to outwardly observable disorders, humoral pathology succeeded in providing explanations for the development of inflammations and tumours and for the formation of pus.

General Surgical Pathology

The following survey is largely derived from the excellent summaries by Adams from the Galenic books *Methodus medendi XIII* and *XIV* and the sequels *De tumoribus praeter naturam* and *Therapeutica ad Glauconem*, concerning Galen's views on aetiology and therapy of a number of common disorders.[45]

Phlegmon is a term which, in Galen's view, indicates either inflammations in general, or, more particularly, a red, firm, painful swelling. It is caused by an accumulation of *blood* of a good quality and moderate consistency. There are many causes, either external, such as contusion, fracture or dislocation, or internal ones. The latter are based on 'the veins being immoderately distended with humours, and the superfluity being cast off upon a part fitted to receive them at the time'. Such places are weaker or laxer than other parts of the body. When the blood is hot and thick, an abscess is probable. The treatment of phlegmon must always consist of direct or indirect evacuation; direct, by the application of cataplasms which are composed of medicines designed to repel the collected fluid, and indirect by venesection. Should the swelling fail to dissipate, but instead start generating pus, it must be opened to evacuate the matter. Pus, as he says elsewhere following Hippocrates, is the product of a change of blood under the influence of the inflammation.

Yellow bile is a particularly thin fluid which enables it to pass through the fleshy and thin parts and accumulate underneath the skin. Accumulation of an unmixed bilious humour leads to herpes. If it is adulterated with blood, the result will be erysipelas. Erysipelas, which is a dangerous disease, has the symptoms of heat and swelling in common with phlegmon, but its colour is paler or may be a little yellow. The treatment of erysipelas should consist of cooling measures, but one must not proceed too far because this would involve the risk of the diseased humour being diverted to an internal, vital part.[46] When erysipelas arises from wounds or sores then a cataplasm of barley flour and early scarification are recommended. It follows that apart from external, local treatment one should initiate an internal, general one with cholagogues.

Cancer is caused by a congestion of *black bile*. Should this be of a sharp nature, additional ulcerations will occur. Through the centuries, black bile in particular was to play a paramount part in pathology. An excess of it would render the blood black and thick. It might erupt either in the skin in which case chronic ulcers and leprosy would ensue, or in the deeper parts, causing carcinoma. Treatment of the latter should be radical excision, without securing the blood vessels by means of ligature, since that would only promote recurrence. Melanogogues should be administered to remove the material cause of the disease. Scirrhus was a preternatural tumour occasioned by a 'thick and slow humour', not primarily malignant although sometimes allied to cancer. It might be an original disease, but was most often iatrogenic, resulting from inadequate treatment of a pre-existing phlegmon or erysipelas.

Oedema, whether it is part of a general disease like dropsy, phthisis or cachexia, or of a localized nature, is imputed to *phlegm*.

Each of the humours then, according to the humoral pathological views of Galen, can give rise to specific complaints. But the live-giving *pneuma* can also cause disease, and it would only seem natural to attribute conditions like emphysema and tympanites to it. Treatment should aim at attenuating the thickened spirit by frictions with calefacient oil.

Bloodletting

For centuries bloodletting was the most frequently performed surgical intervention, it was also often applied in so-called surgical complaints as a supportive measure. The great importance which Galen attached to phlebotomy is amply demonstrated by the fact that he wrote no less than three treatises on this subject.

By drawing blood Galen aimed at either *revulsion* or *derivation*. In the former instance the intention was to divert humours from that part of the body in which they were in excess. This revulsion (e contrario) had to be performed far from the diseased part; one could also use cups or leeches for this purpose. Derivation aimed at the resolution of accumulations of fluid which had already formed outside the blood vessels, by means of venesection in the immediate vicinity of the diseased part, in any case on the ipsilateral side of the body.[47] Venesection in accordance with these principles was practised in clinical medicine well into the nineteenth century. The use of bloodletting in the treatment of fresh wounds or after surgery, should be seen as an attempt to prevent congestion.

Particularly under the influence of the Arabs, astrological elements crept into the practice of bloodletting in the Middle Ages (Fig. 23): they disappeared again in the seventeenth century.

Some Aspects of Galen's Surgery

It seems that Galen's familiarity with surgery was more theoretical than practical. It is questionable whether he ever personally practised the art.[48] The only treatise in which he deals at length with surgical pathology and operative therapy is the voluminous *Methodus medendi*. We will therefore at least glance through it, because mediaeval surgeons — who also called it *Megatechne* — repeatedly refer to it.[49]

Books III to VI concern injuries and their treatment. The optimal way for a wound to heal is by 'prima unio' or 'prima scopus', i.e. without the formation of any intermediary substance. The edges of the wound should be united either by means of a double-headed bandage, with a suture, or with a fibula. Everything that is 'desiccative' promotes healing, because in the body whatever is dry most closely approximates to that which is healthy, while whatever is wet approximates to that which is not healthy, Galen writes after Hippocrates (IV, 5). Wine is therefore an excellent medicament for the treatment of wounds without contusion, (IV, 4), as it desiccates and cleanses and because its penetration is deep.

Severe haemorrhage impedes the agglutination of the wound edges. This may be arrested by bringing together the wound margins with one's hands and then applying a bandage, or by using cold or astringent medicines.

Bleeding arteries and veins can be seized with a small hook and be torsioned or ligated. If a bleeding artery has not ruptured completely, it must be cut. In such a case it is safest to ligate the vessel on both sides of the injury before dividing it (V, 3). Further on, in book XIII, Galen recommends as material for the ligature a special kind of yarn which does not decay quickly. It is imported from Gaul and is for sale in Rome on the Via Sacra. Otherwise, silk may be used, which can be obtained in all major cities where rich women live, or finally thin strings which quite contrarily disintegrate easily and thus soon fall off the vessels. With veins haemostatic medicaments may serve the purpose. Galen mentions several such styptics. They are compounded of boiled resin, wheat flour, woolly hair and plaster; elsewhere it says that they may also contain incense, aloe, white of egg, chopped hare's fur, vitriol, alum, and other substances. If the bleeding is the result of a septic erosion Galen strongly recommends the use of corrosives and the red-hot cautery (V, 4).

Syncope is the subject of no fewer than three chapters in book XII. According to Galen, syncope is the result of a sudden prostration of the vital spirits without a suspension of the respiration. As the entire system is apparently overloaded, evacuation is of prime importance in the therapy. Venesection, however, is not allowed here so that this therapeutic aim must be realized by means of frictions. When the pulse rate drops and becomes irregular, the patient must be given wine. Syncope can, moreover, ensue from causes such as violent pains, insomnia, copious evacuations and fevers.

Book VI treats, among other things, penetrating wounds of the abdomen with prolapse of the intestines or omentum. When the intestine is dilated the surgeon must first apply a sponge soaked in hot water before he makes an attempt at reposition. If necessary the wound must be enlarged. A skilful assistant is needed to expose the wound edges for the surgeon. The gastrorrhaphy — as the abdominal suture was called — can be performed in two ways. The first consists of a running suture, in which on the one side the needle pierces the skin and the muscular layer excluding the peritoneum, while on the return from the opposite side the peritoneum is included (Fig. 6.I). Centuries later, Albucasis compared this suture with the stitch used by furriers for sewing skins. The second method involves a running suture in two layers. It is performed by passing the needle from without through the skin and the muscle, leaving out the peritoneum at the first stitch. Then the needle is turned and from without the surgeon pierces the opposite peritoneum in an inward direction. Finally, in a third bite the thread is passed from

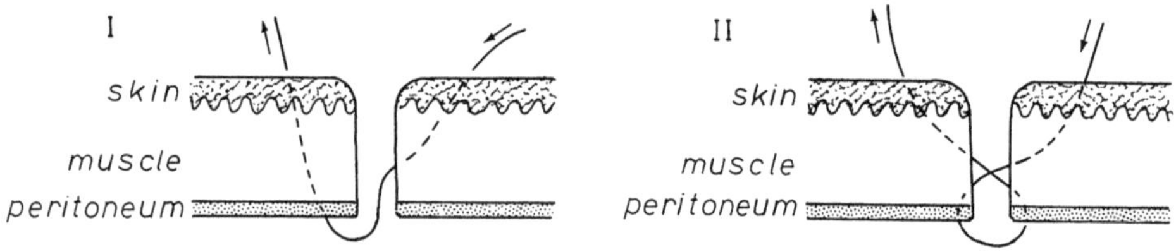

Fig. 6. Two types of abdominal suture according to Galen. *I*: The furrier's stitch; *II*: Running suture in two layers.

within through the opposite muscle and skin outwards, thus completing a figure-of-eight (Fig. 6.II). Both methods have become traditional.

Wounds of the large intestine are easily cured by suture, but those of the small gut heal only with difficulty. The jejunum cannot be cured at all for its walls are thin and, being next to the liver, it receives the bile in an undiluted state. It is not quite clear from his description how Galen treats wounds of this part of the intestinal canal, and those of the stomach (VI, 4).

The next chapter in the same book deals with the treatment of fractures. Since it does not contain much that is new, we had better pass it by.

Much attention is paid to head injuries. As appears from another, probably pseudo-Galenic work — *Definitiones medicae* — in Galen's day eight different types of skull fractures were distinguished. It was already known that paralysis caused by cerebral lesions affect the opposite side of the body, whereas those originating from the spinal cord are ipsilateral.[50] Galen's treatment of skull fractures is somewhat aggressive: even when there is only a simple fissure, he grabs the raspatory and traces the fracture down into the bone by chafing. His motive is that should the fracture appear to extend down to the cerebral membrane, this approach would provide an outlet for any accumulated pus. Galen does not mention here the relieving of a haematoma as an indication. If fractures of the cranium are depressed, he prefers the use of the trephine to drill out a circular section around them continuing with a gouge, apparently to remove the depressed part. Drilling is a risky operation, however, because there is the danger of injuring the cerebral membranes. On the other hand, the disadvantage of using the gouge is that the head is shaken vigorously by the hammer strokes precisely when it is in need of rest. It is safer to use the abaptiston, a perforator which has a circular collar projecting above the point which prevents it from penetrating too deeply. Once a small opening has been made it can be enlarged by means of the lenticular knife. This is provided with a blunt, lentiform point and a curved blade, while the back is blunt and straight. The point is placed through the opening on the cerebral membrane and by hitting the back with a small hammer the skull can be cleft without the danger of damaging the meninges. This method is particularly recommended by Galen. Bone forceps are also suitable for removing bone through a small hole. All of the crushed bone must be removed but it is not necessary to trace each fissure to its very limit. The after-treatment consists of promoting granulation, after the period of the inflammation is over (VI, 6).

Other books by Galen with surgical subjects are his *Commentaries* on Hippocrates' books on fractures, dislocations, the consulting room of the physician and on the Aphorisms. There is furthermore his work *On anatomical procedures* where he discusses the importance of anatomical knowledge for surgeons; he illustrates this with a case of resection of the sternum from his own practice.[51] As regards Galen's *Preternatural tumours*, it should be pointed out that the word 'tumor' in the Galenic context not only signifies 'tumours' in our present sense, but may refer to all swellings, such as inflammations, fistulae, skin diseases, oedema and the traumatic aneurysm which was probably discussed in some detail for the first time by Galen.[52] After Galen's example it would remain customary up to the early eighteenth century to group together disorders accompanied by some kind of swelling. [53] *On affected parts* I, Cap 6, includes the perceptive statement that extirpation of cervical glands may result in a double-sided injury to the recurrent nerves — first described by him — and lead to aphonia, while an injury to one side causes only hoarseness. Finally, the *Ars medica* or *Ars parva* contains a summary of the entire Galenic system of anatomy and physiology, as well as chapters on the treatment of wounds and fractures. This book was used during the Middle Ages at the European universities as well as outside the academic world.

In conclusion it can be said that although his surgery was clearly based on that of Hippocrates, Galen's anatomical knowledge was much greater. For a number of fundamental surgical disorders he gave a rational explanation based on humoral pathology. He had at his disposal better means of wound treatment and employed the vascular ligature. His directions for the treatment of skull injuries were more elaborate than those of Hippocrates, although his fracture treatment did not differ greatly from that by the patriarch of Cos. He said little about herniae, and amputation was mentioned only in passing, where he agreed with Hippocrates that it must be performed through the necrotic part, preferably at a joint. He appears to have had at his disposal an array of instruments.

Because his work exerted such a great influence on the European surgeons of the late Middle Ages and the Renaissance, the last representative of Hellenistic surgery to whom attention must be paid is Paul of Aegina.

1.1.2.4. Paul of Aegina

Little else is known of the Greek physician Paul other than that he was born on the isle of Aegina, that he practised during the first half of the seventh century in Alexandria, and was the author of several works. Of these only a compendium remains, the *Epitome*, dealing with all branches of medicine and made up of seven books. This work, originally written in Greek, was translated into Arabic in the ninth century and into Latin at the end of the ninth or the beginning of the tenth century. It is not likely to have had an immediate large circulation in the West. Only a very incomplete manuscript from the early Middle Ages is extant and the surgeons of the Salernitan and Bolognese schools, to be discussed in Chapter 2, do not mention him. He is first quoted on several occasions by the French surgeon Guy de Chauliac, which leads one to assume that a Latin translation must have been available in the fourteenth century. In the sixteenth century his work made its first appearance in print, in two different Latin editions published rapidly one after the other, besides two editions in Greek, and book VI, which is particularly important for us, in a separate French issue. By that time Paul had become a widely read author in the West. The surgery of Fabricius ab Aquapendente (1533—1619), who was Harvey's teacher in Padua, is made up largely of his work, although this author also borrowed from Celsus and Albucasis. A complete Dutch translation never appeared.

Indirectly Paul had already left his mark much earlier. Much of what the Arabic authors, Haly Abbas, Albucasis, Rhazes, and Avicenna had to say about operative surgery was derived to a considerable extent from the sixth book of Paul of Aegina.

Paul's *Epitome*, as he himself states, is largely derived from the compilatory writings of Oribasius, who greatly relied on Galen.[54] Unfortunately, in most cases Paul fails to identify either his own sources or those of Oribasius. Neither does he ever quote the works of Celsus. The frequent resemblances between Paul and Celsus are probably because both authors took their material from the school of Alexandria. Paul appears to be well acquainted with the work of Hippocrates and Galen.

The sixth book of Paul's compendium provides a complete survey of the state of operative surgery towards the end of Antiquity. In view of its important contribution to the flourishing of surgery during the late Middle Ages and the Renaissance, it deserves to be recognised as one of the seminal works in the history of the craft: it is therefore appropriate to analyse it in more detail here. Our review will be based on the English edition with a commentary by Francis Adams of 1845—47.[55] We will not consider further those aspects which Paul borrowed from Hippocrates or Galen, and which have been referred to above.

The 122 chapters into which book VI is divided treat surgical therapy from head to toe. The author does not deal here with surgical pathology; his few observations on this subject, entirely along Galenic lines, are to be found in the preceding books.

To a large extent the chapters dealing with the head are concerned with eye surgery and ear, nose and throat diseases. Paul is the only Greek writer to give a detailed description of the cataract operation. Chapter 33 contains a description of tracheostomy — which he called laryngotomy or pharyngotomy — borrowed verbatim from the Alexandrian surgeon Antyllus, who was active in the second century. The indication for operation is an inflammation and swelling of the tonsils, causing danger of suffocation. The opening is made by a transverse incision between two rings of the trachea. As soon as the trachea is open, air escapes from the wound and the patient loses his voice. When all danger of the suffocation which formed the indication for the operation is past, the surgeon sutures the skin wound, after it has been pared to roughen the edges.

Indurated glands, especially if they occur in the neck, in the armpits or in the groins, must be considered carcinomatous if they are painful to the touch, but in such cases they must not be operated upon. In the absence of this symptom they may be removed, by separating them from the surrounding parts, the surgeon taking care to avoid blood vessels and nerves, such as the carotid arteries and the recurrent nerves in the neck. Bleeding arteries should be ligated if they obscure the view. Although the surgeon could use forceps, it appears from many sources that it was customary to fix and present tumours and the like with a sharp small hook.

In Chapter 37 Paul discusses aneurysms. Here he quotes Galen's description of this vascular disorder, but he elaborates by distinguishing those caused by dilatation of the artery and those resulting from damage to the vascular wall.[56] The treatment consists of an operation in which a ligature is applied over and under the swelling and the sac is opened by incision.

In bronchocele — goitre — Paul also distinguishes two varieties: a steatomatous and an aneurysmal type. The latter, which can be recognized by the usual symptoms of an aneurysm, must not be operated upon because of the size of the arteries they contain. The former variety can be removed, if one takes care to avoid the vessels.

The chapter on venesection is comparatively extensive (VI, 40). With regard to this, Paul's views are largely in accord with those of Galen, and the same applies to the technique. The most important indication for it is 'a fulness of blood' which may have been caused by all kinds of diseases, primarily of an inflammatory nature. In the case of an acute inflammation bloodletting must be performed on the opposite side; in the case of a chronic one on the same side. From Francis Adams' approving commentary, it appears that in the 1840s classical bloodletting had lost little or none of its therapeutic importance!

Cancer is described by Paul, in Adams' words, as 'an uneven swelling, rough, unseemly, darkish, painful, and sometimes without ulceration (which Hippocrates also called a concealed cancer), and if operated upon, it becomes worse, and sometimes with ulceration, for it derives its origin from black bile, and spreads by erosion; forming in most parts of the body, but more especially in the female uterus and breasts'. As to its treatment he concurs with Galen, who dismissed burning it out with a glowing cautery and advocated operating with a knife.

Following Hippocrates he does open the hepatic absecess and the thoracic empyema by means of slender cauteries (VI, 47).

Since the days of Hippocrates it was customary to drain ascites via a copper tube through a stab incision (VI, 50). The fluid should be tapped only very gradually. Umbilical hernia or exomphalos, of which a fine description is given, differing in that they contain either protruded omentum or bowel, is dealt with in a separate chapter (VI, 51). Prior to the operation the patient must stand up and press so that the circumference of the swelling can be marked on the skin with ink. Next, after having placed the patient on his back, the skin is cut along the ink line and the empty swelling is lifted with a small hook. As in Celsus, the base is provided with a strong cross-stitch, making sure that no fold of the intestine nor part of the omentum is included. The constricted swelling is left until it falls off on its own. An interesting admonition is for the surgeon to abstain from any treatment if the 'exomphalos' is caused by an aneurysm. From this it may be concluded that at least some of the classical authors were familiar with aneurysms of the abdominal aorta.

In the treatment of perforating abdominal injuries (VI, 52) Paul closely follows Galen's recommendations.

The introduction of a metal bladder catheter is conducted in a manner with which even today one could hardly find fault with (VI, 59).

Paul's description of lithotomy is largely in agreement with that of Celsus and probably represents the operation as it was done by the Alexandrian lithotomists, who had a great reputation.[57]

The treatment of scrotal hernia — enterocele — and inguinal hernia — bubonocele — are the subjects of chapters 65 and 66. The cause of both is either a rupture or a stretching of the peritoneum. This double possibility is first mentioned by Oribasius, from whom Paul, as said above, derived much information. The hernia caused by stretching develops gradually, the one caused by rupture suddenly. Retention of faeces in the region of the scrotum brings on dangerous symptoms with pain and rumbling of wind on palpation. His operative treatment of scrotal hernia was as follows. Through a transverse incision in the groin he freed the spermatic cord and the testis from the scrotal skin using his index-finger and brought these structures outside the body. After replacing any abdominal contents he applied an X-shaped stitch ligature high up on the 'extremity of the peritoneum' (hernial sac). Subsequently he laid another lower ligature around the spermatic cord, after which he cut the latter between the two ligatures and removed the distal part of the cord together with the testis.

In the treatment of inguinal hernia the testis was spared in principle. He suggests two operations for this. The 'classical' operation consisted of clearing the hernial sac, or stretched peritoneum as Paul called it, and then invaginating it with a probe. The prominences thus formed on either side of the probe are united by sutures, thereby inverting the sac. 'Most of the moderns', however, preferred the application of cauteries to the skin over the swelling, carefully avoiding burning of the peritoneum. The aim was to produce a scar which might keep back the protruding peritoneum. Paul does not say anything about the treatment of the incarcerated hernia. This complication had not been treated operatively by any of the surgeons of Antiquity. Its mechanism did not become clear until the sixteenth century, after Falloppio had described the anatomy of the inguinal canal.

The anal pathology confronting the surgeon includes fistula-in-ano, haemorrhoids, condylomata, fissures, and imperforate anus (VI, 77—81). The appearance of a fistula is usually preceded by an abscess. By introducing a sound, or a swine's bristle, the surgeon may discover whether the fistula is blind or runs into the anus. The treatment of a fistula consists of incision over a probe, or by introducing and tying a ligature, as recommended by Hippocrates. Haemorrhoids should be ligated, though some surgeons cut them off with a scalpel, applying styptics afterwards. The application of caustics was a third option in the therapeutic approach. Varicose veins of the leg, which are caused by a melancholic humour, are excised by some surgeons between ligatures, whereas others cut out the vessel without ligatures, 'or stretch it from below and tear it out by force' (VI, 82). In this Paul differs from Hippocrates, who was against operating, and also from Celsus, who besides excision obliterated the vein by means of the cautery.

The chapter on amputation of the extremities is remarkably brief. Once again, the only indication offered is mortification, resulting either from a fracture or some internal cause. Following the directions given by the surgeon Leonides, the first part to be severed is the one in which few large veins or arteries are known to be situated. Then the bone is sawn 'applying a linen rag to the parts which have been cut lest they be torn by the sawing and occasion pain'. Finally the remaining soft parts are cut. Red-hot irons are applied in order to effect haemostasis. Paul did not express an opinion on the exact site at which a limb affected by gangrene should be removed.

War surgery, on the other hand, is represented by a sizeable chapter, as it was in Celsus (VI, 88). The importance of extraction of missiles is illustrated by Paul with a well-known quotation from Homer:

For a leech is of the worth of many other men
For the cutting out of arrows and the spreading of soothing simples.[58]

If the weapon is lodged in an important part of the body and fatal symptoms have already manifested themselves, the surgeon had better abstain from treatment, for not only can he do no good, he can but expose himself to the scorn of ignorant people. But if the patient's fate is in doubt he must make an attempt, having first given fair warning of the danger. Paul subsequently gives an extensive account of the symptoms indicating an injury to the brain, the heart, the lungs, the diaphragm, the abdominal organs and the bladder. A serious loss of blood leads to coldness, sweating, loss of consciousness, soon followed by the death of the patient. If a projectile becomes lodged in a large artery, when extraction would cause dangerous bleeding, then the vessel must first be ligated before its removal is attempted.

The final 35 chapters, almost a quarter of the entire book, deal with fractures and dislocations. Paul again chooses the order from head to toe.

Just like Hippocrates he devotes a great deal of attention to injuries of the head: apart from the chapter on blood-letting, it is the longest of book VI. Fractures of the skull bones may occur in various shapes and with different degrees of severity. He denies, however, the existence of the fracture by repercussion which was mentioned by Hippocrates. Skull fractures provide not only local signs and symptoms but are often accompanied by general symptoms, as the result of compression of the brain. His diagnostic approach corresponds to that of Hippocrates and Celsus. In order to assess the seriousness of the trauma it is important to determine whether the cerebral membranes are still adherent to the bone. The occurrence of a wound abscess is much more dangerous if the meninges have been separated from the bone than if they are still attached to it; in the case of the former the surgeon must intervene. The injured part of the cranium is laid bare by two intersecting cuts, one of which can be the wound itself. The four corners which are thus created in the scalp are pried loose from the bone. The blood flow is checked by pledgets moistened in oxycrate — water mixed with vinegar — and a compression bandage. The skull itself is not opened until the next day. In this he follows the procedure outlined by Galen. During the removal of the tabula interna — Paul does not use this term — the cerebral membranes must be protected by means of the meningophylax, a flat metal instrument. The 'moderns' reject the operation with the crown trephine or with a small saw, according to Paul.

With regard to the treatment of other fractures, Paul offers little new compared with Hippocrates and Galen. He differs from Hippocrates when he writes that 'the moderns' apply a splint bandage directly after the reduction, instead of after a lapse of seven days. His description of fracture of the upper leg is limited largely to its reduction. For treatment of fractures of the lower leg it appears that there is no unanimity about whether the leg must be splinted or be placed in a wooden or earthenware box-splint. Paul was the first to describe the fracture of the patella. In common with the authors mentioned above he mistakes fractures of the wrist and the ankle for dislocations. Paul wants compound fractures to be treated either on the first day, prior to the occurrence of inflammatory symptoms, or else not until the ninth day, when the inflammation has subsided. Concomittant wounds must be sutured straight away; once they are inflamed a treatment with cleansing ointments is required.

Unlike his illustrious predecessors Paul does not hesitate to remove any redundant callus with a chisel and a hammer through an incision. If a fracture had healed in a faulty position Paul again brings out his hammer and chisel; he dismisses the practice of refracturing a bone with brute force, as Celsus advocated. Non-union can be the result of insufficient immobilization of the leg, of inappropriate bandages, or of general weakness. The treatment must consist in the elimination of all causal factors and a generous diet.

Paul's general wound treatment is not to be found in the sixth, but in the fourth book of the *Epitome*. Simple wounds can easily be treated by bandaging the wound in such a way as to bring the edges together. Any contaminants such as hair, sand, oil, dirt, etc. must first be removed. If the wound is too large to be closed by a bandage, it must be sutured. Paul does not give any special directions for the methods of suture. As wound remedies he recommends agglutinants which have the power of drying the moisture collected. He lists quite a number of such agents. Painful and inflamed wounds are best treated with anti-inflammatory remedies like wine and oxycrate, and with diluted hydromel — honeyed water — in the case of foul inflammation.

When comparing Paul's surgery to the surgery practised at the time of Celsus and Galen, at first sight little advancement seems to have been made during the intervening centuries. It needs a closer look to ascertain, that any advances have indeed been made at all. They bear mostly on refinements of surgical techniques and such details. Paul of Aegina himself was evidently quite aware of progress being made: on several occasions he mentions 'the ancients' as distinct from 'the moderns', apparently the surgeons of his own generation.

1.1.3. *The Byzantine Empire*

The division of the Roman empire in 395 A.D., which was intended only as an administrative measure, practically amounted to the creation of two independent states, the West-Roman empire and its East-Roman counterpart, which not much later took on the name of its capital, Byzantium. Great cultural differences soon became apparent between these two empires. In the East, where the common language was Greek, there emerged an unique culture which persisted until Constantinople was captured by the Turks in 1453. In the former territory of Byzantium impressive churches with their characteristic round domed roofs sometimes, as in Ravenna, ornamented with splendid mosaics, are to this day reminders of the Byzantine civilization; this is also witnessed by the products of a refined tradition of iconic painting as well as by numerous codices, many of them beautifully illustrated and well preserved. In the medical field, however, the Byzantines made no original contributions. Their medical literature is characterized by voluminous anthologies like the ones by Oribasius and Aëtius, briefly referred to on page 10. On the other hand, the Christian spirit of life led to the emergence of the hospital.[59]

The history of the Byzantine empire is characterized by continuous religious battles. An opinion, deviating from the orthodox, was stated by Nestorius, the patriarch of Constantinople, who preached the duality of Christ. In 431 this doctrine was denounced by the council of Ephesus, and Nestorius was banished into exile. His followers fled from Eastern Syria, where most of them had lived, to the East, and particularly to Persia. There they founded flourishing communities and undertook many missionary activities.

Among the Nestorians there were numerous scholars, not only theologians, but philosophers, linguists and physicians. Their cultural importance is not least revealed by their translations of Greek scientific and philosophical writings, first into Syrian and subsequently into Persian, later also into Arabic. An important centre for translation was the medical school of Jundishapur in Western Persia, founded around 550 A.D. This was still flourishing when, between 637 and 660, Persia was captured by the Arabs.

1.2. THE MUSLIM WORLD

1.2.1. *Cultural Setting*

The teachings of Mohammed (570—632) had united the inhabitants of the Arabian peninsula, formerly a loose conglomerate of nomadic Bedouin tribes, into one people from whom emanated a tremendous expansive force. During the first century after the Prophet's death, the Arabs conquered an area that stretched from the river Indus, across the Near East, the coast of Northern Africa and Spain to the Pyrenees. Around 750 A.D. this large empire fell apart, basically into the Eastern Caliphate with Baghdad as its capital, and the Western Caliphate, of which the seat of government was Cordoba in Spain.

In the territories subjected to the Arabs there soon emerged a characteristic culture, which revealed itself in its architecture, literature, music and in the study of philosophy and various branches of science, which included medicine. A binding element in all this was the Arabic tongue. Since it was permitted to read and study the Koran only in this language, Arabic soon became supra-national and thus the language of Muslim science. Cairo, Baghdad and Damascus in the East, as well as Cordoba, Seville and Toledo in Spain became important scientific centres. From the thirteenth century onward Toledo became a treasury of Arabic culture and exerted a strong attraction for young scholars from all over Europe. Around 1150, the Italian Gerard of Cremona (1114—87) established a reputable translation institute in that city.

The Caliphate of Baghdad existed until the capital was captured by Mongols in 1258. The Western Caliphate did not disappear until two centuries later, when Granada fell to Isabella of Castile and the Moors — so called because the Spanish Mohammedans were in fact mostly dark-skinned Berbers — were ousted from their last Spanish stronghold.

1.2.2. *Arabic Medical Scholarship*

The Arabic practice of science initially consisted in the study of the scientific literature which had been produced by the Indians, Persians and particularly the Greeks. This led to the industrious undertaking of translation into Arabic of those Greek texts which already existed in a Syrian or Persian edition. From the tenth century onwards, however, Arabic scientists published important works of their own, some of which for many centuries were of the greatest value to both the East and the West. It is through Latin translations, many of them produced in Toledo, that these works were made available to Western Europe, and this applies to quite a number of medical and scientific writings from previous centuries.

1.2.2.1. Johannitius

Among the early translators of medical texts was Ḥunain ibn Isḥāq, who lived in Baghdad in the ninth century. He was the translator of a surprisingly large number of writings by Hippocrates and Galen, as well as the *Epitome* by Paul. He is usually identified with Johannitius, the writer of a concise, very schematic outline of the Galenic principles, meant as an introduction to the *Ars parva* by Galen. This *Isagoge* was already available in Latin around 1100 and was used in the teaching of medicine at European universities throughout the Middle Ages.[60] It appears from a catalogue preserved from the first half of the thirteenth century that a copy of the work was amongst the possessions of the library of the abbey of Rolduc in Limburg.[61]

1.2.2.2. Rhazes

Of the Arabic physicians whose works have exerted a great influence on the medicine and surgery of the West, the first to be mentioned must be Rhazes (Abū Bakr Muhammad ibn Zakarīyā' ar-Rāzī, c. 850—923).

His huge opus magnum *al-Ḥāwī* ('the comprehensive book') came to be known in the West as *Liber continens.* An abbreviated version of it, however, has been more influential in the form of the *Liber medicinalis ad Almansorem,* a book which Rhazes dedicated to al Mansur, viceroy of Chorasan. This compilation from Greek, [62] Indian and Arabic sources was translated into Latin at the Neapolitan court of Charles I of Anjou, who reigned from 1266 to 1285.[63] The seventh book of the latter work, which after 1481 went through several printed editions, deals with surgery. The author more than once consults Paul of Aegina.[64]

1.2.2.3. Haly Abbas

A book often quoted in the mediaeval medical literature of the West is *al-Malakī* or *Liber regius* by Haly Abbas ('Alī ibn al-'Abbās al-Majūsī, 930—994). It was already rendered into Latin in the eleventh century by Constantinus Africanus and published as his own work, entitled *Libri Pantechni* — 'books concerning the entire art'.[65] In 1127 it was translated once again, this time by Stephen of Antioch, and it was this translation which was the first to appear in print in 1492. The *Liber regius* ('the royal book': so called because its author dedicated it to the prince 'Aḍud ad-Dawla), gives a systematic survey of the entire science of medicine at the time. It was very popular and it took a century before it was superseded by Avicenna's work. It is made up of two parts, 'Theorice' and 'Practica', consisting of ten books each. The ninth book of the practical part contains surgery. Apart from a few personal additions it is largely derived from Paul of Aegina.

1.2.2.4. Avicenna

The zenith of Arabic medical literature is represented by *al-Qānūn fī 't-ṭibb* ('the canon of medicine') by Abū 'Alī al-Ḥusayn ibn 'Abd Allāh ibn Sīnā or Avicenna (980—1037) (Fig. 7). Like the two authors previously mentioned Avicenna was a Persian. The *Canon medicinae* is one of the most infuential medical books ever written. It does not contain epoch making innovations, but it provides a complete system of medicine according to the principles of Galenism.[66] There is an affinity with Aristotle, while at the same time including new empiric facts. For centuries the book had an enormous impact on medicine both in the East and the West: between 1473 and 1658 Choulant reported at least 29 printed Latin editions, the

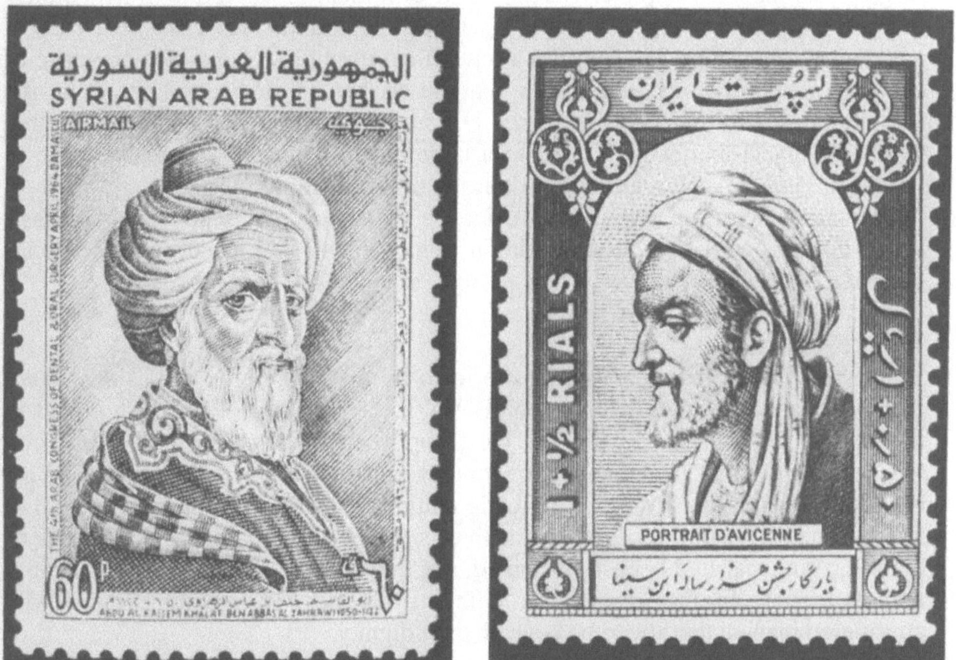

Fig. 7. Albucasis and Avicenna.

first of which was a translation by Gerard of Cremona.[67] The best translation — although incomplete — is the one is 1658 by the Dutchman Vopiscus Fortunatus Plemp, who lived in Louvain. To a considerable extent Galenism was only able to play its dominant role during the late Middle Ages and the Renaissance through the medium of Avicenna.

As far as surgery is concerned the *Canon* is of less importance than the work of Albucasis, to be discussed below. Much can be found on surgery and on external diseases in the third book. This explains why Avicenna is also often quoted by surgeons. His surgery, however, is not very original and largely depends on the surgery of the Greeks, and of Paul in particular.[68]

1.2.2.5. Albucasis

As a writer on surgery, the most important Arabic author was Abū 'l-Qāsim Ḵalaf ibn 'Abbas az-Zahrāwī (936—1013) of Cordoba, better known as Albucasis (Fig. 7). He wrote a very extensive work covering all branches of medicine. The last of its thirty treatises is devoted to surgery. It was translated into Latin in Toledo in the second half of the twelfth century by Gerard of Cremona and appeared under the title of *Liber Alzaharavii de cirurgia.* It soon became a standard textbook throughout Europe, probably because of its eminently practical character. The work is copiously illustrated with drawings of instruments.[69]

In his introduction to this treatise, Albucasis complains that during his day, surgery had almost completely disappeared as a medical discipline in his country of Spain. Proficient surgeons could no longer be found, the result of a lack of anatomical knowledge. He supplies a few salient examples of the incompetence of contemporary surgeons and writes that he wishes to dedicate himself to the resuscitation of the science of surgery. His surgery is nevertheless not an original work, its subject-matter is derived to a large extent from the classical writers, in particular Paul of Aegina, although Albucasis never mentions his name.

Mediaeval Western writers give evidence of acquaintanceship with Albucasis long before his work appeared in print in Venice in 1471, especially Guy de Chauliac often quotes him.

1.2.2.6. Avenzoar

The last physician from the Islamic world to be treated briefly here is Avenzoar: Abū Marwān 'Abd al-Malik ibn Abī 'l-'Alā' Zuhr (c. 1090—1162), who lived in the vicinity of Seville in Spain. His most important work *at-Taysir fī 'l-madāwāt wa-'t-tadbīr* ('Practical manual of treatments and diets') sive rectificatio medicationis et regiminis, according to the Latin edition of 1490, is primarily a manual of internal medicine, but also discusses subjects of a surgical nature.[70] As he tells us himself, Avenzoar had been well trained, not only in medicine, but also in surgery and pharmacy. In this respect he differs from most Arabic physicians, who considered manual therapy to be beneath their dignity.

1.2.3. *Aspects of Muslim Surgery*

For reasons of space several aspects of Arabic surgery, taken from the works of the authors mentioned above, of Albucasis and Avicenna in particular, will here be considered together. This is justifiable, for all of them largely depend on Paul of Aegina. It must be noted that, with the exception of Albucasis and perhaps Avenzoar, these authors probably never practised surgery themselves. In Arabic practice the most important places were occupied by therapies using medicines, by bloodletting, cupping and cautery.

The frequent use of the last mentioned therapy is most striking. The entire first part of Albucasis' book, which altogether consists of three parts, is devoted to this subject. Cauterization, according to this source, can be performed either by the red-hot iron, or by corrosive agents: the 'cauterium actuale' and the 'cauterium potentiale' respectively. Often the indication is an internal disease, and then cauterization is meant either as a revulsive or derivative mode in treatment.

The surgical application of the cautery can serve various purposes. For instance, it can be applied with the intention of producing cicatrization so that any unwanted mobility is limited such as in recurrent dislocation of the shoulder or reducible inguinal hernia. The red-hot iron can also be useful when opening abscesses and empyema, when burning out skin tumours and haemorrhoids, and when searing bleeding arteries. All these applications we met already with the Greek authors. Albucasis gives detailed instructions on its precise use. Avicenna too, is in the front rank when it comes to the use of the ferrum candens.

The treatment of wounds first of all requires careful haemostasis. In explaining the difference between arterial and venous bleeding, Albucasis compared the bleeding artery to the jet of water produced by a urinating child. The haemostatic methods used by the Arabic authors were in no way different from those practised by the Graeco-Roman surgeons. Thus we encounter in Rhazes the styptic agents recommended by Galen — according to Avicenna cobweb is another good agent — while torsioning and ligating too, seems to have been generally known although the use of the cautery was preferred. In wound treatment bloodletting occupies an important place. In the chapter on the care of wounds Albucasis recommends that if the formation of an abscess is feared, one should carry out bloodletting on the opposite side. When there is no inflammatory swelling and when the wound is unadulterated by air contact, a powder consisting of frankincense, dragon's blood and quicklime must be applied, before the wound can be dressed. Should the air have already affected the wound, the generation of pus must be promoted by means of suitable ointments.[71] The belief, held for centuries, that atmospheric air has a deleterious influence on wounds, may well have been instigated by this passage in Albucasis.

A fine description of penetrating abdominal injuries can also be found in Albucasis. He mentions five different methods of gastrorrhaphia: the pin fixed by a figure-of-eight thread, already encountered in Celsus; a continuous over-and-over suture through all layers; the furrier's suture and the closure in two layers as described by Galen; and finally a method which employed a thread passed through two needles. The last method, which Albucasis describes as the shoemaker's stitch, differs from the double-needle technique by Celsus in that each needle is passed straight through the whole thickness of the abdominal wall from within outwards at opposite sides. The shoemaker's or cobbler's suture remained popular well into the nineteenth century; it was recommended by Boyer as late as 1821. As was the case with the Greeks, the stitches apparently were not removed but allowed to come out spontaneously.

For closing intestinal wounds with a needle and thread Albucasis uses fibres from the taenia coli of animals, without specifying which animal. Suturing such a wound can only be attempted in the large intestine; injuries of the small intestine are invariably lethal.

Avicenna was the first to devote a separate chapter to ulcers.

Avicenna and Albucasis pay particular attention to fractures and luxations, as well as to the non-traumatic bone disorders. In the third book of his *Surgery*, which deals exclusively with skeletal traumatology, Albucasis complains that the treatment of fractures is often left to ignorant surgeons or even to laymen 'who have never taken even a quick glance at the books of the Ancients'. Just like Hippocrates, he does not apply the definitive splint bandage until after the fifth or seventh day, when inflammatory symptoms have subsided. On the whole, his approach to bone lesions is comparable to that of the classic authors. But there are dissimilarities too. Thus we encounter in Albucasis for the first time the fenestrated fracture bandage: it enables the surgeon to tend the wound in cases of compound fracture, without having to unfasten the wrapping. Avicenna points out that it is important to provide good aftercare in order to prevent the joints from stiffening. It is somewhat surprising to find in Albucasis' chapters on fractures, a description of fracture of the penis. It is splinted by means of a goose neck which is pushed over the member.

The Arabs were familiar with chronic osteomyelitis. Avicenna is probably the first to have used the expression 'ventositas spinae et corruptio ossis'. The treatment consists of excochleation, cauterizing or even wholly removing the affected bone. Multiple interventions may be necessary to achieve this. On this indication Avicenna did not hesitate to perform the resection of a rib or even of a complete long bone of the forearm or the lower leg.[72]

Albucasis considered an amputation imperative in case of serious necrosis, but only if it was limited to the lower arm or lower leg. He made the incision through the proximal joint. Haemostasis was effected by means of the cautery, and the wound was not sutured. Amputations above the knee and above the elbow were considered impossible.

On the subject of specialised surgery mention should be made of laryngeal intubation with a gold or silver cannula which Avicenna performed to relieve breathing difficulties from strictures of every aetiology. Albucasis writes that he knows no one in his country who has performed tracheostomy. But he was aware that the trachea may heal spontaneously because of an unsuccessful suicide attempt by a slave: the trachea, severed by herself (air was escaping from the wound), healed satisfactorily after a simple suture of the skin. Avenzoar, too, writes that he has never seen this operation performed. He demonstrated its feasibility by means of an experiment on a goat.

Rhazes claims that objects impacted in the oesophagus may be pushed further down with a flexible instrument made of lead. Avenzoar describes the palliative treatment for a stricture of the oesophagus; it consists of introducing a long silver or tin catheter into the gullet past the narrowing, in order to feed milk or a thin pap into the stomach. Avenzoar does not set great store by another method of artificial feeding which was apparently in use and consisted of placing the patient in a bath of warm milk or a thin broth. In contrast to Galen it is Avenzoar's view that food which is administered through the rectum can rise through the intestines to the stomach.

Those herniae that can be reduced are treated by Rhazes preferably with a truss; furthermore he gives a recipe for a suitable emplaster derived from Paul of Aegina. Both Avicenna and Albucasis cauterise the hernial orifice after reduction.

The Arabic writers differ only slightly from Paul in their description of lithotomy.[73] Among the causes of retention of urine, mentioned by Albucasis, are included a stone, a clot of blood or pus, and a fleshy tumour: the last may well have been a case of hypertrophy of the prostate.

CHAPTER 2

The Western Middle Ages

2.1. THE EARLY MIDDLE AGES

2.1.1. *Social Setting*

The political downfall of the Western Roman empire in 467 at first did not bring about many changes in the economic life of Western and Southern Europe. This changed when in the seventh century the advancing Arabs had occupied the eastern, southern and western shores of the Mediterranean. Their advance brought to a virtual halt the old trade relations between Western Europe and the Near East. The little trade that remained in Western Europe was terminated not much later by the predatory raids of the Vikings and by the invasions of the Huns and the Hungarians which cut off the old trade routes between the Baltic Sea and the Black Sea and those in the Danube valley. Northwestern and Central Europe were consequently more or less cordoned off and trade came almost entirely to a standstill: only via Italy, which had remained a part of the still extant Eastern Roman empire, were commercial relations with the East maintained. From the eighth century onward agriculture occupied the most important place in economic life. The significance of the countryside increased while the cities fell into decline.[1] It is understandable that this more or less isolated society, which relied so heavily on agriculture and which was almost continuously in a state of war, showed little concern for science. Only the Church and the royal Chancelleries could provide people who were able to read and write, and consequently it was mainly servants of the Church who had access to the written legacy of previous centuries.

2.1.2. *Monasteries*

That legacy was preserved in monastic libraries. The monastic library, or occasionally also a court library, was from the sixth to the tenth centuries the only place in Western and Central Europe where the theory of medicine could be studied. Some of the cathedral schools which came into existence in the tenth century included medicine as a theoretical subject in their curricula.

During the period which we call the early Middle Ages (c. 500—c. 1100 A.D.) there existed therefore a close relationship between the Church and Medicine, as most theoretically trained physicians were also members of the clergy. The radius of action of these clerical physicians, often monks, was only limited. The 'medical care' of the population at large traditionally remained in the hands of popular healers, illiterates whose inherited skills were handed down from generation to generation, just like any other craft. As might be expected, they have left only few traces. We may assume, however, that the barber-surgeons who started to appear in the Netherlands during the thirteenth century were descended from this group of folk-healers.

The involvement in particular of the regular clergy with medicine had originated in the monastic rule laid down by Saint Benedict (c. 480—547), which set monks the task of the care of the sick.[2]

2.1.3. *Medical Literature*

The medical literature available during the early Middle Ages was of modest proportions.[3] It was written in Latin because Greek had lost its role as the language of science soon after the Great Migration. It consists of texts originally recorded in Latin — often collections of recipes — which are a heritage of late Antiquity, of fragments from Byzantine authors and of a number of works from the prime of Greek medicine, in Latin translations.[4] Among these one does not find the surgical works of Hippocrates, nor the *Methodus medendi* of Galen. There do exist, however, brief excerpts of other classical and late-classical works.[5]

Typical for the Middle Ages is also the fanciful attribution of all sorts of texts to celebrated personalities from Antiquity. Some of these are completely or partly devoted to surgical matters. Examples of this are the *Liber cyrurgie Ypocratis* which I came across in a tenth-century codex which is kept in Paris, and the final chapters of the pseudo-Galenic *Introductio sive medicus*, in a manuscript from the ninth century, to be found in the Badische Landesbibliothek in Karlsruhe. The former text has nothing to do with Hippocrates. It begins with the demands enumerated in the *Prooemium* from Celsus' seventh book, which must be met by a good surgeon (see page 12). Otherwise it appears to be a manual for the use of the cautery, based on the surgeon Heliodorus of the Alexandrian school. Texts dealing with the use of the cautery are typical indeed for the period. The *Introductio* is essentially a survey, being no more than an enumeration a capite ad calcem, in telegraphic style, of surgical disorders and their treatment. In spite of their conciseness, the surgical chapters of the *Introductio* are very reminiscent of those in the sixth book of the *Epitome medica* by Paul of Aegina. However, they do not directly derive from them.

Among the recipes mentioned there are a few medicaments with which patients who had to undergo a painful operation could be anaesthetized.[6] The first consisted of a sponge, drenched in the juice of opium, mandrake, hemlock and henbane and subsequently dried in the sun. Prior to its use the sponge was put into warm water, after which it was kept under the nose of the patient, who had to inhale the vapours deeply, until he fell asleep. To wake him again he was made to breathe the vapours of hot vinegar. The name of this anaesthetic, *Ypnoticon*, indicates that its origin was Greek, and that it had therefore been handed down from Antiquity. This is certainly true for the second medicine, consisting of an extract of mandrake root in wine, as this was mentioned in express terms by Dioscorides and by Pliny, both of whom lived in the first century.[7] The recipe for the soporific sponge and, to a lesser degree, for the mandragora wine turns up over and again in surgical literature, only to disappear quietly in the sixteenth century. Whether such medicines have actually ever been used in practice cannot be determined with certainty. There are indications, however, that this has been the case, certainly in relation to the sleeping draught.[8]

In all probability the literature mentioned thus far was available only to monastic physicians. We are given an insight into the work of the abovementioned folk-healers by three Anglo-Saxon *Laece Books*, instruction manuals from the tenth century, written in the vernacular language. Besides various expressions of superstition, they contain numerous medicinal prescriptions and in a few instances also instructions for surgical treatment, which bear witness to practical experience. It is striking, for instance, that an amputation for gangrene was carried out through healthy tissue.[9]

In the medical writings of the early Middle Ages no actual surgical case reports can be found.

2.2. THE LATE MIDDLE AGES

2.2.1. *Social Setting*

From the eleventh century onward many changes occurred in the situation sketched above. The Normans had been converted to Christianity and had founded flourishing states along the coasts of the North Sea and the Baltic as well as in Sicily and Southern Italy. Sicily had been conquered from the Saracens, and Southern Italy taken from Byzantium. In these regions there was a fertile mingling of Arabic, Byzantine and Western European civilizations. A graphic example of this is visible to the present day in the cathedral of Monreale near Palermo, an incredibly beautiful Norman church with striking Moorish and Byzantine stylistic influences.

More and more the West abandoned the defensive attitude which it had thus far adopted towards Islam. It succeeded in defeating Arabic superiority at sea. The successful First Crusade (1069—99) contributed to the full restoration of relations with the East. In all of Europe this was followed by a revival of trade and by the emergence of industries, such as the cloth mills in Flanders and England. Money again became a major factor, the cities flourished and there was an increased need for people versed in the art of reading and writing. There also occurred a strong revival in the pursuit of knowledge and education; in Italy the first universities were founded at the beginning of the twelfth century. Particularly after the Great Plague of 1347—50 great social changes took place in which commoners increasingly gained influence, while the political powers of the pope, emperor and feudal nobility gradually waned.

The resurgence of theoretical surgery in the late Middle Ages originated in

Italy, in Salerno in the south and in Bologna in the north. This is undoubtedly related to the cultural blossoming which occurred during the twelfth and thirteenth centuries in the south under the rule of the royal House of Hohenstaufen and later the House of Anjou, and in the north from the beginning of the twelfth century in the free city of Bologna under the protection of the Guelphs.

Since in Italy the old trade relations with the East had remained intact and to a certain extent also the social structure as it had existed since late Antiquity, it is understandable that the revival of surgery, indeed its Renaissance, originated in that country.

2.2.2. *Salerno*[10]

We are completely in the dark, however, as to when and how the medical school of Salerno — the oldest of the Christian Occident — came into being, but already by the beginning of the tenth century there was unequivocal proof of its existence. Its literary production did not start until two-hundred years later, inspired by the Latin adaptations of Arabic medical works by Constantinus Africanus (1015—87), who lived in the Benedictine monastery of Monte Cassino. Among these works were *al-Maliki* by Haly Abbas, which appeared in Latin as *Libri Pantechni* (see page 29), a more or less free adaptation of Arabic versions of Hippocrates' *Aphorisms*, including Galen's commentary on them, and *Ars Medica* by Galen.[11]

The Salerno school acquired a special significance because it was there that for the first time in almost 1000 years anatomy was again studied in practice. Even though dissections were carried out only on animals, especially pigs, and in spite of the fact that it produced little original thought because it anxiously conformed to what classical writers had written, yet it shows that there existed a genuine interest in the structure of the body. Such an interest is always coupled with a flourishing of surgery, as we saw in Alexandria and as we shall see later in several other instances.

The first surgical manual to originate from the Salerno school dates from the second quarter of the twelfth century: it is also the first surgical book of the entire mediaeval Occident. Its author is unknown. The book was named the *Bamberg surgery* by Sudhoff, after the city where the oldest remaining manuscript is kept. However, it is not an original work, but a compilation of the chapters on surgery from Constantinus Africanus' *Pantechni* and of a number of early mediaeval texts, including the recipe for the soporific sponge, which does not occur in the *Pantechni*. It does not have a systematic structure. The few descriptions of operations it contains, such as those for intestinal hernia and goitre, are derived from the *Pantechni*, or else they follow a tradition which goes back to Antiquity. It is worthy of note that in the treatment of goitre there is reference to the internal use of the ashes of sponge and seaweed, which we now know to contain iodine. The latter prescription cannot be traced to classical or Arabic sources. Although four copies from the twelfth and early thirteenth centuries of the *Bamberg surgery* remain — which may indicate that the text enjoyed some popularity — it is not referred to by subsequent authors, nor has it ever appeared in print.[12]

A much more systematic composition was the *Practica chirurgiae* (c. 1175) by Ruggero di Salerno, often called *Post mundi fabricam* after its incipit. This work had a large circulation and was highly respected. It was soon adapted and enlarged with notes and comments by several authors, both in Italy and Southern France. The most important commentators were Rolando di Parma, about 1230, and a little later, the 'Quattuor Magistri', whose identities have remained a mystery. While Roger's original does not reveal any Arabic influence — apart from what was handed down via the *Pantechni* — we find more and more commentaries quoting Arabic authors as time goes by: the Latin translations by Gerard of Cremona had apparently found their mark.

Separate and joint manuscript editions of Roger's work and of his commentators' have been preserved in Latin, French, Provençal and Italian, mostly from the thirteenth century. The Royal Library in The Hague holds a late fifteenth century manuscript which contains among other treatises a surgical tract, consisting of a 'Rogerinus' together with doctrines of Avicenna and an explanation of the four elements, epitomized from the *Four Masters* by a certain Jan Bertrand, who is otherwise unknown to us.[13]

The *Glossulae quattuor magistrorum super chirurgiam Rogerii et Rolandi* are considered the highlight of Salernitan surgery. The book is quoted repeatedly by others, including Jan Yperman and Guy de Chauliac but, unlike the *Practica chirurgiae* and the *Rolandina*, it did not have a Renaissance print.[14] Numerous references to Roger and his school can be found in later literature, even as late as the seventeenth century. Following Gurlt, we will consider Roger, Roland and the Four Masters together as the most important exponents of the Salernitan school.[15] They all treat surgical pathology and therapy in four books a capite ad calcem.

Like the authors of Antiquity and the Muslim world, they devote much space to the treatment of injuries of the head. Viewing the high incidence of war wounds of the skull inflicted by weapons such as clubs, battle axes and stone missiles of the type then in vogue this is only a natural sequence. There is an instructive observation concerning a young man who was hit by a sling stone; the resulting cranial wound seemed trifling but nevertheless the boy died the day after. Autopsy — at that time still very unusual — revealed a large quantity of coagulated blood on the dura mater.[16] The Salernitans were familiar with the fracture by contre coup and to determine whether in a cranial fissure the fracture penetrates to the inner surface of the bone, the patient should blow air while keeping his nose and mouth closed: in the case of a penetrating injury a liquid will emerge from the fissure. The palpating finger may provide much more information about the presence of a fracture than the use of a probe. A fissure is unlikely if the patient is able to crack a nut with his teeth, the Four Masters add.

Treatment should consist of removing impacted bone fragments or, if that is impossible, by making burr holes in the surrounding area (Fig. 8). No particulars are given about the indications and methods for trepanation. However, it is demanded of the surgeon who is going to perform the operation that he abstain from intercourse and from the use of strong-tasting food like garlic and onions beforehand, and refrain from talking to a menstruating woman; he must also have washed his hands.[17].

With regard to the Salernitan way of wound treatment it is frequently stated in secondary literature that it aimed at suppuration.[18] A closer study of Roger, however, gives a more balanced picture. It appears that the treatment differed depending on the location and the nature of the wound. Head wounds with or without a fracture, were merely covered with compresses drenched in white of egg until suppuration occurred, after which the wound was dressed with dry linen. On the other hand, wounds of the soft parts were primarily closed (Fig. 9), leaving one end open in order to allow pus to escape or for the insertion of a small drain, in the manner already described by Celsus. The fact that the Salernitans probably were not aware of that author, although using a similar method, illustrates once more how much the practice of surgery was based on tradition. The sutured wound was dusted with red powder.[19] Into the track of an arrow wound the surgeon must insert, after having removed the projectile (Fig. 10), a tent smeared with animal grease. Serious venous or arterial bleeding in the neck was stopped by undersewing, after which the wound, instead of being sutured, was treated with a dessicative powder. Vascular ligature was also a well-known procedure.

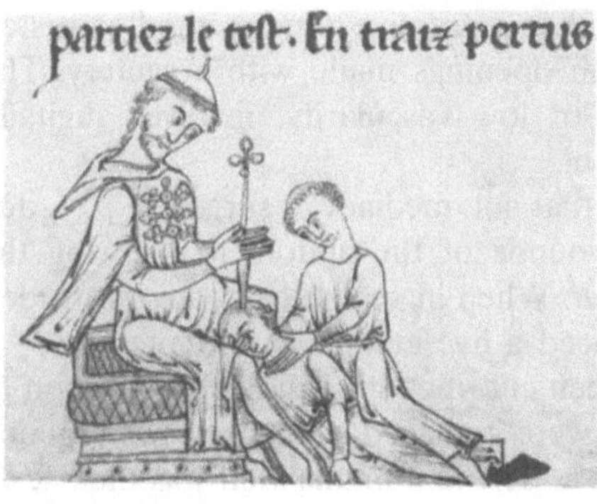

Fig. 8. Salernitan surgery: trepanation of the skull.

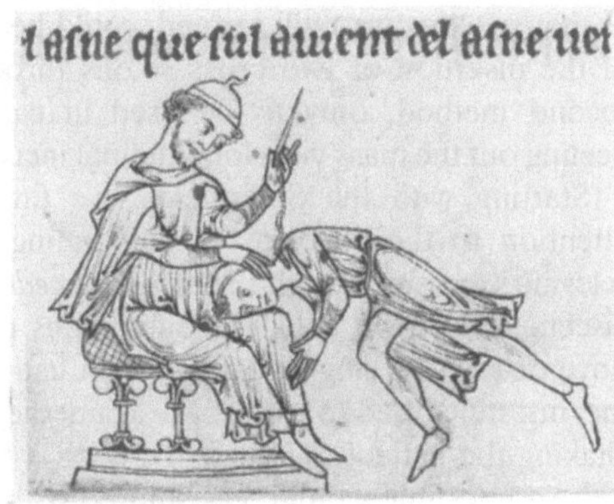

Fig. 9. Salernitan surgery: treatment of a wound in the neck.

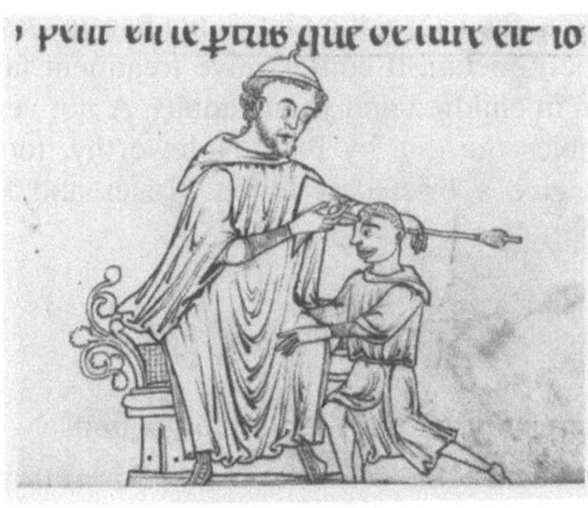

Fig. 10. Salernitan surgery: a serious case.

If the wound was old it had to be washed out until it started to bleed prior to suturing. Suturing was done with silk and a square needle. If the injury had perforated the capsule of a joint the wound was filled with lint drenched in white of egg 'to provoke suppuration'.

Roland explained the preference of the Salernitans for the use of egg-white in bleeding wounds in particular, by its cold nature: it reduced the natural warmth and also checked the generation of pus. Such an explanation does not indicate that the Salernitan school necessarily aimed at healing wounds by suppuration.

Immobilization of fractures was achieved with roller bandages impregnated in white of egg, which hardens somewhat as it dries, with splints applied over the dressing. Another hardening substance was flour mixed with albumen. In the case of a compound fracture a fenestrated bandage was called for. The Four Masters mention breaking the callus in order to reset a fracture which had healed in an unsatisfactory position. In the bandage that Roland used for a collarbone fracture we can already distinguish the principle of the well-known Desault bandage, see Fig. 73.

If conservative methods were of no avail the treatment of goitre or bronchocele as that swelling was still termed, could be rather aggressive. One method consisted of the insertion of two cross setons through openings made with a cautery. The second method, only to be used in case of low vascularity, involved digitally peeling out the mass via a longitudinal incision.

Starting with the Salernitans, we find that all mediaeval surgeons pay due attention to the problem of penetrating wounds of the abdomen following the relevant exposition in the *Methodus medendi.* When in such a case, any protruded viscera had grown cold, the Salernitans placed a live animal on the intestine — a dove or a young dog or cat — which had been cut open longitudinally. As soon as the intestines had warmed up again they were replaced, if necessary by gently shaking the patient as he was lying on a table. The abdominal wall was then sewn up. An intestinal wound was sutured over a small tube of elder or over a length of animal trachea which were placed in the lumen. In such a case the surgeon must first await the healing of the intestinal wound before he could think of closing the abdomen.

As in Paul of Aegina, the cause of an intestinal hernia was attributed to either a torn or a stretched peritoneum. If conservative treatment failed, one could resort to a radical operation in children and young adults. A not very clear description of this operation resembles the one by Paul. Noteworthy, too, is the lithotomy, of which these authors give a brief description. Roger and his successors do not mention the soporific sponge.

2.3.3. Northern Italy

2.2.3.1. Bruno da Longoburgo; Theodorico Borgognoni

Salerno did not long remain the scientific centre for European medicine. In the thirteenth century the focus moved to the Po valley, to Padua and Verona and in particular to Bologna, which had had an important university since the middle of the twelfth century. Among the surgeons who were active in this region we have in the first place to mention Master Bruno.

About the life of this Bruno we know little more than that he came from Longoburgo in Calabria and that he worked in Padua and Verona. In 1252 he completed his *Chirurgia magna*, a work which, as he himself indicated, he had compiled from Hippocrates, Galen, Avicenna, Albucasis, Haly Abbas and other Arabic authors. It appears, however, that this well-arranged book also contains many original observations and remarks. Only a single copy of a Middle Dutch translation has survived.[20] Yet the Flemish surgeon Jan Yperman, to be discussed later, quoted him nine times. The book must therefore have been known in the Netherlands prior to its appearance in print in the 1498 edition of the Venetian surgical collection.[14] This author, too, will be treated here by means of the excerpt in Gurlt.[21]

In his introduction Bruno makes a few important remarks about the way in which surgeons ought to be educated, and about some qualities they must have. Concerning the former, they must watch experienced surgeons at work as often as they can. With regard to their personality he demands that they be neither fearful nor reckless, that they perform their task with great care and, particularly when they operate on risky locations like the brain, they be not drunk. They must be familiar with the most important surgical writings. If they are not, let them at least learn the craft from someone who is. This statement suggests that apart from literate surgeons, by which Bruno probably means university men, uneducated persons were also admitted to the profession. Much of what Bruno writes on matters like this can later be found in Henri de Mondeville.

Bruno defines the scope of surgery as uniting that which has come apart, separating that which has come together in an unnatural way, and taking away that which is superfluous.[22] Bruno's treatment of wounds is based on the principle of dessication. Before the wound can be sutured or dressed it must be cleansed carefully of contaminations like hair, oil or ointment. Large wounds are to be sewn up with a fine, square needle and with a silk or linen thread. The individual sutures must be placed at intervals of the size of a finger top, but the ends of a wound must be open so that pus can escape. A mode of proceeding which ever since the Salernitans was adopted by almost all mediaeval surgeons when they had recourse to wound suture. To dress the wound the use of wet medicaments is not allowed, because that may cause disruption. In the healing process Bruno like Galen distinguishes between a 'prima intentio' and a 'secunda intentio'. The latter must be the aim in case of deep wounds in which wound drainage is inadequate. Such wounds must either be enlarged, or the secretion must be drained via a counter incision.

In cases of penetrating abdominal wounds, if the fallen down and swollen viscera cannot easily be replaced, Bruno follows the advice of Galen and Haly Abbas and suspends the patient by his hands and feet in a hot tub while shaking him gently. Any darkened omentum is simply snipped off. Small intestinal wounds must be repaired with a very fine needle and a silk thread. After the viscera have been returned, the ends of the sutures are left dangling outside — as was done by the Salernitans. The abdomen must not be closed until after the intestines have healed. Such a patient must be nursed with a flexed back in order to relieve the abdominal wall; the diet must not contain food productive of intestinal gas.

Bruised wounds require a treatment with suppurative medicaments.[23] Haemostasis is achieved in the usual manner by elevation, the application of cold substances, the use of red powder, undersewing or cauterization. Much attention is paid to fistulae. They are incurable if they originate from the intestines, the bladder, the ribs, the vertebrae or the joints. He also discusses osteomyelitis in this connection. In his extensive exposition of head injuries Bruno draws on Hippocrates and Galen; an observation of his own is that many have recuperated from an injury of the dura mater. Bruno is in favour of early reduction of fractures; in applying splints he follows classical prescriptions, a broken lower leg may be placed in a wooden box-splint. Much attention is paid to 'apostemata'. By an aposteme he means a 'tumor vel inflatio preter naturam'. He distinguishes between four types: 'phlegmon, erisipela, zinia and zephiros aut cancer', respectively caused by blood, yellow bile, phlegm and black bile; in short, by one of the four 'humores'. In this we recognize the surgical pathology as expounded by Galen, the words 'zinia' and 'zephiros' betray Arabian influence. The symptoms of phlegmon — inflammation — are the same as those summed up by Celsus, although Bruno does not quote him. An abscess must be opened as soon as it is ripe.

The treatment of intestinal hernia and bladder stone does not differ from Paul and Albucasis; from Bruno's description it is not clear whether he removes the testis during an operation for scrotal hernia. Bruno does not discuss amputations.

First among the Bologna surgeons ranked the Borgognonis. Father Hugo, also known as Ugo de Lucca,[24] a physician and surgeon who in 1218 accompanied the army with which Bologna participated in the Fifth Crusade. Hugo himself did not leave any writings but his son Theodoric (1205—98) recorded many of Hugo's principles and experiences in his *Cyrurgia*, which he completed around 1267. As a student Theodoric had entered the Dominican order, but apparently this was not an obstacle to his practising medicine. He had an excellent clerical career, and finally became bishop of Cervia, near Ravenna. The other sources to which Theodoric refers in his book are Hippocrates and Galen — the *Methodus medendi* and the *Commentary on the Aphorisms of Hippocrates* — and, of the Arabic authors, Avicenna, Albucasis, Haly Abbas, Rhazes and a few others. He mentions Roger and his school only occasionally. On the other hand he derived much from the work of the slightly older Bruno da Longoburgo,[25] from whom he copied large excerpts almost verbatim though without ever mentioning his name.

Of Theodoric's *Surgery* fourteen complete and incomplete manuscript editions have been preserved. The copy in the possession of the University of Leyden, with its beautiful illustrations, is world-famous. It dates from about 1400 and appears to originate from Italy, but it is not possible to circumscribe its provenance more precisely. There exist besides eleven manuscript copies translations into Catalan, Spanish, Italian, French, English, German and Hebrew: many of them incomplete. This work, too, appeared in print in Venice in 1498, in the surgical collection mentioned before.[26]

In Theodoric's *Cyrurgia*, the sections on wounds and their treatment are especially of interest.[27] The proper treatment of wounds is by desiccation: Galen had written that everything that is dry promotes the healing process.[28] Wine is the best medicine for all wounds: its penetration is deep, it dries and cleanses, he says after Galen. Used internally it promotes the production of new flesh. His father Hugo treated almost any wound with only wine and work and skilfully applied bandages and he procured excellent scars without resorting to any ointment. Theodoric disapproves of the suppurative type of wound treatment. In the chapter on head injuries, which he prefers to treat by suturing and dry dressings, he writes:

> For it is not necessary, as stupid men do, to place a wick at the end of a suture line; nor . . . is it necessary to generate bloody matter in a wound, as Roger and Roland and many of their disciples teach, and as almost all modern surgeons continue to do. For there can be no error greater than this, and nothing else which impedes nature so much and prolongs the sickness, prevents uniting and consolidating of a wound, deforms the part and impedes cicatrization.

Head injuries receive much attention from Theodoric. He extensively discusses the diagnosis, prognosis and treatment of wounds of the soft parts, the various types of cranial fracture, injuries of the meninges and of the cerebral substance. An interesting observation of his father Hugo concerns a patient who suffered a loss of cerebral matter at the site of the 'cellula memorativa'.[29] Repair took place by producing flesh instead of cerebral matter. Nevertheless, to Hugo's great surprise the patient's memory was unaffected.[30]

The chapters on penetrating abdominal wounds and intestinal injuries are entirely in the Galenic tradition and bear a strong resemblance to those by Bruno. Theodoric's enterorrhaphy, however, is the Salernitan method over a length of elder introduced into the lumen of the gut.

Theodoric's treatment of fractures and dislocations show little originality. Like Hippocrates, he is aware of neurological complications of lesions of the vertebrae. For the prognosis of those of the neck the surgeon must examine the hands: if these are limp and senseless and immobile, the situation is serious. In case of damage to the lumbar vertebrae the same signs must be looked for in the feet. Faecal incontinence, a distended abdomen and the inability to control urination indicate that the disorder is fatal: such symptoms implied damage to the spinal medulla. In the chapter on fistulae, cancers and other swellings such as warm and cold abscesses, furuncles, carbuncles, goitre, ascites, herniae, haemorrhoids and other anal disorders, and skin diseases, we come across an explanation of what is understood by laudable sanies.[31] Such matter is white, gleaming and liquid, and has no bad odour, Theodoric writes after Hippocrates. The white colour shows that nature has succeeded in her attempt to eliminate the disease by a process of coction. The smooth consistency indicates that a 'digestive virtue' is operative, and the absence of a fetid smell is a sign that there is no putrefaction.

In his pathophysiological explanation of various tumours and swellings, Theodoric shows himself a faithful follower of Galen. Gangrene may necessitate an amputation, taking away part of the live and healthy flesh: the wound surface must be cauterized. He does not give further details about this operation.

As regards the diagnosis and treatment of herniae and bladder stones, Theodoric does not differ from his contemporaries. In the fourth book of his *Cyrurgia*, which deals with headache, eye diseases, gout, paralysis and other afflictions, we come across the recipe for the soporific sponge. This recipe does not occur in Bruno. Unlike Hippocrates, Theodoric recommends a strengthening diet for the wounded.

2.2.3.2. Guglielmo da Saliceto

Living at about the same time as Theodoric was Guglielmo da Saliceto, born in Piacenza (c. 1210—80). Most of his life he lived and taught in Bologna. He was considered the most competent surgeon of his day. His *Cyrurgia*, written in 1275, is, just like the writings of his contemporaries, of a compilatory nature. It does not contain any major innovations but the subjects are excellently arranged and the text is enlivened by numerous instructive examples. He quotes relatively few other writers: Galen, a few Arabs and contemporaries. Diagnosis and therapy are lucidly expounded, in a manner which conveys great practical experience. It is therefore understandable that William's surgical text was widely appreciated at the time.

As this author is not quoted by the Flemish surgeons of the late Middle Ages, we will refrain from a discussion of his work: suffice it to say that the fourth book concerning anatomy is probably the oldest treatise of surgical anatomy. The new element in it is its topographical approach, but apart from that the anatomical descriptions are as awkward as those of his predecessors.

William was the teacher of Lanfranc of Milan, to whom we will turn our attention presently.

2.2.3.3. The Rise of Human Anatomy

The first dissection of a human body to have taken place since the days of the Ptolomies in Alexandria was conducted in 1302. This was a forensic autopsy and it was probably no coincidence that it occurred in Bologna, as its university had a very important law school. It was also in Bologna that in 1315 a modest start was made with the teaching of anatomy using human subjects. Mondino di Luzzi, the professor in charge of this teaching, had only very few cadavers available for his demonstration lectures. But apparently they were sufficient in number to enable him to write a book about the structure of the human body, which appeared in print in 1478 — 150 years later! — and which was to be a standard work at many universities for almost two centuries. In 1512 a Dutch translation was published in Antwerp.[32] The anatomy which Mondino expounds, in spite of the fact that he had had the opportunity of dissecting a few cadavers, is wholly derived from Galen. In the late Middle Ages the dissection of the human cadaver did not in the first place aim at conducting independent research but rather at visualizing what Galen had said (Fig. 11).

Bologna's example was soon to be followed by other Italian universities, which were founded in great numbers during the thirteenth and fourteenth centuries.[33] By including anatomy and surgery in the curriculum the medical faculties contributed considerably to the profession's development and to the important social status which surgeons held in Italy at that time.[34] The prominent surgical authors of this period, beginning with Roger, had had an academic background or even taught at universities. Because the professors and students at most mediaeval universities belonged to the clergy, we find that a number of the writing surgeons had received holy orders.

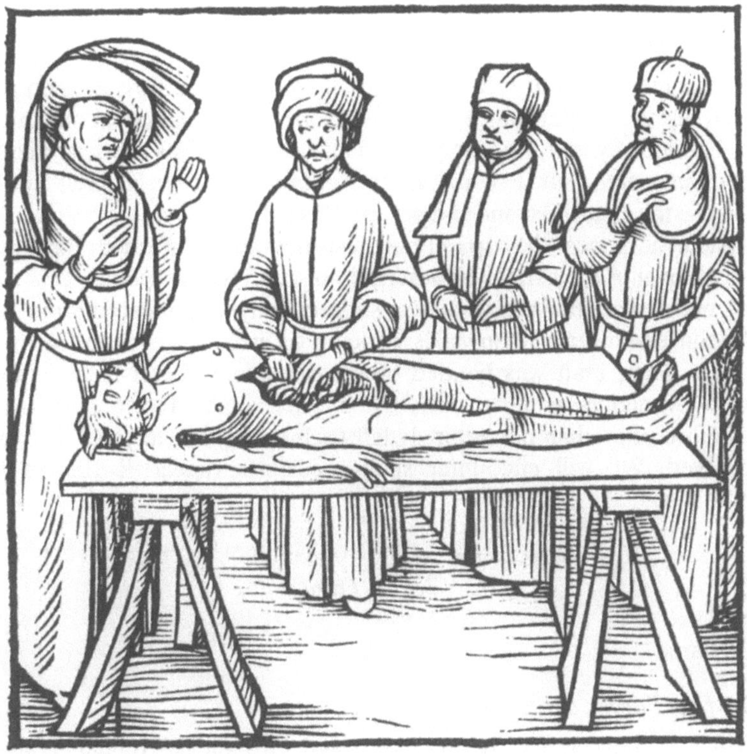

Fig. 11. Anatomical dissection in the 15th century.

2.2.3.4. Surgery and the Church

This brings us to the question how the latter can be reconciled with the famous dictum 'Ecclesia abhorret a sanguine' (the Church abhors blood) which many textbooks of the history of medicine wish us to believe were the words used by the mediaeval Church when she prohibited the clergy to practise surgery. This phrase is a literary ghost, as Talbot pointed out: it is not to be found in the text of any of the several Councils to which it has been attributed nor in the Decretals of the Popes.[35] This does not alter the fact that a binding prohibition to that effect was elaborated by the Fourth Lateran Council in 1215. The interdict, formulated in decree no. 18, stipulates that no member of the clergy is allowed to become involved with anything that has to do with the shedding of blood, whether it concerns pronouncing a capital sentence in a court of law or supervising judicial tortures, or engaging in a duel. No sub-deacon, deacon or priest, it continues, is allowed to practise any form of surgery which involves cauterizing or cutting. It was apparently not too difficult, however, to get dispensation, as the clerical surgeons of the thirteenth and fourteenth centuries — Theodorico Borgognoni, Bruno da Longburgo, Guglielmo da Saliceto, Lanfranchi — all practised after 1212. The interdict, which is apt to have contributed much to the laicization of medicine, is still in force.[36]

2.2.3.5. Itinerant Empirics

Until the eighteenth century there existed all over Europe travelling empirics who specialized in the performance of certain operations, mainly couching for the cataract, herniotomy and lithotomy. Specialized lithotomists are first mentioned in the Hippocratic oath, but it seems as if from time immemorial such 'cutters' have been active in the Near East and India.

In Hellenistic times the operations just mentioned formed part of regular surgery as shown in their detailed descriptions by Celsus and Paul. This apparently does not mean that traditional cutters subsequently disappeared from the scene. From the thirteenth century onwards we learn of their existence in Europe as well, first in Italy. Their craft was handed down as a family secret from father to son, taught and learned in practice only.[37] For quite some time to come established surgeons more often than not willingly left such operations to them, because of the risks involved. We will encounter such specialists repeatedly in the following chapters.

2.2.4. *France*

2.2.4.1. Paris

Position of the Barber-Surgeons

If in the thirteenth century surgery flourished only on the Italian peninsula, one hundred years later it had spread to France, where Paris and Montpellier established themselves as medical centres of European renown. In Paris there had existed a medical faculty since the early thirteenth century, but, unlike the Italian universities, surgery did not have a structural place in the curriculum.[38]

Around the middle of the century the barber-surgeons had united in a guild, the 'Confrérie de Saint-Côme', for the furthering of their interests.[39] An ordinance of 1311 — which was renewed several times — shows that in Paris, after taking the appropriate examinations, admission to the practice of surgery was also open to women.[40]

Lanfranc (Lanfranchi, Lanfranco)

The bridge between the Parisian surgeons and Italian surgery was made by Lanfranc, a pupil of William of Saliceto. Lanfranc had been forced to leave Milan, the city where he had practised medicine and surgery, as a result of the feuds between the Guelphs and the Ghibelines. In 1295 he established himself in Paris. There, he writes, he found surgery to be lingering in a deplorable state. He joined the Confrérie de Saint-Côme and began delivering lectures to its members, and giving clinical demonstrations, which were quite novel at the time. These were a great success. Hundreds of interested people flocked from afar to his lectures, possibly including Jan Yperman, with whom the history of Dutch surgery proper begins. Lanfranc also appears to have taught at the medical faculty. His activities form the basis of French surgery, which was in course of time to flourish so brilliantly with Paris as its centre.[41] He is thought to have died in 1315.

Lanfranc's written legacy consists of his masterly *Chirurgia magna*, which he finished in 1296, and a *Chirurgia parva*, edited somewhat earlier. Both writings had a large dissemination throughout the mediaeval Occident, as is evidenced by numerous manuscripts and many incunable editions and translations. They have strongly influenced later manuals, especially those which appeared in vernacular languages.[42] Unquestionably Lanfranc would have ranked high in late mediaeval and renaissance citation indexes. Of both the major and the smaller work there have appeared Middle Dutch translations, which are older than those in Middle German. The library of the Royal Dutch Society of Medicine possesses a very handsome paper manuscript of a Flemish edition of the *Chirurgia magna* from the fourteenth century, but also in Ghent and in Uppsala there are complete copies, while fragments are held in Darmstadt, Cologne and London.[43] Dutch manuscripts of the Lanfranc *Parva* are in London and in Paris, while incunables of this work date from 1481 (Louvain) and 1529 (Antwerp).[44]

The *Chirurgia magna*, which will again be discussed following Gurlt,[45] is made up of five tracts. In the second chapter of doctrine I of the first tract Lanfranc enters at length into the demands which a good surgeon must meet. These are substantial. His temperament must be balanced, his hands be well-shaped, with long, slender fingers, and his body not tremble. He must be humble, of a strong mind but not overconfident. He should be versed in all sciences, not just in medicine, but in all branches of philosophy, in logic, grammar and dialectics.[46] He must also have a knowledge of ethics and live a virtuous life without greed or adultery, jealousy or avarice. In the home of the patient he shall not look at any woman, nor quarrel with the patient's family, reassure the patient in all respects but inform his kindred in time if the case is serious. He must not concern himself with hopeless cases. He shall give assistance to the poor for whatever they are able to pay, but he is at liberty to ask 'bona salaria' from the rich. He shall honour all physicians and clerics and he shall not antagonize any surgeon if he can help it.[47]

The second doctrine briefly deals with anatomy and physiology.

Lanfranc's approach to the treatment of wounds is described in the third doctrine: it is similar to Bruno's. He gives an elaborate explanation of how to close a wound with sutures and about how to tie a surgical knot. The triangular needle should at its blunt end beyond the eye have a slot by which the thread is prevented from offering resistance when the needle is pulled through the tissues. The wound heals most handsomely if the edges are not approximated too tightly. With deep wounds deep stitches must be used, because if a cavity remains under a superficial closure, blood and purulent matter may gather there, which impede the process of repair.[48] There is no question of suturing a wound that has suffered a substantial loss of tissue; such an injury must be kept clean and allowed to heal by regeneration and cicatrization.

The chapter on peripheral nerve injuries is interesting. When a nerve has been divided completely, Lanfranc writes, the extremity loses its sensibility and mobility, which that nerve had conducted from the brain. In contrast to Theodoric he considers this an indication for surgical repair. This is sought by applying the wound sutures in such a way as to approximate the nerve's ends. Like the other Italian surgeons mentioned so far, Lanfranc describes rabies and its treatment.

First he sucks out the wound by means of a cupping glass, then cuts it open, cauterizes it and dresses it with medicines which attract the poison.

He gives an elaborate account of haemostasis, enlivened by case histories. Besides arterial and venous bleeding Lanfranc mentions bleeding 'a venis capillaribus parvis'. If the haemorrhage cannot be stopped with a simple white of egg bandage, he advises the surgeon to compress the bleeding vessel with his finger 'for well over an hour', after which he must cover the wound with a paste consisting of incense powder, aloe, chopped fur of a hare — haemostatic components that we have met already with Galen and some thousand years later with the Salernitans — mixed with white of egg so as to give it the consistency of honey. If this does not help or if it cannot be used the surgeon must pull out the end of the blood vessel in order to twist it or to tie it with a silk thread — once again a recommendation we met with in Galen — or otherwise sear it with a very hot cautery. One had better leave open cancers alone if they cannot be removed root and branch, because the more cancers are attacked by violent means, the more malignant they become. If bloodletting, cupping, administering enemas, suppositories, salving the neck, armpits and groin are of no avail, tetanus must be treated by cutting a nerve or even the main nerve. This admittedly leads to the loss of sensation and mobility, but it is better to live with a handicap than to die. Lanfranc does not say anthing about the results of his energetic neurosurgical approach to tetanus.

The second tract discusses various bodily injuries a capite ad calcem. In this Lanfranc does not essentially differ from his predecessors. He recognizes 'motio cerebri ex concussione' without a fracture or external wound, but expresses his reservations about trepanation. He does not lend credence to the stories of cut-off noses which were successfully sewn back in their place. If one is able neither to locate an arrowhead nor remove it, one has to wait patiently until the body expels the foreign body. He is familiar with the incisional hernia, which can be the late result of an otherwise healed abdominal wound.

The third tract expounds — at times elaborately — congenital and acquired skin diseases, abscesses, cancer, goitre and others. For the treatment of ruptures he prefers trusses. Cutting for the stone is conducted according to the method of the classical authors. As an early complication of lithotomy Lanfranc mentions the occurrence of severe pains below the navel, high fever with rigors while the extremities grow cold, and hiccups. He does not explain these symptoms, but is well aware that death will not be long to follow. Some patients have to pay for this operation with impotence.

The third tract expounds — at times elaborately — congenital and acquired abnormalities of the genitals, as well as various types of dropsy, haemorrhoids, peri-anal abscesses, fistulae and condylomata, leg ulcers (which must be treated with white-hot cauteries), varicose veins and elephantiasis, which we will not detail here. It is noteworthy, however, that in the sixteenth chapter, which deals with bloodletting, Lanfranc expresses his displeasure over the practice of leaving this minor operation to barbers 'propter nostram superbiam': because of our pride. This statement shows that he looked upon himself as a physician. He challenges the opinion that it is impossible for a single person to be proficient in both medicine and surgery: those who know nothing about operative surgery cannot possibly be good physicians and the surgeon for his part must be familiar with the various branches of internal medicine. As does Albucasis, Lanfranc knows thirty veins in the head, neck, arms, hands and legs which are eligible for bloodletting. He agrees with Avicenna that the use of the cautery is one of the great and noble operations of sugery. However, inspired perhaps by his teacher, who restricted the use of the cautery in favour of the knife, he reduces the numerous types of cauters which Avicenna described to ten.

The subject of the fourth book is fractures and dislocations. Lanfranc is the first to describe the ingenious method of tightening multiple splints by means of two or three small wooden tubes. These tubes are inserted under the cords that fix the splints to the limb. By giving the tubes one or more turns as one does with the handle of the corkscrew, the cords are caught in a loop. With each turn that loop is twisted further, thereby tightening the cord around the splints. Once the fixation of the splints seems satisfactory, a rod is inserted into the lumen of the tubes which should be lying in line. In this way the tension of the cords is retained and they are prevented from sliding down. This method of fixing splints was also used by Guy de Chauliac and others (Fig. 12).

The fifth and final tract contains an antidotary.

2.2.4.2. Montpellier

The Barber-Surgeons' Guild

As early as 1252 the existence of an organization of barber-surgeons at Montpellier is apparent from ordinances, in which regulations can be found concerning statutory closing hours of shops, admission of new members and the rights of widows.[49] The organizational structure of this 'Confrérie de Saint-Côme et Saint-Damian' corresponded in a great many respects to that of the subsequent Dutch guilds, which will be discussed in the next chapter. There was none of the animosity in Montpellier that marked the relationship between the university and the guild in Paris. This may be related to the fact that unlike the majority of other mediaeval universities, including that of Paris, the university of Montpellier was not exclusively a clerical institution.

The geographical situation of the city was conducive to contacts with Italy. Of the surgeons who made extensive acquaintance with Italian surgery two must be given further consideration here.

Henri de Mondeville

Born in Normandy around 1260, Henri de Mondeville probably studied medicine in Montpellier and Paris. He was a cleric. After having obtained the degree of Master of Medicine,[50] he made a study tour in Italy where he was for some time under the tutelage of Theodoric. Later he became physician to the king and taught anatomy and surgery at the medical faculty of Paris.

When he died around 1320 — he was 'asthmaticus, tussiculosus, phthisicus' — his great textbook, on which he had worked intermittently for years, was not yet finished. It nevertheless became very popular and many manuscript editions have been preserved either entirely or in part. The book was soon translated into

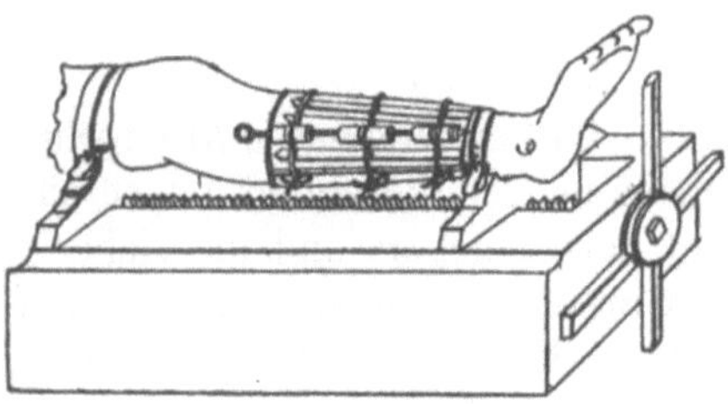

Fig. 12. Lanfranc's method of applying splints to the leg.

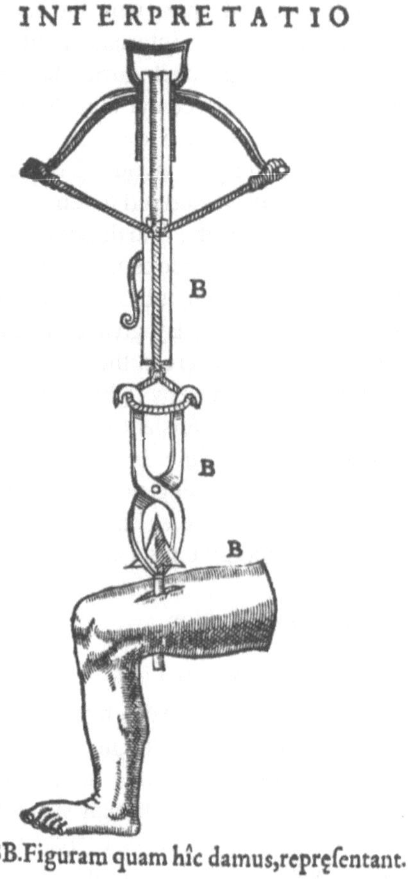

Fig. 13. Arcubalista: pincers combined with an arbalest for forcible extraction of foreign bodies.

French out of the original Latin. The British Museum holds a Middle Dutch translation — without illustrations — of Henri's surgery dating from the beginning of the fifteenth century.[51] It seems as if Henri de Mondeville, apart from the Latin and French, only exists in Dutch translation. In view of the fact that this, the only surviving Dutch manuscript, was severely affected by fire and water damage, we will consider the work by means of the excellent French edition by Nicaise of 1893.[52]

The first tract is on anatomy, which Henri seems to have largely derived from Avicenna. He was strongly convinced of the advantage of anatomical knowledge for the surgeons. It was he who made the well-known comparison with the blind woodcutter, who works his material in the same way as does a surgeon not acquainted with anatomy.[53]

The second tract contains surgery. It is once again largely a compilatory work. For didactic purposes the very detailed text is written after the manner of scholastic didactics.[54] The numerous quotations reflect the typically mediaeval belief in authority.[54] Mondeville proves to be not only an erudite physician, for he was also well read in literature and particularly in philosophy: his entire work bears the stamp of logic and Aristotelian philosophy. This tract is attractive to the modern reader especially for the extensive information it contains on contemporary professional matters: how to become a good surgeon, how to deal with fellow-surgeons, physicians and patients, how to make sure one gets one's fee. This book also shows how widespread was the practice of quackery.

According to Henri, the art of surgery can only be mastered by watching others perform operations, then by operating in company with other surgeons for a considerable time before attempting independent practice oneself.[56] A great deal of attention must be paid to theory, not concentrating only on anatomy and the principles of operative surgery, but also considering general pathology. Every surgeon ought to know something about medicine. The pathology of Mondeville is entirely that of Galen, as it is formulated in his *Ars medica*.[57] Surgery is both a science and an art. Surgery is surer, more preferable, noble, perfect, necessary and lucrative than treatment with regimens of diet and drugs and therefore it is superior to medicine.[58] His deontological comments bear a strong resemblance to Lanfranc. He argues moreover, that it is not a good thing when several physicians treat simultaneously one and the same patient, who will then have many different drugs prescribed for him. None of the surgeons will then be able to act exactly as he thinks fit on the basis of his experience, for no surgeon is willing to reveal the personal tricks which he feels ensure his success. As a result rich patients often receive worse treatment than the poor who can only afford the services of one physician.[59] Mondeville carefully describes how medical men ought to behave when they are in consultation.

The relationship between surgeons and physicians was often anything but congenial. Mondeville illustrates this by means of the following example. When a physician is summoned in the first instance to attend a surgical case other than a wound, dislocation or fracture, he will seldom immediately refer the treatment to a surgeon. Instead he will cunningly say:

> My dear man, it is a known fact that surgeons are arrogant and utterly ignorant, and the little knowledge they may have, they have obtained from us, physicians: besides they are malicious and cruel people. You are truly better off with a physician, it is not for nothing that a physician asks a high fee. For the love of you I will treat you to the best of my abilities, even though I am not a surgeon.

If all ends well, that is the end of the affair. But if there is no improvement the physician will say at a certain point:

> Sir, I told you at once I am not a surgeon. Nevertheless I have treated you according to the rules of the craft. Now in the meantime I have become so busy, that I can no longer care for you; I advise you to take a surgeon from now on, and you had best take so and so.

He then sends for an ignorant surgeon, who will not be able to recognize any mistakes the physician may have made. If the patient recovers, the physician can still claim all the credit, but in the opposite case he can easily blame the stupid surgeon. Conversely, many surgeons meddle with internal diseases without involving a physician.[60]

That Henri de Mondeville is not without a trace of cynicism is apparent from his summary of surgical savoir-faire: not to shrink from stench; to know how to cut or destroy like a butcher; to be able to lie courteously; and to know how delicately to wheedle gifts and money from patients.[61] The matter of the fee seems to have preoccupied him greatly: he repeatedly points to the fact that patients, once recovered, will try to back out of their financial obligations. The surgeon is therefore advised to insist on advance payment.[62].

Of the actual surgical portions of his tracts, we will deal mainly with his treatment of wounds. In this, Mondeville follows Theodoric's method, which he introduced in France together with his Paris teacher Jean Pitard and which was tested to his great satisfaction during several military campaigns.[63] The principal differences between the traditional wound treatment and that of Theodoric and himself, is explained in detail in his discussion of injuries of the head. The adherents of the current method, which goes back to Antiquity, he calls 'les ancients', while he calls Theodoric and his school the 'moderns'. He does not exactly reveal whom he considers 'ancients' but since he repeatedly appeals to the *Methodus medendi* by Galen, they are apparently not the classical authors in general. It is clear though that he includes the Salernitans in this category.[64]

The moderns aim at a wound healing without suppuration. They do not consider pus a normal product of the process of wound repair, but as something which is brought about as the result of some five different factors. The first one is deterioration of the wound caused by open air: this can be prevented by closing the wound as soon as possible. The second cause is an excessive influx of juices, which can be countered with measures enhancing the drainage, elevating the afflicted part, wine compresses, and a light diet. The third factor lies in the weakness of the afflicted part, which can be combated with an appropriate bandage together with internal and external use of wine. An unsuitable diet can also bring about suppuration, as well as, finally, the application of digestives.[65]

Unlike Hippocrates, Henri recommends haemorrhage to be staunched as soon as possible, because loss of blood can lead to 'syncope'.[66] Wound treatment must not be conducted in the vicinity of red objects — such as blankets of that colour — because there exists attraction between equals: the blood would then flow more forcefully or afresh.[67] If possible the surgeon must close the wound immediately after the removal of impurities. When dressing the sutured wound hot wine compresses must be used. For local treatment only wine need be considered and even then only in the case of suppuration and wounds which are healing by granulation. One should never pour wine into fresh, clean wounds.[68]

The technique of wound closure Henri describes in detail but we will only reflect that like Celsus he recommends refreshing older wounds by chafing the edges until they bleed slightly. [69]

Of the major operations De Mondeville only discusses amputation, which he performed in cases of gangrene in order to call a halt to further decay. But when the gangrene had already progessed above the knee, he considers the patient doomed. The amputation can be performed most easily in the proximal joint, if one wants to perform the operation lower down it must be done precisely at the boundary between the healthy and the sick parts with a large red hot iron or a golden knife.[70] Henri de Mondeville does not mention the soporific sponge, which his master Theodoric seems to have used.

The third part of his great work is only half finished. Mondeville never got round to the fourth book, which was to include fractures and dislocations. The fifth tract, however, being an antidotary, was completed.[71]

Guy de Chauliac

This physician and surgeon, about whom comparatively little is known, appears to have been born in the small village of Chaulhac in the present Département de la Lozère in 1298 and then to have studied in Toulouse and Montpellier. Like Henri de Mondeville, he spent some time in Bologna, where he attended the anatomy lessons of Nicolo Bertuccio, the pupil and successor of Mondino. He was both personal physician as well as commensal chaplain to three successive popes in exile at Avignon. Guy was already in his sixties, when 'ad solatium senectutis', as he explained, he wrote his *Inventorium sive Collectorium artis chirurgicalis medicinae* or *Chirurgia magna.* He died around 1368. A *Chirurgia parva*, previously attributed to him, which is really not much more than a formulary, was apparently not written by Guy.

Guy's *Grande chirurgie* is one of the highlights in the history of surgery. The author proves himself to be a man of incredibly wide reading; there are more than 3000 references in his book to more than a hundred authors, in particular the Arabs. The name of Avicenna appears no less than 661 times, that of Albucasis 173 times and to a lesser degree those of Rhazes, Haly Abbas, Avenzoar and others. Of the ancient authors mentioned, Galen tops the list: Guy appears to have known no fewer than 31 works by him.[72] He mentions Lanfranc most often of the Western authors (102 times), although he reproaches the Italian for having based his work largely on that of William of Saliceto. And yet the *Grande chirurgie* is not primarily a 'scholarly' book. Like all the works of the great mediaeval surgeons it is also based on an extensive practical experience, for the author tells us he has attended 'quantité d'opérations', and has performed, over long periods of time, operations in the various places where he has lived. He does not however introduce intrinsic innovations of any importance.

Unlike that of Henri de Mondeville, Guy's work stands out for its harmonious structure, a clear and succinct style and a critical treatment of the subject matter, so that Nicaise rewarded him with the title of 'Father of didactic surgery'. He was praised as: '. . . cet excellent auteur, que tout le monde reconnait pour le premier qui ait reduit la chirurgie en art' by the Parisian surgeon Laurent Verduc, who published a textbook in the form of questions and answers in 1691, based on the *Grande chirurgie*, for the benefit of contemporary students of surgery.[73] For centuries, *La grande chirurgie* had a large circulation in many languages. At the end of the last century Nicaise counted 34 surviving manuscript editions in Latin, French, Provençal, Catalan, Flemish,[74] English and Hebrew, written between 1368 and 1478. Some of them are beautifully illustrated. After the invention of printing it appeared in several languages in at least 56 printed editions; one, in French, was as late as 1683.[75] The catechetic adaptation of Verduc went through eight editions, the last one in 1744. Guy or Guido was frequently quoted in the surgical literature all over Europe far into the eighteenth century. Even his great compatriot Ambroise Paré has not quite been able to eclipse his reputation. *La grande chirurgie* passed through four editions in Dutch between 1509 and 1646. In view of the considerable direct and indirect influence which Guy de Chauliac's work had on surgery, including that of the Netherlands, we shall go into it in greater detail.[76]

The work consists of seven 'traités', preceded by a prologue and a 'chapitre singulier' in which Guy reflects on the art of surgery and its practitioners. His deontological precepts do not differ greatly from those of Bruno, Theodoric, Lanfranc and Henri. In the prologue can be found the famous, often quoted statement: 'Scientiae enim per addimenta fiunt' (the sciences are made of additions) '. . . we are as children on the shoulders of a giant for we can see all that the giant sees and a little more besides'.[77]

After a short but valuable historical survey the author continues with a division which he believes can be made amongst contemporary surgeons. First of all he distinguishes two major 'sects': the logicians or rationalists — those who have studied the works of the Ancients — and the empiricists. In this he apparently follows Galen, who heartily disapproved of the latter category. By and large, the division between surgeons with some kind of scientific background and empiricists remained valid until the early nineteenth century. Next to this, Guy makes a second division with reference to:

- those who treat all wounds with poultices in order to cause suppuration. In doing so, these men appeal to Hippocrates' aphorism: softness in wounds is favourable, hardness is bad. He includes Roger, Roland and the Four Masters in this group.
- those who aim at a dessicative treatment in all cases by using wine compresses only, following Galen's statement in the fourth book of the *Methodus medendi*: what is dry is closer to that which is healthy, and what is moist is closer to that which is unhealthy. Both Bruno and Theodoric belong to this category.[78]
- those who, based on the fourteenth book of the *Methodus medendi*, in which it is stated that treatment must be sure and painless, adopt a middle course by dressing all wounds with salves and soft plasters. They are represented by Guglielmo da Saliceto and Lanfranchi.
- two groups of laymen who, like soldiers, dress wounds with oil, cabbage leaves and linen while uttering magic formulae, or who, like women, entrust recovery entirely to God's saints.

From what we have summarized of the work of Roger and his school it may be clear that Guy does not quite do justice to the wound treatment of the Salernitans who in a Hippocratic way adapted their approach to the situation, type and condition of the wounds.

In the seven books now following, Guy always offers a general survey of the subjects and afterwards discusses them with reference to specific locations.

The first book (traité) deals with anatomy. As for the use of this science, Guy quotes a statement by Galen in which the latter enumerates four advantages: the first and most important advantage of anatomy is to demonstrate God's omnipotence, the second advantage is to be able to distinguish the afflicted parts, the third is to be able to foresee the future dispositions of the body, the fourth and last advantage is to know the diseases.

There are no indications in Guy's work, that he ever practised anatomical dissections himself. His scientific method is strictly theoretical, whereby, in a typically mediaeval way, he advances the opinions of several authorities and then tries to reconcile them. If synthesis proves impossible, he choses from amongst the divergent opinions the one which seems to him most plausible. In doing so he always attempts to follow in Galen's tracks: to Guy, Galen's statements are a parameter, against which the opinions of others ought to be measured.[79] The connection which Guy de Chauliac would wish to have seen established between the science of anatomy and the practice of surgery, he himself failed to bring about.

The books which come next are arranged in a particular sequence, first noticeable in the fourth book of the *Canon* of Avicenna and often found afterwards: *tumours* — which includes all conditions that are accompanied by swelling — *wounds, ulcers, fractures* and *dislocations*. Following Fabricius ab Aquapendente — who in turn was probably inspired by the five Mosaic books — this quinquepartition was termed 'pentateuch' in the sixteenth century.[80]

Guy's second book accordingly deals with such things as abscesses, cysts, furuncles and a variety of skin diseases. The subject of 'buboes' inspired him to write his famous description of the plague of Avignon. Guy also included in this book scirrhus and other 'melancholic abscesses' and goitre, as well as elephantiasis, varicose veins and a number of other outwardly visible conditions with the exception of intestinal hernia.

Book three discusses wounds and their treatment. This book is one of the most important of his entire oeuvre. In it he gives a good classification of wounds with a detailed description of their aspects, of the complications which may arise and of the prognosis of injuries of the separate tissues and organs. His approach relies on that of Galen to a very great extent. For the removal of foreign bodies Guy had at his disposal quite an assortment of specially designed instruments of different kinds, including the spectacular arcubalista for the extraction of arrows which had penetrated into the body (Fig. 13)

His methods for haemostasis are those of Galen and Avicenna. Differing from Henri de Mondeville, he adheres to the Hippocratic custom of first letting a certain amount of blood escape: this prevents fever and inflammation which impede the process of repair. After a flowing away of blood the wound will furthermore be drier. 'Dryness is nearer to what is sound, and moistness to that which is not sound', Guy points out, referring to the fourth book of Galen's *Methodus medendi.*

When the wound is small and uncomplicated, a simple dressing is sufficient. Usually, however, a light compress drenched in white of egg is applied first of all. Galen had already pointed out that beaten white of egg stops bleedings, soothes pain and prevents or eases inflammation. If the wound is larger, suture is often necessary. Guy is familiar with five different methods of closure. The first one is the interrupted suture. For this he uses long needles with a triangular point and silk thread. The second method is that of the 'fibula', which can already be found in Celsus. The third mode of closure is the quilled suture, in which a double thread is tied over quills on both sides of the wound. Guy furthermore mentions the use of small metallic clasps, in fact a forerunner of Michel's clips. The fifth method is the dry one, whereby the sutures are placed in adhesive plaster strips which are stuck on the skin on either edge of the wound.

It is customary to dust red powder on the wound afterwards, which has an incarnative and conservative effect. The wound dressing consists of white of egg compresses. Oil of roses or other greasy substances can be applied around the wound, but not on the wound itself as it slows down the healing process. This dressing must be left for four days. If the wound has failed to consolidate by then, it is rinsed with warm wine and dressed with compresses drenched in wine which must be renewed daily. The wound will then be healed in a few days. Wine is an excellent medicament for all wounds because of its astringent quality. Arnold of Villanova (c. 1234—1311), a prominent Spanish physician who taught at Montpellier amongst other places, advocated alcohol for the same purpose, which would have an even more astringent effect.

Guy apparently does not sew up deep wounds. He points out that it is highly important to enable an easy drainage of wound secretion, which can be brought about by putting the patient in a suitable position and if necessary by applying a counter-incision. He does not favour the use of tents, such as Bruno used to insert at each end of the wound, but instead prefers a seton. Deep wounds must be dressed twice daily with a purifying agent. They must be left to heal from within and suturing should only be opted for when the cavity has filled.

Medical-historical textbooks often reproach Guy for the fact that his treatment of wounds was retrograde, insofar that he advocated the use of salves and plasters rather than simple dressings. But the above gives ample proof to the contrary. Among the possible wound complications Guy mentions shock, as described by Galen.

In the more specific part of this chapter Guy, like the other mediaeval authors, pays considerable attention to injuries of the head. Like William of Saliceto — and long before-hand Galen — he explains the contralateral paralysis which can accompany a cranial trauma by the anatomical fact that the nerves which run to the right half of the body have their roots in the left hemisphere and vice versa. He draws up careful indications for trepanation and gives detailed descriptions with drawings of the required instruments.

The fourth book deals with ulcers. Guy, like the surgeons after him, not only included chronic wounds in this category, but also fistulae, haemorrhoids and such like disorders.

The fifth book is concerned with fractures and dislocations. It contains a critical survey of the relevant works by mainly Arabic and Italian authors. The general treatment of the subject contains careful instructions for the application of immobilizing bandages. As regards the fracture of the shaft of the femur, Guy rejects Albucasis' method, in which the leg, bent at the knee, is firmly tied against the back of the upper leg by way of a splint. Like most other authors, he immobilizes the broken leg in the extended position by means of splints. It is worth noting that he also exercises a form of continuous traction by means of a leaden weight. This weight is suspended from a cord which runs over a pulley, and is fastened to the patient's foot. Such patients ought to be nursed on a mattress with a central opening to enable defaecation. Above them should be hung a cord, by means of which they can pull themselves up.

The voluminous book six deals with sundry diseases — many of which are included by other authors within the bounds of the pentateuch instead of being annexed — and their treatment. It is a motley crew, consisting of gout, skin diseases, burns, eye diseases, tooth diseases, crooked back, whilst in the first part is also included a treatise on amputation. The most important indication for it is once again necrosis. If the decay has reached a joint, the member can be separated by simple exarticulation without making use of the saw. But if the gangrene is contained within a certain distance of the joint, one must amputate where the flesh is still firm and alive. To carry out that operation both the healthy and the affected part are bandaged separately, the limb is grasped firmly by assistants, and the flesh cut between both bandages with a razor. The wound edges are then protected with cloths and the bone is sawn through. The stump is cauterized or treated with boiling oil.

Amputation is apparently an operation which Guy is reluctant to perform because the patient is often left with feelings of resentment and regret. Like Hippocrates, he would rather wait for the moment when the decayed part drops off spontaneously at the level of a joint. Guy relates that some surgeons, including Theodoric, use soporifics in case of an amputation; either the narcotic sponge or an opiate potion. He rejects the use of opium, however, because of the danger of addiction: mediaeval doctors were aware of that problem. He does not appear ever to have administered narcotic drugs himself.

Passages on intestinal hernia and renal and vesical calculus are also to be found in this treatise. Both are relatively large in scope but not very innovative. Here Guy's most important sources are Galen, Avicenna, Haly Abbas, Albucasis and the Italian masters. Amongst the conservative methods of treatment of hernia can be found the recipe for a plaster, having ship's pitch as one of its ingredients, which must be applied to the groin before fastening on the truss. He describes no less than six different operations for this condition, of which four involve hemicastration. The first one, based on Albucasis and performed by surgeons of the Salernitan and Northern Italian school, consisted of tying the spermatic cord as high as possible via an incision, and the removal of the part distal to the ligature together with the testis. The second one, also performed by Albucasis and the Italians, amounted to cauterizing the spermatic cord from the outside at the pubis with a red-hot iron. For a variant of this method, proposed by Theodoric, an escharotic — cauterium potentiale — was used, preferably arsenic. This was the method advocated by Guy. The fourth manner, which was supposed to have been practised by Roger, implied the placing of a thread around the spermatic cord from the outside by means of a needle and firmly tying it to a piece of wood. This was then left until the cord was cut. A fifth way, such as Lanfranc was said to have taught, was to expose the os pubis via an incision and to singe it with the cautery deep to the spermatic cord; the intention presumably being to induce a cicatrization which would prevent the contents of the hernia from sliding down. The sixth method which, like the preceding one, did not involve a hemicastration, consisted of applying a golden thread around the spermatic cord and to tie it only so as to close the entrance to the hernial sac. According to the authors quoted by Guy cauterizing the hernial orifice was the surest method. 'He who has a hernia, does not live without danger', Guy affirmed. This danger lay in a possible descent of a loop of intestine, filled with indurated faeces, which, if it could not be restored, would be fatal. The treatment of bladder stone was according to the precepts of classical authors. Like other 'periti' Guy never performed this operation himself, instead referring it to 'cursores', travelling empirics who have already been briefly discussed on page 46.

Book seven, finally, entitled *Antidotarium*, describes medicines and minor therapeutic operations to be used for the various surgical complaints. It is concerned with bloodletting, applying cupping glasses and leeches, administering enemas, actual and potential cauteries, poultices and with drugs.

From the above it may be gathered, that in the thirteenth and fourteenth centuries a class of sugeons arose in Italy and France which had managed to go far beyond the level of the simple artisan through extensive knowledge of scientific literature — embodied in the works of the ancient and Arabic authors — and with an interest in the theoretical backgrounds of operative surgery without having lost touch with actual practice. These surgeons usually held an academic degree in medicine. This explains why in contemporary manuscript illustrations surgeons are generally depicted in dress appropriate for scholars rather than for artisans. Their pathological, therapeutic and deontological conceptions show a considerable measure of agreement.

2.2.5. *The Netherlands*

2.2.5.1. Economical and Cultural Setting

In the Southern Netherlands trade and industry already flourished early in the twelfth century. Bruges and Antwerp developed into major staple towns for overseas traffic from the north, west, and south. The transit trade with England too was of prime importance. In Bruges, Ghent, Yper and Louvain English wool was manufactured into cloth, which clothed three quarters of the population of Europe. Many cities attained great wealth and with it a certain degree of autonomy. The cities of Liège and Tournai, and a number of abbeys including those of Stavelot, Lobbes and Rolduc, were important centres of culture and education. The production and trading of cloth, which in the twelfth and thirteenth centuries brought prosperity to so many of the towns and cities of Flanders, Hainault, Northern France and later also to Brabant, did not achieve such importance in other provinces until the fourteenth century. Holland was economically insignificant in the twelfth century. There was neither trade nor industry, and as yet not even a town of any importance. The major trading centres of the Northern Netherlands in the twelfth and thirteenth centuries were Tiel and more especially Utrecht, as well as the Hanseatic towns along the river Yssel. These cities were also the most prominent as centres of education and learning. None of their schools played a direct part in the history of surgery in the Low Countries, but may well have contributed indirectly by producing translations.

2.2.5.2. Evidences of Surgical Practice

Evidence of the existence of skilled surgeons — or rather lithotomists — in the Low Countries can be found in the hagiography of Saint Gerard, written in the middle of the twelfth century. In this we find the story of count Arnold I of Flanders who suffered badly from a stone in the bladder. When this became known, a great number of surgeons hastened to his court, offering to rid him of his affliction by means of an operation. Although they operated publicly on eighteen other sufferers from the stone to demonstrate their skill, with only one fatal accident, the count could not bring himself to undergo the treatment.[81] In later centuries, lithotomists were still active in the Netherlands. Amongst the sick who in 1383 went on a pilgrimage to the miracle working statue of Our Sweet Lady in St. John's Cathedral in 's-Hertogenbosch, there was one sufferer who was miraculously cured of an urinary fistula resulting from a bladder operation which he had undergone five years before.[82]

The city archives of Utrecht preserve a certificate of the city council, for a lithotomy successfully performed in 1497 by one Master Steven Rycoutszoon of Haarlem.[83]

Mediaeval surgeons may have left other traces in the Netherlands. The story goes that the skull of Geert Groote (1340—84), founder of the Modern Devotion movement, when exhumed around 1450, showed an artificial opening, possibly the result of a trepanation. The cryptic statement which he used to make during his life: 'Habeo caminum in capite' (I have a chimney in my head), may well refer to this.[84]

Barber-Surgeons in Civic Service

From civic accounts which have been preserved, it appears that in the thirteenth and fourteenth centuries the city authorities began to feel a greater sense of responsibility for the general health conditions within their jurisdiction. This is shown by the appointment of physicians and surgeons, charged with the medical and surgical poor relief. The town surgeon also had to treat those who suffered the rack and other corporal punishment, and accompany the city militia in time of war. Like the town physician, he usually received an annual salary, not only in coin but in kind with fabric for his clothing, he also benefited in the shape of exemption from excise on spirits. The city surgeon in Deventer in the fourteenth century received about the same salary as the under-bailiff, the city carpenter and the city clerk. His duties, however, did not occupy him full time, allowing him to conduct sufficient private practice to provide the major part of his income.[84] The office of town surgeon and town physician persisted until well into the twentieth century, at least at Utrecht, with essentially the same commitments towards poor relief.

2.2.5.3. Surgical Literature

A thirteenth century catalogue of the library at Rolduc near Kerkrade reveals that that abbey held several medical manuscripts in Latin. Amongst these were three books on medicine by Constantine the African,[86] suggesting possible contacts with Italy. The abbey architecture showing Northern Italian stylistic features further strengthens this impression.

Dutch civilization of the late Middle Ages did not only find expression in architecture and the plastic arts. Middle Dutch literature was of great account and Middle Dutch was indeed the first vernacular into which the Latin artes-literature was translated.[87] It will be remembered that many surgical texts, originating in Italy and France appeared in the Middle Dutch vernacular. But there were also a number of homegrown products in that language such as the treatises of Jan Yperman and Thomas Scellinck as well as minor texts by unknown authors.

Yperman and Scellinck

Little is known about the lives of Yperman and Scellinck. Jan Yperman was born in the second half of the thirteenth century and probably died around 1330. According to some sources he attended the lessons and clinical demonstrations of Lanfranc in Paris. He lived and practised in Ypres, which during his life-time with some 28 000 inhabitants was one of the three largest towns in Flanders. From 1304 onward he was charged with the care of the surgical patients in the hospital founded by Christina Belle in 1276, for which he received an annual salary from the city government.[88] On two occasions, he accompanied the Yper militia on campaigns. Jan Yperman enjoyed a proverbial reputation throughout all Flanders.

In 1310, for the benefit of his son who apparently did not know any Latin, he wrote his textbook of surgery in Flemish, taken from the Latin and 'uyt syn selves verstandnisse' (from his own knowledge, Fig. 14 and 15). Like its Italian and French counterparts this work is largely a compilation. Yperman quotes at least thirty authors: ancient Greeks as well as Arabs and Italians. He mentions Galen and Avicenna most often, followed by Lanfranc. The Salernitan influence is striking.[89] It is not very likely that Yperman really read all these authors himself, but it is evident that he drew on a wide personal experience. His book is richly illustrated with sketches of instruments, affording the modern reader a good idea of the tools of the mediaeval surgeon. With the exception of Albucasis and later in the fourteenth century Guy de Chauliac, such depictions are nowhere to be found in early surgical works, either in such large numbers or in such great diversity.

Four manuscript copies have been preserved of Jan Yperman's *Chirurgie* which, as orthographical differences show, appeared in several parts of the country until the close of the fifteenth century.[90]

Even less is known of Scellinck's life. It is not clear when or where he was born, although his birth-place may have been Tienen. Nor is it known when he died. He was a sworn master of surgery in Namur.[91] His book contains indications that he travelled. In 1343 he finished his *Boeck van surgien* (Book of surgery), dedicated to his 'lieven kinderen Thomas ende Jan Scellinc sinen broeder' (dear children Thomas and Jan Scellinc his brother).

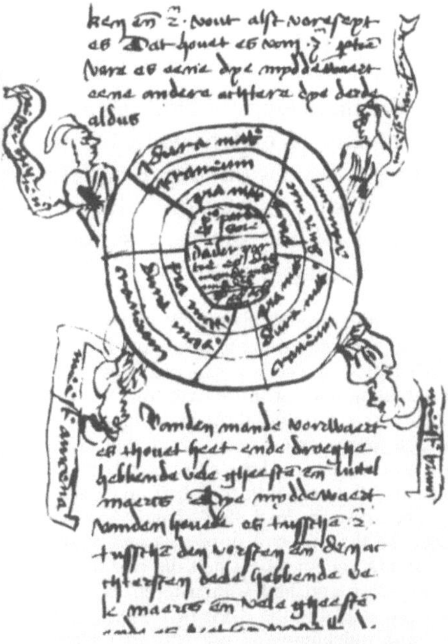

Fig. 14. Jan Yperman: a schematic cross-section of the skull, showing the cranium, dura mater, pia mater and the brain matter consisting of three parts. The anterior part is warm and dry and has little marrow, the middle part being warm has much marrow and spirit, the posterior part is cold and dry and has little marrow. Master Galienus, Master Lancfranc, Master Brunus and Master Avicenna seem to approve of this diagram.

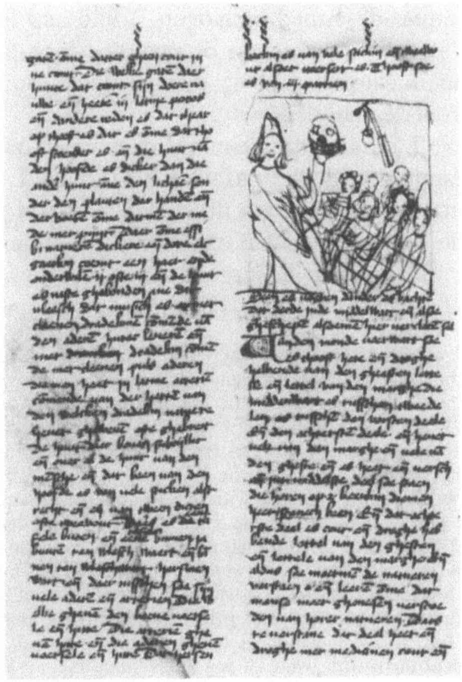

Fig. 15. Jan Yperman: 'Anatomical lesson'.

This work too, is largely a compilation of the now familiar Italian, Arabic and Greek authors, commented on from the vantage-point of an extensive personal experience and enlivened with examples from his own practice. It is striking that Scellinck does not mention his compatriot Yperman. The work is preserved in two manuscripts, both dating from the late fifteenth century.[92]

Any likeness between the texts of Yperman and Scellinck is due to their having used the same literary sources, be it not always to the same extent: Yperman appears to have relied more heavily on Lanfranc than did Scellinck. The arrangement of their works is quite dissimilar. Whilst in Scellinck the surgical 'pentateuch' more or less stands out, Yperman rigorously adheres to the 'a capite ad calcem'-principle even to the extent that cranial fractures and head-lice are treated in one and the same book on the head. In contrast to Yperman, Scellinck touches anatomy but lightly. He is on the whole somewhat more conservative in his therapeutic approach and seems to have preferred actual and potential cautery to the knife. In their wound treatment the Flemish do not differ from their Italian and French predecessors, aiming at healing by first intention wherever possible, using techniques described by Roger, Bruno and Henri de Mondeville. Due attention is paid to the phenomenon of pus, of which Scellinck with reference to Albucasis, Hippocrates and Galen, distinguishes four different kinds, representing four different degrees of gravity.

Like Lanfranc, the Flemings distinguish between the three types of bleeding and are familiar with the vascular ligature and the technique of undersewing. Their styptics are the same as those which were found in the authors discussed earlier, on the basis of personal experience Yperman adds the patient's own dried blood. That the mediaeval surgeon was at times hard pressed to control a serious haemorrhage, is illustrated by the following anecdote by Scellinck.

> Now I want to tell you what happened to me once at Gemblies. I rode through the town on my horse, near the Meat-hall, when a great many people suddenly came up and begged me to dismount and go with them. And they took me to a hall which was already full of people, where a man was lying who had a wound in his hand. Master Jan of Gemblies had been treating him for more than four weeks. And that hand had rotted so far that one of the veins was already rotted through. And it was bleeding so vigorously that the blood sprang up as high as a man making water. And three old masters were standing there with three hot cauteries and burned the vein. And the more they burned it, the harder it bled, and the man seemed almost dead because the vein was scorched and overheated because of the burning, and it looked as if the man's hand was a dead man's hand. And he was as pale as ashes. Then I went up to him and put my finger on the vein and stopped it and made haste to send for two priests with the holy sacrament and extreme unction and I had the one priest stop the vein until the other priest had heard the man's confession and had administered the last rites. And in the meantime I sent for quicklime and pulverized it and made a lot of plasters and drenched them with white of egg and I filled the wound up with quicklime and put plasters on the wound which were soaked in white of egg. And I dressed the wound neatly and the man recovered and if I had not been there that man would surely have died before you could have said three or four pater nosters.[93]

Both Yperman and Scellinck appear to have performed intestinal repair for which Yperman made use of an intraluminal stent, a practice which Scellinck, like Lanfranc, rejected.

Like the other mediaeval books on surgery the Flemish works show that surgery was primarily concerned with traumatology (Fig. 16). As to selective surgery we find that both authors present a detailed description of the couching operation. They also give an outline of the conservative and operative treatment of hernia, whereas Scellinck enters fully into lithotomy according to Arabic descriptions.

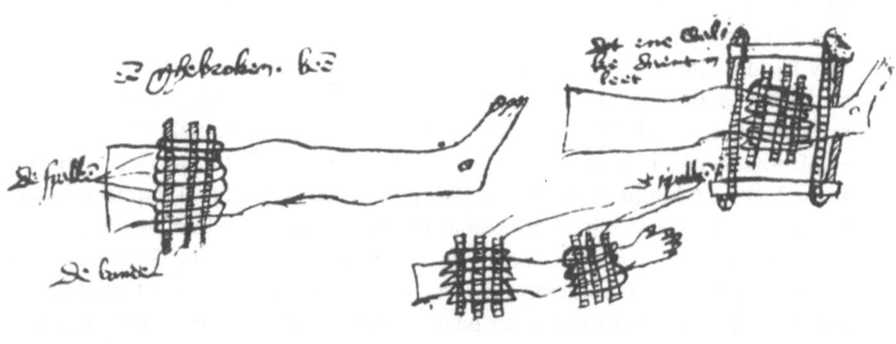

Fig. 16. Splint bandages for fractured ams and legs. The right upper drawing probably represents a suspension bandage.

Yperman initially confines himself as far as the latter operation is concerned, to a reference to *Post mundi fabricam* by Roger the Salernitan: this work was apparently easy to get hold of in the Southern Netherlands in the thirteenth century, probably even in the vernacular. But at the end of his book he describes a method for a hernia operation performed with a knife and a cautery, however, 'I master Jan Yperman never did this because it is too hazardous for the patient'. The Flemings do not discuss amputation, nor for that matter did Bruno and Lanfranc.

Both Yperman and Scellinck show familiarity with Latin, while they demand of the 'ideal surgeon' that his reading is not confined to medicine only. Jan Yperman even argued in favour of a combination of medicine and surgery in one person. That he was serious about this demand is apparent from the fact that he wrote a Flemish textbook of medicine as well.

Unlike the prominent surgeons of Italy and France, Jan Yperman and Thomas Scellinck had no university degree. They nevertheless represented a superior class of surgeon. The existence of such a class of surgeons in the Netherlands too is moreover suggested by the fairly extensive literature which was available in the Dutch vernacular. Yperman and Scellinck both make clear in their writings that the majority of the contemporary surgeons were still illiterate empirics without proper training. It is somewhat surprising to find that Yperman and Scellinck whose works were copied again and again for a period of some 150 years, are never quoted in the early editions of Renaissance authors, and did not themselves appear in print until the twentieth century. This may be due to the fact that about the time of the invention of printing, Guy de Chauliac was already dominating the field in the Netherlands too: Middle Dutch translations of his *Chirurgia magna* were available as early as the mid-fifteenth century. Guido's ascendancy, from 1507 onwards he had repeatedly appeared in print in the Dutch vernacular, might also explain why three centuries had to elapse after Yperman and Scellinck before Dutch surgery in the person of Baten again produced a textbook of note.

Minor Surgical Texts

Behind the name of *Jonghe Lanfranc* is concealed the unknown author of a modest work on treatment of wounds and apostemes; external diseases caused by any of the four humours as explained by Galen. It is mainly a collection of recipes for salves, plasters, powders and wound potions. Although the name suggests otherwise, this treatise is not an adaptation of any of Lanfranc's works. Instead it goes back to older sources, mainly to Roger and the Roger adaptations, occasionally also the *Liber Avicennae*, a Middle Dutch formulary, which must have been compiled around 1340.[94] Until recently the *Jonghe Lanfranc* was taken for a translation of the *Chirurgia parva*. Eight copies of this work have been preserved entirely or in part, dating from the period of the mid-fourteenth to the mid-sixteenth century.

Jansen-Sieben and Keil called attention to an alphabetically arranged collection of fifty-two surgical glosses from the fourteenth century, occurring in a codex which originated in the Hanseatic town of Deventer.[95] It is to be expected that even more Middle Dutch surgical texts are still dormant in the manuscripts.

CHAPTER 3

The Renaissance

3.1. THE RISE OF THE REPUBLIC OF THE UNITED PROVINCES

In 1433 the powerful duke of Burgundy, who possessed not only the duchy of Burgundy but also Flanders and Franche-Comté, managed to wrest from Jacoba of Bavaria the counties of Holland, Zeeland and Hainaut. He also acquired Namur, Brabant, Limburg and Luxemburg through inheritance and purchase, while his son and heir Charles the Bold forcefully took possession of Guelders, Lorraine and a part of Switzerland, before losing his life in the battle of Nancy in 1477. The technique of warfare had undergone fundamental changes by then as a result of the introduction of firearms. It was during the battle of Crécy in 1346, in the Hundred Years' War between the English and the French, that guns are said to have been fired for the first time.

In the Burgundian period some important socio-economic developments took place. Holland and Zeeland experienced a strong economic boost in the fifteenth century due to the increasing participation of the cargo ships from those provinces in the traffic between the agrarian countries around the Baltic and the industrial West of Europe. Amsterdam in particular, which was still an insignificant fishing village in the twelfth century, was to benefit from this development. The Hollanders were increasingly successful in outstripping the trade of the Hanze. In Zeeland the city of Middelburg flourished, the result of the acquisition of the staple right on English cloth.

In the Southern Netherlands the economic centre gradually moved from Flanders to Brabant, in particular to Antwerp and Bergen-op-Zoom, which became major transit towns for all of Germany via Cologne.

The flourishing of trade and industry led to the rise of an upper middle class in the wealthy cities. Land ownership was no longer the only source of wealth, as money became increasingly important. The Burgundian period witnessed a tremendous flowering of music, architecture and painting, and also education, testified to by the foundation of the university of Louvain in 1425.

Charles's daughter Maria the Rich had to cede Burgundy to the French king. Her son Philip the Fair, born out of her marriage to Maximilian I of Austria, married the Spanish princess Joanna of Castile. Charles V was born out of this union, he successively inherited from his parents and his Habsburg grand father the Dutch provinces which had been part of the Burgundian realm, Spain and the Austrian Succession States. The Dutch provinces in the North which were not yet under his domain were forced to acknowledge Charles V as their sovereign. The Reformation, which began around 1500, was forcefully suppressed by him.

His son and heir Philip II aimed at an absolute integration of the Low Countries with the Spanish-Habsburg monarchy. He appointed stadtholders over the several provinces, and as such William of Orange, a favourite of his father, became stadtholder of Holland, Zeeland and Utrecht. Like his father, Philip actively persecuted the adherents of the new faith.

The stern measures against the protestants, and the presence of Spanish troops, led to an increasing disaffection. 1566 was the year of the iconoclastic fury, as a result of which Philip sent a strong army to the Netherlands under the duke of Alva who instituted a reign of terror which claimed many victims. But he really became unpopular when he introduced a new system of taxes, of which the sales tax of no less than 10 percent, the so-called 'tenth penny' in particular was an annoyance.

The prince of Orange, the chief leader of the rebellious citizens, managed to avoid persecution by a timely escape to Germany. From that country, he organized raids into the Netherlands in several places, thus hoping to realize a large-scale rebellion, which, however, failed to take place. But when in 1572 the Sea Beggars, sailing from England, captured Holland's coastal town of Brill, a number of cities in Holland and Zeeland soon declared themselves for the prince of Orange. Some of those cities were forced to submit again to the authority of the king, but in 1574 Alkmaar and Leyden managed to withstand the Spanish besiegers. Leyden was rewarded with a university, the first one in the Northern Netherlands.

Large-scale pillaging by the poorly-paid Spanish soldiers in the Southern Netherlands, in spite of their predominantly Catholic sympathies, led to their unification with the protestant rebels in the North, having the common goal of ousting the royal troops. But the religious differences proved too great for the continued success of the union. After several Southern provinces had once more accepted the authority of the governor, the Northern provinces, together with a few Flemish towns, concluded the so-called Union of Utrecht in 1579. This Union formed the foundation for the Republic of the Seven United Provinces which came into being in 1587, after the rejection of Philip II as sovereign in 1581 and the assassination of William of Orange three years later.

This Republic bore the character of a federation, in which each separate state was to retain its own administrative independence. The rather weak central government lay with the States-General and the Council of State. The stadtholders of the provinces acquired a few sovereign rights. The stadtholder of Holland, the major province within the Republic, was also commander-in-chief of the army and the navy. This stadtholdership — which was to become hereditary — was held by members of the House of Orange, descended in direct or indirect lineage from William of Orange, the 'pater patriae'. The separate provinces did not possess a powerful central government either, and the cities enjoyed a high level of autonomy. This political organization continued to exist until the close of the eighteenth century.

The war with Spain was immediately resumed after the foundation of the Republic, until by the end of the century the entire territory of the Seven United Provinces was free from enemy troops. It was not until 1648, however, after 80 years, that the war with Spain reached a final conclusion.

After the Portuguese had discovered the sea route to the East Indies at the end of the fifteenth century, Lisbon had become the most important European staple town for spices. In the subsequent distribution of that much sought-after merchandise over Western and Northern Europe, Dutch cargo ships played an important role. After the annexation of Portugal by Spain in 1580 the Dutch trade encountered so many obstacles that the Hollanders decided to find their own route to the Indian Spice Islands. Near the end of the century they indeed succeeded in finding the route, which laid the foundation for the colonial empire which the Dutch were to possess for three centuries and which contributed greatly to their wealth.

3.2. MEDICINE

In the Northern Netherlands, medical authors first appear in the early sixteenth century. They may have taken their medical degree either at the University of Louvain or at some French or German university if not at Padua or Bologna in Italy. They were international in outlook: some of them had travelled widely or even practised for some time abroad. Galen and the Arabian authors were their chief authorities. These early works are of no importance for our subject.

3.3. THE SURGEONS

3.3.1. *The Forming of Guilds*

Surgeons were already known to be practising in the fourteenth century, for example in 1351 at Rotterdam and in 1380 at Utrecht. It is, however, only since the middle of the fifteenth century that we find indications of their organisation in the trade guilds for artisans customary in the Middle Ages in large parts of Europe. Trade guilds were occupational associations with obligatory membership, which protected the interests of the members.[1] They were organised by the town council who also acted in a supervisory capacity. In the province of Holland it appears that various surgeons' guilds were founded in the 1460s. Such confraternities were recorded in Leyden in 1466, in Rotterdam in 1467 and as early as 1465 in Gorkum. In Amsterdam and Middelburg guilds were not heard of until 1497 and 1501, respectively. Those early surgeons also acted as barbers.

Early guild charters, such as those from Gorkum, mainly set out the financial obligations of the members. The contributions served in the first place for maintaining the guild's own chapel or at least its own altar in an existing church, dedicated to the patron saint of the corporation. Barbers and surgeons frequently placed themselves under the protection of the Holy Cosmas and Damian (Fig. 17).[2] In some cases the barbers and surgeons formed guilds with men of completely different trades, for instance with the cloth-merchants in Utrecht or with the clog-makers in Amsterdam.[3] Physicians, who were few and far between in the fifteenth and sixteenth centuries, did not belong to the surgeons' guilds nor did they have any organisation of their own.

The regulations from the fifteenth century also mention the annual celebration of the name day of the patron saint as a formal church ceremony followed by a feast, the obligatory participation in the obsequies of a deceased guild-brother and other such activities. Even after the Reformation, when the religious element moved into the background and the corporation clearly took on the character of a statutory trade organisation, these traditions were upheld and the guilds continued to carry the name which had been derived from their — Roman Catholic — patron saint.

Our knowledge of day-to-day routine in the surgeons' guilds in the fifteenth century has many gaps. This also holds true for the non-university trained practitioners of the sixteenth century, although of late we have come to know more about that age thanks to the indefatigable researches of professor M. J. van Lieburg from Amsterdam. Van Lieburg collected together the decrees promulgated between 1513 and 1597, with reference to the practice of surgery, from the city archives of sixteen towns in the North Netherlands. The autonomy, which the Dutch cities in large measure enjoyed until the end of the eighteenth century, was the reason why legislation with regard to public health fell under the competency of the local government. It was therefore only valid for the jurisdiction of the separate cities and did not have a national character. From an article in which Van Lieburg gives a provisional conclusion on the analysis of this material we derive most of the following.[4]

The proclamation of city ordinances regarding medicine and surgery was usually justified by referring to its importance for the citizens. Then followed in the text a definition of the competencies of physicians, surgeons, barbers, pharmacists and drug vendors. The ordinances which bore special reference to surgeons' guilds contained stipulations over their form of organization and management, prerequisites for admission, examinations, the apprentices and their training, the required term of apprenticeship, obligations including those for meetings, processions and funerals of guild members, codes of behaviour, competencies and protection against unlicensed practitioners (Fig. 18).

3.3.2. *Examinations*

It was only possible for a person to join a guild if he had passed the master's examination. Entry was obligatory for everyone within the jurisdiction of the city who wished to engage in surgical practice, including hairdressing and barbering. In so far as the terms of examination are incorporated in the successive ordinances of the surgeons' companies, they are a reflection of the scientific development which gradually came about in the course of the fifteenth and sixteenth centuries among the barber-surgeons. The oldest ordinances from the middle of the fifteenth

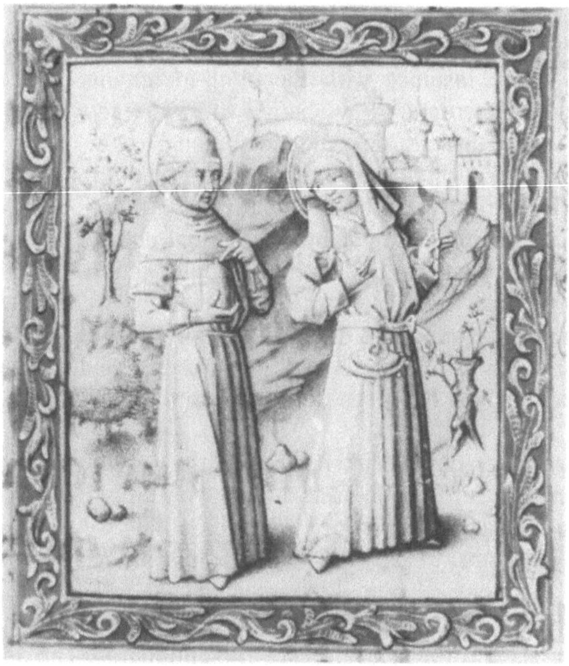

Fig. 17. Saints Cosmas and Damian.

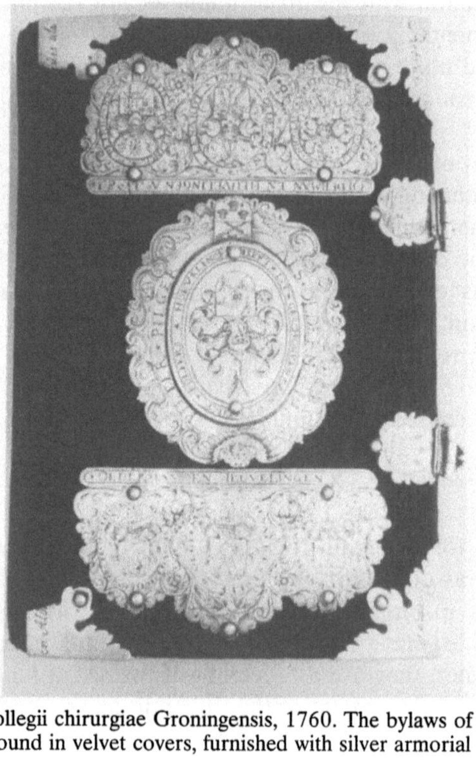

Fig. 18. Liber legum collegii chirurgiae Groningensis, 1760. The bylaws of the Groningen Surgeons' Guild, bound in velvet covers, furnished with silver armorial engraving.

century were aimed at the barbers in a narrower sense and limited to the requirement that the candidate should be capable of conducting blood-letting in the proper manner and manufacturing a lancet from raw preformed iron and be able to sharpen it,[5] whereas as ordinance of Amsterdam in 1552 also required knowledge of the theoretical background of blood-letting. This theoretical background was probably provided by the short tract *Fleubotomia of Master Avicenna*, described below. There the matter rested for the barbers. For the surgeons, however, the phlebotomy test was a preliminary step in the master's examination, whereby theoretical knowledge was also required of unnatural growths, wounds, ulcers, fractures, dislocations and materies chirurgica, as was stipulated in the 1552 ordinance.[6] Also the candidate had to be able to evaluate some cases correctly and prove his practical ability to perform trephination on a skull. This meant the beginning of a division being made between barbers in a narrower sense and barbers with a knowledge of surgery.

The fact that we can recognize the 'quinquepartition' of Guy de Chauliac in the arrangement of the theoretical requirements is no coincidence. Guy de Chauliac had a pre-eminent influence on surgery in the Low Countries at the time, as is evidenced by the various Dutch editions of the *Chirurgia magna* which appeared in the sixteenth century and by the terms in which the Amsterdam surgeons framed their request to king Philip II: into that request we will enter more fully below. Research carried out by Van Lieburg into the terms of examination in ordinances from all over the country between 1552 and 1590 permit the conclusion that sixteenth-century surgery everywhere in the North Netherlands remained in the Chauliac tradition.

3.3.3. *Surgical Practitioners*

It appears that the professional group of those engaged in some kind of surgery cannot be sharply defined. Especially since the middle of the sixteenth century it was far from homogeneous. Between the medical upper stratum of doctors holding university degrees who as a rule did not engage in practical surgery, and the low-ranking barbers in a more restricted sense, a middle group gradually formed, partly from physicians who did not wish to limit their theoretical interest to their proper sphere,[7] and partly from barber-surgeons with some knowledge of medicine. A proportion of these surgeons had received basic academic schooling in the 'liberal arts', in which case they must have been conversant with Latin. One or two of them had even obtained a degree in medicine and were therefore entitled to engage in the practice of internal medicine.

The existence of the various groups is nicely illustrated by the subtitle of the Dutch edition of Lanfranc's *Chirurgie* of 1529, in which the book is recommended as being 'very useful and profitable for all doctors, and masters, learned or simple. And also for all barbers' (Fig. 19). City ordinances dealing with the regulation of surgery — for example the one mentioned above promulgated in 1552 in Amsterdam — sometimes enumerate various subgroups: those of the 'pox-masters, cancer-masters, whitlow masters, masters of scrofula, nodules or any type of pustules or excrescences' and operators on bladder stones, herniae and cataracts,

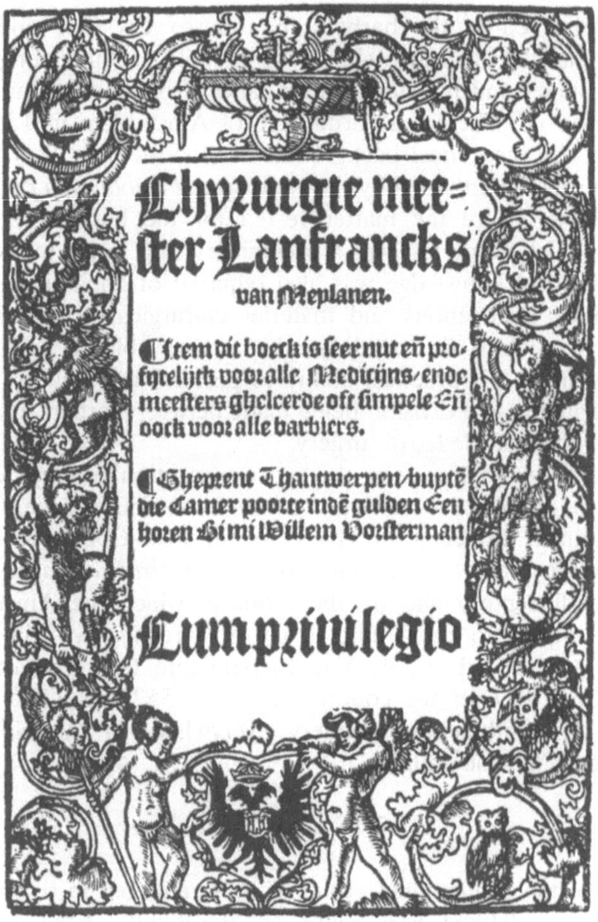
Chyrurgie mee-
ster Lanfrancks
van Meylanen.
¶ Item dit boeck is seer nut eñ pro-
fytelijck voor alle Medicijns/ende
meesters gheleerde oft simpele En
ooch voor alle barbiers.
¶ Gheprent Thantwerpen/buytē
die Camer poorte indē gulden Een
horen Bi mi Willem Vorsterman
Cum privilegio

Fig. 19. The elegant title page of the Dutch edition of Lanfranc's *Chirurgie* of 1529.

whom we have already met in the Middle Ages as a special class of unorganized practitioners. The first subgroup, after proving their competence, were allowed to practise freely in the city. The latter category, common throughout Europe where the representatives led an itinerant existence, were only permitted to conduct their dangerous operations in the presence of a master-surgeon and a town physician. It was not possible for them to become members of the surgeons' guild. Charlatans — kwakzalvers — were only permitted to practise in the cities for limited periods of time — for example during weekly or yearly markets — after paying a certain subscription to the surgeons' guild.

From 1597 onwards barbers in Amsterdam who were only capable of shaving and bloodletting were in fief to but no longer members of the surgeons' guild. Their exclusion did not imply that barbering as such had disappeared from the guild for the surgeons retained their right to exercise that trade: until the beginning of the nineteenth century hair dressing and shaving contributed important additional earnings or even the principal income of many a master-surgeon.

From the material collected by Van Lieburg it would appear that at the beginning of the sixteenth century women could still be mentioned in the same breath as the male barber-surgeons, but in the second half of the century they were no longer present in the middle group which had developed in the meantime. Besides the tasks of acting as midwives or treating specifically feminine ailments, they were otherwise only marginally active surgically in cupping and administering clysters. The same development occurred in France — at least in Paris — where qualified women surgeons, spoken of more than once in the ordinances of the fourteenth century, were almost to disappear in the sixteenth century (see p. 46).

3.4. ANATOMY AS A BASIC SURGICAL SCIENCE

3.4.1. *The Relevance of Anatomical Knowledge to the Surgeon*

It is striking that in the conditions of the examinations between 1552 and 1570 referred to above, anatomy was not specifically mentioned. Yet Guy de Chauliac had underlined the importance of practical anatomical knowledge in surgical practice as follows:

> Surgeons who do not know anatomy make mistakes very often and cut through nerves and ligaments. When one is dealing with a wound, it will be easy to determine through one's knowledge of anatomy, whether a nerve has been cut, or a tendon or even a ligment.

In the discourse on the build of the human body at the beginning of his *Chirurgia* in which he wrote these words, Guy refers to similar statements made by Galen, Haly Abbas, Avicenna and Henri de Mondeville.

3.4.2. *Royal Privilege for the Surgeons in Amsterdam*

Guy's incitement to study practical anatomy resounded in various places. In 1556 king Philip II, in his capacity of count of Holland, granted the barber-surgeons' guild in Amsterdam, recently detached from the clog- and pattenmakers with whom it had formerly been associated under one organization, the annual privilege of dissecting a human cadaver. For this purpose the judicature had to place at its disposal the mortal remains of a criminal who had been executed.[8]

In the text of the privilege the surgeons' request — to which it was the answer — was quoted in great detail. It may be concluded that the surgeons had alleged that the 'art of surgery and anatomy' cannot be gained only from books, but that 'dissecting an anatomical subject . . . is of great advantage and enlightenment to physicians, but also particularly in the instruction of surgeons and barbers . . .'. If this dichotomy directly reminds us of what Guy de Chauliac wrote about the study of anatomy, further comparisons of the text of the privilege, casu quo the surgeons' request, with the 'apology of anatomy' as it appears in the Dutch edition of Guy's *Chirurgie* of 1507, confirms that the Amsterdam barber-surgeons derived their arguments from Guy de Chauliac. It is clear therefore, that the Italian anatomical tradition of the late Middle Ages had not only reached this country via the Dutch edition of Mondino, but also particularly through the apparently well-read work of Guy de Chauliac.

The pursuit of a medical discipline, which indeed anatomy was, could not simply be left to the surgical craftsmen. It would appear from the stipulation included in the privilege of king Philip that dissections which were for the benefit of the surgeons, must take place 'in the presence of and with instruction from expert physicians'.

3.4.3. *The Tardy Rise of Modern Anatomy*

It is remarkable that Galenic and mediaeval anatomical traditions should live on through Guy's mediation, the more so as Andreas Vesalius (1514—64), a native of Brussels, had already laid the foundations for modern anatomy in 1543 with his famous folio *De humani corporis fabrica libri septem*, illustrated with superb woodcuts from Titian's studio in Venice.[9] Towards the end of the sixteenth century, several surgeons' guild-halls had a Vesalius in their bookcase. However, the catalogues concerned do not always state which particular work of Vesalius was involved. In 1543 the same publisher also produced a concise adaptation of the *Fabrica*, entitled *Epitome anatomica.*

According to Vesalius the latter edition was intended for beginners, being a summary of his great work. This is certainly not the case, 'at best it is a compression of selections from the *Fabrica*'.[10] Due to its elementary character and its brevity, the *Epitome* was a popular work. Two Dutch translations were published in short succession, one in 1568 in Antwerp (Fig. 20) simultaneously with a translation of the *Vivae imagines* by the Spaniard Juan Valverde d'Amusco — an anatomy book which was strongly influenced by Vesalius — and one in Bruges a year later. Professor Pieter Pauw at Leyden edited the *Epitome* once again in Latin, with notes and comments in 1616. One may well wonder what the direct impact was of both the *Fabrica* and the *Epitome* on surgery at the time. The *Fabrica* definitely offered far more than a surgeon would have required for his daily practice whilst the epitomized edition was not particularly useful as a surgical-anatomical text either. This is somewhat surprising because Vesalius himself was an active surgeon.

The Montpellier professor Barthélemy Cabrol apparently had a better understanding of the needs of surgical apprentices and medical students. For their benefit he published his *Alphabet anatomique* in 1594, in which the material was arranged in tabular form, supplemented by 34 interesting surgical case reports. This book, which had no illustrations, was translated into Dutch in 1630 by Dr. Caspar Nollens. Three years later a new Dutch edition appeared, rewritten by Vopiscus Fortunatus Plemp (1601—71), a friend of Tulp.[11] Plemp did not closely follow the original in his revision: he avoided the tabulation and replaced Cabrol's case histories with parts of Pieter Pauw's commentary on Hippocrates' book on head injuries. The volume was now provided with illustrations taken from the anatomy books of Juan Valverde, Giulio Casserio, Caspar Bauhin and Andreas Vesalius. It was instrumental in coining a Dutch anatomical vocabulary. It was

DAT EPITOME OFTE CORT BE-
GRIIP DER ANATOMIEN, ANDR. VESALII. WT HET
Latijn in neder-duudſch naer den oprechten zinne ouer-gheſtelt, door
M. Ian Wouters, ghegagiert Medicijn ende Chirurgijn der ſtede vander
Vere in Zeelãt: eñ wort ghedeelt in zes capittelen met zijn additië.

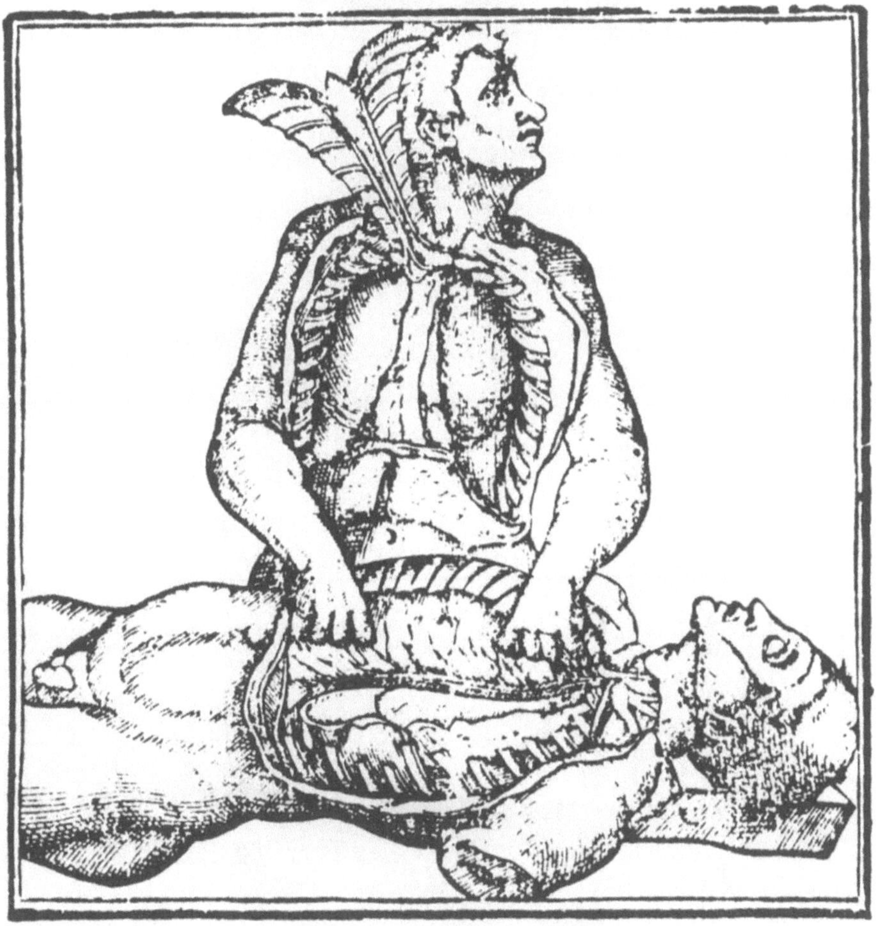

TE BRVGGHE,
Inde peerde ſtrate bij my Pieter de Clerck, Ghezworen Drucker der
Con. Maieſteyt. Anno 1569. Eñ daer vijntmenſe te coopen.
Cum Gratia & Priuilegio.

Fig. 20. Title vignette of the Dutch edition of Vesalius' *Epitome* of 1569. This remarkable representation, taken from Valverde's *Historia de la composición del cuerpo humano* (Rome, 1556), is a humorous combination of two separate woodcuts from Vesalius' *Fabrica*, both showing the position of the thoracic viscerae.

published once more in 1663, together with Aquapendente's *Operative surgery* and Fernel's *Anatomy* (Fig. 21).

It was probably mainly through the surgery books by Paré and Guillemeau,

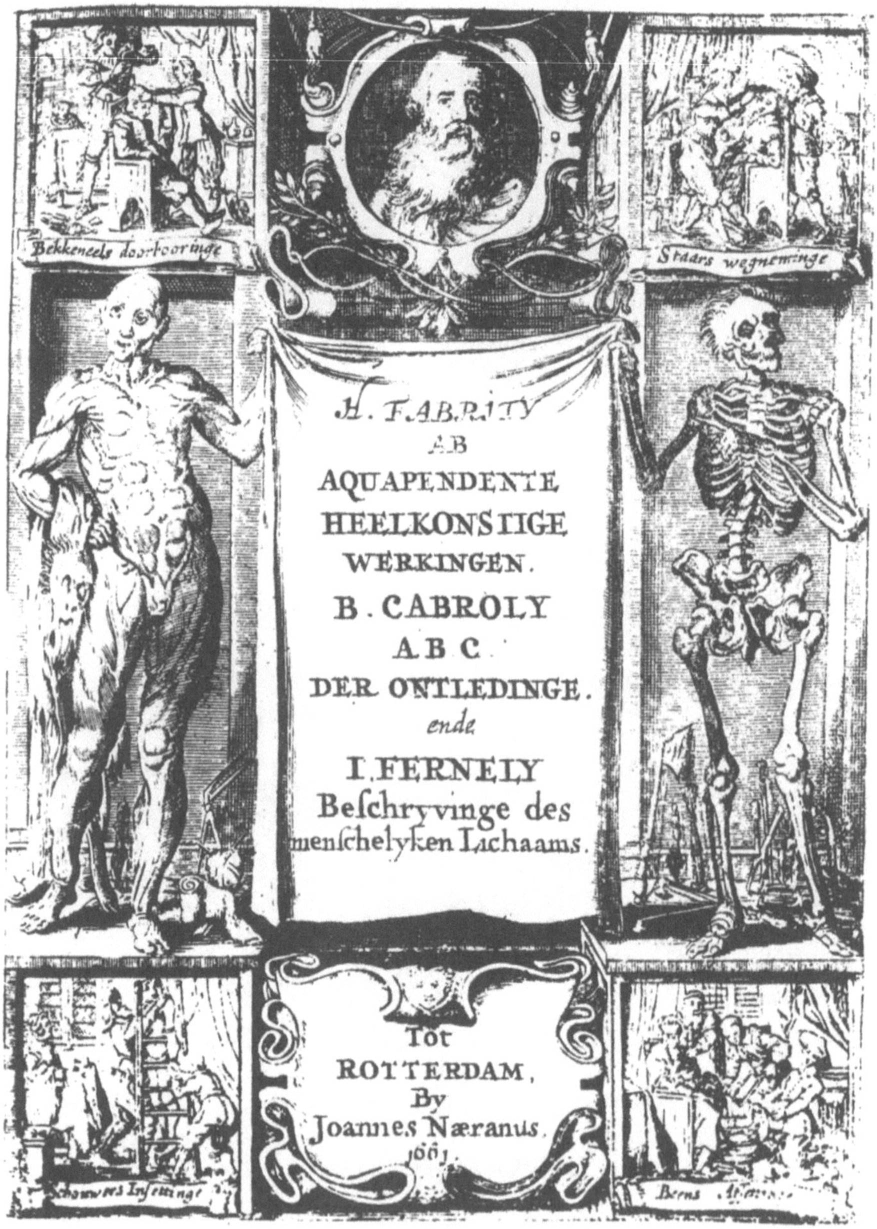

Fig. 21. Frontispiece of a collection of three useful works for surgeons. The portrait at the top represents Fabritius ab Aquapendente. The muscle man carrying his own skin reminds one of St. Bartholomew: this might be an allusion to the Christian name of the second author.

which will be discussed later, that Vesalian anatomy gained a firm footing in this country. In their work, both authors actually derived the chapters on anatomy, including the illustrations, from Vesalius.

The slow acceptance of the new anatomy finds its reflection in the lists of subjects on which candidates could be tested for the master's examination, which hung in the Amsterdam guild-room. These lists, which also included details of the literature in which the correct answer could be found, were renewed from time to time. Even the list from 1622 scarcely refers directly to Vesalius as far as anatomy is concerned. It refers more to Guy de Chauliac, Johannes de Vigo and Ambroise Paré.[12]

Who would have formulated those questions in the year 1622? We may safely assume that the 'praelector anatomiae' had a hand in this. In Amsterdam anatomy was at first taught by an officer of the surgeons' guild. As this took place in a less orderly manner than could be wished for, the city fathers appointed a medical doctor of good repute as praelector to the surgeons and their apprentices in 1587. The first two lecturers in Amsterdam, Maarten Coster and Sebastiaan Egbertsz, were still faithful followers of Galen. In the very large library of the former, there were no books by Vesalius. Egbertsz held his position until his death in 1621. Both instructors were not known to engage in much dissecting (Fig. 22). It was only towards the end of the century that the need of accomodations meeting the specific requirements of the teaching of anatomy was felt and the first anatomical

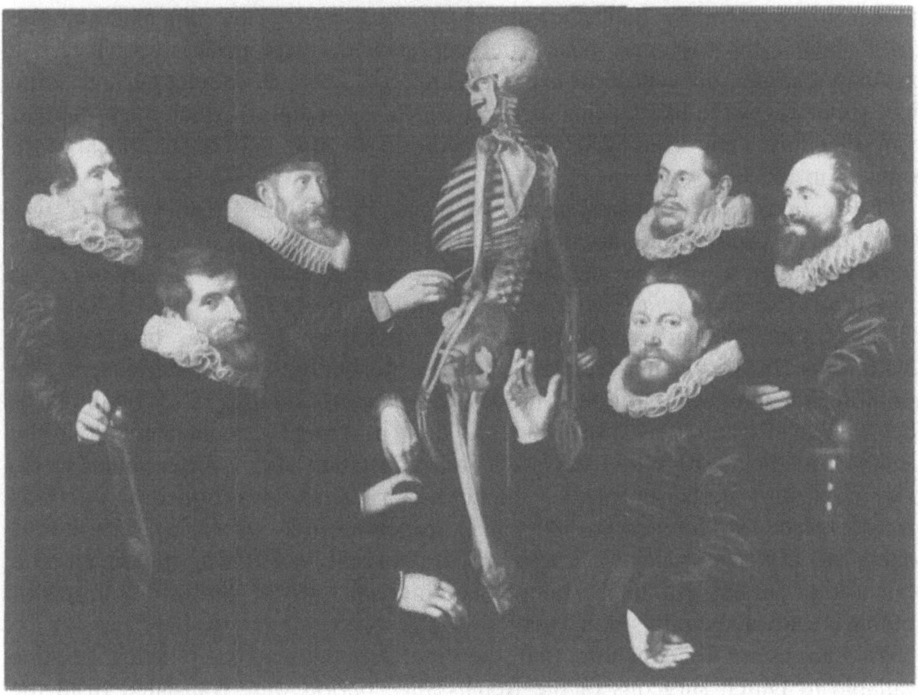

Fig. 22. Anatomical lesson of Dr. Sebastiaan Egbertsz. The lecture is on the subject of Adam's rib.

theatres appeared in the Netherlands following the example of Montpellier (1530), Ferrara (1588) and Basle (1589). We will go more fully into these theatres in Chapter 4.

3.5. SURGICAL LITERATURE

3.5.1. *Translations*

The invention of the art of printing is one of the most remarkable achievements in the cultural history of the West. One may marvel at the high quality of the product which the early printers quickly achieved and at the large number of works which went to press. Twenty-five printers in the South Netherlands produced some 900 titles before 1500.[13] In Antwerp the foundations were laid for the great flourishing period which the printers were to experience there in the sixteenth century. In the North Netherlands the first publishers to be mentioned by name were established in Utrecht in 1473.[14] Fours years later the first book to be published in Dutch was issued in Delft with a translation of the Old Testament. Outside the Netherlands the cities of Nuremberg, Strasbourg, Basle and Venice had printing-shops of European renown.

Amongst the early Dutch printed books we encounter two surgical incunabula. The first, which was published in Louvain in 1481, is a collection of three treatises: the *Chirurgia parva* by Lanfranc, the *Anathomia* by Guy de Chauliac and the *Fleubothomia* by Avicenna. The latter represents a very brief abstract of the extensive chapter on venesection in Avicenna's *Canon*: it enumerates on some eight small pages the likely veins together with the conditions which might benefit from bleeding them (Fig. 23). A new edition of this collection appeared in Antwerp in 1529.

The second is the *Tractaetken van cyrurgien* by Guy de Chauliac, which was published in Delft round about 1480.[15] It was probably a translation of his *Chirurgia parva*, a work wrongly attributed to Guy and containing only notes on dispensing. The *Chirurgia magna* from this author appeared in Dutch in Antwerp in 1507 (Fig. 24) and in Ghent in about 1553, both editions had woodcut illustrations. In 1560 and even in 1646 yet further editions materialized. The tradition of 'Guido' was continued in *De chirurgica institutione* (1543) by the Paris doctor Jean Tagault (?—1545) who, as 'docteur régent', taught surgery at the faculty of medicine for many years. A Dutch translation of this very popular work, to which a surgical pharmacology — 'materia chirurgica' — was added by the Paris professor Jacques Houllier (1498—1562), appeared in Antwerp in 1559. It was edited as *Der chirurgijen instructie* by Lambrecht van Tuylt, 'physician and prelector of surgery within the famous commercial town of Antwerp'.[16] Little or nothing is known about this Van Tuylt.

We can therefore conclude that the first printed textbooks which became available to Dutch surgeons of the Renaissance period were translated from the French.

A further volume which came off the press in Antwerp in 1533 was *Dat*

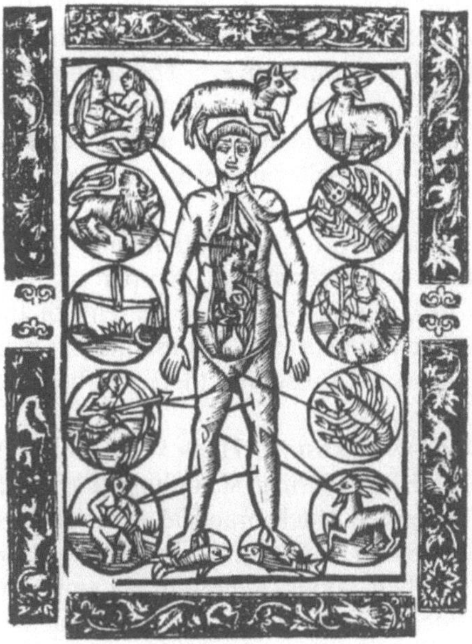

Fig. 23. Frontispiece of pseudo-Avicenna *Fleubothomia.* The diagram explains the influence of the constellations on the different parts of the body.

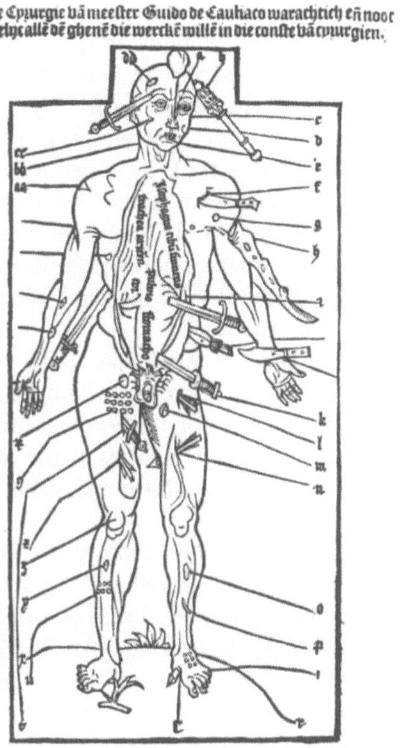

Fig. 24. Wound man: frontispiece of the 1507 Dutch edition of Guido de Cauliaco's *Cyrurgie.* The wound man, showing on his body all sorts of injuries caused by widely diverse agents, was a popular figure in Renaissance surgery (Cf. the cover illustration).

chyrurgylick werck. In fact it contained a translation of two different works by Giovanni da Vigo (1450—1525), the *Practica in arte chirurgica copiosa* and the *Compendiosa*, the latter is an abridged version of the first but goes more fully into the use of instruments.[17] The author, according to Nicaise the last of the Arabists,[18] was a surgeon at the Pontifical Court in Rome who lived from circa 1460 to 1517. The larger book, which first went to print in Latin in 1514, was an enormous success. It appeared in many languages and editions, including various Dutch ones up until the middle of the seventeenth century (Fig. 59). For almost two centuries it was one of the most popular surgery textbooks in Europe. It was eminently practical, presenting a succinct survey of the essentials of the craft in clear language with numerous prescriptions and other useful information. However, the text contains very little original information and makes repeated referrals to ancient Arabic and mediaeval authors, in particular to Galen and Avicenna. Both works are arranged according to the pentateuch.

In his treatment of wounds Da Vigo does not distinguish himself from others: if it appears that the wound is going to heal primarily, suturing should be considered.

Lacerated wounds should be treated by inducing suppuration. We also encounter the concept that wounds may 'decay' under the influence of air.[19] Among his haemostatic measures he mentions the ligature.[20] Amputatuion for gangrene should take place between the healthy and mortified parts.[21] Da Vigo was one of the first to write about wounds from firearms, of which — so he wrote — he had seen many. As he took these wounds to be poisoned, he considered that burning them out with red-hot irons or with boiling oil was imperative.[22] This author was very conservative in his treatment methods. He reluctantly took up the scalpel and was happy to leave operations on calculi, cataracts and herniae to the itinerant operating surgeons.[23] A mercury plaster which bears his name was used well into the nineteenth century.

A few German works as well found their way to the Netherlands in the sixteenth century. Two of them originated in Strasbourg, a prosperous, free reichstadt, famous for its book printing works as said before. At the end of the fourteenth and the beginning of the fifteenth century surgery, represented by men such as Jerome Brunschwig and Hans von Gersdorff, prospered there too, be it for only a limited span.

Brunschwig and his somewhat younger fellow townsman Hans von Gersdorff, who called himself Schylhans,[24] probably had little formal schooling: they both wrote in the vernacular. Each of them had acquired much practical experience in the field during the war against Charles the Bold. The battlefield has been of old an important training school for surgery.[25] In their books, they both lay emphasis on all sorts of injuries, on fractures and dislocations and on interventions such as trephination and amputation. This holds true for Brunschwig's book in particular. Gersdorff's work, although less voluminous, deals also with a few subjects of a non-traumatic character including leprosy and ergotism. Both works are embellished with very fine woodcut illustrations, Brunschwig's publication contains the first picture of surgical instruments in the history of printing.[26] The illustrations in Gersdorff reveal more details of several surgical methods of treatment than the stately ones in Brunschwig, which for the greater part represent a party of physicians and surgeons visiting a patient in his Gothic abode (Fig. 27). Both authors quote classic and Arabic authors, and to a lesser degree the famous mediaeval surgical authors among whom Lanfranc occupies a prominent place. It seems that they both also relied on an unidentified German edition of Guy de Chauliac.[27]

The texts of Brunschwig and Gersdorff have much in common. They both present an overview of the anatomy of their days which was still quite bizarre and fanciful. Brunschwig stresses particularly the importance of familiarity with anatomy for the surgeon: we encounter in his line or argument Henri de Mondeville's parable of the blind wood carver.[28]

In their wound treatment, Brunschwig as well as Gersdorff make use of sutures in appropriate cases.[29] The different ways of suturing which we met with in Albucasis, we encounter once again in these Renaissance authors: Gersdorff appears to be acquainted with the intestinal suture as indicated by Roger of Salerno. Their wound powders and salves too, appear to be compounded from constituents which were traditional ever since Galen. For haemostasis they utilise the whole scale of the expedients familiar to us now, including undersewing.[30]

When haemorrhage might frighten a patient, he should be blindfolded (Fig. 29) or be made to believe that such bleeding can only be beneficial.

The removal of arrowheads still presented the surgeons with serious problems, and since the introduction of firearms they were faced with the additional difficulty of extracting bullets (Fig. 25). Brunschwig, like Da Vigo, regards the latter type of wound as poisoned because of the powder that was supposed to have tainted the bullet.[31] Just as in shot wounds inflicted by poisoned arrows, boiling oil should be poured into the wound track. If in spite of this the wound does not become subject to suppuration, the surgeon should introduce a lint greased with pork fat to extract the poison.[32] Gersdorff does not express a definite view on that matter. He states that in the war against the Burgundians he often had to cope with shot off extremities. In such cases he cleared splinters from the bone ends, using a saw or tenaculum forceps, staunched the haemorrhage and covered the wound with a thick layer of lint saturated with hempseed-oil which was kept in its place by a stocking.[33]

Head injuries receive the customary attention in the course of which Brunschwig remarks that in his compatriots' skulls fractures occur less frequently than in those of Italians, for the reason that Germans have a thicker brain pan.[34] He closely follows Guy de Chauliac in his classification of head injuries and indications for applying the trepan. Gersdorff makes no reference to that operation. He does, however, describe an instrument consisting of a little tripod with a pointed screw in its middle which can be moved down and up, to pick up and raise an impacted bone fragment (Fig. 26). The treatment of fractures and dislocations in Brunschwig is on traditional lines but contrary to most of his predecessors he is ready to correct fractures that have healed in an unsatisfactory position. The bone is first softened by bathing the patient for two or three hours twice daily for a week in a decoction of various herbs. Then the callus is refractured either by vigorous pulling or by bending over a knee or a cushioned wooden wedge or by having an aid stand on the limb which is supported by two padded logs (Fig. 27).[35] In Gersdorff we find an illustration of the splinting of the leg as described by Lanfranc (cf. p. 49).

Unlike Brunschwig, Gersdorff also concerned himself about ankyloses and contractures for the treatment of which he devised hinged iron gutters which could be flexed or extended by means of a screw arrangement (Fig. 28).

In accordance with the time he lived in, Brunschwig, in the fourth tractate of his book which treats of all sorts of injuries, also gives directions for the treatment of those who suffered judicial torture or corporal punishment. Should for instance somebody survive being broken on the wheel, he should be buried in warm horse dung for twenty-four hours before receiving treatment for his fractures. Such a patient requires absolute rest in a large guttered body splint with an opening which enables him to defaecate without moving. Those who were whipped should be bled and anointed.[36] Surgeons could be summoned to be present when by judiciary order somebody was having a hand or a foot chopped off. In the case of a hand, Brunschwig recommends thrusting the bleeding stump into the inside of a black hen cut open alive.[37]

Both our authors lay down detailed directions for amputation. Amputations

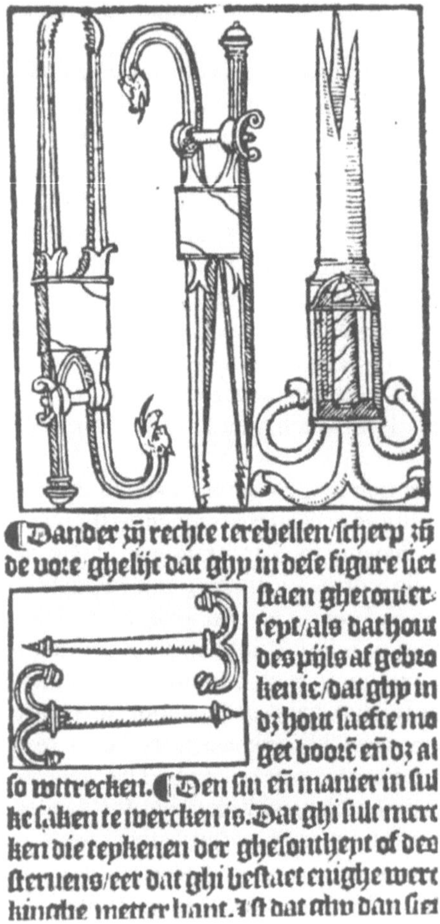

Fig. 25. The introduction of firearms is reflected in the surgeon's armamentarium. The two upper right instruments serve to extract arrows, but the left one is designed to remove bullets. The two pointed screws below are also for the extraction of leaden bullets.

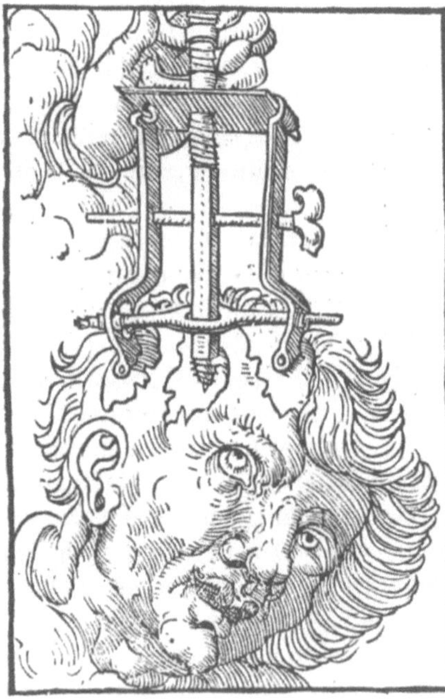

Fig. 26. Screw for raising an impacted bone fragment in the skull.

should, according to Brunschwig, neither be done in the gangrenous part nor just at the line of demarcation, but at some distance higher up, preferably through a joint or at least through healthy parts. Haemostasis is quite a problem here: the red-hot iron and boiling oil are the means most frequently resorted to. The undersewing of blood vessels, although well-known, is not mentioned in this context. Gersdorff covered the wound with lint and a wet pig's or cow's bladder. Healing should take place by granulation.

The indication for this operation was gangrene in the great majority of cases, usually resulting from Saint Anthony's fire (ergotism: Figs. 29 and 30).[38] The frequent occurence of ergotism is suggested by a casual remark by Gersdorff that

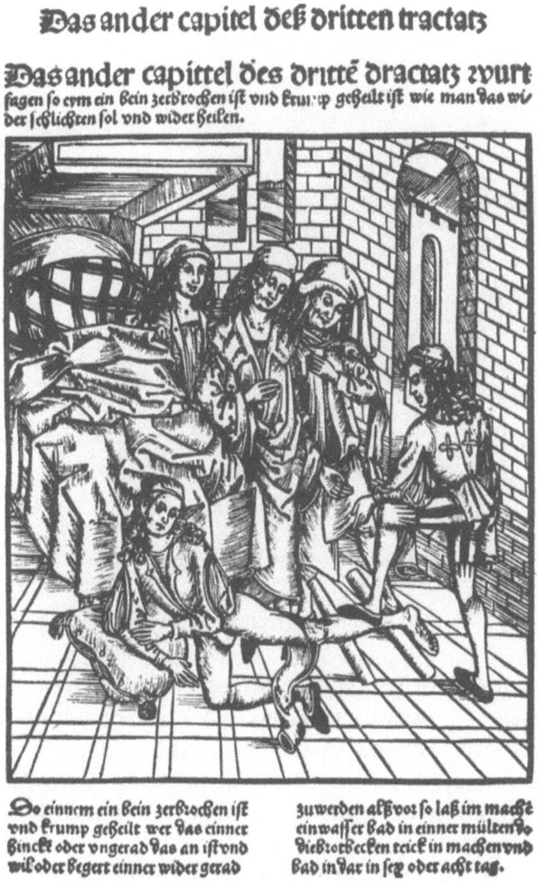
Das ander capitel deß dritten tractatz

Das ander capittel des drittē dractatz zwurt sagen so eym ein bein zerbrochen ist vnd krum p geheilt ist wie man das wider schlichten sol vnd wider heilen.

So einnem ein bein zerbrochen ist vnd krump geheilt wer das einner hinckt oder vngerad das an ist vnd wil oder begert einner wider gerad zuwerden alß vor so laß im machē ein wasser bad in einner multen do die brotbecken teick in machen vnd bad in dar in sey oder acht tag.

Fig. 27. Refracture of a lower leg.

he had performed maybe a hundred or two-hundred amputations in St. Anthony's Hospital in Strasbourg, in his civilian practice, therefore.

Brunschwig as well as Gersdorff makes mention of a potion consisting of root of salatrum mortale, semen hyoscyami, white poppy, black poppy, opium, saffron, mandragora and the like, which may be used to put patients asleep before an operation.[39] Gersdorff claims never to have used this potion nor to have heard of somebody else ever having used it.

Gersdorff's book appeared in a Dutch translation in 1593.[40] It must have been quite popular in this country for it went through at least four editions, the last one in 1651. The Dutch edition yields in quality to the German original: the quality of the woodcuts is as inferior as the print, and the anatomical folding plates have been reduced.

Some sixty years before, another Dutch translation from the German had appeared which, in spite of not bearing any author's name on the title page, has always been regarded as an adaptation of Brunschwig's text (Fig. 31). In the 'Totten beminden leser' (to the beloved reader), the author does in fact introduce

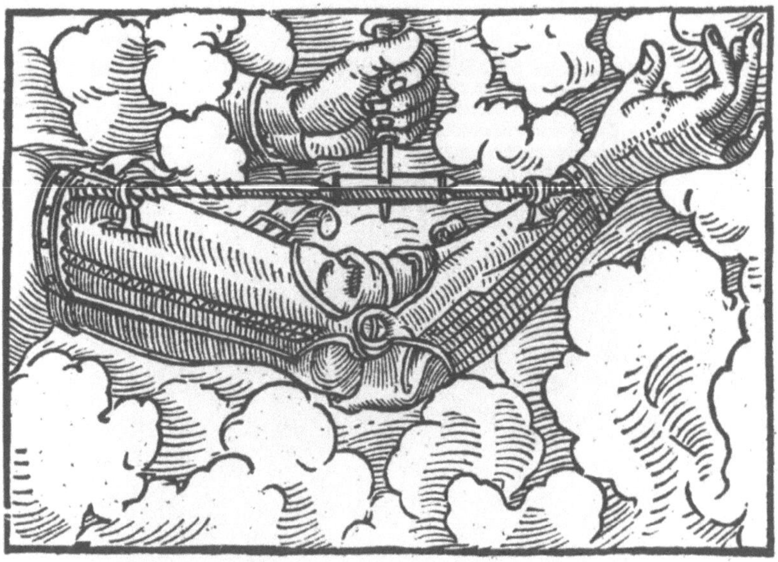

Fig. 28. Forcible correction of a contracture.

himself as 'ic Jeronimus bruyswyck te Straesborch geboren wten geslachte van Salernen'.[41] It appears, however, that this work is actually a free and abridged adaptation of Gersdorff. Several of the well-known Gersdorff illustrations have been included. Conversely, the typical Brunschwig pictures are absent.

The English translation of Brunschwig in 1525 is the first printed book on surgery in that language.[42]

Another German work which was — partly — turned into Dutch in the middle of the century (1556) in Antwerp is *Die Grosse Wundarzney* from Paracelsus' original edition of 1536.[43] Paracelsus, or Aureolus Philippus Theophrastus Bombast von Hohenheim (1493—1541) which was his actual name, is one of the most controversial figures in the history of medicine. Some considered him to be a renovator of medical science through his introduction of chemical notions, while others saw him as a fantastic figure or even a charlatan. Entering into his imaginative world of neoplatonism, theosophy and alchemy is far from easy. Luckily we do not have to set foot in that world to examine his views on surgery. Where and by whom Paracelsus, who was a physician, was trained in surgery is unknown. He probably gained much of his surgical experience during military campaigns in the Netherlands, Denmark and Italy, in which he took part as an army doctor.

From the *Wundarzney* we come to know Paracelsus as an extremely conservative surgeon, even more so than Da Vigo. With regard to treating wounds he had great faith in the healing force of nature. 'It is not the surgeon who cures wounds, it is the natural balsam in the body'.[44] This trust went so far that he mostly refrained from stitching wounds and sought support for the body's own healing powers in the use of internal and external medications, such as wound salves, balsams, plasters and powders, for which he gave the formulae.[45] It is essential to

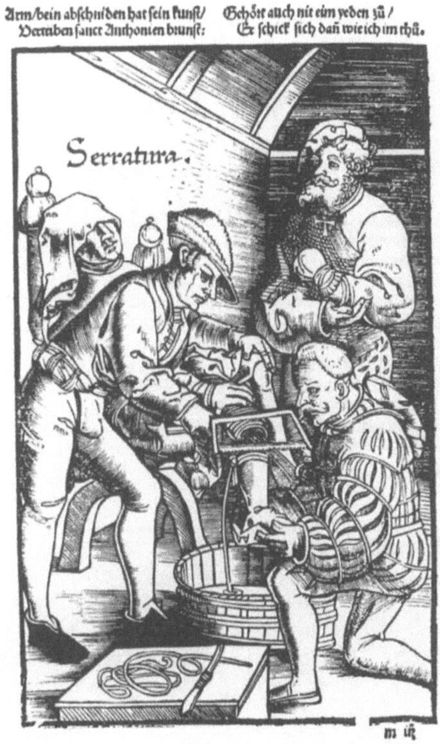

Fig. 29. Lower leg amputation in a case of 'St. Anthony's fire' (ergotism). To prevent the splashing of blood, a tub partly filled with water or sand is placed under the bleeding limb. Such tubs were used until the introduction of antiseptic surgery made it safe to use ligatures. The man standing in the background is probably suffering from gangrene of his hand.

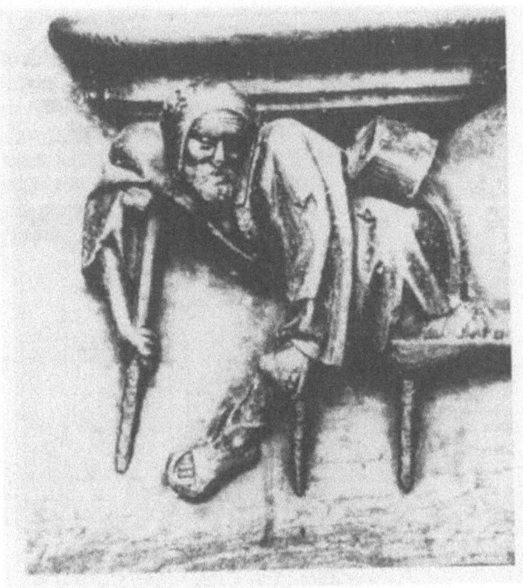

Fig. 30. Lower leg amputee moving on knee crutch.

keep a wound clean. He also had a number of remedies at his disposal to staunch bleeding, such as 'white hair of hare, from beneath the tail', ashes of frogs or even costly carnelian, the latter to be held by the patient or hung around his neck, but we read nothing about vascular ligatures or other mechanical devices. Foreign bodies, such as arrowheads and bullets, should not be removed with instruments but treated with external medication and wound potions until it is possible to extract them with the fingers.[46] For the immobilization of fractures Paracelsus used an extension device consisting of rings and screws, but he was not willing to reveal the details in print.[47]

Paracelsus showed no appreciation whatsoever for the Greek-Arabian traditions: quotations from other authors in his work are therefore few or absent. He impressed upon his readers that science must not consist of copying the texts of our predecessors but must be based on one's own investigation of nature. He flatly rejected Galenic humoral pathology, but the theory of the 'three principles' which

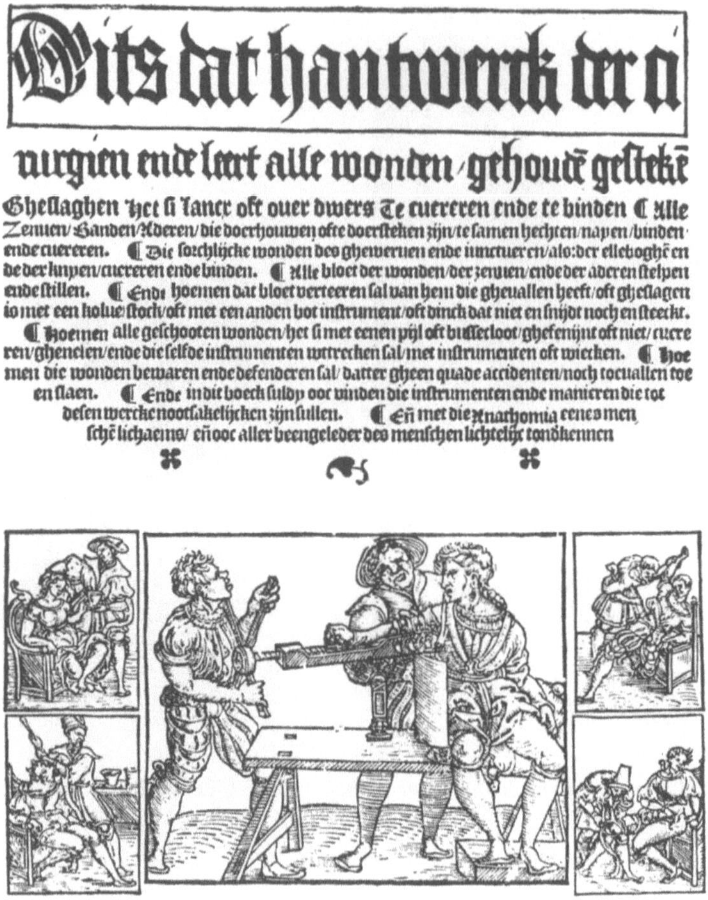

Dits dat hantwerck der ci
rurgien ende leert alle wonden / gehouwē gestekē
Ghestaghen het si lancx oft ouer dwers Te cureren ende te binden ¶ Alle
Zenuen / Banden / Aderen / die doorhouwen oftte doorsteken zijn / te samen hechten / nayen / binden
ende cureren. ¶ Die sorchlijcke wonden des gheweruen ende iuncturen / als: der elleboghē en
de der knyen / cureren ende binden. ¶ Alle bloet der wonden / der zenuen / ende der aderen stelpen
ende stillen. ¶ Ende hoemen dat bloet verteeren sal van hem die gheuallen heeft / oft ghestagen
is met een kolue stock / oft met een anden bot instrument / oft dinck dat niet en snijdt noch en steeckt.
¶ Hoemen alle geschooten wonden / het si met eenen pijl oft busseloot / ghefenijnt oft niet / cure
ren / ghenesen / ende die selfde instrumenten uuttrecken sal / met instrumenten oft wiecken. ¶ Hoe
men die wonden bewaren ende defenderen sal / datter gheen quade accidenten / noch toeuallen toe
en slaen. ¶ Ende in dit boeck sulby ooc vinden die instrumenten ende manieren die tot
desen wercke nootsakelijcken zijn sullen. ¶ Eñ met die Anathomia eenes men
schē lichaems / eñ ooc aller beengeleder des menschen lichtelijc tondkennen

Fig. 31. Pseudo-Brunschwig, really an adaptation of Gersdorff.

he substituted for this was derived from alchemy and therefore was not less speculative. Paracelsus did not so much seek the 'light of nature', which he wished to see shine upon medicine, in scientific research as we know it today, but sought it in natural philosophy.

He repeatedly stressed the value of personal experience: 'One must write and record the truth yet where one questions and also does not know the cause, refrain from writing . . .'.[48] Paracelsus strongly expressed his opposition to cautery and the knife.

The therapeutic reticence which he exercised in a time when surgeons generally had few leanings towards bloody interventions, must have met with the approval of many. In Dutch literature from the sixteenth and seventeenth centuries it is by no means rare to come across references to Paracelsus.

One might expect to find that the Spanish domination of the Netherlands had also made its influence felt on medical literature. This is indeed the case: we already cited the anatomy book by Valverde d'Amusco. Among the Dutch publications in the sixteenth century another important Spanish work should be noted, this one written by Francesco Arceo (c 1493—post 1574) who lived and worked in Llerena in the province of Badajoz and enjoyed an excellent reputation throughout his country. Through the mediation of doctor Alvaro Nuñez (Alvarus Nonnius), a Spanish physician who practised in Antwerp, Arceo's book was published in that city in 1574. The first part of the Latin treatise is about the healing of wounds; the second part deals with fevers. Its title is *De recta curandorum vulnerum ratione, et aliis eius praeceptis libri II . . . De febrium curandarum ratione.* This dichotomy can be explained by the fact that the author was a physician as well as a surgeon. The book must have been greatly appreciated inasmuch as it was soon translated into English (1588) and a new Latin edition was brought out in the seventeenth century in Amsterdam (1659). Various German translations were published (the last as late as 1717), besides Dutch ones in Roermond in 1667 and in Leeuwarden almost simultaneously, to be followed by a reprint only a year later.

The preface contains some interesting comments about the daily practice of surgery in those days. What was once the surest and safest branch in the whole of medicine and was practised by the greatest, was now said to be in a state of abjection and near-extinction through the ignorance and low-descent of almost all who engage in it. This being the fault of the doctors themselves who, in declining manual work, relegate it to empirics and even to the most incapable of barbers. They furthermore allow books, written by recent authors, to be perverted, rather than converted, into vulgar tongues.

In the book on wound treatment, head injuries traditionally occupy a prominent place. Arceo adopts a strong stand against 'beard scrapers or unlearned chirurgeons', who consistently enlarge all head wounds with a firm cross incision, subsequently to fill them with cotton and wool drenched in white of egg. They are also very lavish in their use of digestives: substances which generate pus.[49] Further on in the book he denounces surgeons as being blown-up and money-grabbing folk who blindly follow their masters' mistakes and do not know how to use their instruments properly.[50] One of his case-histories bears upon an intracranial haematoma with a closed skull fracture, requiring evacuation through trepanation.[51] For the actual burring and the after-treatment he describes the methods of Guy de Chauliac and Giovanni da Vigo.

In the case of penetrating injuries of the chest he recommends that the patient should be placed on the affected side, making sure of a free evacuation of blood and other discharges by keeping the wound open through the use of drains. Strips of surgical dressing were used for the latter purpose and apparently also mallow stems wrapped with yarn.[52]

Although this book chiefly deals with wounds, as the title indicates, we also find detailed instructions for the treatment of breast cancer.[53] This should consist of excision via a longitudinal incision. In order to be able to manipulate the tumour after it has been exposed, it should be pierced with a length of strong thread, the ends of which must be held in the hand.

As far as penetrating abdominal wounds are concerned, Arceo could boast of four cases of injuries to the colon, including one where it was wounded in three places, which he treated successfully with a 'suture such as glovers use'.[54]

In the chapter on the treatment of fresh wounds Arceo once again enumerates a number of errors which the lower sorts of surgeons were particularly apt to make: the use of only one type of wound salve, diachylon[55] or whatever, the taking of unnecessarily deep bites with too thick a needle and thread and poor apposition of the wound edges. The scars were therefore often unsightlier than the wound itself. If bone fragments were even partly loose they were removed because it was held that bone did not regenerate.[56]

Arceo mainly follows Da Vigo's instructions in his treatment of wounds and is therefore rather polypragmatic. Wounds are indeed to be stitched, but subsequently smeared with balsam of his own invention,[57] using a cock's feather. This is then covered over with Da Vigo's 'emplastrum basilicum, magistrale dictum'.[58] The application of these medications is aimed at forming laudable pus. In his suturing Arceo does not appear to strive after healing by first intention.

In the treatment of fistulae and abscesses, Arceo describes as his own invention, a hollow lead drain.[59] In the chapter about ulcers of the head, which were most often caused by syphilis, he goes into luetic bone necrosis of the skull cap and its treatment.[60]

Amputations of the extremities are not included in this book. In the history of orthopaedic surgery Arceo occupies a special position through his treatment of club-foot. This entailed redressement forcé and continous fixation using an iron splint, later followed by special foot-wear. His description was the first to appear on this subject since Hippocrates.

Modern French surgery made its entry into Holland towards the end of the sixteenth century in no less a person than Ambroise Paré, whose collective works were published in Dutch in Dordrecht in 1592. In 1547 a translation of his book on the treatment of shot wounds caused by hand firearms, which had been completed two years previously, had already been published in Antwerp.

Ambroise Paré (1510—1590) belonged to the category of barber-surgeons. He took part in many military campaigns and sieges during the wars of the French kings. He recorded the experience he gained in this way in a large number of books. His *Apologie et traité contenant les voyages faits en divers lieux* (1580), in which he included his experiences on the battle-field, is one of the most delightful accounts of personal recollections ever committed to paper by a surgeon. As Paré was not on good terms with Latin, he wrote in French which rather went against the grain of the faculty of medicine and the learned surgeons in Paris. Even so he was very well read in the classics and in contemporary literature, having had translations made of books by ancient authors which were not already available in French.[61]

Paré was a transitional character with great respect for ancient and Arabian authors, whereas his surgical writings were chiefly based on practical experience. Amongst the authors he quoted we find many names of his contemporaries. The chapters on anatomy no longer reverted to the mediaeval tradition such as that handed down by Guy de Chauliac, but were based on the modern anatomy of Vesalius.[62] He observed his patients better than his predecessors and his operative treatment showed much more daring.[63]

The 1592 Dutch translation of the fourth French edition, comprising twenty-eight books, is a magnificent volume containing all the numerous illustrations Paré had included in the original work. It appeared long before German and English translations saw the light of day. This edition contains no fewer than 1130 pages in folio, not to mention the index.

The first book is a general introduction. Here we find definitions of the objectives of surgery, followed by an exposition of the classic humoral pathology and the way in which the surgeon may recognize diseases due to vitiated body fluids using his own five senses. The six non-naturals (cf. p. 357 note 57) are duly heeded. Anatomy, covering no fewer than four books, receives much more attention than was normally the case with surgical textbooks. The illustrations, derived from Vesalius, are rather coarse and cannot by a long way bear comparison with those of the *Fabrica*.

From the seventh to the sixteenth book inclusive, the subject matter is arranged according to the well-known quinquepartite division.

The book on unnatural tumours — in which swellings such as phlegmon and oedema are traditionally included — falls back on classical, mainly Galenic, notions: a local accumulation of healthy blood results in phlegmon, vitiated blood causes carbuncles, gangrene and necrosis, corrupted bile various types of herpes, unnatural phlegm, 'watery and flatulent swellings', black bile scirrhus and cancer.[64]

Paré also included herniae among the unnatural swellings.[65] He preferred to treat these conservatively with a truss. Strangulated herniae, which surgeons in Antiquity and the Middle Ages had been powerless against, he treated surgically by notching the hernial orifice using a grooved sound, as his countryman Pierre Franco, to whom we will return presently, had done before him. Contrary to the itinerant herniotomists, Paré performed radical operations without castration. For this purpose he employed the 'punctum aureum' or 'golden stitch', already described by Guy de Chauliac and more recently by Franco. He moreover reminded his readers — again following in the footsteps of Franco — that a swelling in the groin could be due to an undescended testicle.

In the treatment of wounds, described in books 9 and 10,[66] Paré proved to be opposed to the use of wicks. Needle and thread were required when it was not possible to approximate the edges of the wound with bandages. He generally employed interrupted stitches but for intestinal wounds the furrier's suture. The edges were not to be pulled too tightly together, to enable any pus to escape more easily. To staunch bleeding he used the traditional astringent, cooling and drying medicaments — like Armenian bole or sealed earth, frankincense, mastic, aloe, hare's fur — mixed with white of eggs. Paré described as wound complications tetanus, paralysis — due to vertebral dislocations for instance — and 'syncope or fainting'.[67] The latter condition was treated by pouring brandy into the patient's mouth, holding strong-smelling flowers or apples under his nose, pulling his hair and shouting his name.

In Paré's treatise on head injuries we come across, for the first time, the liver abscess as a complication of such lesions, which has been mentioned so often subsequently in surgical literature.[68] In the general treatment of head injuries it is notable that Paré had patients suffering from insomnia inhale the vapours of a warm sponge soaked in narcotics: extract of poppy, mandragora, henbane, etc. The soporific sponge of the Middle Ages, although no longer used to anaesthetize patients before an operation, was apparently still being employed as a remedy for insomnia!

In the local treatment of head lesions Paré gives a thorough exposition of the application of the trepan of which instrument he had designed his own variant.

In his comments on injuries of the chest he describes rents in the diaphragm and subcutaneous emphysema which may arise after damage to the lungs and airways.

The book on gunshot wounds is amongst the best of his entire oeuvre.[69] In this he opposes the general notion that wounds inflicted by hand firearms ('handbossen') constitute a special form of burn, caused by the supposedly red-hot bullet, moreover poisoned with gunpowder. Paré no longer treated such wounds with boiling oil, as Da vigo had advised, but with suppurating agents. He highly valuated 'oleum catellorum' which consisted of oil in which two puppies had been cooked, earthworms, turpentine and brandy. Gunshot wounds had a high secondary mortality. In this connection he noted that the wounds of those who had died some time later after sustaining this type of injury, had exuded large quantities of evil-smelling pus, sometimes even with worms. In all cases pus collections also arose in other parts of the body, including the internal organs. The cause of all this was corrupted air for 'it is not possible to fight against God or against the air'.[70]

Another credit which should be given to Paré apart from his abandoning the use of boiling oil, is the improved amputation technique.[71] He conducted this operation through healthy tissue. After having placed the patient in the proper position, he pulled the skin and muscles as high up as possible and tied a strong cord around the limb just above the site of amputation. This served to keep the muscles in their raised position, would limit haemorrhage, and moreover reduce sensibility. Then he cut circularly through the soft parts to the bones, severed the structures between them and applied the saw. He did not use a red-hot iron to stop the bleeding, as was common practice in those days, but ligatures. The way he used to tie the bloodvessels was rather coarse and better is referred to as massligation. In cases of severe post-operative bleeding he recommended the undersewing of the main artery percutaneously higher up. After removal of the cord used as a tourniquet, the skin and muscles of the stump were pulled together loosely by four deep stitches. His cases mainly involved the lower leg: he does not seem to have performed amputations of the femur. He does have claim to being the first to perform an exarticulation at the elbow.

What he had to say about fractures and dislocations was mostly derived from Hippocrates. His own additions were an extension device for reducing femoral shaft fractures (Fig. 32) and a guttered splint made of tin for the lower leg. Paré was probably the first to describe the femoral neck fracture.[72]

In the seventeenth book 'dealing with a diversity of occurrences and particular operations',[73] Paré gives a thorough account of lithotomy according to the method described by Mariano Santo in 1522 and afterwards explained more fully by Pierre Franco, without mentioning their names. He apparently never conducted this operation himself.

Special mention should be made of the prostheses and orthopaedic and other

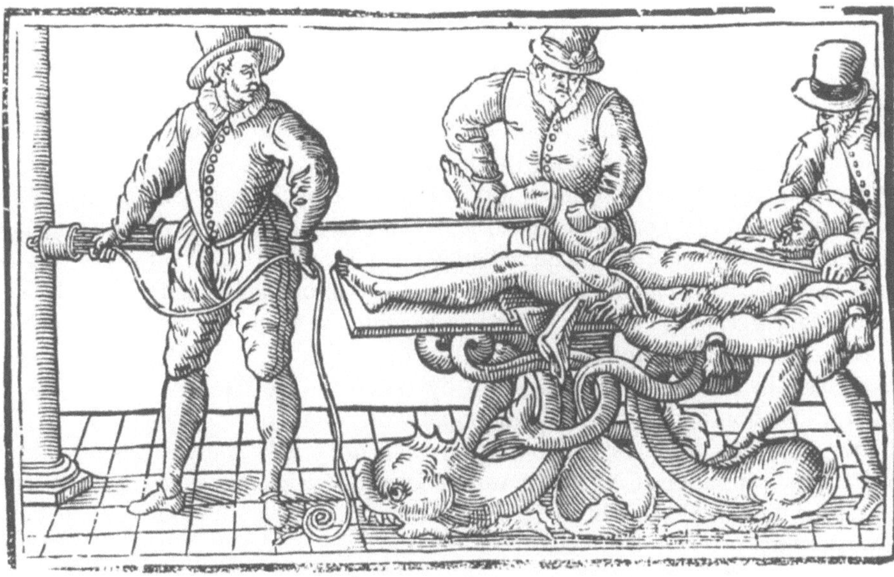

Fig. 32. Reduction of a dislocated hip using a mechanical device designed by Paré.

devices which Paré invented and illustrated. These not only include the wooden legs and crutches of old, but also artificial hands, arms and legs, apparatus for correcting club-feet, contractures and paralysis, urine receptacles and several more.

The books about venereal diseases, the plague, obstetrics and reproduction from Paré's collective work, will not be dealt with here. It is curious that in the treatise on reproduction the Dutch translator left the paragraph concerning intercourse in the original French 'for the sake of modesty'. There remains to be said that Paré wrote the first book on forensic medicine in which he included directions for issuing medical attestations. A fantastic book about monsters demonstrates that even this great Renaissance surgeon was by no means free from superstition. On the other hand he had never believed in the healing powers of bizarre drugs like mummia — human mummy material imported from Egypt, recommended by Paracelsus — or unicorn's horn.

Professional experiences, personal recollections and case histories, which he presented in profusion, greatly enhance the appeal of his writings. From his work he not only emerges as a conscientious surgeon and an inspired investigator, but also as a pious man: 'Je le pansay, et Dieu le guarist'.[74]

The Dutch translation of Paré's work ran through nine new editions in the seventeenth century, which is conclusive evidence of its popularity in the Netherlands. Even as late as the eighteenth century, Paré was frequently cited in surgical literature.

His translator was Carel Baten M.D. (c. 1540—1617), a native of Ghent who, after touring France and Germany, settled in Antwerp. As a protestant, he was forced to leave the city following its capture by the Spanish army under Alessandro

Farnese in 1583. Baten was town physician in Dordrecht until 1602 and presumably left for Amsterdam after that. His rendering of Paré's work found its way to Japan via the Dutch trade settlement on Decima in the bay of Bagasaki. Narabayashi Eikyu Chinzan (1643—1711), a Japanese student of the Dutch surgeon Hoffmann, translated it into his mother tongue.[75]

Carel Baten or Carolus Battus also had some other translations to his name, including in 1598 the beautifully illustrated *Francoijsche chirurgie*, ofte de manuale operatien der chirurgie by Jacques Guillemeau (1550—1613), who was one of Paré's students. This Dutch edition was translated into English under the title *The Frenche chirurgerye* ... It was, according to Billings, much the best work on this subject which had as yet appeared in English.[76]

Likewise in Dordrecht, although not by Baten but by Pieter van Nieustadt, a Dutch translation appeared of the principal work of Pierre Pigray (1533—1613), another of Paré's students: *Epitome praeceptorum medicinae, chirurgiae* (Paris, 1612). This translation, *Cort begrip van de leere der medicijne ende chirurgie* after its first printing in Dordrecht in 1623, ran through at least five more publications in Amsterdam.

3.5.2. *Original Publications Printed in Dutch*

The first printed medical publication of Dutch origin appeared around 1530. It was written in Antwerp by a certain Petrus Sylvius, about whom we know nothing further, under the title *Tfundament der medicinen ende chyrurgien* ... This book is an amalgamation of classical, Arabic and mediaeval writers — including Lanfranc — with Da Vigo as the only 'modern' author. It contains many woodcut prints, some of which are very fine indeed, none of them, however, having a bearing on surgery. The contents are richly variegated; in the prologue the writer expresses his hope to gratify *all* doctors, surgeons and pharmacists with this book. Thus one finds chapters on medical astrology, blood-letting, uroscopy, botany, diseases of women and infants, the plague, anatomy, surgery and finally an antidotarium. In the chapter on uroscopy the illustrations of the urine in the half-filled urinals are painted by hand in the relevant colours. The surgical section deals mainly with traumatology but there are also chapters on fistulas and ulcerating cancer.

Baten's *Secreetboeck van veele diversche en heerlijcke konsten* (Dordrecht, 1594) was original too. It comprised a collection of remedies against diseases in man and animals and household tips and was also translated into English.

Much more important, however, is his *Handboec der chirurgyen*, first published at Dordrecht in 1590, which went into its seventh edition in 1662 in Amsterdam. This book, as the author clearly indicates in the preface, was written directly in the vernacular for the benefit of the surgeons, who generally were unfamiliar with Latin. It follows the usual arrangement of swellings including syphilis, wounds, ulcerations, fractures and dislocations and is clearly based on Paré. For haemostasis Baten describes the customary methods of suturing the wound, the application of styptic medicaments or if needs be the red-hot iron. In cases of profuse haemorrhage, however, it is a certain remedy once the wound has been dressed to apply continuous digital pressure on the bleeding artery or vein day and night until the danger has passed. The author had experienced one such case where it had been necessary to maintain the compression for eight days and nights.[77] The book is free from scientific frills and is lacking in details of surgical therapy.

In the works by Dutch physicians and anatomists of the sixteenth century, including those by Pieter van Foreest (1522—97), Boudewijn Rouss (?—post 1590), Volcher Coiter (1534—76), Jan van Heurne (1543—1601) and Pieter Pauw (1564—1617), one finds a fair number of surgical case histories.

The fact that surgical case histories flowed solely from the Latin quills of academically educated physicians in those days, indicates that the barber-surgeons still stood closer to the barbers in a narrower sense than to the learned doctors. Writing on surgical subjects was apparently the business of physicians.

3.6. TOWARDS A MORE OPERATIVE FORM OF SURGERY

The literary works of Paré and his school testify to a certain change of mentality which in the second half of the sixteenth century became apparent in European surgery. Previously even prominent surgeons such as De Vigo, whom we met already in this chapter, or Fabricius ab Aquapendente and Fabricius Hildanus, to whom we will return in the next one, had preferred to work mainly with plasters and salves. Surgical therapy now became clearly more active. It was not only that operations were performed earlier, but some surgeons even ventured to carry out types of surgical treatment which had hitherto been left to cutters: herniotomy and — albeit with diffidence — lithotomy. One of those daring surgeons was Pierre Franco, a contemporary of Paré.

3.6.1. *Franco*

Pierre Franco (c. 1500—61) was a man of some education and one of the ablest surgeons and most original surgical authors of his age. He was born in Provence where he spent the first part of his life and later moved on to settle in Switzerland. He is the author of two books in the vernacular. The first one, *Petit traité contenant une des parties principalles de chirurgie*, appeared in 1556 under the motto: 'Il faut endurer pour durer'.[78] It was a modest volume, meant for professional lithotomists and herniotomists. The second, published in 1561 under the title *Traité des hernies, . . . et autres excellentes parties de la chirurgie*, was a more complete manual of surgery. In both treatises he accurately described a number of surgical procedures, mainly concerning hernia, bladderstone, cataract and also amputation, evidently from extensive personal experience.[79]

Franco distinguished eight different types of hernia: three true herniae and five 'herniae par similitude'. True herniation, resulting either from stretching or tearing of the peritoneum, was divided into enterocele, epiplocele and bubonocele or inguinal hernia. The first two varieties were apparently scrotal herniae. As to inguinal hernia — a name which had not yet appeared in Guy de Chauliac or Henri de Mondeville — it appears from his description that he was either referring to the present day small or medium sized indirect hernia, or to the direct inguinal variety: 'and this type of hernia is round'. This sort was thought to be caused by stretching of the peritoneum.[80]

False hernia included hydrocele, sarcocele, varicocele, pneumatocele and humoral hernia.[81] True hernia could be treated conservatively, using an emplastrum and a truss after reduction. Radical surgical treatment of the most common form, being intestinal hernia or enterocele, usually entailed hemicastration. After pushing back the contents of the hernia the scrotum was opened at the distal end. This incision, 'qui est de mon invention', comprised less risk for the patient because any pus could run away freely after the operation. After the testis had become visible the hernial sac was cut away from the scrotum as far up as possible and clamped — apparently together with the spermatic cord although this is not mentioned — with a specially designed clamp. Above this the hernial sac was run through with a stitch ligature after which the parts under the clamp were cut away. Adhesion of a bowel loop to the peritoneal pouch, a situation which Franco had not encountered in descriptions of other authors, could make manual replacement impossible. In these cases — which nowadays we would call 'sliding hernia' — it was necessary to separate the adherent viscus from the wall of the hernia sac digitally via a small opening made very close to the intestine.

Franco was one of the first — if not the very first — to treat the strangulated hernia surgically. The operation was carried out using a rod of about the thickness of a goose quill. One of the ends was flattened and rounded. By way of an incision high up in the scrotum the hernial sac was located. Against the flat end of the rod which was inserted via a small stab wound, this structure was incised until the abdominal opening had been reached through which the intestinal loop protruded. The reduction could subsequently be effected. The notching of the ring is not explicitly mentioned. It was thought best to conclude this procedure with the radical operation.

In the case of epiplocele it was possible to perform a radical operation without removing the testicle. After the hernial sac had been opened, the protruding omentum was secured as high up as possible, then excised and the proximal part repositioned. Franco also gave details of the surgical treatment of a scrotal hernia without removing the testis. By way of a small incision high on the scrotum, the hernial sac was dissected from the spermatic cord in the direction of the 'trou' (hernial orifice), taking care to save the spermatic vessels as much as possible, and closed by a suture ligature. This operation was particularly indicated if the patient only had one testicle left. The hernial sac might also be carefully cauterized in situ. Another method in which the testis is spared is the one 'avec le fil d'or', called 'point doré', which we have already encountered in Guy de Chauliac. Gold — 'or de ducat' — was chosen, Franco informs us, as this metal is 'amy de la nature' and therefore well tolerated. We will not discuss his methods of treating false herniae.

What Franco had to say about lithotomy was also important. He knew of four variations. The first operation was the ancient method of Celsus, in those days still the one most in use. He entered into more practical details aimed at the prevention of complications than had any author before him.

In the second procedure he made use of a round curved metal 'staff' with a groove in its side. This sound was introduced into the bladder via the urethra. An assistant held the handle and moved it to the patient's right, turning the sound somewhat to the left, at the same time pressing it lightly into the perineum so that its tip could be felt projecting against the pelvic floor at the left buttock. An incision was then made in the direction of the tip of the staff until the wall of the bladder was reached. This structure was punctured and then the neck of the bladder subsequently incised by cutting along the groove of the staff. A pair of forceps of Franco's own invention was then used to take hold of the stone and extract it. This approach became known as lateral lithotomy. If it was not found possible to retrieve the stone easily the operation was discontinued. After a few days, a second search for the stone usually achieved the desired end. Franco was the first to describe suprapubic cystotomy as an alternative approach. Although he had once used it successfully in a child, he did not really recommend it. He was also well acquainted with the more current Marian technique to which we will refer presently.

Franco's book apparently did not have a wide distribution in the Netherlands. Petrus Camper proudly stated in 1777 that he possessed a copy presented to him by the late professor Roëll, but that there were none to be found in the great library of Leyden University, nor in the university collections in Franeker or Groningen.

3.6.2. *Santo*

In Italy, lithotomy began to be accepted as a regular surgical procedure mainly through the efforts of Mariano Santo, a student of Johannes da Vigo. Mariano Santo (1498—post 1550), Dr. med. et phil., who lived and worked in many places in Italy, wrote a *Libellus aureus de lapide in vesica per incisionem extrahendo* in 1522. The first Roman edition was soon followed by several others in Venice and Paris. The tract also appeared in surgical collective works printed elsewhere. In this small monograph, he divulged a method of lithotomy which soon became universally known. It is described by Franco as follows. The patient was placed in the lithotomy position and a grooved metal staff, shaped like a male catheter, was introduced through the urethra into the bladder. Its convex part was used to push out the urethra on the left side of the perineum, where an incision was made through the skin, subcutaneous fat and muscles, in the direction of the urethra. The urethra was then incised in its membranous part over the staff. Guided by the groove of the staff, an 'exploratorium' — a shorter and straight grooved sound — was pushed into the bladder through this incision. The staff was now removed and a pair of 'ductores' were introduced over the 'exploratorium'. Whereupon the latter instrument was taken out in its turn, allowing a dilating instrument to be inserted between the two rod-shaped 'doctores' or conductors. Using this instrument, the prostatic urethra and the orificium urethrae internum were carefully dilated until the opening was sufficiently large to pass a scoop or pair of forceps for extracting the stone. Since quite a few instruments were required for this operation, it became known as 'lithotomy by the greater apparatus' in distinction to the Celsian method 'by the apparatus minor'.[82]

3.7. SURGICAL PHARMACEUTICS (MATERIA CHIRURGICA)

Leafing through the surgical literature of Antiquity, the Middle Ages and the Renaissance described thus far, we find that a striking amount of attention was paid to the drugs with which surgeons were required to be acquainted. Johannes da Vigo called surgery a therapeutic instrument besides diet and potions.[83]

Since the old days surgeons, as well as doctors, have compounded their own medicines and the relevant chapters in textbooks not only outline the application but also describe the preparation of medicaments.

The different fields of activity of a physician and a surgeon find expression in the prevailing pharmacy of each profession. In the ordinances of the surgeons' guilds in the sixteenth century it was clearly formulated — in accordance with the traditional assignment of tasks — that surgeons were permitted to administer or sell 'external remedies' but only internal medicines such as wound-potions, which would serve as supportive measures in the treatment of external afflictions.[84] Internal therapy belonged in principle to the domain of the doctor. From the examination requirements laid down in ordinances of various surgeons' guilds, it appears that the prospective surgeon was expected to demonstrate his proficiency in the practical preparation of a number of medications which were mentioned by name. Questionnaires which have been preserved from this period as well as compendia in the form of questions and answers, offer further insight into what the surgeons in the sixteenth century were required to know about pharmacy. A comparison of the *Examen chirurgicum anno 1595*, a handwritten document which can be found in the records of the surgeons' guild of St. Cosmas and Damianus in Rotterdam, with the current Dutch literature of that time, shows that the examination requirements including pharmacy, formulated in that document, were based on *Der chirurgijen instructie* by Jean Tagault with which we are already familiar.[85]

In the sixteenth century the dispensing of medicines became more and more the work of pharmacists. But as the times at which the pharmacists in the various cities received their own ordinances were rather divergent, this development did not take a synchronous course in the North Netherlands. City surgeons therefore continued to compound their own medicines until way into the seventeenth century and those in the country, of course, for very much longer.

CHAPTER 4

The Golden Age

4.1. POLITICAL AND ECONOMICAL HISTORY

In the seventeenth century the Republic of the Seven United Netherlands experienced a remarkable period of prosperity in many respects. The war with Spain ended in 1648, when a peace was concluded, whereby Spain acknowledged the Republic's independance. The Republic had long before established itself as a free and sovereign confederate state and was playing a more and more important role in European politics.

Shipping and trade had been important pillars of country's economy ever since the latter part of the Middle Ages (Fig. 33). In the first half of the seventeenth

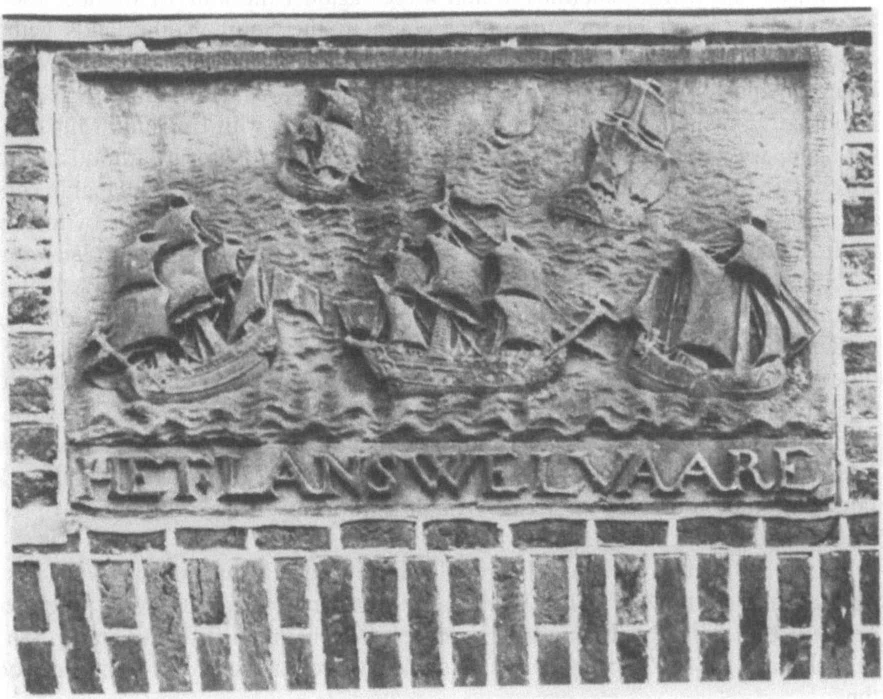

Fig. 33. The way Holland became wealthy.

century nearly all continental trade with the Baltic countries and even that with England was in the hands of the Netherlands, while the Dutch East-India Company, established in 1602, more or less held the European monopoly of the trade in spices. The commercial relations of the East-India Company not only stretched to the East Indies but also to the Levant, to India, China and Japan. The Dutch trading fleet consisted of more than 11 000 freighters. The West-India Company, established in 1621, made great profits during the war with Spain by capturing the richly loaded galleons sailing home from South and Middle America. Trade and shipping contributed in bringing prosperity to industry.

It is understandable that England, which also had large shipping interests, endeavoured to check the strong position of Holland on the seas. In 1651 the British parliament enforced the Act of Navigation for this purpose. This meant that merchandise from the European continent could only be imported into England via British vessels or ships from the countries of origin.

This law meant a very serious trade barrier for the Dutch Republic and led to the outbreak of the First Anglo—Dutch War (1652—54). Mainly due to the poor state of its navy, this war went badly for the Netherlands. After peace had been declared the fleet was, therefore, completely reorganized.

The continuous trade rivalry with the English gave rise to another appeal to arms with the Second Anglo—Dutch War (1665—67). It ended in a much more honourable manner for the Netherlands than the first, thanks to a well-equipped navy, commanded by capable admirals such as Tromp and De Ruyter. Shortly afterwards, the former enemies joined forces against the king of France when he attempted to assert his presumptuous claim to the South Netherlands with the power of arms. This war did not go too badly for the allies. A second war with France, which broke out in 1672, seemed to take a catastrophic course for the Republic. Louis XIV, who had managed to join forces with England, Munster and Cologne, was able to occupy a large part of Dutch territory without any great effort. The following year, stadtholder William III, who was both a capable general and a diplomat, managed to drive the war into the South Netherlands by forming a triple alliance with Spain, Brandenburg and the German emperor, coupled with the execution of a lucky campaign. Throughout the last quarter of the seventeenth century William III remained the main political opponent of the king of France. Holland behaved as a great power and was more or less accepted as such by the other countries. This was due not only to its own internal strength but also to the weak positions in which Germany, England, France and Spain found themselves during the final decades of the century. William's influence increased even more when together with his English wife, daughter of the duke of York, later king James II, they were crowned as William and Mary, king and queen of Great Britain and Ireland in 1689.

From 1688 onwards under his leadership a new European coalition took the field against Louis XIV. This War of the League of Augsburg was fought once again in the South Netherlands. The defeat which the British inflicted upon the French navy in 1692 brought them dominion over the seas for a long period of time.

In the seventeenth century, Dutch internal politics were sometimes characterized by heavy religious quarrels between protestant groups as well as by long-winded and deep-seated differences of opinion between supporters and opponents of the stadtholdership. It was in itself a most remarkable thing that the Republic, which had abjured its sovereign, should formally maintain the royal delegate, the stadtholder, in its body politic.

4.2. CULTURAL LIFE

It was not only as a trading power that Holland held a dominant position in Europe. As cultural centre it could hold its own against any other nation. Dutch civilization, which at that time had its own distinct character, amazingly reached its climax almost immediately after the birth of the nation, as Huizinga has observed:

> In the narrow territory (of the Republic) directly after its birth, great achievements and great figures came together in the space of less than a century, the statesmen, the generals, the naval heroes, the painters, the poets and the scholars, the founders of world trade and power in East and West. Is it possible to name one other country in which the national culture matured so quickly after its nativity?[1]

All this was achieved in spite of the warfare. As the hostilities mainly took place either at sea or outside the national borders with an army consisting chiefly of mercenaries, the average Dutch citizen was seldom directly involved in the war and social order was able to carry on undisturbed. Even scientific contacts remained intact with the enemy: the Third Anglo—Dutch War (1672—74) did not impede Jan Swammerdam, Reinier de Graaf and Antoni van Leeuwenhoek from keeping up their correspondence with the Royal Society in London.

Unlike France, culture in the Netherlands was not concentrated in a royal court, but could be found in the residences of the city merchants, particularly of Holland and Zeeland, the provinces in the Republic which predominated in every respect. Amsterdam actually stood in the forefront; with about 200 000 inhabitants it was one of the largest cities in Europe.

In cultural life, literature held its prominent position through such writers and poets as J. van den Vondel and P. C. Hooft, but this age was also the era of the jurist H. de Groot, the philosopher B. Spinoza and the composer J. P. Sweelinck. The memory of the Golden Age of the Netherlands is best preserved through its fine arts, paintings and engravings, Rembrandt being the most outstanding representative (Figs. 34 and 35), but also through its typical architecture Dutch influence stretched from Germany to the Baltic countries.

In the seventeenth and eighteenth centuries the largest concentration of publishers and printers in Europe was located in the Dutch Republic.

4.3. UNIVERSITIES

Each province of the confederacy was allowed to have one university. Accordingly, there were such institutions in Franeker (1585), Groningen (1614), Harderwijk (1645) and Utrecht (1636). Amsterdam, although by far the most important

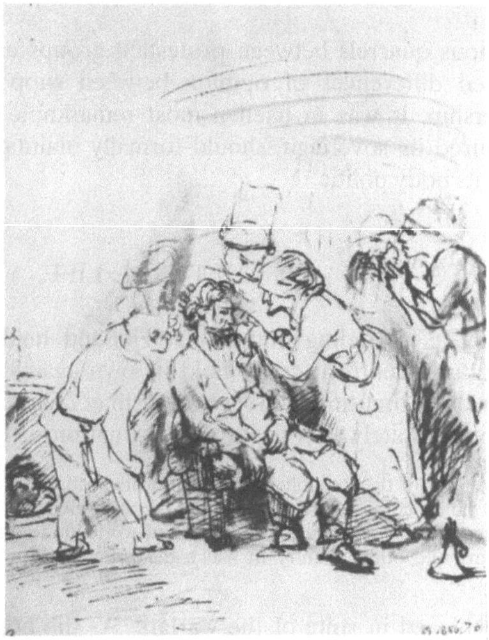

Fig. 34. A man suffering from a head injury is being assisted by a woman and a surgeon. The surgeon keeps an elongated instrument (a probe?) between his teeth ready for use. Holding an instrument, such as an amputation knife, between the teeth to leave the hands free was customary in the pre-antiseptic era.

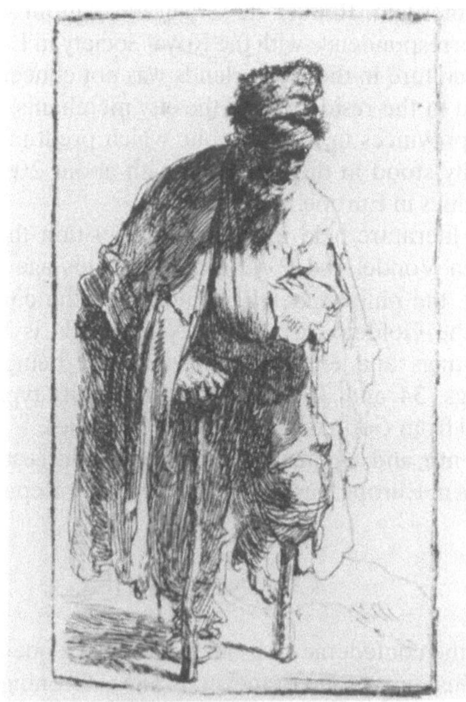

Fig. 35. Beggar with a wooden leg.

cultural centre in the whole country, could not boast its own university because the province of Holland already had one in Leyden (see p. 65). However, it had an Athenaeum Illustre since 1632 — an institution for further education, but without the authority to grant academic qualifications. Similar Athenaea could be found at a few other places in the country. A university being purely an educational institution, its reputation depended entirely on the tuition it offered and the fame of its lecturers.

The natural sciences, which about this time became detached from the traditional 'Liberal Arts', received less consideration than either — protestant — theology or the humanities, for it was not yet considered to be a profession.

As far as medicine was concerned, in the sixteenth and seventeenth centuries it was not so much a question of teaching a certain subject as explaining a certain book.[2] In the first years after the foundation of the university of Leyden, texts by Hippocrates, Paulus Aeginata, Aristotle, Galen and Celsus occupied the timetable. At the examination which preceded graduation in medicine, candidates had to explain two aphorisms of Hippocrates. It was not until late in the seventeenth century that changes came about in Leyden, due to the ideas and modern views brought forward by Sylvius. Clinical instruction at the bed-side, introduced by him and continued by Boerhaave, became customary especially in Leyden and attracted scholars from all over the world. Scientific research was conducted for the greater part outside the universities.

4.4. TRENDS IN MEDICINE

In the seventeenth century, medical thinking no longer displayed the coherence which had been characteristic since late Antiquity. The discoveries of Vesalius and the post-Vesalian anatomists had demonstrated that Galen was by no means the infallible source of medical knowledge and the dismantling of Galenism proceeded steadily on.

Apart from humoral pathology, which continued to find fervent adherents, two other schools of thought were arising. The first was the so-called iatrochemical or chemiatric school which attempted to explain physiological and pathological phenomena on the analogy of the processes that take place in chemical retorts. The most prominent representative of that school in Holland was the Leyden professor of medicine François de le Boë Sylvius (1614—72). Sylvius did not aim at the construction of an entirely new system, but tried rather to supply traditional Galenic notions of humours and spirits with a modern chemical foundation.[3] He explained body heat as the product of a chemical reaction, brought about by the mixing of blood which contains alkaline bile, with blood containing acid chyle. He had demonstrated in the laboratory that by adding potash lye to acids, there was a development of heat. By placing the encounter between acid and alkaline blood in the heart, the antique view of the heart as the source of body heat could remain.

The new chemical notions appeared to be very acceptable for pathology and physiology as well. Bile of old was a potentially dangerous body humour. Its black variety in particular could cause disease when it was no longer alkaline, as was normally the case, but when it had taken on acid properties. For the assessment of 'acid' or 'alkaline', chemists of the time of Sylvius only had their tongues at their disposal. In his patho-physiological considerations, Sylvius attached great importance to lymph.[4] The lymphatic system had only recently been discovered (1653) and the function of its clear, watery contents, not described by Galen, was raising quite a few questions. Lymph, as Sylvius had established by tasting, was a 'succus subacidus', a subacid juice. Should its slightly acid nature turn into acrid acid, the ensuing 'acrimony', sharp and biting as it was, would predispose to morbid conditions such as cancer: 'ab acido enim acri cancrum generari'.

To the opposing iatrophysicists, who tried to explain the processes of life by means of the laws of physics and mechanics as they were known at the time, the body appeared as a machine. This school of thought, which originated in Italy, received in Holland a strong boost from the ideas of the French philosopher, natural scientist and mathematician René Descartes (1596—1650).[5] In his *Traité de l'homme*, which appeared posthumously in 1662, he described the body as a sort of engine, composed of solid parts and kept in operation by the blood and the nerve spirits moving in the blood vessels and nerves. Man, however, is not only a machine for he has a conscious mind as distinct from animals which were thought to be merely automatons. Animal experimentation, which was rapidly coming into vogue in the seventeenth century, found its ethical justification in the latter presumption.

The views of Descartes led to much controversy. On theological grounds, their exposition was forbidden at the universities of Leyden and Utrecht, but this did not prevent quite a few doctors from accepting a technomorph model of the living organism. The rise of iatrophysics or iatromechanics was greatly influenced by the theory which William Harvey (1578—1657) made public in 1628 regarding the circulation of the blood. In this Harvey compared the action of the heart with a double action pump and by means of a simple calculation he had shown that the total amount of blood which leaves the heart per hour would weigh thrice as much as the total body weight of the experimental animal. It was therefore out of the question that blood, after having been turned out by the liver, could be promptly absorbed and assimilated by the other organs, as Galen had taught. Harvey's theory initially met with strong resistance in several countries but it was very soon accepted in Holland through the intermediary of Descartes and a number of prominent physicians including Sylvius and Van Beverwyck.

The discovery of the blood circulation meant the beginning of modern physiology, just as the work of Vesalius and his contemporaries in the previous century had paved the way for modern morphology. Harvey's investigations moreover proved to the hilt the value of a quantitative approach toward physiological problems, and of the expression of the findings in measure — by volume, weight and number; whereas Galenic physiology had only had qualitative descriptions to offer.

4.5. ANATOMY

The Dutch took an active part in the further development of both the basic sciences of medicine in the seventeenth century. As far as anatomy was concerned their interest was particularly directed at the lymphatic and chyliferous vessels. It was Johannes van Horne (1621—70), professor of anatomy and surgery at Leyden, a student of Pauw, who discovered the thoracic duct in humans in 1651, while Frederik Ruysch was to reveal the valves in dried lacteal and lymphatic vessels.[6] Ruysch proved himself to be a master in another much used anatomical technique, namely the injection of coloured, setting liquids into blood vessels. This procedure enabled him to demonstrate the vascularization of the heart muscle. We will return to Ruysch later in this chapter (see p. 141).

Other well-known anatomists were Reinier de Graaf (1641—73) from Delft, who discovered the ovarian follicle named after him and Nicolaas Tulp from Amsterdam. Jan Swammerdam (1637—80), also from Amsterdam, best known as an entomologist, must also be mentioned here for his discovery of the processus vaginalis peritonei in 1672 from which he concluded that a hernia was never the result of a tear in the peritoneum.[7] The persistent tubular prolongation of peritoneum which favours the formation of an inguinal hernia in the female is named after Anton Nuck (1650—92). who taught anatomy and surgery in The Hague before becoming a professor at Leyden.

Antoni van Leeuwenhoek (1632—1723), a fellow-citizen of De Graaf, was not a doctor. He achieved international fame through his investigations with simple microscopes constructed by himself. He was able clearly to describe the capillary blood-flow, the erythrocyte, the spermatozoon and the striation of striped muscle. Moreover, Van Leeuwenhoek is considered as the discoverer of the infusoria and bacteria.

4.6. PHYSIOLOGY

Dutch scientists were also active in the field of physiology. Professor Jan de Wale (1604—49) at Leyden described experiments which demonstrate that arterial blood passes into the venous system while the above mentioned Johannes van Horne discovered that chyle was not transported directly to the liver, as Galen had proclaimed, but entered the bloodstream via the thoracic duct. Jan Swammerdam investigated the respiratory mechanism, and Reinier de Graaf examined the action of the pancreas. All these experiments were conducted on live animals: through Harvey's discovery the significance of animal experiments had clearly come to light. From experimental physiology to experimental surgery is only one step: this step was taken in the seventeenth century but it should be noted that those who engaged in it were physicians rather than surgeons.

4.7. EXPERIMENTAL SURGERY

The discovery of the blood circulation in the sixties led almost simultaneously to animal experiments in England, France, Germany, Italy and Holland, involving the intravenous administration of drugs and even the transfusion of blood.[8] The first intravenous injection administered to an experimental human subject was carried out by Johann Sigismund Elsholtz in 1660 in Berlin. An illustrated report was published in his attractive little book *Clysmata nova*.

In England, several members of the 'Invisible College' — precursor of the Royal Society — actively occupied themselves with such experiments. Richard Lower (1631—91) described the details of experiments with direct blood transfusion in dogs together with a case in which a human subject was used, in his *Tractatus de corde* from 1669.[9] The human experiment dealt with a bachelor of divinity, whose brain was sometimes a little too warm. He was transfused with lamb's blood without suffering injury. In Paris Jean-Baptiste Denis (c. 1625—1704), personal physician to king Louis XIV, conducted seven blood transfusions from animal to man with the assistance of the surgeon Paul Emmerez after completing a number of preparatory experiments on animals. Lambs and calves served as donors (Fig. 36). Twice the transfusion was carried out on a healthy subject who was especially engaged for the job. The other five were conducted on three patients who were suffering respectively from fever with anaemia due to repeated bleeding, diarrhoea which at autopsy appeared to have been caused by intussusception, and mental disturbance. In the last case the patient complained of pain in the loins directly after treatment and produced blood-stained urine, which was later followed by a nosebleed. When this patient died several months later, it was decided to discontinue what was in effect an experimental mode of treatment. Denis made a thorough report of what had happened in which he included a description of the work of Lower.[10] In the same year, 1667, a Dutch translation of Denis' account was published by J. H. Glazemaker.[11]

In Holland it was Reinier de Graaf who took an interest in experimental blood transfusions. Personal contacts with Denis whom he visited more than once during a stay in Paris, probably gave him the inspiration. The equipment he used for the purpose consisted of a length of bird's intestine with well-fitting duck's quills at both ends so that they could be inserted into the veins of both donor and receiver at the same time. This piece of equipment proved to be much more practical than the rigid silver and copper tubes in use abroad.[12]

Before going on his study tour to France in 1664, De Graaf together with a fellow student at Leyden, Joachim Georg Elsner from Breslau, subjected a bitch to a splenectomy, an experimental operation which the latter had carried out once before. Elsner was led into doing so by a statement made by the very well-known physician Jean-Baptiste van Helmont (1577—1644) living in the South Netherlands, who had said that the spleen was the organ from which the desire to have progeniture originates.[13] Both dogs survived the operation. The first came into heat after a time but did not conceive, whereas the second splenectomized bitch produced two healthy puppies.[14]

Experimental splenectomies in dogs appear to have been popular in Holland at the time, as indeed it was elsewhere in Europe.[15] Barbette, for instance, gave an account of six such experiments in his *Praxis*.[16] With the exception of the first dog, all animals had survived. These operations must have been performed in Amsterdam prior to 1665, the year in which Barbette died. Frederik Dekkers, the editor of Barbette's *Praxis*, stated in his comments that he too, had removed dogs' spleens. One bitch could no longer conceive afterwards, 'which is why some

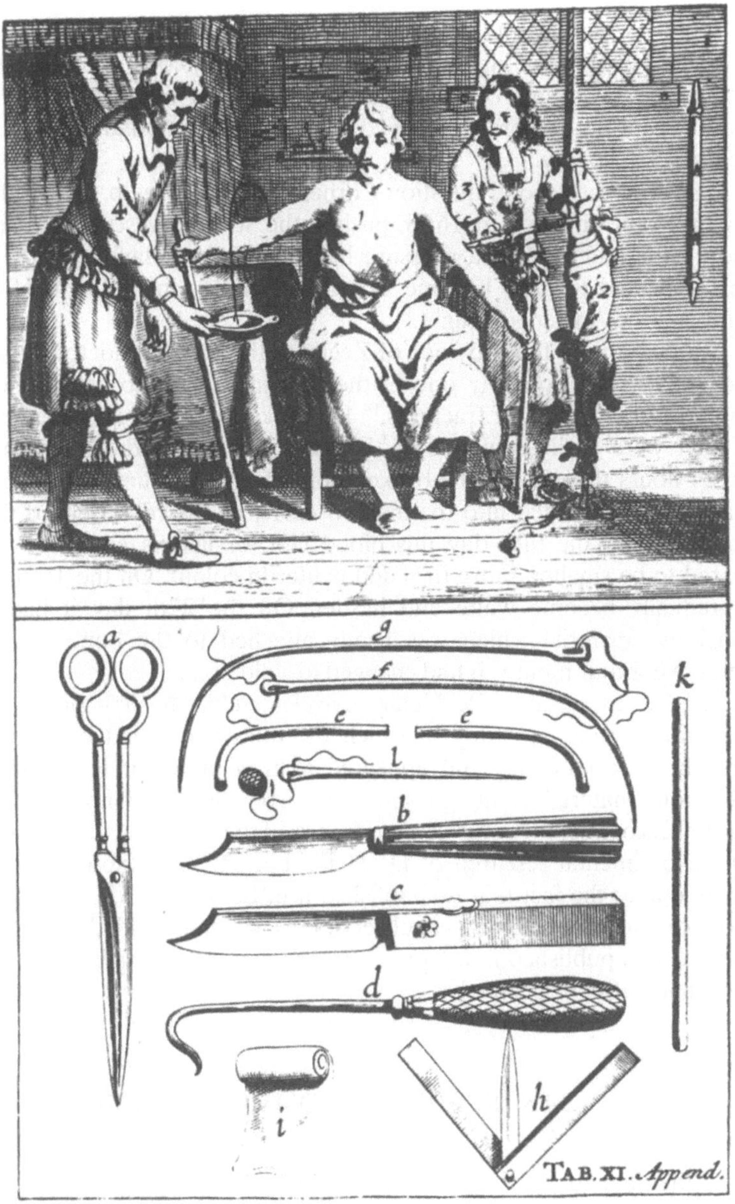

Fig. 36. Simultaneous bloodletting and blood transfusion using an animal as donor.

ascribe to the spleen a virtue of producing blood suitable for procreation'. Job van Meekeren (see p. 142) also reported on one such experiment which was successfully carried out by one Henricus Balsy, M.D., and so did Frederik Ruysch.

Other examples of experimental surgery in Holland's Golden Age were concerned with questions of tracheostomy, of how haemorrhages come to a spontaneous arrest, and of the healing of fractures.

In 1670 or thereabouts Johannes Baptista van Lamzweerde (1630?—17?), a doctor who set himself up as defender of the physiological ideas of Aristotle, demonstrated by means of animal experiments that a tracheostomy was not as dangerous as it was generally believed. A dog which had undergone this operation made a quick recovery.[17]

In answer to the second question Cornelis Solingen (see p. 132) cut the femoral artery and vein of a dog in 1668, pushed the severed vascular stumps back into the soft parts and applied a pressure bandage. Eleven days later the ends of the vessels appeared to have become closed with 'fibres in the form of a node', not with flesh as the Ancients thought.[18]

In Middelburg, in the province of Zeeland, the medical doctor Anton de Heide (1646—169?) was probably one of the first in Europe to conduct experimental research on the healing of fractures.[19] He broke the hind legs of large numbers of frogs that were easily available at the time and followed the process of repair. After 24 hours the ends of the broken bones were surrounded by a haemorrhagic effusion which extended into the marrow cavity and partly involved the surrounding muscles. On the fifth day this blood clot, or lamina cruenta as he called it, appeared to be smaller, more firm and lighter in colour. On the 16th day the crust had gradually become white and harder. On the 27th day it had turned into cartilaginous material which was firmly attached to the bone and surrounding muscles. After four months it had changed to solid bone.

In another experiment De Heide investigated the healing process following a trephination wound in a dog in which the dura mater had been cut. After two weeks, the defect in the skull appeared to have more or less closed over with cartilaginous material, although somewhat irregularly and not right to the bony edges. In his comments the researcher discussed the phenomenon of proud flesh.

The experimental research of De Heide became well-known abroad. This was not only due to the fact that he published it in Latin in 1683, but also through the 'anatomical, medical and surgical observations' which he added to a pharmaceutical text which was published in a German translation in Leipzig by two different firms in 1690 and 1700, respectively.

4.8. SCIENTIFIC COMMUNICATION

Before the invention of the art of printing, exchanging letters was the only possibility for scholars to notify each other of their findings. Even after the introduction of the printing-press, letters remained the pre-eminent means of communication for some time, supported by the fact that Latin continued to be the language of science. It became customary for authors of textbooks or more specialised monographs, then coming into the vogue, to have letters, which they had exchanged with correspondents at home and abroad, printed in their works. In this way the learned correspondence has been partially preserved, but as it sometimes lies hidden in books where such letters would not normally be expected, it is poorly accessible to historical research.

The seventeenth century was also the time that periodicals made their appearance in the form of printed proceedings and reports, published by the Academies of Science which since the sixteenth century had come into existence in many countries. The Dutch Republic did not have such an institution which is the reason why one more than once comes across Dutch contributions in the *Philosophical Transactions of the Royal Society in London* established in 1666, or in the *Ephemerides* published since 1670 by the German 'Academia Naturae Curiosorum', better known as 'Leopoldina'.

Clinical case histories frequently saw the light of day as compilations, often batched in tens — *decades* — or even in hundreds — *centuriae.*

4.9. SUPERSTITION

From what has been said above about anatomical research on the human cadaver and about experimental physiology and surgery, it must not be concluded that medical science had now taken a determinedly positivistic direction according to the guidelines traced out by Francis Bacon.[20] The Renaissance was a period in which all sorts of superstitions were flourishing, as shown by the persecution of witches, and from which medicine had not been exempted.

In the field of surgery, weapon salve and sympathy powder became well-known, and both were used for treating wounds. Weapon salve, which is often attributed to Paracelsus, was actually conceived by Rudolf Goclenius (1572—1621) who was a professor of physics at Marburg.[21] This salve was composed of usnea — moss which had grown on the skull of a hanged man, or at least on the pan of someone who had not died of natural causes — human blood, lard, mummia, linseed oil, turpentine and bole.[22] It was not applied to the wound but to the weapon which had inflicted the injury. The wound itself was left alone or, at the most, bathed in wine or water.

The powder of sympathy was introduced in 1661 by Sir Kenelm Digby (1603—65), who was chancellor to the king of England and no more a doctor than Goclenius.[23] The powder consisted of vitriol. After dissolving it in warm water, the linen which had been used to dress the wound was soaked in the solution. At the moment the bandages having the patient's blood on them came into contact with the dissolved powder, the patient was supposed to experience great relief. According to Digby this effect was due to the astringent action of vitriol, particles of which he thought to have been transported to the wound by blood atoms set free from the bandages as they were being soaked. Attracted by a mysterious but natural force of sympathy, these atoms would return through the air to their place of origin. Again the wound itself was not interfered with. A variety of other sympathetic wound treatments 'at a distance' has also been described which, in retrospect, had the great advantage that local treatment with salves and other medicaments was dispensed with.

Weapon salve and sympathy powder found great credence with Johan van Beverwyck, a well-known physician in Dordrecht.[24] Yet the same Van Beverwyck was one of the first continental advocates of the theory of blood circulation!

We must therefore view theoretical surgery in the seventeenth century against a chequered background of fading Galenism, the appearance of a new form of empirical pursuits of science and the belief in magic powers.

4.10. SURGERY AS A SOCIAL PHENOMENON

4.10.1. *General Survey*

It can be stated in general that the development of surgery, certainly in the first half of the seventeenth century, lagged behind anatomy — particularly microscopic anatomy — and physiology.[25] As before, the great proportion of surgeons received an artisan form of training consisting of an apprenticeship, and had little inclination or aptitude for a more scientific application of their craft. Doctors therefore still held the most prominent position among the authors who wrote on surgical subjects.

In Italy the situation was more favourable. Besides the barber-surgeons and the itinerant empiricists there were proportionally many university trained doctors who practised surgery. A combined professorial chair for surgery and anatomy existed at all the universities in that country. All this, however, could not prevent the main focus of European surgery from moving more and more towards France at the end of the century, particularly to Paris.

Two different surgical companies had been in existence in Paris since at least the early fourteenth century. One, which was known as the community of Saint-Côme, consisted of pure surgeons, i.e. those who only practised surgery and did not engage in barber's work. The other was the barber-surgeons' guild. In 1655 both companies united.[26] Although the amalgamated community of Saint-Côme was subordinate to the medical faculty, it gradually grew more and more independant. Moreover, surgery had been considerably raised in social prestige through the successful operation for fistula-in-ano, which Charles-François Félix (1650—1703), the king's first surgeon, had performed on his royal patron in 1687.

As before, surgical education still consisted almost entirely of apprenticeship training, although during the latter part of the century the community of Saint-Côme instituted several demonstration lessons. These became extremely popular, necessitating the erection of a new amphitheatre in 1694 (Fig. 37). This magnificent building, which still stands today on the Rue des Ecoles, could accomodate some 750 persons. At the beginning of the eighteenth century, Saint-Côme organized courses in anatomy, osteology and operative surgery.[27] This 'School of Surgery', as it was sometimes called, was not the only location in Paris where public lessons and demonstrations of surgical interest were given.

At its foundation in 1635, the Jardin du Roy, the botanical garden which still exists today as Jardin des Plantes, was provided by the king with non-university professorial chairs for botany, chemistry and anatomy. In 1673, this last chair was extended to one for anatomy and surgery. Its first occupant was Pierre Dionis (16?—1718), an outstanding Paris surgeon. His lessons and practical demonstrations in surgical anatomy and operations were so popular that the large

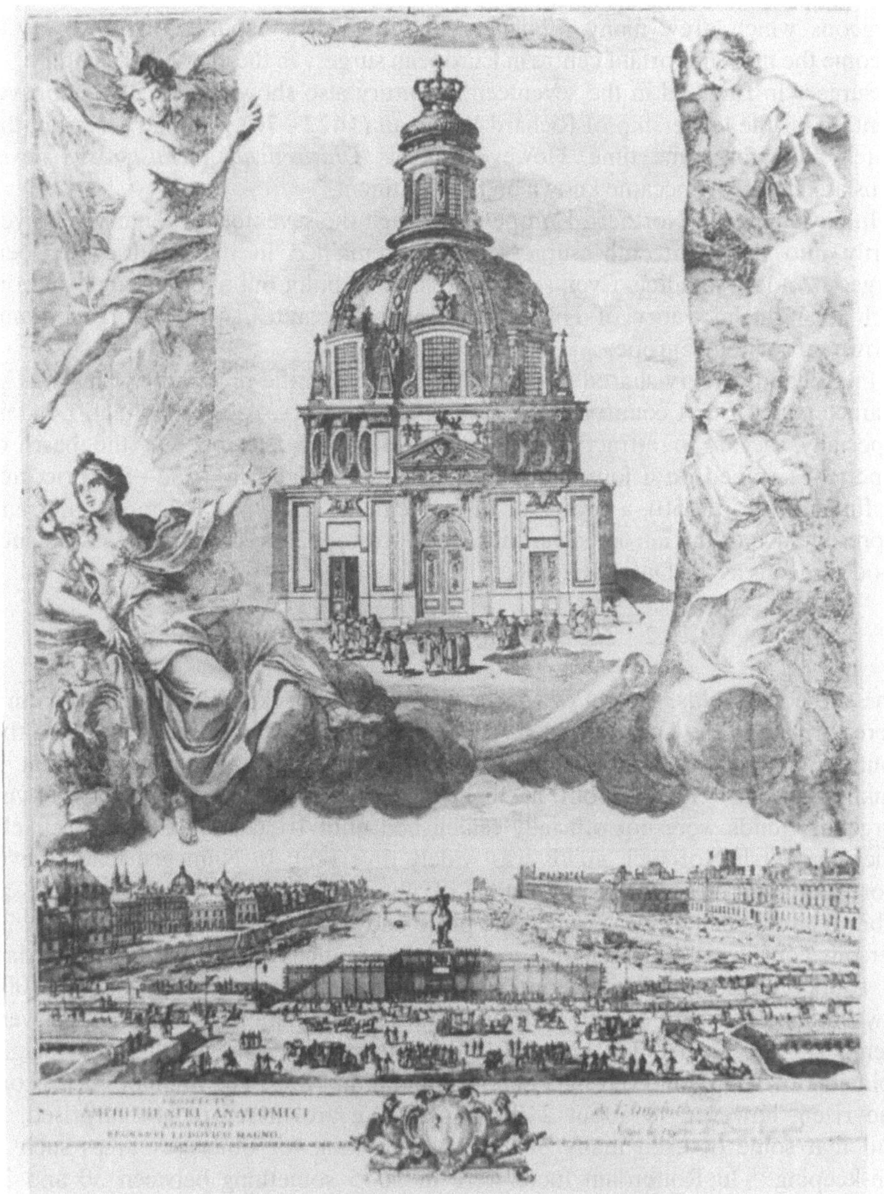

Fig. 37. Paris: Theatrum anatomicum of St. Côme, constructed in 1694.

hall in which they were held could not contain even half of the persons interested. Dionis' *Cours d'opérations de chirurgie*, based on his lectures, remained a popular textbook until late in the eighteenth century throughout the whole of Europe. It was translated into several languages including Dutch. Towards the end of the century it was especially the private surgical tuition offered by prominent Paris surgeons which drew many foreigners to the French capital. This city was to become the most important centre in European surgery in the eighteenth century.

Surgery in England in the seventeenth century also showed a decided improvement under the leadership of Richard Wiseman (1622—76) who had served in the Dutch navy for some time. However, as his *Chirurgicall Treatises* was never translated, it hardly became known on the Continent.[28]

In Germany and Northern Europe all through the seventeenth century and even partly into the eighteenth, surgery mainly remained in the hands of barber-surgeons of low standing. Even so, it is possible to point out a few German authors such as Wilhelm Fabry of Hilden and Johann Schultes, whose works became known throughout Europe.

In Holland surgery shared in the cultural and scientific prosperity which was so characteristic of that country in the seventeenth century. Amsterdam and Leyden, especially, began to attract students from all over Europe. On the basis of experience gained on a journey to Holland and England in 1682—83, Friedrich Hoffmann (see p. 150), a professor of medicine at Halle and the most important representative of the iatromechanical school, wrote that no country possessed such good surgeons as the Dutch Republic.[29]

4.10.2. *The Surgeons' Guilds in the Netherlands*

The surgeons' guilds, several of which can be traced back to the fifteenth century, were thriving in the Dutch Golden Age. Such guilds existed in many places in this country, and not only in the more important ones.[30] It is noteworthy that in Enkhuizen and Gouda, both at the time prominent and prosperous towns, surgeons' guilds were not officially established until 1636 and 1660 respectively. The membership of such guilds was widely divergent. In Nijmegen it was never more than ten in a town population of about 13 000.[31] In Delft, to take an arbitrary year such as 1642, when the place had some 25 000 inhabitants, only 37 persons constituted the surgeon's company, apprentices included.[32] In Amsterdam in 1600 only 28 master-surgeons were available for rather more than 100 000 townsfolk.[33] This city experienced an explosive population growth in the seventeenth century: in 1670 it had 200 000 inhabitants in spite of the great plague epidemic of 1635, followed by a minor outbreak in 1655. The number of surgeons had risen, however, to about 240 in 1688. We are therefore not surprised, to find that some or even many of them had to look for other resources such as inn-keeping.[34] In Rotterdam there were in 1675 something between 30 and 35 surgeons to 45 000 inhabitants.[35] The separation from other craftsmen, with whom the surgeons had previously been united in one guild, had been completed everywhere by the end of the sixteenth century.[36] Nor did the barbers in the strict sense any longer form part of the surgeons' guild after the early years of the seventeenth. The Amsterdam regulation of 1597 recognised only qualified surgeons as members. Those surgeons, however, were granted the right of barbering, and this privilege was perpetuated in ordinances of later date. The barber was licensed only to set up a business of haircutting and shaving on payment of a yearly contribution to the treasury of the surgeons' guild. Wigmakers too, were liable for contribution without being able to join. Membership was moreover only open to freemen of the town. Women could not be members. A surgeon's widow, who wished to continue the business of her late husband was only allowed to do so if she had an experienced 'knecht' (mate) on the premises who would do the actual work. From the archives of the Amsterdam surgeons' guild it appears that in the eighteenth century women were occasionally granted permission to establish themselves as dentists ('tandmeesteres'). Roman Catholics were not admitted to membership either. In Nijmegen the law even provided that no one would be allowed to sit for the surgeons' examination, without having submitted an attestation of his having been confirmed in the true reformed religion ('attestatie van syn belydenis, dat is van de ware gereformeerde religie').[37] Amongst the seventeenth-century surgeons one occasionally meets with a protestant minister.[38] Such a dignitary was invariably a Mennonite: the Mennonite ministers did not receive any salary from their parish and therefore had to make other provision for their income (Fig. 38). Only in the second half of the eighteenth century were Jews, by way of exception and on certain terms, admitted to a few craft guilds including that of the surgeons.[39] Jews were treated in Amsterdam as quacks, for they were allowed to practise surgery, without being able to join the surgeons' company, and then only if they paid a certain tribute to that corporation. If they were accepted at all, they had to pay a higher tribute than their Christian colleagues while they were forbidden to operate a barber's shop. In 1674 the city fathers decided that two Jewish surgeons whose proficiency was beyond doubt, should be admitted to the guild. One of them, Samuel Leon Bonavente, enjoyed a great reputation as a lithotomist. He had learned the art from François Colot in Paris (see p. 243) and had many non-Jews amongst his patients: nor did indeed other Jewish physicians and surgeons limit their practice to their coreligionists. But only the Emancipation Decree issued by the Batavian Republic in 1786 gave Jews the right to join the guild.

The board of the guild consisted of officers, probably varying in number relative to the membership of the local company. The definition of the board's members, was not everywhere identical.[40] It was not uncommon for medical doctors to sit on the management board, often indeed as president as was the case in Enkhuizen, Haarlem and Delft. Municipal praelectors, almost always M.D.s, held a seat qualitate qua. In Leyden, where special relations existed between town and university, the guild had been presided over by the professor of medicine, later of anatomy, since the early years of the century. Two more M.D.s had served as assessors.

Usually the wardens were elected by the members of the guild but sometimes the town authorities had some considerable say. In Haarlem, for instance, the governing body was appointed by the city fathers, whereas in Amsterdam new officers were appointed by the burgomasters on the nomination of the board. The responsibilities of the board implied supervision over the observance of the regulations ('articulen'), attention to finances and tuition and repression of interloping ('beunhazerij') and other undesirable competition. One of the wardens, the examination master ('proefmeester'). was entrusted more particularly with the organization and the holding of the examinations.

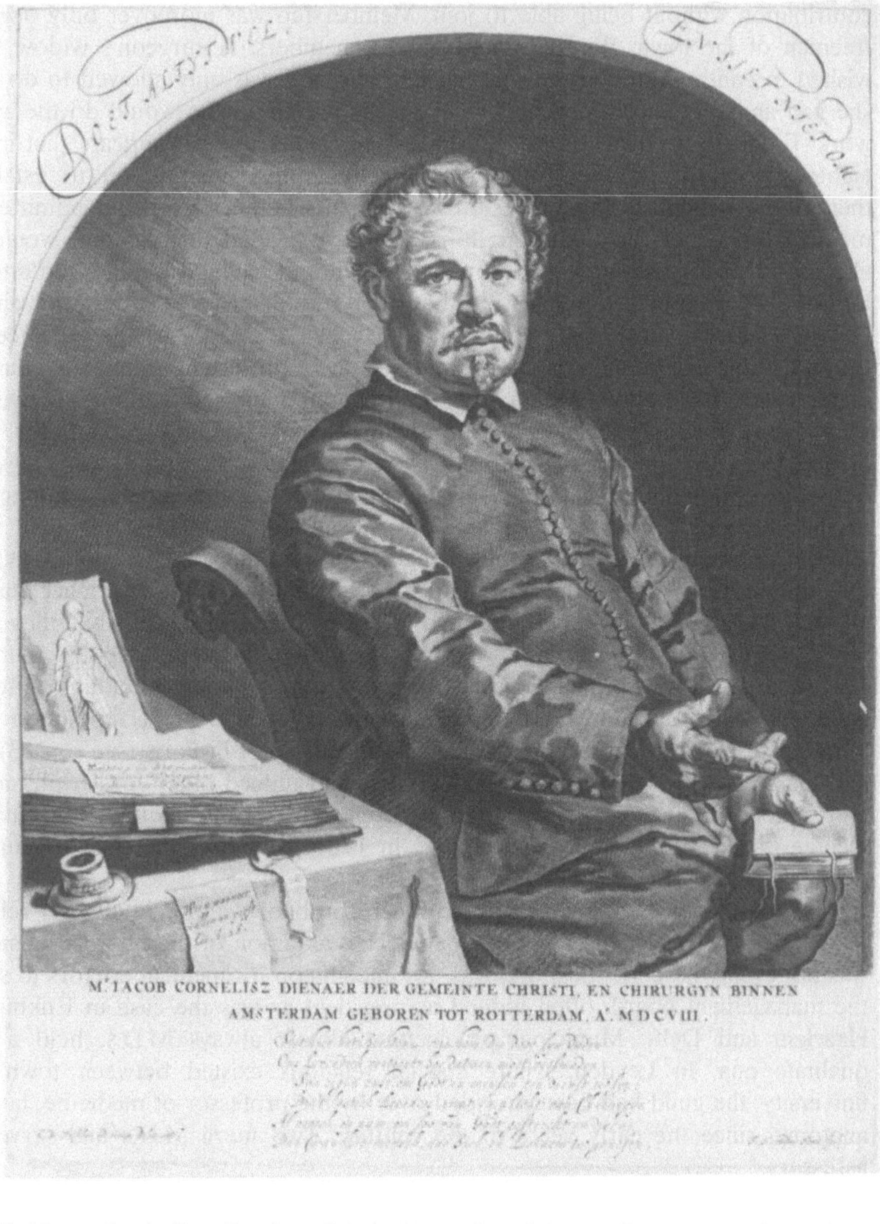
DOET ALTYT WEL.
EN SIET NIET OM.
M.r IACOB CORNELISZ DIENAER DER GEMEINTE CHRISTI, EN CHIRURGYN BINNEN
AMSTERDAM GEBOREN TOT ROTTERDAM, A°. MDCVIII.

Fig. 38. Master Jacob Cornelisz (van Dalen), Mennonite minister and surgeon at Amsterdam. Cf. Fig. 85.

The revenues apart from subscriptions and entrance fees, consisted of fines and examination fees. Part of the income was diverted to the poor relief fund ('armenkas') of the city, but the surgeons' guild, just like most other similar corporations, also kept an assistance fund of its own for needy guildsmen and surgeon's mates ('chirurgijnsknechten') and for destitute widows of colleagues. The guild assembled at regular intervals, and absence or lateness was punishable by fine. The duty of collecting fines and giving notice to the guild members of meetings or other gatherings of a different character was usually imposed upon the youngest member. Only prosperous companies could afford a paid servant. Ever recurring items in the expenses account of the Nijmegen guild warrant an assumption that the meetings of that venerable body must have passed off pleasantly.[41] They relate to wine, beer, tobacco, smoked herring, black radish and other refreshments while glassware had to be replaced regularly. It would not have been much different elsewhere.

Yearly changes in the board took place on September 27, the feast day of the patron saints Cosmas and Damian. This was particularly the day on which the guildsmen took some recreation with dining and wining ('mit een onder hen eenige recreatie mit eten ende drincken nemen').[42]

There were no guilds in the rural areas of the country. Yet there were surgeons practising there too. They were bound by similar regulations to those of their colleagues in town, enacted however by the bailiff or by the polder boards which had wide administrative powers.[43] Country surgeons were often former ship's surgeons who had only taken the 'zeeproef' (see p. 114). Space does not permit us to enter into the picturesque history of Dutch naval surgery.

4.10.3. *Surgeons' Halls*

At first the guilds in Holland did not have their own, regular meeting-places. They assembled at inns and the examinations were held at either the residence of the dean or one of the other officers. Only at Amsterdam did a surgeons' guild-hall already exist in 1597, as may be inferred from an ordinance of that year. From about 1640 onward, the surgeons' guilds in other towns had the use of their own halls.

The dimensions of such halls differed widely. They were usually situated on the upper floor of a large public building: a meat-hall (Amsterdam prior to 1619, Rotterdam), a weighhouse (Amsterdam 1619, Enkhuizen 1636, Leyden 1669), a gateway (Nijmegen 1614). a hospital warehouse (Middelburg 1656), a hospital (Gouda, 1699), a church (Amersfoort 1648 or before). Delft formed an exception since in 1656 the hall was installed on the ground floor of a former convent. Sometimes they adjoined the municipal anatomical theatre (cf. p. 117). The appointments of these rooms reflected the degrees of prosperity of the guilds.

In the centre usually stood a table with chairs (Fig. 39). Then there was a cupboard, often with glass doors, containing the surgical instruments which were the property of the corporation (Figs. 40 and 61). Every corporation had a smaller or larger collection of instruments, specially for use in major operations such as trepanation or amputation, which were no daily occurrences: master-surgeons could borrow them when the need arose.[44]

The remaining furniture might consist of a chest to keep the archives and other valuable possessions, glazed cupboards for the display of anatomical specimens or curiosities and a bookcase. Some guilds, by the standards of the time, had fairly large reference libraries. The Middelburg company had according to a printed catalogue no less than 145 books in 1746. The Rotterdam surgeons were likewise the proud possessors of an important library containing works by Paré, Battus, Pigray, Fabricius Hildanus, Spigelius, Bartholin, Van Beverwyck, Würtz, among many others. New members had to pay an entrance fee of ten guilders for the upkeep of the library and the instrument collection. The book case in the Gouda hall contained Vesalius' *Fabrica*, the textbooks of Guy de Chauliac and Brunschwig and many others.[45] Even the simplest hall contained a human skeleton for teaching and the examination in osteology. The chimney-piece might incorporate an oil-painting. Coats of arms of the town and the family arms of officers, either carved in wood or painted, might embellish either the mantelpiece or the instrument cabinet, or be woven into the cushions of the chairs. In Enkhuizen they were displayed in stained glass fitted into leaded casements. Some guilds in the course of time came into possession of important collections of painted portraits. In Leyden these paintings represented individuals, usually deans, elsewhere the lecturer of anatomy together with the other officers. We will go into a fuller consideration of these group portraits or 'anatomical lessons' when considering the anatomical theatres (see p. 119). The guild-wardens in Gouda had two spectacular surgical specimens, an enormous nasal polyp and a large mandibular bone sequestrum respectively, represented in oils and hung on the wall where they may still be admired. Some guilds could boast silver utensils such as inkstands,

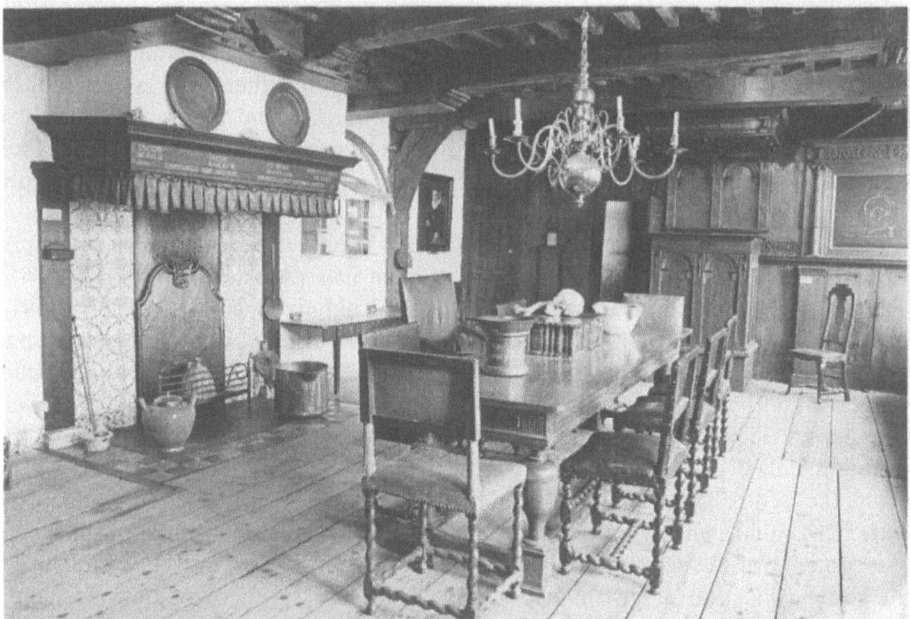

Fig. 39. Surgeons' Hall, Enkhuizen, 17th century. On the mantelpiece names of wardens together with the device 'Omnibus hic mutae praecellunt artibus artes': Here the silent arts (i.e. medicine) exceed all (other) arts. At the back a lectern.

representative badges or tableware. The surgeons' halls in Gouda, Enkhuizen and Amersfoort have been restored to their original state and are open to the public.

4.10.4. *Vocational Training*

Anyone who wanted to settle down and practise surgery in a Dutch town was required by law to join the local guild. One could, however, only enroll after passing the examination for master-surgeon. To be granted permission to take such an examination, one had to be a freeman of the town and had to have completed an apprenticeship with an established master.

The two years of apprenticeship in the early period were being extended in 1479 in Utrecht to three for the barber-surgeon's examination and four for the master-surgeon's.[46] Only in the seventeenth century were other towns to follow: Middelburg increased the time of apprenticeship to three years[47] and Amsterdam in 1664 even to five.[48] There was no uniformity throughout the country.

Entering into an apprenticeship was a formal affair which was fixed by contract: in the Amsterdam municipal archives one finds in the notarial protocols quite a few such agreements.[49] In contrast to what was customary in other craft guilds, the apprentice-surgeon had to pay a fee for his tuition, at least for the first few years, particularly when he came to board with his master as was common practice. The contract had to be registered in the files of the guild's board who demanded an entry-fee for it. The apprentice was provided with a 'lesbrief', a document which granted him free admission to lectures and demonstrations, except for public dissections on a human subject when apprentices too had to pay for admission. During the first two or three years the apprentice served as a 'leerknecht'. Within that time he was not allowed to change his tutor.[50] Then came a period of three or two years — in an apprenticeship totalling five — for which the trainee had to register again. During this second phase, in which he received a modest wage, he was designated as 'knecht', when he enjoyed somewhat more liberty and was allowed to change his master. Contrary to the practice in other guilds, the surgeons' companies did not have 'gezellen' (journeymen or mates): for the surgeons this place in the guild's hierarchy was supplied by the 'knecht'. When the 'leerknecht' had served his time, his master had an obligation to provide him with a testimonial ('leerbrief') which had to be presented at the examination for master-surgeon. Apart from practical tuition in his master's shop, the apprentice, at least in the larger towns, had the opportunity to gain theoretical knowledge by attending the lectures and demonstrations of anatomy and descriptive and operative surgery given by the local 'praelector anatomiae' or by other doctors of medicine or master-surgeons: the attendance at such lessons was obligatory. There were also demonstrations in the Hortus botanicus when such existed. We will discuss the recommended books on p. 136.

By no means all candidates succeeded in passing their exams at the very first opportunity after having fulfilled the appointed apprenticeship. This could often be blamed on deficient coaching by the masters, who were rather wont to restrict their 'leerknechts' and 'knechts' by keeping them mainly at work in their barber shops ('scheerwinkel'). The masters' wives, moreover, knew very well how to exploit boarding apprentices for odd jobs about the house. Critical remarks on this state of affairs were not withheld by contemporaries. Cornelis Bontekoe (1647–85), a physician who had started his medical career as a surgeon's apprentice, expressed them in the following words.

> Still being boys, they go into a shop, often not being able to read or write. There they learn to scrape beards, powder hair, turn up moustaches, smear plasters, make lint and they walk the streets for a few years (presumably running errands), sometimes (dipping into) five or six books full of errors, by authors whom they mostly are unable to understand. Meanwhile they observe the practice of their masters, who oftentimes themselves are not of the best kind, or should they chance to be, take good care that their pupils never quite find out the secrets of their art. Thus the apprentices never become such skilful doctors as they should be, in turn leaving their pupils without instruction, not disclosing to them their remedies . . . .[51]

The age at which the master's examination was taken, varied from twenty to forty years. Fourteen or fifteen was the youngest age at which a 'leerknecht' could begin.[52]

The master's examination ('meesterproef' or 'huysproef') consisted of several parts. One of them, as of old, was the art and theory of phlebotomy, in which the candidate also had to display his practical skill in sharpening lancets. Practical bandaging also formed part of the examination, as did the application of the trepan to a skull. The theoretical part concerned anatomy and — according to the pentateuch of the textbooks — tumours, wounds, ulcers, fractures and dislocations. Materies chirurgica, with its repercussives, resolutives, maturatives, abstersives, incarnatives and consolidatives — all external medicines — was not wanting either.[53] The panel of examiners was constituted from the guild's officers with the examination master ('proefmeester') if such an official existed, together with the 'praelector anatomiae' or in his absence one of the town physicians.

Taking this examination was a costly affair. The pitiable candidate not only had to pay a substantial examination fee for each of the different components and to settle any unpaid fines, but he had also to present a certain amount of money to all the doctors and surgeons present. Then, too, there was a charge for the diploma — which was only valid for the area of jurisdiction of the town — and he was finally expected to have a feast prepared for the examiners and their spouses. The examination took place in the surgeons' hall or in the hospital or even in the anatomical theatre if the town could boast one (Fig. 40). By the sixteenth century the candidate had to take an oath upon his promotion to master-surgeon.[54] Many apprentices never got as far as taking the master's examination. For those who did not, there remained the choice of taking the much easier examinations for either ship's surgeon ('zeeproef') or surgical attendant ('meesterknecht'). The 'zeeproef' could be taken — at least at Enkhuizen — after an apprenticeship of only two years.[55] A 'meesterknecht' was allowed to conduct a surgical practice on his own account for a limited term, usually by way of locum tenens.

4.10.5. *Anatomical Theatres*

Instruction in anatomy occupied a place of increasing importance in the seventeenth

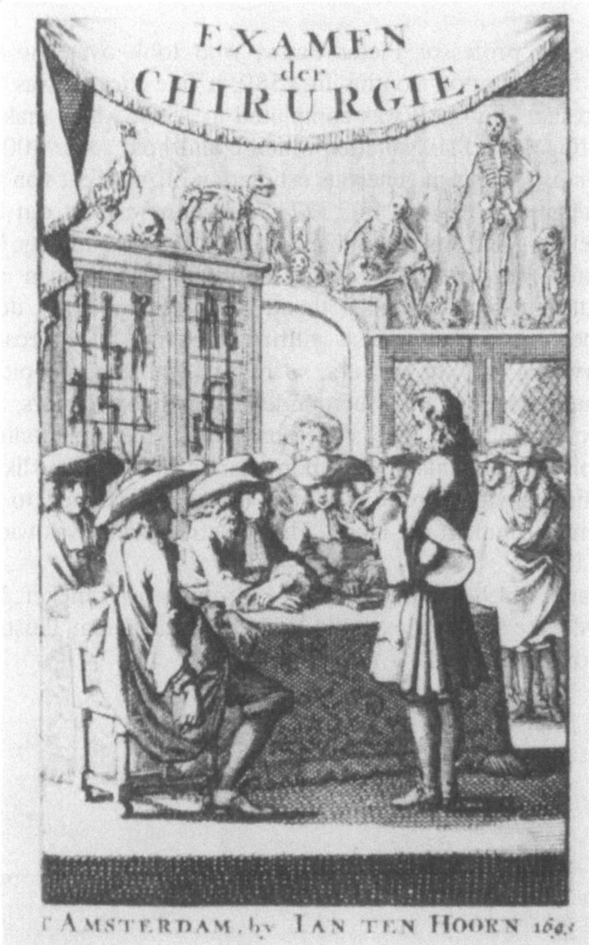

Fig. 40. Examination in surgery. The examination takes place in a surgeons' hall as evidenced by the instrument collection in the cupboard and the osteology collection. Such examinations were apparently held in public.

century, in the medical curriculum at the universities as well as in the more practically directed education of the surgeons. The great number of anatomical theatres which were established in our Golden Age testify to that. The most famous also abroad, was the one in Leyden. Here the university, which was founded in 1575, was responsible for establishing the theatre and introducing anatomy into the programme of medical students. It appears that partly at the instance of the medical students one of the two professors of the medical faculty, Gerardus Bontius, received an assignment to lecture on anatomy in 1587.[56] This subject formed part of the 'institutiones medicae': the theoretical basis of medicine. The anatomical demonstrations included in this preliminary teaching were to be held in the secularized Faliede Bagijnenchurch.

On the initiative of professor Pieter Pauw, who took over the teaching of anatomy from his former tutor Bontius in 1589, a fine theatre was built in the chancel of the aforesaid church. It was completed in 1593, which makes it earlier than the one in Padua. It had six galleries which could hold some 400 spectators, according to a perhaps somewhat generous estimation of Albrecht von Haller, who took his doctor's degree at Leyden in 1727. A section was cut out for the two steps leading to the rows and for a cupboard holding the instruments. When there were no dissections, the balustrades were adorned with human and animal skeletons.[57] The interior of the Leyden theatre was several times depicted and engraved in copper by various artists during the first two decades of the seventeenth century (Fig. 41). In that era, so rich in emblems, people saw in the dead subject on the dissecting table, surrounded by living spectators, a symbol of the transitoriness of earthly life. The skeletons, two of them personifying Adam and Eve, others holding pennants in their bony hands with mottoes like 'memento mori' or 'mors ultimum vita brevis' or 'homo bulla', also served to remind the visitors of the vanity of human existence. This theatre, which was widely copied, was demolished in 1822.

Between 1615 and 1649, the universities of Groningen, Franeker, Utrecht and Harderwijk followed the Leyden example and the Athenaeum Illustre at Breda was provided with one in 1646.

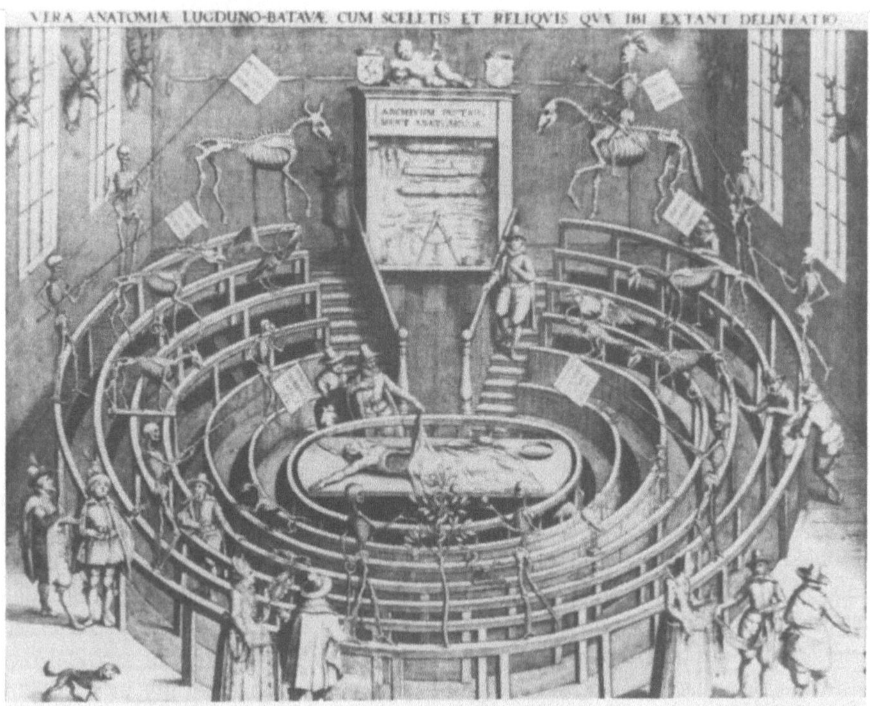

Fig. 41. Anatomical theatre at Leyden, 1610. At the bottom right a young lady is being shown a stripped human skin.

For the extramural tuition of surgeons and midwives, theatres were established by city governments in no less than eight places: Amsterdam (1550), Delft (1614), Utrecht (1621, later on taken over by the university), The Hague (1628), Dordrecht (1634), Leyden (at the Caecilia Hospital, 1696), Rotterdam (1642), Middelburg (1658), 's-Hertogenbosch (1662, subsequently taken over by the Athenaeum Illustre).[58] The expenses of the equipment of these theatres were sometimes borne by the surgeons' guild, sometimes by the town.

At the St. Pieter's or Inner Hospital ('Binnengasthuis') in Amsterdam a dissecting room was available to physicians and surgeons recognised by the burgomasters as competent to work and give private lessons there.[59]

All these theatres were accomodated in existing premises, apart from perhaps Harderwijk where the modest little building which contained the anatomy dissecting room — it still stands — may have been erected for the purpose. Some of the municipal theatres made available to the surgeons were housed in church buildings (in Delft in the Old Church, later moved to the chapel of the former Magdalen Convent, in Utrecht in the Pieter's Church, subsequently in the present-day Lutheran Church) or in an adjoining structure (to the Main or Jacob's Church in The Hague) or on the upper floor of a fair-sized secular building like the Meat Hall in Rotterdam, the Iron Weighhouse ('IJzerwaag') in Dordrecht, one of the city gates in 's-Hertogenbosch ('Vuchterbinnenpoort') and — after 1691 — the Weighhouse in Amsterdam. In Middelburg the anatomical dissections took place in the attic of a warehouse belonging to the hospital, where also the surgeons' hall was accomodated. In Delft, Amsterdam, Rotterdam and a few other places, the anatomical theatre and the surgeons' hall were also adjoining. None of these theatres survived. Only the ceiling of the Amsterdam theatre in the attic of the Weighhouse, painted with the coats of arms of leading surgeons and provided with several skylights, has been preserved until this day.

The theatre in the proper sense consisted of mounting concentric circular wooden galleries as were those in Leyden. Except for the front row they offered standing room only. The number of rows varied. The Amsterdam theatre at the Weighhouse was the largest in the Republic, having eight galleries. It was followed by that of the University of Leyden with its six galleries. In The Hague, Delft and Rotterdam the theatres consisted of four rows. As the diameters of the ground rows were everywhere more or less identical, the Dutch theatres could roughly hold some 200 to 400 spectators.[60] This is much more than the number of the local master-surgeons and their apprentices. The attendance at anatomical demonstrations on human objects was, however, by no means limited to this group. Such dissections were usually open to the general public on payment of an admission fee to meet expenses. These expenses were incurred by the procuring and afterwards the burying of the subject, the payment of a consideration to the persons — usually guildsmen — who lent assistance, the expenditure on candles and other materials and on a festive dinner for the anatomist and the sitting officers to end up with.[61]

The frequency of public dissections, however, was low: human objects were apparently hard to get. They were no longer exclusively supplied by the judicial authorities but now more often obtained from the hospitals:[62] the most important supplier for the entire territory of the United Provinces in the eighteenth century was the Inner Hospital in Amsterdam.[63] Owing to the shortage of human cadavers the lecturers often-times had to rely on animals. The theatre also served as a classroom for the regular theoretical lessons in anatomy and surgery.

Anatomical research did not primarily take place at the theatres but in the dissecting rooms of hospitals like the Caecilia Hospital in Leyden, the St. Pieter's or Inner Hospital in Amsterdam and the 'Gasthuis' at Middelburg, or even at private residences.[64]

Each theatre gave accomodation for educational purposes to a smaller or larger collection of sometimes very cleverly made anatomical, embryological and pathologic-anatomical preparations in spirits or other preservatives. Human and animal skeletons too, formed part of it, as well as mounted exotic animals and minerals. Although in such collections the desire of the day for the extra-ordinary or for the rarity clearly manifested itself, they yet constituted the precursors of our present-day anatomy and natural history museums.[65]

4.10.6. *Guild Lecturers of Anatomy*

Experienced masters of the guild itself initially acted as lecturers of anatomy, but starting about 1578 at Amsterdam, the civic authorities in Delft, Utrecht, The Hague, Dordrecht and Rotterdam in the course of the seventeenth century appointed only doctors of medicine as special '(prae)lectors' of anatomy. In Delft, this dignitary was entitled 'doctor anatomicus' until 1770; in Amsterdam, starting with Frederik Ruysch in 1668, even elevated to professorial status. Elsewhere too, as in The Hague, the lecturer was sometimes called professor.[66] Their lessons were, unlike those at the universities where Latin was the medium, given in the vernacular as they were meant primarily for the surgeons and their apprentices, who were under obligation to attend on pain of fine. Their teaching commitment towards prospective surgeons — and sometimes also towards the midwives and their apprentices — included the examinations. Their obligations were laid down in a sometimes elaborate instruction which was at the same time a set of regulations for the proper working of the theatre. Praelectors usually also held the position of town physician and conducted a private practice besides. Their salaries varied in the middle of the century between 100 guilders (Rotterdam) and 350 guilders (Amsterdam) a year. In Amsterdam the salary of the lecturer was charged to the surgeons' guild, but as a rule it was the responsibility of the town.[67]

The Leyden surgeons never had a praelector of their own. The municipality, which was represented in the university curatorium, decided that the barber-surgeons should be admitted to the anatomy lessons in the Béguine church.[68] Since these lectures were held in Latin, they would have eluded the surgeons and their apprentices. However, they were welcome 'to behold and regard', to quote the words of Orlers who reported on the Leyden theatre in 1614.[69]

This could not have been very satisfactory, so it does not surprise us to note that the surgeons still tried to obtain their own dissecting room. In 1636 they were offered the autopsy room in the Caecilia Hospital, which was to achieve international fame at the end of the century through the bedside instruction by Sylvius and later by Boerhaave. In this room, the interior of which seems to have been copied from the one in the Faliede Bagijnenkerk, they held their meetings, dissections and examinations until 1669 when the surgeons' guild was given its own facilities on the top floor of the Waag (Weighhouse).[70] The Waag, a charming medium-sized building designed in 1629 by the renowned architect Pieter Post, still stands today (Fig. 42). It was here on very rare occasions that anatomical dissections took place for the sole benefit of the Leyden surgeons and their apprentices, the demonstrations being given by the praelector from The Hague or by the professor who lectured on anatomy to the medical students.

Some lecturers have been recorded in paintings, portrayed in their role of teaching. World famous of course is the 'anatomical lesson' of Dr. Nicolaas Tulp, painted in 1632 by no less a master than Rembrandt. The anatomical lesson of Dr. Joan Deyman of 1656, was also put on canvas by the same artist but seriously damaged by fire. Those of a long line of Amsterdam lecturers were portrayed by Aert Pietersz, Thomas de Keyser, Adriaan Bakker, Jacob van Neck, the younger Jurriaen Pool, Cornelis Troost and Tibout Regters and are deserving of notice. These so called 'anatomical lessons' are really group portraits in which the wardens of the guild had themselves pictured together with the lector anatomiae, who in the medical and surgical life of the Dutch towns in the seventeenth and eighteenth centuries, occupied such a prominent place.[71] The Delft guild too was in possession of some fine group portraits of this kind: these were painted by Pieter van Mierevelt, Cornelis de Man, Thomas van der Wilt and Nicolaas Reynenburg (Fig. 43).[72] Even from Hoorn such an anatomizing group portrait has been preserved, made by Christiaan Coevershoff.[73]

4.10.7. *The Surgeon's Shop*

Once the surgeon had gained the master's diploma, he was at liberty to establish himself in practice within the area of jurisdiction of the town. It appears from advertisements in the *Amsterdamsche Courant* that this often happened by taking over a shop and paying a 'goodwill'.[74] A contract from 1698 found in Schoonhoven appears to contain the same elements as similar agreements of today, viz. the transfer of the data of patients ('het scheerboek') for a payment and the pledge of the seller not to practise for the first few years in his former district.[75] A surgeon's shop in which one could as a rule also have a shave or a haircut, distinguished itself by a brass barber's basin hung out as a shingle (Fig. 44). One of the punishments that could be imposed on a barber-surgeon was the order to 'take in his basin': this implied the closure of his shop.[76] Later the surgeons left the 'sign of the basin' to barbers in the narrower sense.

In Friesland the spirally white and red striped barber's pole was the official doorway sign. In Holland and England and much more recently in America too, such poles became the distinctive designation of barber's shops. Their significance is not entirely clear: perhaps it symbolizes the stick which the patient undergoing venesection had to squeeze so as to make the arm veins stand out (Fig. 36). The red stripes would then represent the outflowing blood. Sometimes a stone tablet in the facade, representing a wound man or the Good Samaritan could symbolize the

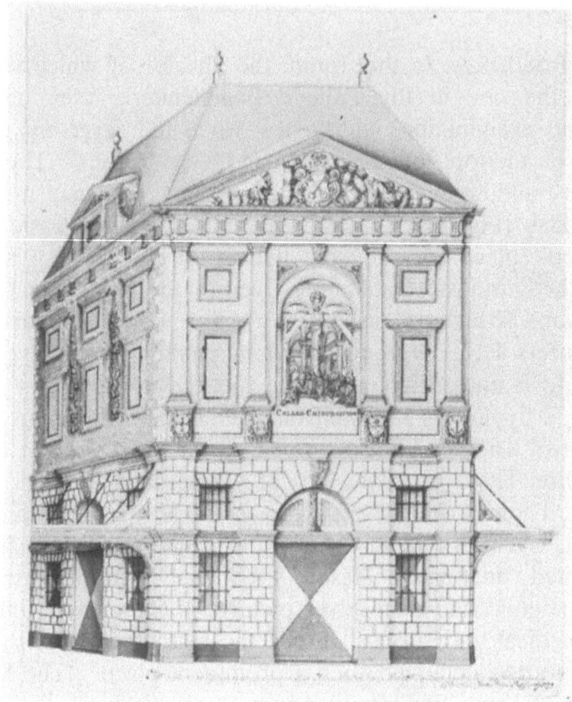

Fig. 42. Surgeons' Hall, over the Weighhouse at Leyden.

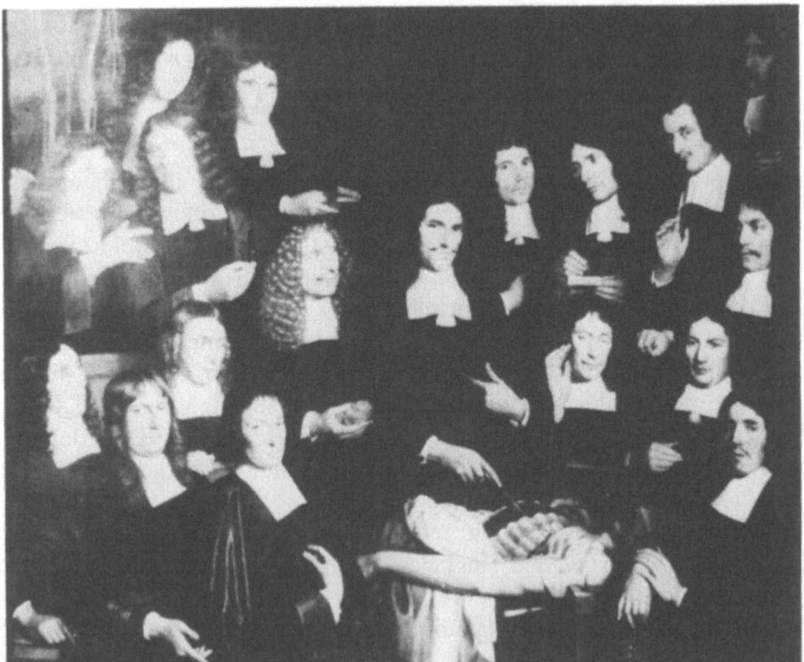

Fig. 43. Anatomical lesson by Dr. Cornelis 's Gravesande at Delft, 1681. The person standing to the left of the dissector in the background, is believed to be Anthony van Leeuwenhoek.

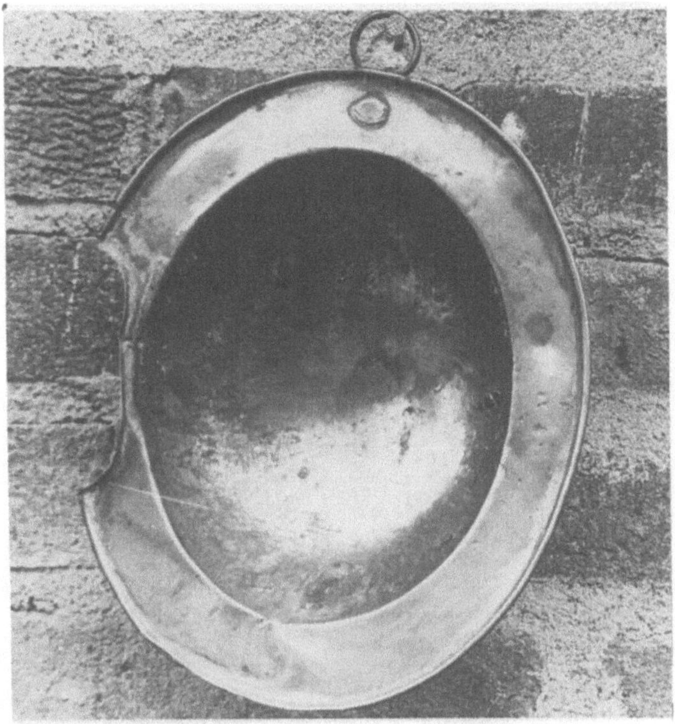

Fig. 44. Brass shaving basin, used as a signboard.

profession of the tenant. But he could also, like any other shopkeeper, call attention to his business by means of a signboard painted with an appropriate representation or by a rhymed legend.[77] A way of advertising which later came to be forbidden by the local authorities was a window display of dishes containing blood as pieces of evidence of the master's proficiency at drawing blood.

Several paintings and prints of the seventeenth century allow us a glimpse of the interior of contemporary surgeon's shops,[78] for instance the picture by Egbert van Heemskerck (c. 1634—1704), representing the shop of Jacob Fransz Hercules at Amsterdam in 1669 (Fig. 45). In the centre the master himself is standing, busy performing a venesection. His ten-year old son is holding the basin in which the blood is being received. In the background an apprentice is shaving another customer, and yet another client is awaiting his turn while reading a newspaper. In the forefront on a wooden platform to protect her from the cold arising from the stone floor, the surgeon's wife is seated with two children at her knee. A cupboard at the back of the room holds pharmaceutical jars. This interior has a more cared for look than that of the village barber-surgeons depicted by a David Teniers or a Cornelis Dussart (Fig. 46).

Patients of means who were in need of constant surgical supervision were sometimes boarded with a surgeon when for some reason or another they could not be tended at home.[79] Until well into the nineteenth century the hospital was only a place for the indigent sick.

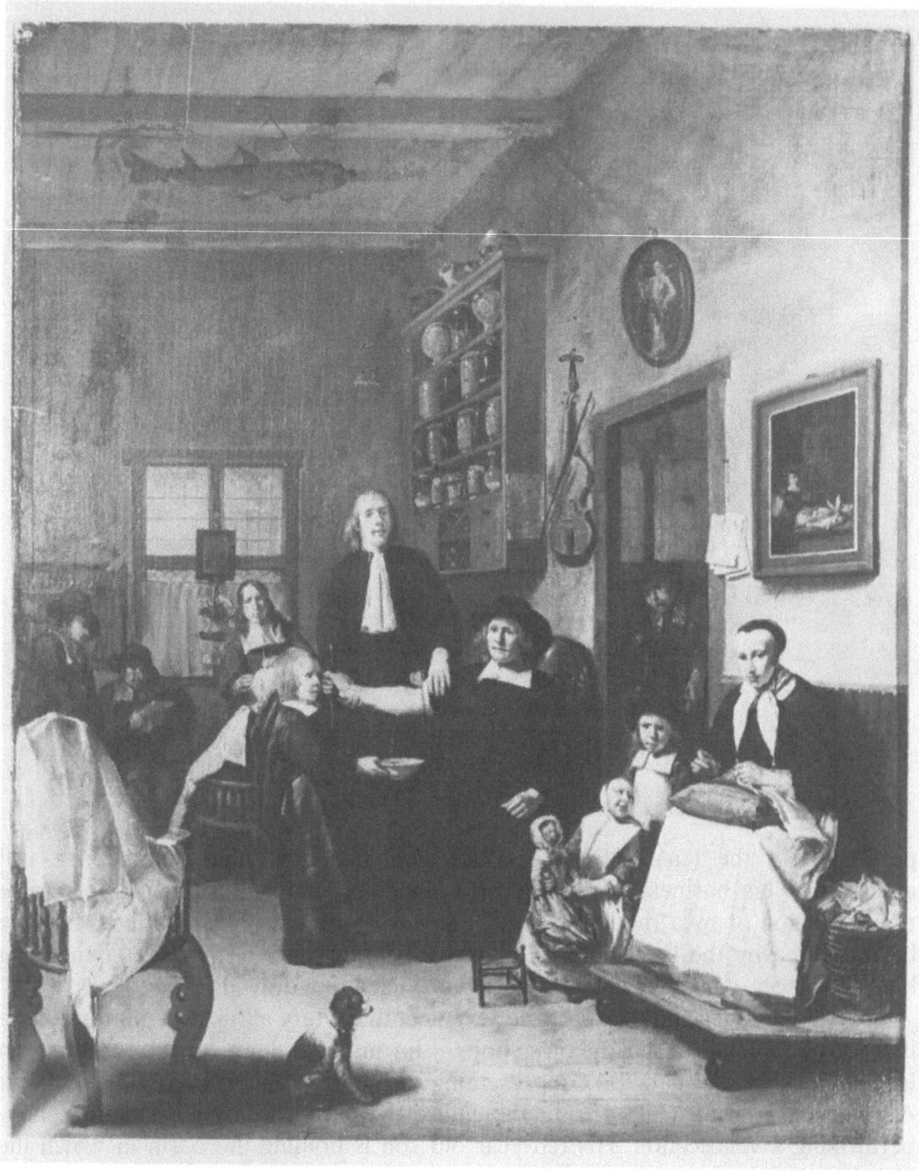

Fig. 45. The surgeon Jacob Fransz Hercules in his barber's shop.

4.11. HOSPITALS AND HOSPITAL SURGEONS

Hospitals were founded in Northern France and the Netherlands in the twelfth and thirteenth centuries in such great numbers, that some authors refer to an 'explosion de charité'.[80] The one at Ypres dating from 1276 has already been mentioned in passing (p. 60). Some of these institutions are still functioning as hospitals today.

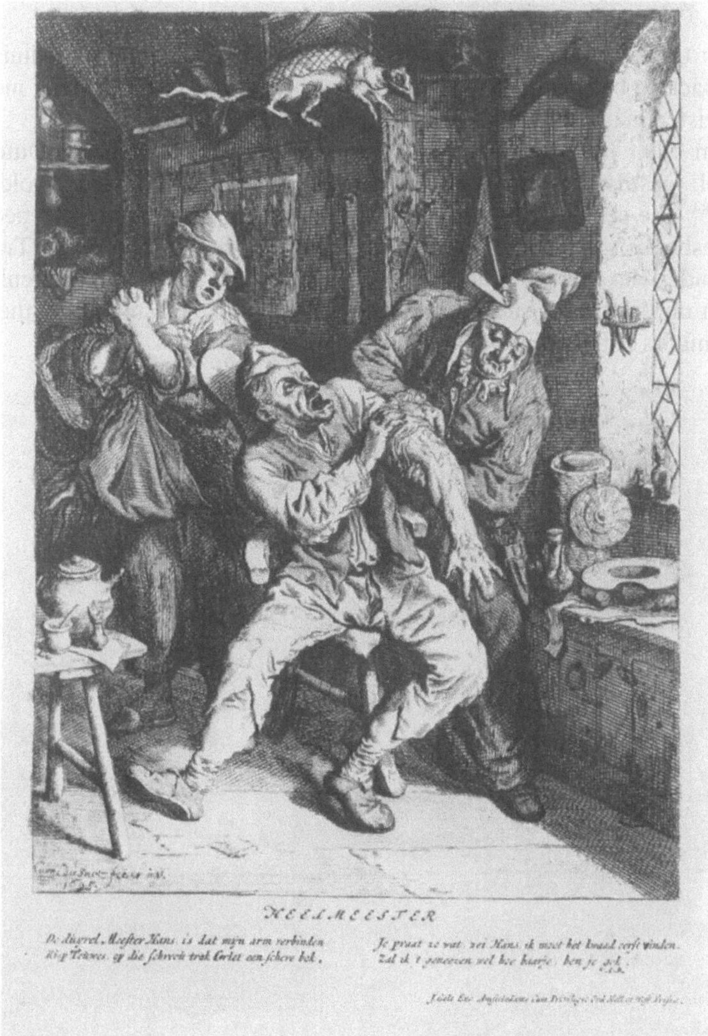

Fig. 46. Surgeon probing a wound. On the window-sill stands a shaving basin and a cylindrical basket in which the flask containing the patient's urine was taken to the practitioner for uroscopy. The animal hanging from the ceiling, apparently a stuffed armadillo, represents the legendary salamander which was said to thrive in fire. Hung in pharmacies or barber's shops, the so-called salamander symbolized chemistry.

To name a few: the St. Jan's Hospital at Bruges that existed already in 1188,[81] the old hospital at Delft from 1252 which fused in 1623 with another one to become the 'Oude and Nieuwe Gasthuis', the one in 's-Hertogenbosch which must have existed long before 1274 and which now as 'Groot Ziekengasthuis' is one of the important provincial hospitals in the country. In Zutphen as early as 1268 mention was made of an establishment which after two amalgamations now lives on as 'Nieuwe Spitaal'. The 'St. Elisabeth's or Groote Gasthuis' at Haarlem appears for the first time in archival documents in 1375.[82] The 'Catharijnegasthuis' in Utrecht dated back to before 1285 but this one was closed in 1812.[83] Many more hospitals have existed in other Dutch towns and also even in villages.

From what has just been said it follows that the mediaeval Dutch name for hospital, 'gasthuis' is surviving even today, but mainly in a few old established names.[84] The seventeenth-century 'gasthuis' was a hospital, an old people's home, an almshouse and sometimes even an orphanage all in one. Travellers and vagabonds who were not ill could stay for a few days. It is difficult to give an opinion on the size of such 'gasthuizen' since it was not customary then to express it in numbers of beds (Fig. 47).

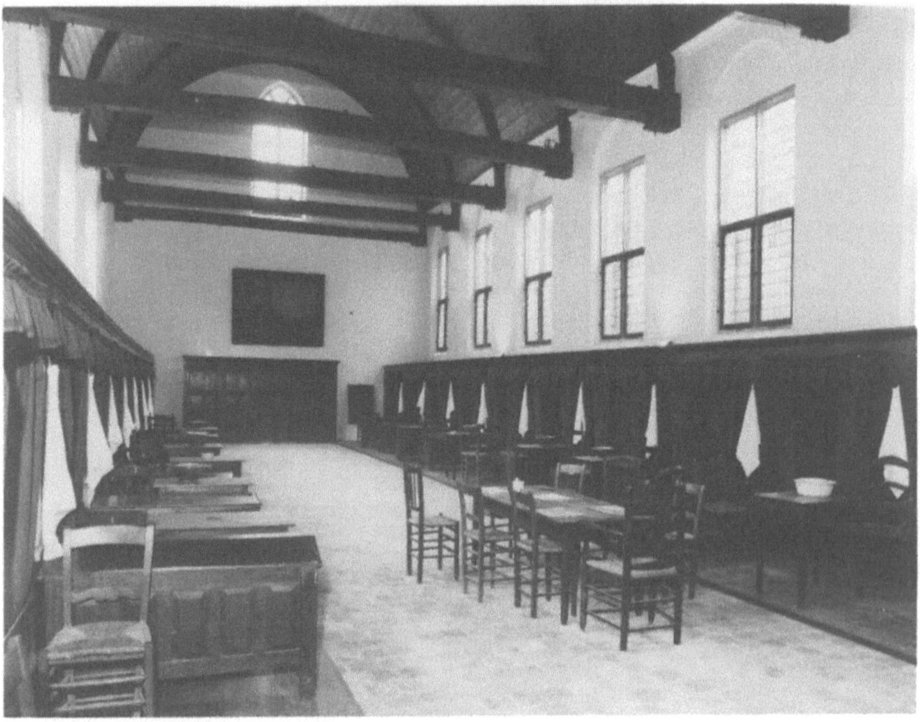

Fig. 47. Restored men's ward of the St. Pieters- and Blokland Gasthuis at Amersfoort, in use from 1535 until 1908.

They had all come into being as charitable institutions, although the founding agencies might have been dissimilar. The 'gasthuis' at Delft for instance arose in conjunction with a Norbertine double monastery whereas the one in Utrecht was founded by the Hospitallers of St. John. In Zutphen the old 'gasthuis' once had been a Hospital of the Holy Ghost.[85] The vast majority, however, were set up by gifts from the faithful, usually private persons of substance, concerned about their own salvation and sympathizing with the distress of their fellow-men. According to the view entertained in the Middle Ages that each charity should be self-supporting, many donations of land and farms fell to them by means of which some hospitals had grown quite prosperous.

The attendants may initially well have been of religious status but this did not alter the fact that the city fathers soon became directly involved in the administration. They laid down regulations and may have appointed one or two from among themselves, or other prominent persons of the community, to the superintendency. When no monastic or conventual group offered itself, the care for the inmates was placed in the hands of 'religious maids or virtuous widows', who put servants to work.

Since the 'gasthuis' was not primarily a hospital in the modern sense, medical attendance remained for quite some time subordinate to the cure of souls. Thus the 'gasthuis' at Delft did not appoint a surgeon until 1450 and the first physician until more than a century later. Shaving the male inmates was part of the duties of the hospital surgeon.[86]

The surgeons in the hospital were definitely subordinate to the physician. For instance they were not allowed to perform any operation or even a venesection without the doctor being present and had to accept that that gentleman at fixed intervals also made the round of the surgical patients. Still the surgeons engaged by a hospital enjoyed a privileged position compared to their private colleagues in having a salary and being able to offer their apprentices far more in the way of patient treatment than ever could be the case in private practice. Being a hospital surgeon was only a part-time employment, leaving time for private practice.

In the seventeenth century, the most important hospitals in the North Netherlands were the Gasthuis in Middelburg and the St. Pieters- or Binnengasthuis in Amsterdam, in the capitals of the two prominent provinces. The 'gasthuis' in Middelburg was already in existence in the fourteenth century. In the early documents it is called 'onser vrouwen hospitale' (Our Lady's Hospital), later St. Barbara Gasthuis and ever since the Reformation just 'Gasthuis'. The account book of 1565 reveals a glimpse of the activities of surgeons, for example the amputation of the arm of a sailor, on another occasion the treatment of a man whose hand had been cut off in public by court order.[87] Four surgeons were attached to the 'gasthuis' at Middelburg, the first one appearing in the records in 1465, appointed on an annual salary.[88] They were alternately on duty in pairs for a month; only when there was a great pressure of work was the presence of all four required. More than once this hospital had to cope with great numbers of wounded at the same time: after the battle of Nieuwpoort in 1600 and the following siege of Oostende for instance, or during the successive Anglo–Dutch sea wars.

The Amsterdam 'gasthuis' after 1579 was housed in two former convents at the Grimburgwal; it resulted from the amalgamation of two older ones dating from the second half of the twelfth century. For more than four centuries it was located at the same site until in 1981 it disappeared into the gigantic Academic Medical Centre in the Bullewijkpolder.

In Amsterdam, even before the fusion, surgeons appointed by the city were working in both 'gasthuizen', the first one being recruited in 1525. An ordinance from 1549 enacted that only town surgeons should be admitted.[89] The first operation of any importance we are aware of was performed on February 17, 1554, by the town and hospital surgeon Mr. Willem Andries with the permission of the town authorities. It consisted of the amputation of four toes of the left foot and three of the right and was done in the presence of two medical doctors and three master surgeons with a chisel especially procured for the occasion at a cost of four pence.[90]

Before 1590, the town surgeon in Amsterdam had had to surrender his 'gasthuis' commitment to two special hospital surgeons.[91] The duties of these surgeons have nowhere been clearly defined but it appears that they were expected to present themselves twice daily in the hospital to visit and bandage the surgical patients. They were apparently appointed for an indeterminate time at an annual salary which after twenty years (1616 to 1636) was raised from 300 guilders for the two of them to six hundred. In 1626 for the first time specialist departments were initiated in the Amsterdam hospital when patients with open wounds and contagious diseases other than venereal ones, were separated from the rest and accomodated in a special 'verbanthuys' ('bandaging-house'). For the severely injured there was a separate little cottage annexed. The stay in the 'verbanthuys' cannot possibly have been an unqualified pleasure, in 1657 the complaint was heard that the house was almost carried away by lice: this was followed by a resolution to have the bedsteads replaced by detached cribs.[92]

4.12. MILITARY SURGEONS

Serving on the General Staff of the army in the field in the seventeenth century were three master-surgeons.[93] They must have been highly qualified experts, shown by their having the relatively high salary of 600 florins a year plus an allowance for expenses as well as free meals. They had the supervision over the surgeons attached to the companies: there were as yet no regimental surgeons in the Dutch forces. The company surgeon or 'veldscheer' (field-barber) stood on a much lower level, being a barber or a surgical apprentice who had joined to gain practical experience (Fig. 48). This opportunity could at times indeed be offered. Already within the first three months of the siege of Ostende by the Spanish in 1601, the zealous surgeons on the Dutch side cut off more than five hundred arms and legs. When the troops were in garrison, quarrels were wont to arise between the town's surgeons and their military counterparts, who although it was forbidden to them were not averse to doing a bit of 'poaching' in the civilian population. The surgeons' guilds archives have preserved numerous documented souvenirs of such quarrels.

4.13. TRADITIONAL CUTTERS

Some 'operateurs', as the traditional herniotomists, oculists and lithotomists are designated in the surgeons' archives, still led, as before, an itinerant existence. They could only temporarily establish themselves in a town to practise their

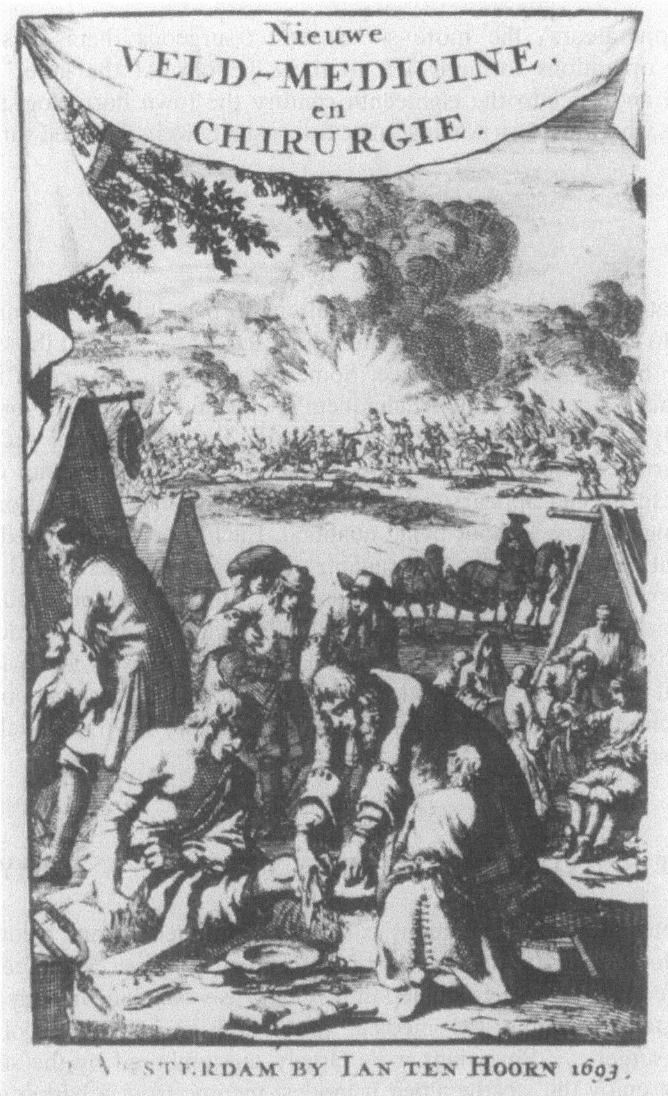

Fig. 48. A military surgeon in action. A shaving basin, hung outside his tent, served as a signboard, as it did in town practice. In the middle background, a wounded man is being brought in on a stretcher slung between two horses.

specific craft by special permission of the local authorities, granted in the presence of a town physician and some of the wardens of the surgeons' guilds. Into the activities of one of them, the lithotomist Frère Jacques, we will enter at greater length below (p. 246). Sometimes they took up permanent residence, in which case they were registered with the surgeons' guild to which they had to pay contribution without having the right to join.[94] Officially the guild had to decide on the admission of such 'cutters', but in practice a written permission issued by the civil authorities often sufficed.[95] As time went by, increasing reticence was exercised in admitting 'operateurs', the more so as master-surgeons themselves started to venture on operations formerly left to these people. At the latter part of the seventeenth and on into the eighteenth century the town herniologists and town lithotomists, who were then coming to the fore, usually were qualified surgeons.

4.14. BONESETTERS

For the treatment of fractures and dislocations in particular, the common people were wont to call in the aid of unqualified bonesetters.[96] Amongst these, the public executioner held a prominent place. Someone who was an expert in inflicting fractures and dislocations upon delinquents subjected to the rack or the wheel, could surely not fail to restore them.[97] From the registers of the Collegium medico-pharmaceuticum at Haarlem until the end of the eighteenth century, the provincial executioner appears to have been repeatedly reprimanded or even fined for practising surgery without being qualified. Each time he defended himself by claiming that he was 'at liberty and capable of acting as bonesetter and surgeon'. In Utrecht, Dordrecht and Leeuwarden as well, the executioner had a surgical practice which after his demise was sometimes continued by his widow.[98] In the village of Jisp in the province of North Holland once lived a whole family of non-medical bonesetters celebrated for their skill in treating dislocations. The most famous amongst them, Mr. Cornelis Ploegh, who died in 1696, also held the office of burgomaster.[99]

4.15. THE RELATIONSHIP BETWEEN SURGEONS AND PHYSICIANS

In the seventeenth century, surgeons as a group continued to rank below university graduated doctors. In the second half of the century, however, we increasingly find master-surgeons who have graduated in medicine as well. Concurrently there was a readiness growing within the medical profession to become involved in the practice of surgery.[100] Physicians were largely outnumbered by the surgeons. As they did not enjoy the steady, albeit it modest income from a barber's shop, they had to depend upon the fees from patients of better means. A few had an additional income by serving as the town doctor. Small towns had but one such an official, larger ones usually more. The institution of town doctors existed in the Netherlands since the late Middle Ages (see p. 59). In the seventeenth century they were moreover appointed to the task of sitting on the commissions for the examination of surgeons, plague-masters and midwives and carrying out other forms of official medical control.

Physicians, although not organized in any guild, were not entirely without supervision. Commencing with Amsterdam in 1637, then in many towns in Holland and Zeeland in particular, there existed supervisory bodies — Collegia medica — consisting of a few physicians and pharmacists. These had to advise the town government on matters regarding public health, verify the medical papers of physicians who wanted to establish themselves, inspect the pharmacists' shops, etcetera. There were no such Collegia in Guelders.

The authority of the Collegium medicum did not extend to the surgeons as the responsibility for the management of affairs within the guild lay upon its own officers. Haarlem formed an exception after 1693 by including surgeons in its Collegium medicum or 'Collegium medico-pharmaceuticum', as it was named in that town.

Indirectly the town physicians of course did interfere with the surgeons in several ways.[90] We have already remarked that in some towns the guild was presided over by a medical doctor.

4.16. PROFESSIONAL LITERATURE

4.16.1. *Foreign Works*

The professional literature which the Dutch surgeon of the seventeenth century had at his disposal, either in Latin or in Dutch, was very extensive. Apart from 'classics' like Hippocrates' treatise on head injuries, his aphorisms and Guido's (de Chauliac) surgery, it consisted of works of authors from various countries in the more recent past. Of French origin were of course the works by Paré and his school and by Barthélemy Cabrol, both already referred to (see pp. 86 and 72). The same applies to the Spaniard Arceo who was also still being repeatedly cited.

A striking feature is the prominent place then occupied by Italian literature. Apart from Da Vigo (see p. 77), we should mention the anatomical and surgical treatises by Gabriele Falloppio (1523—62), one of the most prominent anatomists of his time. There were also those of Leonardo Botallo (1530—?), presumably Falloppio's pupil, whose *Opera omnia* appeared in 1660 in Leyden, edited by Van Horne,[101] and the surgical books of Fabricius ab Aquapendente,[102] professor at Padua and founder of the magnificent anatomical theatre which still commands the admiration of the visitor; as well as the finely illustrated *De recondita abscessuum natura* by Marcus Aurelius Severinus (1580—1656) from Naples. The latter work which first appeared in 1632, was re-edited in Leyden in 1724: it is looked upon as the first textbook of surgical pathology. The relatively large interest in Italian literary works may have been created by the study tours made to Padua and other scientific centres in Italy, perhaps even more so in the seventeenth century when anatomy and surgery in that country were represented by many outstanding men.

Amongst German authors we may add to those already enumerated in the previous chapter, Wilhelmus Fabricius Hildanus (1560—1634) whose numerous publications were extremely popular in Holland[103] and Johannes Scultetus (Johann Schultes, 1595—1645) celebrated for his *Armamentarium chirurgicum*, a book on operative surgery with numerous illustrations which after its first appearance in 1655 passed through many editions and translations all over Europe. In 1621, a Dutch translation was published of *Practica der Wundartzney* by the Swiss surgeon Felix Würtz (1518—74) which was reprinted repeatedly after it was first issued in 1563.

Another author popular in Holland at the time was the Dane Thomas Bartholinus (1616—80), principally because of his *Historiarum anatomicarum centuria*.[104] From references in Dutch literature to works by the above mentioned authors — and to quite a few more — it appears that literary productions of French, Italian and German origin were being widely read in this country.

4.16.2. *Dutch Literature*

4.16.2.1. Three Popular Textbooks and Their Authors

Amongst the Dutch textbooks those by Jan van Beverwyck, Paulus Barbette and Cornelis Solingen should be cited in particular. Of these three medical doctors, only the last actually practised surgery. Books on surgical subjects were as before mostly being written by doctors of medicine, just as experimental surgery was usually conducted by physicians.

Jan van Beverwyck, M.D. (1594—1647)

Jan van Beverwyck occupies a prominent place amongst the medical authors of the seventeenth century. He was a very cultivated man, with a wide knowledge not merely of Latin and Greek, but was conversant with no fewer than five modern languages, which was far less common. After his medical studies at Leyden he made a 'peregrinatio academica' through France, Italy — pausing to take his doctor's degree at Padua — and Switzerland. He then established himself at Dordrecht where he became town physician and 'praelector anatomiae' at the municipal anatomical theatre. He wrote several treatises on sundry subjects of which *De calculo renum et vesicae* (*Steen-stuck*) of 1638 and *Heelkonste* (Surgery) of 1645 are the most important to us. They both appear in his collected works in one volume, numerous editions of which were published after 1651, illustrated with copper-plate engravings after 1672. In 1672 and 1674 two different German editions of the collected works appeared, and a German translation of the monograph on calculus in 1671. The text is elaborate but elegant, interspersed with statements of ancient and contemporary medical authors, with verses by classical poets in particular. Beverwyck gives anecdotes and case histories out of his own practice, or drawn from others, and quotes poems by the popular poet Jacob Cats, some of which were especially composed for *Steen-stuck*.

Scientifically his monograph on renal and bladder stone is the by far most important, and in it, he was one of the first on the European continent to recognise the accuracy of Harvey's theory of the blood circulation. Beverwyck formed his own theory on the genesis of urinary stones.[105] Such concretions could not possibly arise from slimy matter, baked to a stony lump by the heat of the kidneys or bladder as was accepted earlier, but rather from an 'earthy and salty substance' ('aerdachtige en saltige stoffe') owing to inefficiency of the kidneys or bladder. It was not correct that *all* bladder stones originated in the kidneys, as Fernel would have it, although this was so in the majority of cases. For the growth of a stone some nucleus was necessary, around which the stony matter accumulated. Clay-like matter could never be baked to stone by the heat of the body, for the moisture which such matter contains, could not be driven out as long as it remained in watery surroundings. It was the mixture of earth and salt in certain proportions which he believed could turn the mud into stone. A third cause consisted in a torpid state of the kidneys or bladder which prevented the water from being voided in good time.

Beverwyck recognized several kinds of stones and gave an excellent description of the clinical symptoms of their presence in the ureters and bladder. Among the foods which caused gravel, milk had always had this reputation as well as cheese.[106] Furthermore, bread not well baked was included and various kinds of fruit, peas, pork, salt or smoked beef, salt or smoked fish, water-birds like swans, geese and ducks, and hard-boiled eggs, but chiefly acrid wines cultivated in stony soil.

The age at which this ailment most frequently presented itself lay between fourteen and fourty-two years. Many assumed the gravel to be hereditary.[107] 'That is why the Greek Aretaeus with no less humour than truth remarks that the tendency to develop stone of the kidneys is more difficult to prevent than the fecundity of the womb'.

Beverwyck introduces his *Heel-konste* by an eulogy of surgery, herein he claims that surgery in respect of diagnosis and treatment was ahead of internal medicine. Unlike most other authors, he treats of surgical pharmacy at the beginning of this work, otherwise the traditional quinquepartition is largely adhered to. Some chapters are introduced by anatomical descriptions. In the chapters on tumours, in which as usual all conditions associated with a swelling are encompassed, Beverwyck once again explains the circulation of the blood, this time with illustrations taken from Fabricius Aquapendente and William Harvey. In dealing with wounds he points out that the seriousness of an injury is by no means always related to its magnitude:

> It happened at Leyden, when I was studying there, that a certain student when sporting with a lass was pricked by her in the muscles with a pin which was quickly followed by an inflammation with great pain, then by gangrene and ultimately by death.[108]

Beverwyck denies the poisonousness of gunshot wounds for the treatment of which he highly recommends Paré's ointment prepared from the flesh of cooked puppies, earth worms and turpentine: he knows of nothing better. For haemostasis he provides several styptic remedies. We have mentioned already his belief in the beneficial action of weapon salve and sympathetic powder (see p. 105). Beverwyck moreover believes in wound potions for which he gives several recipes according to the part of the body wounded. Pus is altered blood, it serves to separate nonviable, contused parts from the healthy flesh. Once the separation has taken place, the moment has come to apply incarnatives and subsequently cicatrizants ('velmakende middelen').

Bandages not only serve to cover the wound, but also to bring the edges together. When no satisfactory approximation can be obtained in this way, the wound should be sutured.

Amputation has to be done through the healthy parts. If the lower leg is involved, it should be performed a handbreadth below the knee even when the condition which constitutes the indication is limited to the foot. Like Paré, he shows reluctance to use the red-hot iron in this operation.[109] Beverwyck's *Surgery* is an erudite compilation of earlier and contemporaneous writers: no original ideas are to be found in this work.

Paul Barbette, M.D. (1619—65)

A further example of a M.D. who wrote on surgery and anatomy as well as on medicine, was Barbette, a physician emigrated from Alsace who had obtained his doctorate at Leyden. He established himself in Amsterdam where he became close friends with François de le Boë Sylvius who practised in that town for a number of years before he became professor of medicine at Leyden. They were both highly interested in anatomy and performed private dissections in the St. Pieters Hospital.

In 1655, Barbette — whose father is said to have been a surgeon — published a compendium of surgery: *Chirurgie nae de hedendaeghse practijk beschreven.* It was followed by a treatise on surgical anatomy in 1659. He wrote moreover a book on medicine, and an account of the plague epidemic which struck Amsterdam in 1655. All his books went through numerous editions in several languages: his *Chirurgie* and *Anatomica practica* were translated into Latin, German, French and English, his collected works into Latin, German and Italian.[110]

His *Chirurgie* consists of four parts. The first part, entitled 'Surgical handicraft' includes short chapters on both surgical techniques as well as chapters on the pathology, diagnosis and treatment of sundry ailments. Comparatively much space is allotted to fractures and dislocations, and to herniae. The chapter on dropsy contains the only illustration in Barbette's *Chirurgie.* It shows abdominal paracentesis using a trocar modified by the author. Parts II to IV inclusive deal with tumours, wounds and ulcers, respectively. These are the first three sections of the traditional pentateuch. The two final sections on fractures and dislocations as such are absent; the author probably felt that they had been covered sufficiently in the first part of the book (Fig. 49).

His *Anatomia practica* deals with anatomy traditionally arranged from head to heels but contains also some pathology and physiology. He paid much attention to the question of the generation of the blood, a problem closely connected with the function of the liver which at the time was the subject of heated discussions into which we will not enter.

In his book on internal medicine, entitled *Praxis Barbettiana*, are some interesting autopsy findings. He came for example across a case of necrosis of the descending colon and another of volvulus of the small intestine in which the bowel had twisted at seven different sites. He explained the aetiology of ileus by too acrid a bile — which shows him to be a partisan of his friend's Sylvius chemiatric pathology — in cases of intussusception he somewhat diffidently proposed laparotomy. He was possibly the first to describe a case of pancreatic necrosis.[111]

In his *Praxis* he moreover described the experimental removal of the spleen in dogs already referred to on page 102.[112] Barbette's books abound with prescriptions, mainly for external remedies. This formulary may well have contributed to the popularity his books enjoyed amongst practitioners.

Cornelis Solingen, M.D. (1641—87)

By the second half of the seventeenth century some surgeons had succeeded in

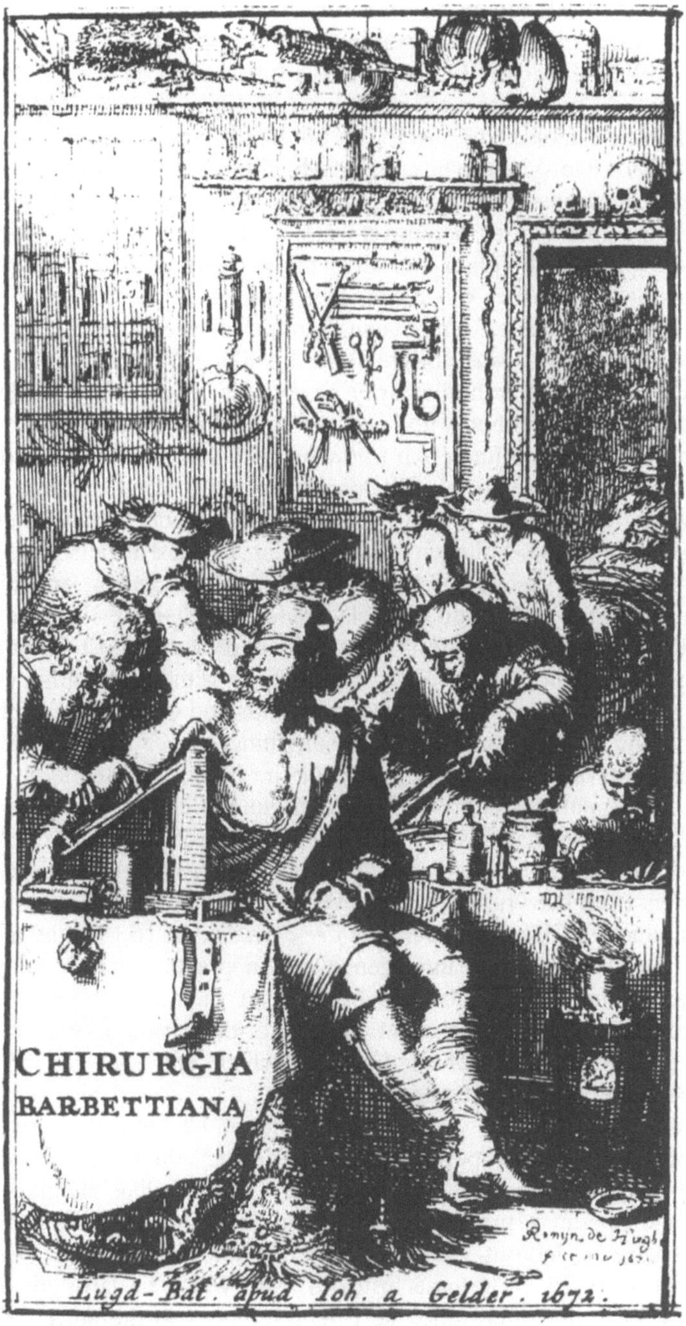

Fig. 49. Reduction of a dislocated shoulder in a 17th century barber-surgeon's shop, according to a method described by Hippocrates. Behind the seated patient a leg amputation is being performed, while a third patient is being carried in. The artist, Romeyn de Hooghe, drew the frontispieces of several other surgical textbooks.

obtaining a medical doctorate. One such was Cornelis Solingen. After eventful years as a surgeon in the navy, serving on the flag ships of the admirals Cornelis Tromp and Wassenaer van Obdam, then in the army, he was accepted as a master-surgeon by the Hague surgeons' guild. In 1677 he received his M.D. from Utrecht, upon which he established himself as a physician, surgeon and obstetrician at The Hague. It was not long before he enjoyed a high reputation.

Solingen must have been quick-tempered. An action by a Hague notary public preserves the memory of a quarrel with a colleague.[113] A consultation should have taken place with Johan and Cornelis Stalpart vander Wiel, both of whom physicians at The Hague. When Solingen arrived for the conference a few hours late, the brothers had left after having already inspected the patient's lesion and bandaged it again. This was not greatly to his liking. When Johan Stalpart had the misfortune to encounter him shortly afterwards in the street, Solingen lost his self-control and went at him with his silver-headed cane. Stalpart ducked under the arm of his assailant and flung him to the ground. The public were delighted by the not exactly edifying spectacle of Stalpart holding his attacker down with his knee, whilst the latter had him firmly by the hair. Bystanders finally separated them. From his writings too, Solingen appears as an aggressive person.[114] He made no concealment of his dislike for lazy and unreliable midwives, greedy, clumsy and conceited surgeons and proud physicians. He thus characterized one of his Hague fellow-surgeons as 'the bluntest, worst, most reckless, most ignorant and most shameless of all, who with his dirty, awful tricks with sharp, biting corrosives like spirit of vitriol and aqua fortis produces wounds and corrosions which at first were not there and, indeed, one who calls anything cancer which happens to come under his observation within the throat or the breasts, subsequently torturing and maltreating the patients badly with his confounded caustic remedies making them believe that it is cancer or some other dangerous condition in order to take large sums and fill his purse by dirty, wicked gain derived from make-believe deceit'.

Solingen, from his writings, was conversant with French and Latin. His books — amongst which his *Manuale operatien der chirurgie* of 1684 is the most important for our purpose — reveal intelligence and a practical mind. Reading them is, however, not unqualified pleasure because of their discursiveness. Apart from surgery, Solingen was also active in the field of obstetrics, on which subject he has written two books. His collected works, which appeared in 1698, were also published in German at Wittenberg in 1712.

Manuale operatien der chirurgie, in spite of its literary shortcomings, is an outstanding textbook of operative surgery in which the author, averse to ostentatious learning, describes in 34 concise and businesslike chapters 'a capite ad calcem' the operative procedures in use at the time. Diagnosis, pre- and post-operative care are left out. He does give a detailed account of the best instruments to use, see page 257. The case histories, with which he lards his text, are quite interesting but only rarely does he give references to literature. He commences with the surgery of the head to which Solingen gives considerable attention.[115] The indications for using the trepan are the presence of blood on the dura mater or of bone fragments or foreign bodies penetrating the skull. In the event of multiple fractures each one should be individually trepanned. Solingen's ophthalmologic operations are not limited to the eyelids, but also pertain to hypopyon, cataract and lacrimal fistula. The chapters on dentistry describe the technique of extraction, the filling of cavities with gold, silver or lead and the securing of wobbling elements ('wiggelende tanden'). Nasal polyps are to be extirpated, oedema of the throat ('watersucht van de keel') requires tracheostomy. Thoracic surgery encompasses paracentesis,[116] the treatment of fistulae and amputation of breasts. For the last operation Solingen too, makes use of a solid traction thread or a big, two-pronged fork to lift the gland from the thoracic wall. For haemostasis he favours styptics. His treatment of penetrating abdominal injuries does not offer new aspects;[117] retention of urine should be treated with a catheter.

Solingen is quite comprehensive in his description of lithotomy and its various methods.[118] Fabricius Hildanus and in particular Pierre Franco are the great authorities for him. For ascertaining the presence of a stone in the bladder it is best to use a metal catheter since by rectal examination there is danger of a tumour being mistaken for a stone. No less than four variations of operation with the staff are explained.

Solingen deals with ruptures ('scheuringen') in extenso.[119] He prefers to treat them conservatively by means of a truss. Good trusses could be obtained from the well-known instrument maker Johan van Musschenbroek at Leyden, but Solingen modestly remarks that he himself could also supply excellent ones, as the Parisian physician De Blegny testified.[120] Operative treatment — Solingen speaks of herniotomy as a 'cruel intervention' — may likewise be done along different lines. The method most commonly used, called the quack's way, entails castration: it appears to be the same as the method advanced by Paul of Aegina some thousand years earlier. Franco's method, which consists of ligating the spermatic cord over something more than half of its width by means of a stitch ligature whilst saving the vessels and abstaining from removing the testis ('zonder de kloot te verwijderen') is a difficult and time-consuming intervention, according to our author. He is familiar with the 'golden stitch' of which he describes three variations. After the operation the patient should lay on his back for twenty days, with his head low and his legs elevated. An incarcerated hernia which cannot be reduced, should be treated by operative enlargement of the hernial orifice on the introduced finger or a flat sound. Solingen is very elaborate too in dealing with extirpation, as he calls amputation of extremities.[121] Like his contemporaries, he confines himself to the forearm and the leg: the amputation above the elbow and the knee is mentioned only in passing. Just like Paré, he favours amputation through healthy tissue. He disapproves of the removal of the forearm and the leg at the elbow and knee joint respectively (as favoured by others including Hildanus, who in his turn relied on the Italian Maggius)[122] because of the inferior skin covering of the stump which results from it. His amputation technique is an improvement on that of Paré, not least by his use of a metal retractor of his own invention for drawing back the cut muscles. For haemostasis he prefers red-hot irons with an olive-shaped head which enables a well-aimed and accurate cauterization of the cut ends of the vessels. The brazier for heating the cauteries should be placed out of the patient's sight 'om d'afschrixwille' (in order not to terrify him).

The treatment of fractures should consist of extension, reduction and 'deligatio'.[123] For carrying out extension, Solingen prefers manual traction, if necessary indirectly by means of napkins fastened over and under the adjoining joints. He is disinclined to employ mechanical extension apparatus as used by Hildanus, because of its being too complicated. Reduction should be performed with greased hands under continuous traction.

After having covered the skin with a cloth smeared over with an 'emplastrum de laudano' of his own composition which marvellously eases the pain, Solingen then proceeds to apply the fixing apparatus. This consists of roller bandages in three layers, with the strongest compression at the fracture site, on which the splints are fastened. These are coated at the inner side with sticky sparadrap as to prevent their slipping off. The best splints are made from the wood used in making lemonboxes. After six or eight hours the surgeon should satisfy himself that the bandage is not too tight. After this continued and continuous supervision is still required: the splints have to be reapplied twice a day but the innermost bandages are allowed to remain untouched for ten or twelve days. It is said that consolidation of a femoral fracture takes forty days, of the humerus thirty, of the radius and ulna twenty, of the phalanges fifteen days, 'but in Holland it usually does not happen that fast'.

Solingen is familiar with continuous extension bandages for the upper and lower leg. Traction should be performed with twisted ribbons stitched through with cotton-wool, while the extremity is resting in an iron or preferably copper guttered splint. Equinus deformity and pressure sore of the heel should be prevented.

4.16.2.2. Books Recommended to Apprentice-Surgeons

Rustingh's Suggestions; Surgical Catechisms

The books recommended to apprentice-surgeons by Salomon van Rustingh (1650– post 1700), a former army surgeon who had established himself as a physician and surgeon at the village of Zuid-Schermer in the province of Holland, were those by Scultetus and Solingen. Ruysch was included probably for his anatomical works, for should they not be available Blankaart's *Anatomie* would do as well. Then there was a book, the author of which Rustingh did not mention 'recently published at Rotterdam in quarto (and everywhere obtainable from booksellers) and treating of all surgical manual operations' and finally 'Acquapendens'.[124]

Curiously, Rustingh failed to refer to the current textbooks especially composed for apprentices in the form of questions and answers. Those written by Cornelis Herls and Cornelis van de Voorde were very popular. Herls as well as Van de Voorde practised at Middelburg where the former was town surgeon and the latter, being a medical doctor, was instructor ('praelector') in anatomy and surgery from 1658.

After Herls' premature death in 1625 two of the manuscripts which he left behind have been edited by others: *Examen der chirurgie* in 1625(?) and *Chirurgijns scheepskist* ('Surgeon's sea chest') in 1672. *Examen* went through three editions within one year. It was reprinted at least five times, German translations appeared in 1676 and 1692 in Nuremberg. Van de Voorde was the author of *Lichtende fakkel der chirurgie* ('Shining torch of surgery', in later printings *Nieuw lichtende fakkel* . . .). This torch was first lit in 1664; it flared up for the last time in 1742. By turning the leaves of such surgical catechisms we acquire a fair idea of the theoretical knowledge which the prospective surgeon in the second half of the seventeenth century was expected to display when presenting himself for the master's certificate. It was certainly not to be sneered at. We will have a closer look at Van de Voorde's book containing the theory of surgery as it was being taught by a municipal praelector at an important town in his public and private lessons.

Cornelis van de Voorde, M.D. (c. 1630—78)

The 1668 edition of the textbook by Van de Voorde which we had at our disposal, is a work in octavo running to 603 pages in small print without illustrations. The style suffers greatly from prolixity. The writer cites a great number of authors from at home and abroad which his young readers at the time might not have particularly valued, but which nowadays allows us to have insight into the current literature of the second half of the seventeenth century.[125] He presents very few case-histories, but gives a good survey of the pathophysiological conceptions then in vogue.

The book has been divided into three parts: anatomy, theory and practice of surgery. Van de Voorde states in the preface that a surgeon should know his anatomy like a sculptor his wood or stone (cf. p. 50). Knowledge of internal anatomy is admittedly of little use to a surgeon practising in a town like Middelburg with many physicians, the treatment of internal diseases being of course the responsibility of the doctors. But it may well happen that the surgeon would have to exercise his craft not in a town but in the country or on board ship where, in the absence of doctors, he would have to officiate as physician as well ('het officium van medicijn moet bedienen').

The first part, dealing with anatomy, runs to 169 pages, but includes quite some physiology as well. It opens with general remarks on the use of that discipline. Anatomy is profitable because it 'vividly brings before us the frailty and vanity of our body' and because it is a guide to surgery. A distinction must be made between simple or 'similar' and 'dissimilar' parts.[126] 'Similar' or simple parts such as fat, fibres and flesh for instance, are always found in the same composition throughout the body. Less simple and therefore 'dissimilar' are skin, bone, cartilage, the ligaments and the membranes, and the vessels which are of three kinds, namely arteries, veins and nerves.[127] Consideration is also given to the generation of simple and dissimilar parts. One of the questions put to the apprentice is: 'Tell us in what way you think that the flesh of the muscles is being generated and produced?' The correct answer should be: 'This way the great anatomist Adr. Spigelius has most clearly taught us by saying that blood settles between the fibres of the muscles, where because of the innate and inflowing heat it comes to curdle just like curdled milk in the little rushed or willow baskets, which is how in Italy and also with us sheep's cheeses are made'.[128]

We are surprised to learn that the spleen serves as a counterweight to the liver. It 'sends' moreover an acid ferment to the stomach to assist digestion.[129] Even more interesting is the function ascribed to the greater omentum. 'It foments those entrails meant for boiling such as the stomach and intestines and aids their action by its warmth, for it is spread over them like a thick, silken blanket and that this is actually the case is confirmed by the observations of learned men, for Galen records that a certain fencing instructor having sustained a wound in the abdomen through which he had lost a major part of his omentum, after having been cured by the art, was forced to wear thick warm clothing on his belly to assist the boiling of his stomach'.[130] This was confirmed by the late Mr. Albertus Kyperus [who reported] that a certain man having lost the greater part of his omentum through an accidental injury but yet was cured, was compelled to keep a live puppy on his abdomen and if he omitted that, his stomach did not boil.[131]

Van de Voorde shows that he is quite conversant with the anatomical literature of his time being aware of the discovery of the lacteals in 1627 by the Italian Gaspare Aselli — Azellius as he calls him — and of the thoracic duct (1651) by the Frenchman Jean Pecquet, or Pekket as Van de Voorde spells the latter's name. The function of lymph still raised many questions and there was a focus of interest in the formation of saliva, tears and liquor pericardii, and the dilution of the coarse blood in the vena cava.[132] Lymph is an excretion of the blood, by its separation it purifies the blood from superfluous saltness. In healthy individuals lymph therefore has a salt taste (cf. p. 100) and to confirm that one only has to taste the saliva or sweat — which are products of lymph — of healthy individuals. A current controversy was whether blood was formed in the liver from the chyle which entered that organ through the mesenteric veins as Galen had written, or likewise from chyle in the heart. Van de Voorde appears to be a partisan of the latter 'modern' conception and ascribes the conversion of chyle into blood to the innate heat of the heart.[133] He holds the theory of the circulation of the blood but denies the existence of anastomoses in the capillary system because nobody has actually ever seen them. Among the approximately fifty authors cited by Van de Voorde in the anatomical part of his work, Hippocrates, Aristotle, Galen and Avicenna still occupy a respectable position although those from a more recent past and from his own days are predominating. Quite frequently we come across references to *De fabrica corporis humani* by Adrianus Spigelius. The French physician and anatomist Jean Riolan (1580—1657), a convinced Galenist whose *Enchiridium anatomicum* in 1649 was edited in Leyden, is also repeatedly met with. It deserves special notice that apart from Dutch, French, German, Italian and Scandinavian authors a few English ones are cited as well, something that only rarely happened at the time.[134].

If in the first part of the book a distinct transition to a more modern organ-physiology may be noticed, in the second part, treating of the theory of medicine, we find a 'general' physiology, still entirely in Galenic-Aristotelian tradition, and based on elements, temperaments and humours set in motion and regulated by vital spirits, innate warmth, the soul and its various faculties and all kinds of nutritive, extending, procreative and other forces.

Causes of diseases may be external or internal or both together in conjunction.[135] External causes are to be found in some disorder of any of the six non-naturals, the indispensable sustainers of life, which we dealt with in Chapter 2, note 57. Air, one of them, may be noxious for its qualities — cold, moist or dry — and by its relative quantity. Too little fresh air results in the pores of the skin becoming clogged with miasmata.[136] No definition of miasmata is given but they appear to be exuded by human beings, even when in good health, by exhalation and insensible perspiration, but may also arise from dead coals, burning candles, pools and marshes, putrifying organic material and the constellations of the planets.

Internal causes consist in either qualitative or quantitative disorders of the spirits or humours.[137] Thus an excess of animal spirits in the blood may engender aneurysm or syncope and apoplexia. Qualitative or quantitative alterations in any of the four cardinal humours entail such specific morbidities quite in accordance with ancient humoral pathology as explained on page 16. In his chapters on venesection as well as on the use of purgatives, Van de Voorde once more shows himself a confirmed Galenist.

The third part of *Lichtende fakkel* is concerned with 'praktyka'. The subject-matter is once again arranged according to the surgical pentateuch. Gangrene — so we read in one of the chapters on tumours or 'aposteumata' — is one of the most difficult diseases the surgeon may have to deal with. It results from a 'decay of the firm parts of the human body, brought about by debility of the innate warmth which constitutes life'. Other causes may be impeded evaporation or poisoning.[138] Its treatment should aim at preventing the development of sphacelus or complete mortification by the use of a diet and sundry medicaments. Once sphacelus has developed, there is no other course but extirpation of the affected part. This should be done through healthy tissue. Removal of a limb is technically feasible up to a hand's breadth below the axilla and right up to the knee, only very few ever surviving an amputation of the upper leg. In preparing the patient for this operation, attention should be paid to his state of mind and a minister of religion summoned. A few hours preoperatively the patient should be given an invigorating cordial, consisting for instance of strong broth with egg yolk and orange juice, or equal parts of wine and beer with egg yolk, some cinnamon, sugar and bread. The operative technique, which Van de Voorde describes in full with regard to the leg, apparently the most common location, need not be laboured since it does not deviate from the conventional method.[139] In his description of cancer, still largely carcinoma mammae, Van de Voorde gives expression to traditional views: this disease originates from black bile being retained in adenomatous and parenchymatous parts. Disturbances in the six things non-natural as well as heredity, contamination and trauma may constitute contributory factors. In his discussion of symptoms he follows Falloppio. Treatment should primarily consist of a regimen to harmonize the non-naturals. Amongst the dietary prescriptions enumerated by our author are the use of goatmilk as was recommended by Fabricius ab Aquapendente and tea, highly lauded by the late professor Kyper at Leyden for its neutralizing effect on melancholy matter. For local treatment we find a number of resolvents. Van de Voorde thinks it best to operate when cancer is still closed. The authors he refers to in his discussion of operative treatment are Fallopio, Fabry of Hilden and even Arceo![140]

When it comes to head injuries, the relevant book by Hippocrates still appears to be a standard work. Trepanation is indicated in cases of extravasation of blood between dura mater and skull and depressed fracture. Van de Voorde elaborately discusses the technical details of the procedure, the trephine devised by Fabricius ab Aquapendente was in frequent use.[141]

In regard to injuries of the thorax, we note that he does not want to see penetrating wounds being sutured straight away as prescribed by Guy de Chauliac, but that he covers them only with protective packs and bandages on the authority of Falloppio, Aquapendente, Paré and others. To prevent the influx of cold air, changing the bandages should take place in a heated room. Fluid in the pleural space is to be sucked out by mouth, using a metal tube interrupted halfway by a hollow copper globe which collects the extracted fluid.[142] A separate chapter deals with the details of thoracocentesis.

We pass over the third section of Van de Voorde's book in questions-and-answers which is on ulcers. As a matter of curiosity we merely record that ulcers which swarm with worms and lice, like the ones that troubled the Pharao of Egypt and king Philip II of Spain, are a vengeance of Heaven and therefore inaccessible to therapy.

The final two treatises, dealing with fractures and dislocations, are relatively very short: only the compound fracture ('gecomponeerde fractuur') of the leg is discussed at length.[143] Reduction should be performed as soon as possible. Considerable swelling and pain may provisionally be treated by wrapping the limb in the warm skin of a sheep or calf or the great omentum of any animal, as was recommended by Scultetus. Sharp bone ends which protrude from the wound are filed or pinched off. Reduction is brought about by pulling by degrees in opposite directions, preferably by apprentices who have already acquired some proficiency. If by pulling in combination with external manipulation no satisfactory position can be achieved, the surgeon should adapt the fracture ends through the wound by means of a chisel-like iron instrument. After reduction has been effected, the wound is dressed using attar of roses. A window is cut in the material to enable daily inspection of the wound. The actual fracture bandage consists of a spiral bandage covered with compresses which lend the leg a uniform thickness so as to enable the hollow wooden splints to rest on it without any free space. These splints numbering seven or eight, are secured to the bandages. Thereupon the leg is placed between two long, stiff bundles of straw reaching up to the knee, and kept together by a cloth. The heel should rest upon a cotton ring and the leg is in its entirety placed in a slightly elevated position. In fractures of the lower limb in particular, one should make every effort to prevent shortening. A Middelburg surgeon used to say — echoing Hippocrates — that no patient could bring more shame on him than by encountering him in the streets having a limp. Van de Voorde does not explain, how to treat a femoral fracture or any other broken bone.

The last chapter on dislocations covers only a few pages. Dislocations may be partial when they are called 'retortio', or present themselves as 'elongatio' because of lengthening of the ligaments and tendons, or as a genuine luxation. Among the signs of a successful reduction one regards the traditional cracking noise heard during the manipulation. According to Van de Voorde this is not caused by the expulsion of air which finds itself in the joint cavity as believed by many, but by the tearing of cartilage or rupturing of ligaments.

In conclusion we may state that Van de Voorde's textbook extensively treats of the theory of surgery with a great show of learning, but as to the practical aspects of the craft only gives outlines with an occasional example. The Middelburg examinee apparently was not required to display his knowledge on how for instance herniotomy or lithotomy should be performed, for descriptions of these two interventions are lacking.

This work confirms once again, that the scientific progress of medicine mainly took place in the field of anatomy and the physiology of individual organs. The pathophysiological conceptions in the second part of the seventeenth century appear not to differ substantially from those of ancient medicine: the discovery of the blood circulation apparently had not been able as yet to lead them into different channels.

4.16.2.3. Collected Case Histories

Collections of medical case histories were much favoured reading in the seventeenth century. Among the Dutch producers of such collections Tulp, Ruysch, Van Meekeren and Van Roonhuyze held a foremost place.

Nicolaas Tulp, M.D. (1593—1674)

Nicolaas Tulp was one of the most prominent doctors in Amsterdam. He took a great interest in anatomy, and from 1628 to 1652 he held the office of praelector anatomiae in his town of residence. In addition he filled several other public appointments including that of burgomaster. After having practised for twenty-five years, he published a book on his medical observations. Editions in Dutch and Latin kept appearing until the middle of the eighteenth century. In the preface Nicolaas Tulp wrote to his son Pieter, to whom he had dedicated the volume: 'but if your inclination induces you to do anatomical dissections, beware of having yourself detained by outer strokes, cut down to the inside and examine not only the nature of the viscera, but especially *the seats and causes of the hidden diseases*' (loca et caussas abstrusorum morborum).[144] These words indicate that the anatomical conception in pathology, which was only to reach its full maturity a hundred years later with Morgagni, awoke as early as the middle of the seventeenth century. It is indeed quite possible that Morgagni derived the title of his famous book *De sedibus et causis morborum* from the words of Tulp just cited. On the whole, however, his medical conceptions still remained within the boundaries of humoral pathology. Tulp did not shrink back from applying the trepan himself in cases of head-injuries (see p. 219).

Frederik Ruysch, M.D. (1638—1731)

Frederik Ruysch, whom we know already as a proficient anatomist and a master in preparing anatomical specimens (cf. p. 101). held the office of instructor of anatomy and surgery at Amsterdam from 1666 until his death, with the personal title of professor (Fig. 50). He was, moreover, supervisor of the municipal botanical garden. Besides his class instruction at the anatomical theatre or in the botanic garden, he gave private lessons to Dutch and foreign students. He has been twice depicted as instructor at an 'anatomical lesson': by Adriaan Backer in 1670 and by Johan van Neck in 1683. Medicine and surgery he practised only as a consultant. Ruysch also achieved merit in obstetrics and botany, but these we have to pass by. His celebrated private anatomical collection attracted visitors from all over Europe, amongst whom was Czar Peter the Great of Russia. The latter purchased the whole collection and had it shipped to St. Petersburg: part of it is still on display in Leningrad today.[145] We are well informed how Ruysch's collection looked and what it contained because of the extensive catalogue he had printed with fine copper engravings after drawings by accomplished artists like C. Huyberts, J. Mulder, J. Folkema and J. Wandelaar (Fig. 51).

From his collected anatomical, medical and surgical works we may draw a few data which are of interest for the historian of surgery. One of them is the tense operation for an aneurysm in a patient from Dordrecht, which we will consider more fully into on page 223. Of considerable importance was his establishment that pulsation is not invariably present in every aneurysmal tumour: when the blood within the sac has coagulated, this sign may be absent as Ruysch once observed in a case of an aneurysm of the aortic arch which had eaten away a considerable part of the ribs and the sternum.[146] He furthermore gave an excellent description of rectal carcinoma. Then again one finds with Ruysch a short treatment of fracture of the femoral neck. This fracture was still little known in spite of its having been described by Paré in 1572. The Amsterdam town surgeon Gerrit Borst (c. 1645—1727) had met with a long established case at the autopsy of an aged woman, who a few years before had had a fall and had been limping ever after. Borst observed eight cases altogether. Some of his autopsy specimens ended in the collection of Ruysch, who described and depicted them (Fig. 52).[147] Not a single one of these fractures showed any bony healing but fibrous union did sometimes occur. Ruysch himself sustained a hip fracture towards the end of his life by falling from a foot-stove. He was treated by Abraham Titsingh, a prominent Amsterdam surgeon whom we will discuss in the next chapter.[148] The latter prescribed a treatment which he had learned from Ruysch himself: two months of bed rest with a large piece of medicated chamois leather on the broken hip and a broad bandage around the pelvis. Thereafter the patient was allowed to walk on crutches 'as well as luck might serve him'. Ruysch apparently never regained the use of his leg but that did not restrain him from continuing his teaching. For that purpose he had himself transported to where he wished to be in a carrying-chair.[149]

Job van Meekeren (1611—66)

In the second half of the seventeenth century some surgeons too, began to edit interesting cases from their practice. One of them was Job van Meekeren who during the course of his life served as town surgeon, surgeon to the admiralty, warden of the surgeons' guild and hospital surgeon at Amsterdam.[150] He was a well-read man and apparently conversant with Latin. In his book he mentions about seventy authors together with references to the relevant sources, and some thirty more without, whom he presumably cites at second hand. The German surgeon Wilhelm Fabry appears to have been Van Meekeren's favorite author, followed by Aquapendente, Paré, Tulp and Thomas Bartolinus. In common with Barbette he had a great interest in anatomy, together they did dissections at the St. Pietersgasthuis. Van Meekeren carefully recorded the remarkable cases he saw in his practice: a number of them have been brought together in his *Heel- en geneeskonstige aenmerkingen* which only appeared two years after his death. A

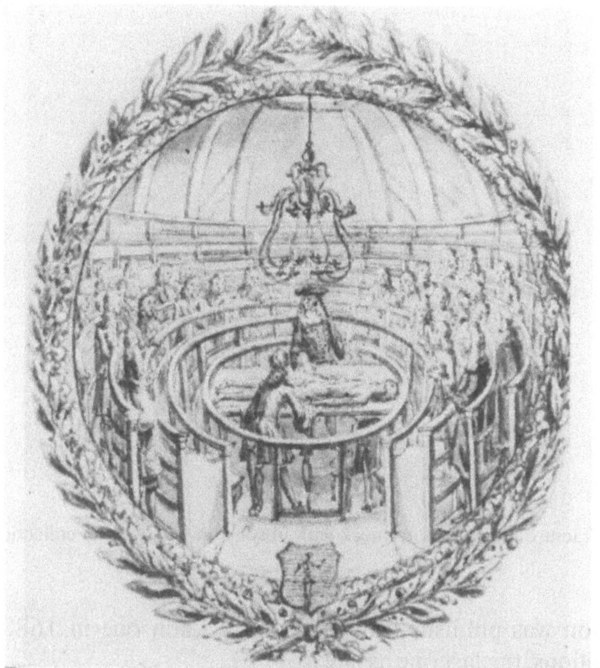

Fig. 50. Anatomical lesson in the Amsterdam theatre. The lecturer is believed to be Professor Ruysch.

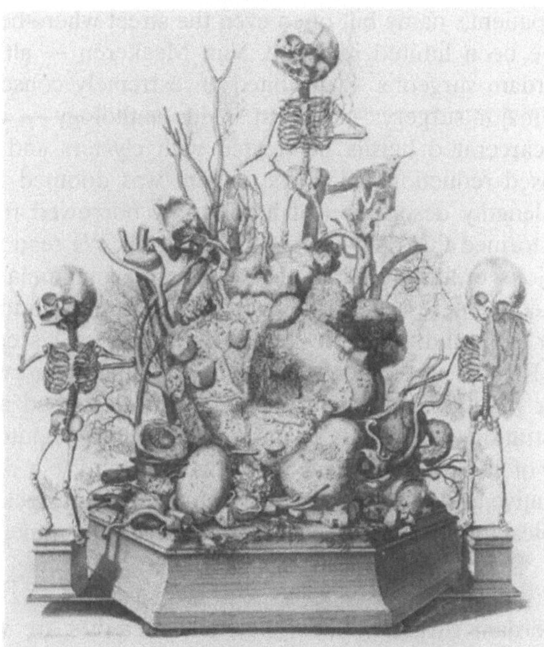

Fig. 51. One of the showpieces of the Ruyschian collection. It is composed of bladder- and gallstones, dried blood vessels, foetal skeletons and a little bird. One of the foetuses is weeping and dries his eyes with a piece of omentum. It is, indeed, a 'mememto mori'.

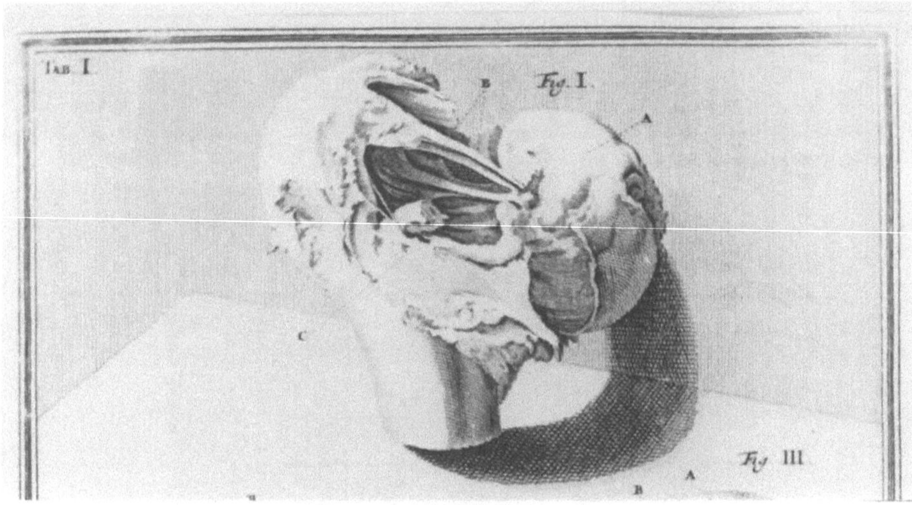

Fig. 52. Fracture of the femoral neck with fibrous union from the collection of Ruysch.

German version was published in 1675 and a Latin one in 1682, as well as two new Dutch editions, the last one as late as 1773.

Professional confidentiality was little thought of in the seventeenth century and this applies to Van Meekeren too. In many of his case-histories he not only mentioned the patient's name but often even the street where he lived. His practice appears to have been limited in scope. Van Meekeren — although in the front rank of Amsterdam surgeons — exhibited an extremely conservative therapeutic approach. His major surgery — at least in his anthology — did not go beyond trepanation. Incarcerated hernia he treated with clysters and plasters but when attempts at closed reduction failed, the patient was doomed to die. Indeed, our author gave a lengthy description of herniotomy borrowed from Pigray without ever having performed this risky intervention himself. We read nothing at all about major amputations or lithotomy or the treatment of mammary cancer. He had, however, a sincere interest in pathology and performed autopsy in uncommon cases whenever he could. Van Meekeren, like many of his contemporaries, still exhibited the Renaissance interest in rare conditions so we find cases like omphalocele or monstrosities such as phocomelia described and depicted in his book. The illustrations of patients or morbid conditions of autopsy findings which embellish many of his vivid narratives are by his own hand (Fig. 53).

The conservative attitude which manifests itself in Van Meekeren's recollections may well be typical for the practice of surgery at large at the time.

Hendrik van Roonhuyze (1622—72)

Another Amsterdam surgeon, whose personal memoirs are well worth reading, was Hendrik van Roonhuyze. His *Genees- en heelkonstige aenmerkingen* which first saw the light of day in 1672, appeared two years later in German at Nuremberg and in 1676 in English in London. He too, was a well-read man with a

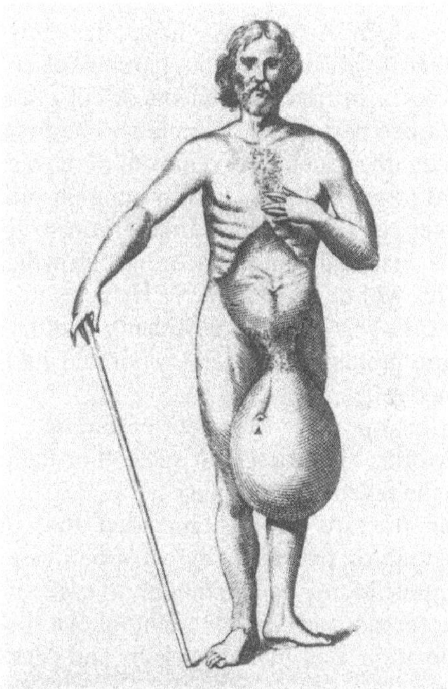

A man with an enormous scrotal hernia.

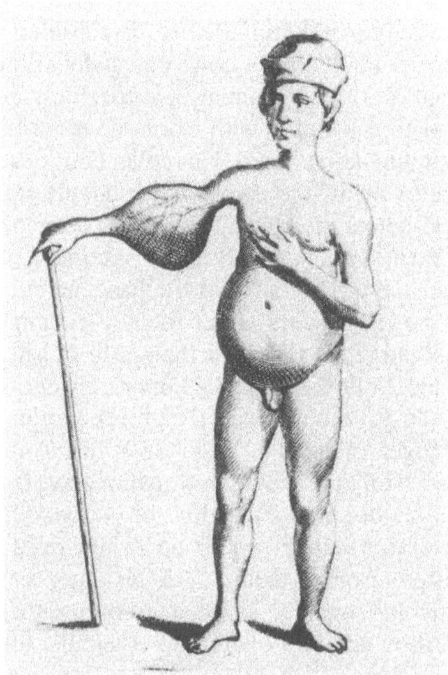

A boy with a malignant tumour of his arm.

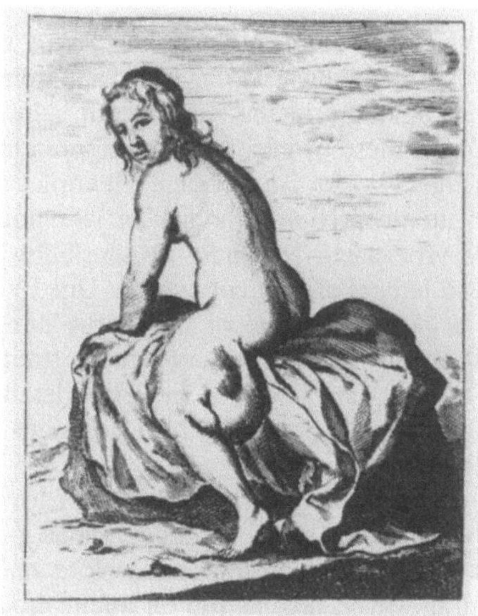

A girl with a fatty tumour on her upper leg.

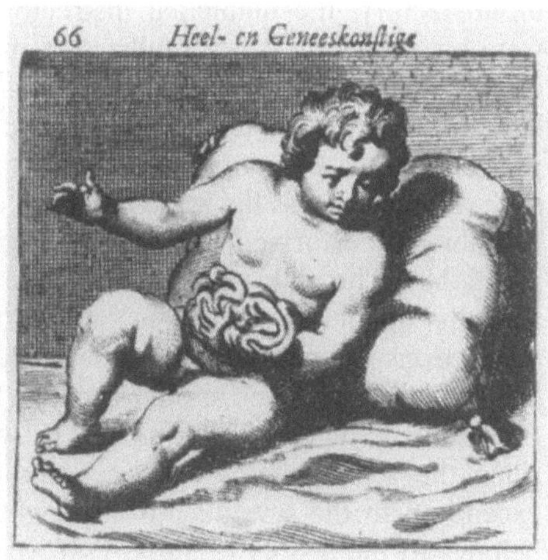

A newly-born baby with an omphalocele.

Fig. 53. Four of the patients seen and drawn by Job van Meekeren.

knowledge of Latin. Before establishing himself in Amsterdam, he made study tours to Paris and — quite unusually at the time — also to London, particularly in order to receive training in obstetrics. He was a professional friend of Job van Meekeren together with whom he more than once performed operations. The first communication from his collection describes the operative removal of a big tumour below the ear, which suddenly started to grow rapidly until it hung on the chest below the clavicle. Its surface was uneven, its consistency variable from soft to hard. Van Roonhuyze considered it as 'a malignant and cancer-like growth'. After having ligated it at the base, he cut it off with a sharp knife.[151] He does not inform his readers about the subsequent course: way into the nineteenth century most surgeons regarded their task finished the moment the operative wound had healed. Follow-up studies were rarely performed (cf. p. 230).

Van Roonhuyze had a high reputation for his operative treatment of harelip.[154] Sprengel referred to it in 1805 using the words: 'The best and most thorough treatise on that operation which we have from the seventeenth century'.[153]

For the immobilization of a mandibular fracture he recommended that a perforated copper splint be firmly fixed to four or five teeth by a copper wire twisted around them.[154] In his later communications we encounter a case of torticollis happily cured by cutting the sternomastoid muscle right above its insertion to the collarbone. A similar observation was made by Tulp and Van Meekeren.

4.17. OBSTETRICS

Roonhuyze was held in particularly good repute as an obstetrician. With the intention of improving the professional level of the midwives, which was apparently unsatisfactory, the municipal instructors of anatomy in the seventeenth century were instructed by the city fathers to enlighten these women and their apprentices on the structure of the female organs (Fig. 54). At Amsterdam, Hendrik van Roonhuyze was the first to receive such an instruction although he was not a praelector, but a town obstetrician ('stads vroevaar'). The main responsibility of such a dignitary was the removal of the dead fetuses of indigent women. Once Van Roonhuyze performed a laparotomy for a case of rupture of the uterus during pregnancy. The child appeared to have died, but the mother survived the trauma and the operation. In the second part of his *Aenmerkingen* he gave detailed instructions for performing caesarian section,[155] an operation which he seems to have conducted himself about ten times (Fig. 55).

The obstetricians ('vroedmeesters') whom we find regularly in the larger towns since the second half of the century, were usually surgeons, Ruysch being an exception. In the seventeenth and eighteenth centuries obstetrics therefore really belongs to the history of surgery. It would, however, take us too far afield should we pay more than marginal attention to this discipline here.

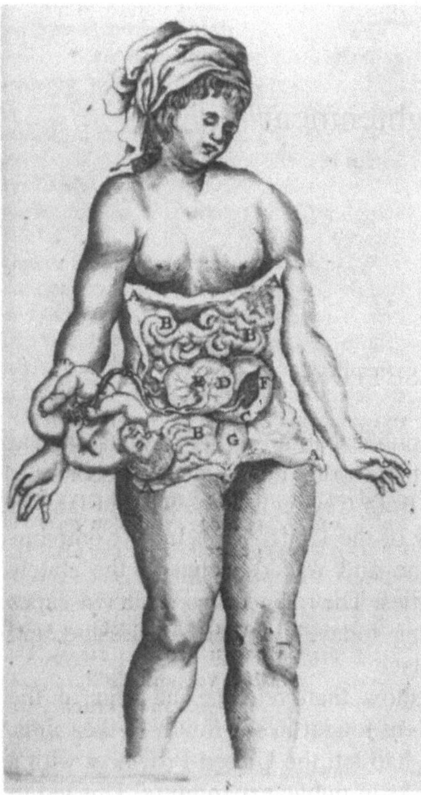

Fig. 54. Autopsy in a case of extra-uterine pregnancy, observed by H. van Roonhuyze.

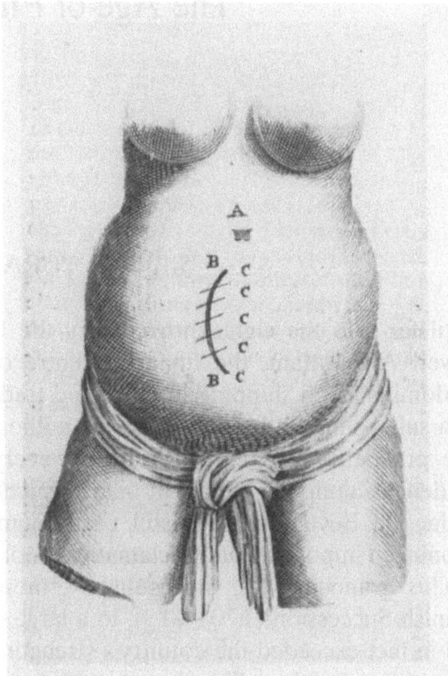

Fig. 55. Incision used by H. van Roonhuyze for the caesarian section.

CHAPTER 5

The Age of Enlightenment

5.1. CULTURAL SETTING

Until far into the eighteenth century the Republic continued to pose as a great power. Amsterdam, the financial centre of the world, maintained its economic predominance in shipping tonnage and trade. Both Ceylon and the whole island of Java subordinated themselves to the authority of the United East-India Company. The prosperity was easily visible to everyone and was reflected in the stately residences along the canals in many Dutch cities. They appear on the townscapes of Jan de Beyer, and are still partly standing today. In Holland, Zeeland and Groningen important land reclamations took place.

This grandeur was, unfortunately, more show than reality. The War of the Spanish Succession (1701—13), to a large extent fought in the South Netherlands, had in fact exceeded the country's strength. It had left the United Provinces with a large national debt calling for rigorous cut backs in public expenditure. This led to neglect of the army and navy which cost the Dutch dearly when they once again took part in a coalition against France in the War of the Austrian Succession (1740—48). Dutch support of the rebellious British colonies in North America resulted in the outbreak of the Fourth Anglo—Dutch naval War (1780—84) which ran a disastrous course for the Republic. England and France gradually superseded Holland in the economic field as well.

Just as happened in the previous century, repeated conflicts arose between adversaries and supporters of the House of Orange. After the death of king-stadtholder William III in 1702, town oligarchies had largely gained control of affairs, breeding all sorts of abuses which in time were to affect the powerful surgeons' guild in Amsterdam. The weak governments of the succeeding Orange stadholders were unable to remedy this. It led to the rising of the Patriots, a new political movement in the seventies, who rebelled against the power of the oligarchic families ('regenten') as well as the stadholdership. The ideas of the Enlightenment, which had blown over from Britain and France, formed the basis of the movement's ideals. The Patriots increasingly gained the upper hand and when in 1795 the armies of the French Revolution marched into the North Netherlands, they took control. The last stadtholder fled with his family to England. By the proclamation of the Batavian Republic after the peace with France, a definite end was brought to the old Republic of the Seven United

Netherlands. The federal structure was replaced by a unified state with a central government in The Hague. Parliament no longer consisted of delegates sent by the separate provinces, but of members elected by a still rather limited voting system. The new Batavian Republic accomplished a great number of reforms. Thus, in 1798 the first constitutional law in the history of the Netherlands was enforced, which guaranteed freedom of religion and equality of all citizens before the law.

The peculiar characteristics of seventeenth century culture had largely been lost much earlier, through the infiltration of French fashion, style and literature. As a result of this Frenchification, eighteenth century culture was more or less out of touch with the common people. Since the seventies, the abundant cultural life induced by the Enlightenment in Germany and Britain, resulted in many German and English literary works being translated into Dutch. The Dutch literature itself of that period makes rather a dull impression. As it gradually adapted to the ideas of the Enlightenment it became more and more didactic, and in the second half of the century also sentimental and romantic. Pictorial art still had the important Cornelis Troost, with his well-known genre paintings and Isaac Ouwater with his cityscapes.

Intellectually and scientifically Holland could still boast quite a few scholars of European renown, especially in physics and chemistry, although it was no longer a leading centre of North-West Europe, as it had been in the seventeenth century. Various societies of science and the arts exercised stimulating influences. The printing presses were operating at full speed: material which could or dared not be printed elsewhere found a publisher here. In part this allowed the Republic to function not only as an international money market but also as an important market for cultural products.

5.2. MEDICINE

The eighteenth century witnessed the further breakdown of Galenism. Discoveries in the field of descriptive and pathological anatomy and physiology provided a large source of new data, some of a very fundamental nature, which could not be fitted into the traditional medical system. The battle between the iatrochemical and iatrophysical schools of thought had not been settled by the beginning of the century, although iatrophysics was gaining the upper hand.

The abundance of new data once more awakened a desire to fit things into a framework or system which allowed a mutual context, and thus increased their use for the development of theories or in practice. In the first half of the century the medical systems of Georg Ernst Stahl (1660—1737) and Friedrich Hoffmann (1660—1742) at Halle in Germany and Herman Boerhaave (1668—1738) at Leyden came especially to the fore.

Stahl held that in all organic actions the 'anima' played the leading role as regulator. His concept of disease was chiefly humoral, with the principal cause of most diseases being an excess of blood or plethora. In its regulating function the 'anima' therefore resorts above all to spontaneous haemorrhages, particularly by way of haemorrhoidal bleeding.[1] Medical treatment too, should aim at neutralizing the fullness of blood, which Stahl apparently considered to be an active process as distinguished from passive hyperaemia.

According to the views of Hoffmann, the human body was a type of hydraulic engine, kept in motion by a 'nerve affluvium', originating in the brain, which filled the nerves at the time generally thought to be hollow. Disease was either due to a hypertonic or an atonic condition. In the moving parts these conditions manifested themselves as cramps or paralyses respectively; in the sensible parts as pain or numbness. Local inflammation, haemorrhage, mucous discharge, neuralgia were expressions of a tonic state, chronic ailments usually those of an atonic one. Treatment should consist of either tone reducing or tone enhancing remedies.

Boerhaave's system, like that of Hoffmann, was of an iatromechanical nature, albeit in combination with iatrochemical principles. The causes of disease could either be found in the solid parts, such as congenital malformations or deviations in mass, size, position or tone; or in the body fluids. Derangements of the humours could be of a quantitative or qualitative nature.

At the bedside, however, Boerhaave did not take much heed of his own theories but let himself be guided by strict objectivity. Here he was clearly influenced by the celebrated London physician Thomas Sydenham (1624—89) whom he held in high esteem. Following Hippocrates' example, Sydenham relied mainly on clinical observation when dealing with patients.

In the eighteenth century, also known as the age of Enlightenment, the consciousness gradually grew that society was collectively responsible for its dependants: women and children, the mentally ill, prisoners and servicemen including sailors at sea. This partly explains the rise of obstetrics as a medical discipline and applies equally to paediatrics, orthopaedics and psychiatry. There also grew an awareness of problems concerning hygiene and public health, while medical ethics received serious attention for the first time since Hippocrates.

Of medical literature it can be said that the traditional authorities of Antiquity were rapidly losing ground, although they were still often quoted. Anatomy unchangingly occupied a prominent place, whilst physiology was adopting modern chemical and haemodynamic principles, but nonetheless retained many elements of humoral pathology. Textbooks often had a long life. It is striking that translations and reprints, which sometimes appeared many years after the first edition, were frequently not adapted to include the intervening developments, with the result that they were already somewhat obsolete when they appeared.

Although there was certainly no lack of discoveries and innovations in the age under consideration, Dutch medical literature from that period on the whole does not strike us as particularly dynamic. The works of authors from the sixteenth and seventeenth centuries lived on and on to be quoted time and time again. Writing in the vernacular was increasingly the fashion. In the Netherlands and in Germany works which had been originally published in Latin often quickly appeared in the native language as well, and especially in surgery. Dutch versions of English, German or Italian books were frequently made from French translations rather than from the original editions, and were, therefore, translations of translations.

5.3. SURGERY

5.3.1. *France*

The French managed to maintain their dominant position, gained in the course of the second half of the seventeenth century, for almost a hundred years. This is partly the result of the many wars of Louis XIV and Louis XV, bringing forth a large number of surgeons with great operative skill. Most of the leading French surgeons had obtained practical experience on the battlefield before establishing themselves in the capital to practise, train students and write books.[2]

French surgery owed its prominent position not least to the fact that it had been able to free itself from obsolete forms of organization at a much earlier date than had other countries. This was favoured by the presence of a powerful central authority. The appointment of the office of 'first surgeon to the king' in 1668, with a supervisory function over the whole kingdom meant that the French surgeons' guilds fell under royal surveyance.[3]

In 1724 Georges Mareschal, personal surgeon to Louis XV, at the instigation of Lapeyronie managed to persuade the king officially to acknowledge the tuition given at Saint-Côme (cf. p. 106) as 'Ecole de Chirurgie' and have it endowed by the government.[4] That meant the liberation of surgery from the tutelage of the medical faculty of the university. In 1775 the school, in the meantime promoted to Collège de Chirurgie, moved into a new building in the Rue de l'Ecole de Médecine, which had been especially founded for the purpose. This building is presently known as the 'Ancienne Ecole de Médecine'.

It was also Mareschal who, together with Lapeyronie, initiated the foundation of a scientific society in 1731, which became known as the 'Académie royale de Chirurgie' in 1748. The best surgeons from the capital of the realm were thus brought together under the chairmanship of the first surgeon of the king. The Academy organized regular meetings and annual prize competitions.

A royal ruling from 1743 stipulated that candidates for the master-surgeon's examination in Paris had to hold the grade of 'magister artium' obtained at one of the French universities.[5] In consideration of the successive enactments being made in aid of the emancipation of surgery as an independant profession, it is somewhat surprising to find that only in that year by the selfsame royal privilege just mentioned, the surgeons in France were divorced from the barbers with whom they had previously formed one guild.

New ideals grew with surgical education. It should not only be practical, but also scientific, as was argued in the preface of the first volume of the *Mémoires de l'Académie royale de Chirurgie*. These *Mémoires*, which appeared between 1743 and 1773 in five thick folio editions, are a portrayal of scientific surgery in the eighteenth century at its best. References in Dutch literature prove that they were also read in this country. The subjects described include the treatment of wounds, the generation of pus, operative surgery also incorporating obstetric, eye, ear, nose and throat procedures, fractures and dislocations and surgical pathology. Some articles are in the form of long essay reviews, but there are also case reports and descriptions of new instruments. A number of contributions are illustrated with fine copper engravings. The award winning entries for the annual competition appeared in *Receuil des pièces qui ont concouru pour le prix de l'Académie royale de Chirurgie.* They too give important information on surgery at that time.

The possibilities of receiving tuition in various surgical subjects gradually increased. The three existing courses at the Ecole de Chirurgie in Saint-Côme: anatomy, operative surgery and 'osteologie and bone diseases', were extended with 'principles of surgery' and 'therapy'. When, in 1750, the school was promoted to Collège de Chirurgie, the courses on 'principles of surgery, osteology and theory' were replaced by physiology, pathology and general therapy. These subjects were subsequently given in three year cycles by professors, paid by the realm. Obstetrics, eye diseases, chemistry and botany were added later.[6]

In the Jardin du Roi, as before, one could follow lessons on anatomy and operative surgery. All tuition was given in the vernacular. The large hospitals, in which a surgical hierarchy was beginning to form, organized practical courses for their students, in anatomy and operative surgery on cadavers.[7]

The actual originator of surgical instruction at the sick-bed, in the outpatient's clinic and at the operation table is Pierre-Joseph Desault (1744—95), surgeon in chief of the Hôtel-Dieu since 1788: he taught hundreds of students a practical and simple surgery which was related to pathology.[8] Apart from a surgical magazine which was only short-lived, Desault himself did not publish any works. His influential *Traité des maladies chirurgicales et les opérations qui leur conviennent* (1799) was written by François Chopart (1743—95) and his *Oeuvres chirurgicales* were edited by his pupil Xavier Bichat between 1798 and 1802.

Foreign students liked to take private courses in anatomy and surgery, given by leading surgeons. These were also of a practical nature and usually lasted three months.[9] But it was, for a fee, also possible to have practical training as a journeyman under a chosen master-surgeon.

The requirements for the master's examination underwent a fundamental change when in 1768 the apprentice system dating back to the Middle Ages was abolished and replaced by the obligation to follow lessons at the Collège de Chirurgie for a given period. Yet prospective surgeons often affiliated themselves to an established master in this period to gain practical experience.[10]

5.3.2. *England*

In Great Britain too, surgery expanded enormously in the eighteenth century, building on the foundations laid in the second half of the previous century by Richard Wiseman. In 1745, the London surgeons separated from the Barbers' Company and established their own surgeons' corporation. Towards the end of the century the training of surgeons who wished to join the Company of Surgeons was excellent, compared to many places on the Continent.[11] It required an apprenticeship of five years to a private surgeon followed by the attendance at two courses of lectures, two courses of dissection and finally by one year of clinical experience on the wards of a hospital in London, Edinburgh, Glasgow or Dublin. The lecture courses were provided by medical schools in a number of large hospitals and, more adequately, by private anatomy schools. An outstanding example of such a school was the one in Great Windmill Street in London, established in 1770 by

John Hunter's brother William. In addition to anatomy and surgery, the Great Windmill Street School also offered courses in physiology, pathology, midwifery and diseases of women and children. In London, medical schools were established in St. Bartholomew's, St. Thomas's, Guy's and The London Hospital. These hospitals likewise offered clinical instruction but this could also be had at the Westminster, St. George's and Middlesex hospitals. Apart from St. Bartholomew's and St. Thomas's, whose origins go back to the Middle Ages, all these institutes were founded in the eighteenth century.

After having 'walked the hospitals' for a year, the candidate was ready to apply for membership of the Company of Surgeons. For this he had to pass a tough examination. There were also less qualified surgeons in Britain since former ship's and army surgeons, after a number of years in the services, were entitled to engage in civilian practice.

There was no lack of surgeons who had earned a good reputation throughout Europe.[12] William Cheselden (1688—1752) for instance, who worked at St. Thomas's Hospital in London, was especially famous for his great skill in performing lithotomies, see page 250. In the second half of the century particularly, England and Scotland brought forth an impressive succession of renowned surgeons. Among them was Cheselden's student Samuel Sharp (1700—78), employed at Guy's Hospital, who was well-known for his handbook of operative surgery which ran through many editions and was translated into Dutch and French. On the staff at St. Luke's Hospital was William Bromfeild (1712—92), the first to resect the head of the humerus.[13] Then there was the celebrated Percivall Pott (1714—88), who was the chief surgeon at Bartholomew's for more than forty years. Pott wrote a whole series of excellent books and monographs on hernias, head injuries, hydrocele and fractures. He gave the first description of a form of occupational cancer — chimney-sweep's cancer of the scrotum — and of the angular spinal curvature which was named after him. And of course we should mention John Hunter (1728—93), one of the greatest surgeons of all time. Hunter was the actual founder of experimental and surgical pathology. In particular his studies on inflammation and wound healing were of fundamental importance. He collected a large number of anatomical, pathological and natural history specimens, some of which have been preserved and can still be seen today in the Hunterian Museum at the Royal College of Surgeons of England. In Edinburgh successive generations of the Monro family, together with Benjamin Bell (1749—1806) contributed to making the Royal Infirmary one of the most outstanding medical centres in Europe.[14] Bell's *System of surgery* was a standard work for many years. It was also published in Dutch.

Since the middle of the eighteenth century England, and London in particular, began to exert some attraction for Dutch surgeons. Of those who — sometimes more than once — crossed the Channel to that country we will portray F. B. Albinus, P. Camper, M. S. du Pui and J. Mulder further on in this chapter.

5.3.3. *Germany*

In the German speaking countries, surgeons from the Prussian army played a large role. Many of them had been trained in France: Frederick the Great of Prussia was a great admirer of French military surgery. These men included Joh. Leberecht Schmucker (1712—86), Joh. Christian Anton Theden (1714—97) and Joh. Ulrich Bilguer (1720—96). They were the authors of textbooks and books containing surgical case notes which attest to great experience, a practical mind and veracity. Their work also appeared in Dutch.

University surgery was represented in particular by Lorenz Heister (1683—1758), professor at Altdorf and later at Helmstedt. His *Chirurgie*, published in 1718 for the first time, was one of the most popular textbooks for three quarters of a century and it was translated into many languages. With this book he laid the foundations of scientific surgery in Germany. We will return to Heister later. The textbooks by Joh. Zacharias Platner (1694—1747), professor at Leipzig, were also held in high regard. Platner received part of his training in France and England.

The second half of the century was dominated by August Gottlieb Richter (1742—1812), professor at Göttingen, and by Karl Caspar von Siebold (1736—1807) at Würzburg. Richter, by his writings, was the first German surgeon to introduce his fellow countrymen to English surgery, after his training in London with Percivall Pott. Like John Hunter, Richter endeavoured to turn surgery into a scientific discipline. His *Anfangsgründe der Wundarzneikunst*, which appeared in seven parts between 1782 and 1804, laid the foundations for a newer form of German surgery, becoming the example for all subsequent textbooks on this subject. He made a very important contribution to the knowledge of hernia. His *Chirurgische Bibliothek*, brought out in fifteen parts between 1771 and '96, was the first journal of surgery in Germany; it also appeared in a Dutch version. Siebold was a field surgeon in the French army in his younger years and spent quite some time in Paris and London. He was a member of a family which produced a number of well-known doctors.[15] Several of the most important German surgeons of the nineteenth century were educated at Von Siebold's Würzburg clinic, founded in 1769.

5.3.4. *Italy*

Among the Italians whose influence was felt all over Europe, we must first and foremost mention Giovanni Battista Morgagni (1682—1771), professor at Padua. His *De sedibus et causis morborum per anatomen indagatis libri quinque*, published in 1761, is one of the most important books in the whole history of medicine. It contains his attempts to correlate the clinical symptoms, manifest during their illness, with the autopsy findings in some 700 patients. In this way he laid the foundations for modern pathological anatomy. It is significant that in his book Morgagni hardly mentions Galen, although he is known to have lectured on Galenic works in his earlier years. In European surgery it was a particular student of Morgagni, Antonio Scarpa (1752—1832), professor at Pavia, who became of importance not only because of his studies in anatomy but especially through his publications on fractures, ophthalmic diseases and herniology. After his death Scarpa's head was preserved in spirit and has been proudly kept in the medical-historical museum of the university of Pavia ever since.

5.3.5.1. General Overview

The French Period

The ample opportunities for making further theoretical and practical studies of operative surgery, anatomy and obstetrics offered in France, were also taken by many Dutchmen. Thus it may be said that many if not most of the surgeons who during the eighteenth century occupied a prominent place in the Netherlands had spent various periods of time in France on completion of their education in their native country: after their homecoming they were often designated as 'French masters'.[16] Besides public lectures and demonstrations many Dutchmen in Paris were drawn to the private courses given by Joseph-Guichard Duverney (1648—1730), Jean-Louis Petit (1674—1750), Jean Astruc (1684—1766), and especially Henry-François Le Dran (1685—1770), Sauveur-François Morand (1697—1773) and René-Jacques Croissant de Garengeot (1688—1759). Later, during the same century, it was Antoine Louis (1723—92), Raphael-Bienvenu Sabatier (1732—1811) and Pierre-Joseph Desault who attracted many students from abroad. Those who intended to practise lithotomy were likely to make for Claude-Nicolas le Cat (1700—68) in Rouen.

However great the number of those who in the course of the eighteenth century spent a study period in France, only a minority of the Dutch surgeons could have been involved: apart from the travelling expenses and subsistence the tuition fees must have been for many a financial barrier. Le Dran charged 4000 livres for a complete three-year course,[17] and Ant. Andouillé in the Charité asked three louis d'or for a three-month 'cours d'opérations' on a cadaver.[18]

The prestige of French surgery led to a great demand for French textbooks. The number of French works published in translation is therefore considerable. This also applies to Holland. Among the works published in Dutch one should mention the well-known book about diseases of the bone — fractures and dislocations — by Jean-Louis Petit, the most prominent French surgeon of the first half of the century. This will be further discussed on page 197.

The book by Pierre Dionis, the well-known teacher at the Jardin du Roi, was published in Dutch in 1710 while a Dutch translation of a commentary on it by Georges de la Faye (1699—1781) appeared in 1740.[19] The extensively illustrated book on surgical instruments by René-Jacques Croissant de Garengeot appeared in Dutch in 1728. The textbooks by Henry-François le Dran appear to have been quite popular: no fewer than five of his works were translated into Dutch, while his monograph on bullet wounds was published in Amsterdam also in French. In 1761, Van der Haar assessed that Dutch surgeons owed a great deal to Le Dran's publications (Fig. 56).[20]

On the basis of what has been said above, the first half of the eighteenth century may well be termed the French period in the history of Dutch surgery. German influence, apart from the works by Lorenz Heister and the still much-read Fabricius Hildanus and Scultetus which will be discussed below, was not very strong, while English influence was practically absent.

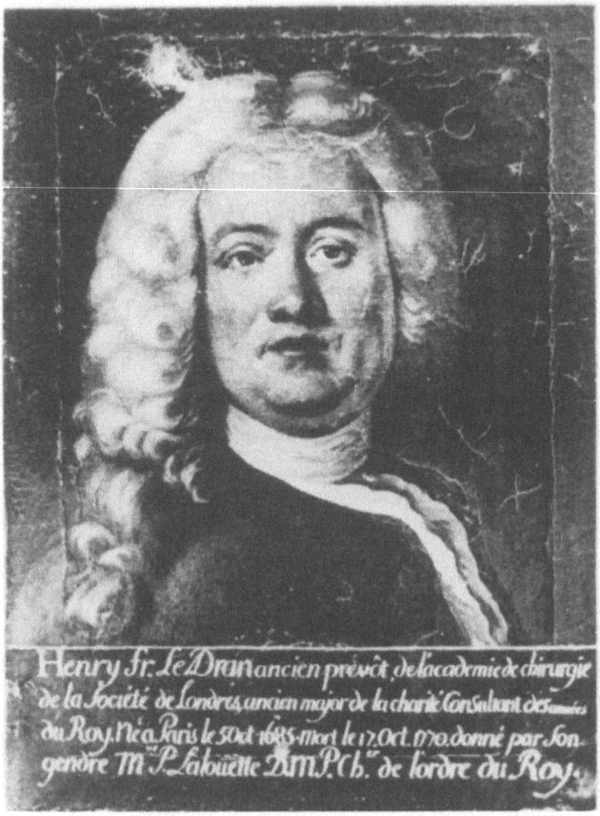

Fig. 56. Henri-François le Dran, an outstanding representative of 18th century French surgery.

This 'French period' did not mean that Dutch surgery had completely lost its own identity. There still existed outstanding surgeons in Holland and as ever Dutch publications found their way abroad. The year 1794 even saw the publication of a periodical, edited by Chr. Fr. Niceus, with abstracts from the Dutch literature, entitled *Holländisches Museum für Deutschlands Aerzte und Wundärzte*; however, only one volume ever appeared. Until well into the eighteenth century German surgeons in particular — among whom the later famous Johann Friedrich Lobstein (1736—84) and Richter — considered it worthwhile to include Holland in a scientific tour.

Not everybody in this country was all that pleased with the predominant French influence in rebus chirurgicis. This became evident when in 1728 three young surgeons were sent to Paris at the expense of the Amsterdam guild, on the advice of the Dutch ambassador in Paris.[21] In a letter to the city council of Amsterdam the diplomat had reported on an operation performed on the municipal secretary in the French capital after he had fainted during a council meeting. The operation had consisted of a laparotomy, in which the abdomen was opened below the ribs. Reportedly two or three ulcers were found in the intestines. The patient survived the intervention, in spite of his sixty years. The ambassador supposed that such a surgical operation would have been unthinkable in the Netherlands. Nevertheless, his proposal did not find favour with the Amsterdam surgeons, because their guild would have had to raise the necessary 1000 guilders yearly. The town surgeon Abraham Titsingh (1684—1776) argued that in Amsterdam enough surgeons were to be found who could hold their own against the French. The Dutch, moreover, conducted their operations more neatly and more accurately yet did not resort to the knife too readily.[21] The Rotterdam surgeon Johan van Wyck (1690—c. 1750), who throughout the country enjoyed a good reputation on account of his private lessons in theoretical surgery and his few textbooks, also expressed unfavourable views of French surgery. This was to counterbalance the words of praise about French surgery written by another Rotterdam surgeon, Pieter Vink, M.D., in the introduction to his translation of *Cours d'opérations de chirurgie par Dionis*, augmenté par G[eorges] de la F[aye].[22] Van Wyck reproached his fellow-townsman for having been in Paris for too short a time to allow a fair appraisal of French surgery on the strength of his own observations. As an illustration of the accidents which may result from the French 'dash' lauded by Vink, Van Wyck published the text of a letter, dated August 23, 1740, which had been sent to him from the French capital by a Rotterdam surgeon, whom, however, he was unwilling to identify. In the letter the unnamed surgeon reported on what he had witnessed in the field of operative surgery in the large Paris hospitals. 'It is indeed true that in Paris one can witness many operations which vary in nature and seriousness', his correspondent wrote, 'but the surgeons are little concerned about a correct indication and a good after-care. Fatal accidents, such as bleeding to death after an amputation, are therefore bound to occur'.[23]

In the second half of the eighteenth century foreign professional literature no longer came predominantly from France. Along with a growing interest in German and English belles letters, there arose an increasing demand for German and English medical books. Thus, in the Netherlands there appeared translations of most of the works of the British and German surgeons mentioned between pages 152 to 154. Of the numerous books by the Austro-Hungarian surgeon Joseph Jacob Plenck (1738—1807), whose publications on all branches of medicine were received with much approbation, quite a few were translated into Dutch, including three on surgery.

But original surgical literature, whether in the form of books or monographs, was not wanting in the eighteenth century. Apart from the works to be mentioned later in this chapter by Boerhaave and Van Swieten, Sandifort, Titsingh, Nuck, Schwencke and De Gorter, Dutch surgeons also had at their disposal numerous other home-made products. For instance the *Genees- en heelkundige waarnemingen* of 1743 by the Leyden surgeon Cornelis Trioen, M.D. (1686—1746), was a work illustrated with very fine drawings by his brother-in-law, the well-known artist Frans van Mieris (Fig. 57 and 58). Later in the century the Amsterdam surgeon David van Gesscher emerged as a productive medical writer. Finally, numerous articles on surgery followed developments which had occurred abroad, in the journals of scientific societies founded in the Netherlands during the second half of the century: the 'Hollandsche Maatschappij der Wetenschappen te Haarlem'

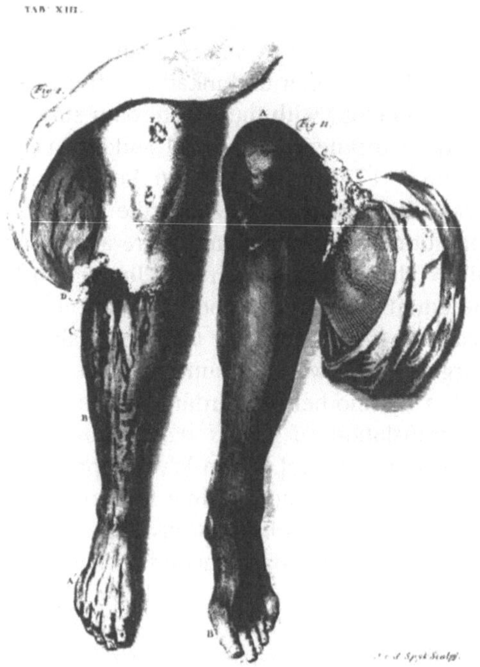

Fig. 57. A fatal case of spontaneous gangrene of both legs in a woman aged 23, observed by Cornelis Trioen and depicted by Frans van Mieris.

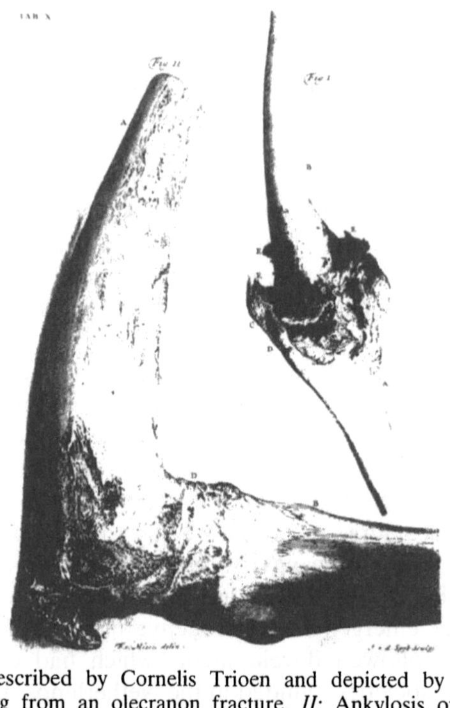

Fig. 58. Bone pathology described by Cornelis Trioen and depicted by Frans van Mieris. *I*: Ankylosis of elbow resulting from an olecranon fracture. *II*: Ankylosis of knee in 90° flexion, following osteomyelitis of the femur.

(Dutch Society of Sciences at Haarlem) (1752), the 'Zeeuwsch Genootschap der Wetenschappen' (Zeeland Society of Sciences) (1768), the 'Bataafsch Genootschap der Proefondervindelijke Wijsbegeerte te Rotterdam' (Batavian Association of Empirical Philosophy at Rotterdam) (1769—1770) and the 'Provinciaal Utregtsch Genootschap voor Kunsten en Wetenschappen' (Society for the Arts and Sciences of the Province of Utrecht) (1778). Arising from the need for the distribution of knowledge and from an optimistic belief in progress through the application of the sciences, they are characteristic of the Enlightenment. The societies pursued their aims by organizing lectures, holding prize competitions and publishing their transactions. These transactions in particular made a considerable contribution to the distribution of professional knowledge among physicians and surgeons. At that time no specific medical periodicals existed in Holland, so Dutch physicians had to turn either to the transactions of these societies, or to journals produced for the educated general public, such as *Algemeene Vaderlandsche Letteroefeningen* (General Dutch Literary Exercises) in order to have their articles published at home.

This was not an ideal situation. On the one hand the 'weetgierige heelmeesters' (inquisitive surgeons) complained that the publications which they considered important were buried among articles of an altogether different nature, while on the other the non-surgical members of those societies were unhappy that their journals were overloaded with treatises and observations concerning the 'akeligste lichaamsgebreken' (the most unpleasant bodily defects).[24] Whoever wanted his scientific efforts to have a larger circulation had to get them accepted by the *Philosophical Transactions*, the *Mémoires de l'Académie royale de Chirurgie à Paris* or the *Ephemerides* (see pp. 105 and 151). Dutch surgeons who used this opportunity were Schlichting — in the *Acta Naturae Curiosorum* and in the *Philosophical Transactions* — and Camper — in the *Mémoires de l'Académie royale de Chirurgie*.

Not everyone could afford a subscription to the relevant foreign periodicals; besides, the foreign language was a barrier to many of them. The Leyden professor Eduard Sandifort (1742—1814), who had a great knowledge of languages, obliged his fellow countrymen by publishing a *Natuur- en Geneeskundige Bibliotheek* (Library of Physics and Medicine), after the example of similar digests which had appeared in Germany. This came out in the vernacular in eleven volumes from 1765 to 1775, containing summaries of works on medicine and natural history from journals published abroad such as the *Philosophical Transactions, Transactions of the American Philosophical Society* and *Medical Observations and Inquiries.* He regularly supplied lists of recently published foreign works.

Training by the Guilds

In the training of surgeons no substantial change occurred during the eighteenth century: it remained the concern of the guilds and followed the traditional apprenticeship. In such a system the quality of the education is totally dependent on what the individual master is able and willing to teach his pupil. The practical experience which an apprentice acquired during his training was basically involved with hair cutting and shaving; only a few pupils were allowed, during the final one or two years, to accompany their masters as they went out to visit their patients in town. Pupils were able to attend only those operations which their teachers hazarded and were therefore only too anxious to be apprenticed to hospital surgeons. In cities which could afford a praelector, in principle a weekly afternoon lecture on anatomy and theoretical surgery was held. However, these lecturers appear often to have failed in the performance of their duties and it therefore depended on the apprentice surgeon himself how he acquired his theoretical knowledge. In the brief autobiography which precedes his Dutch translation of Smellie's well-known *Treatise on the theory and practice of midwifery* (London, 1752) Matthijs van der Haage (c. 1723—86) of Nijmegen gives a delightful description of his 'education' in various cities, under several masters. None of them ever bothered to teach fundamental theory. He was therefore forced to buy an arbitrary selection of books on medicine, surgery and anatomy, which, on account of his poor schooling, he found himself at first unable to read. When as a result of sheer persistence he had increased his knowledge sufficiently to understand what was in his books, he was finally able to pass the master's examination.[25] Johannes de Gorter also expressed his scorn for his pupilage 'indien het leren mag genaamt worden' ('if it can be called an education at all').[26] Most apprentices prepared for the theoretical part of the examination with the learning by heart of Herls' *Examen* and similar compendia.[27] It is obvious that such an educational system hardly promoted progression. This is also shown by the failure of eighteenth-century examinations to improve substantially on the standards of the preceding century.[28]

It is therefore understandable that after the completion of his training the new surgeon was happy to spend some time abroad — particularly in Paris — in order to acquire a greater proficiency in operative surgery and practical obstetrics. The fact that many young physicians and surgeons included anatomy in their study period abroad, indicates that the teaching at home of this pre-eminently Dutch subject — where nota bene it was flourishing at the time — was considered insufficient both by students of medicine and of surgery. Pieter Vink attributed the shortcomings which he noticed in Dutch surgery to an inadequate knowledge of the structure of the human body. Even for the treatment of an everyday complaint such as whitlow most surgeons had too little ready knowledge of anatomy to distinguish between the various types in which this affliction might manifest itself.

Private Courses in Anatomy and Surgery

Private courses with practical exercises on a cadaver, so-called 'collegia anatomico-chirurgica', had ever since the second half of the seventeenth century been given by prominent surgeons at Paris and London, at Amsterdam and Rotterdam, and probably at other large towns throughout Europe. They usually took three months. These courses represented a higher surgical education which, particularly in the eighteenth century, greatly contributed to the rise of a surgical elite: an elite which was also capable of performing those major operations, which had always been the domain of the specialized cutter: lithotomy, couching of the cataract and herniotomy.

Social Status

The education described above, its quality being primarily determined by the practical and theoretical qualifications of the master together with the student's financial resources for supplementing his training elsewhere, further increased the differences in the professional status of individual surgeons. In the second half of the seventeenth century, a small group began to specialize in difficult operations such as lithotomy. At the same time, the general educational background of some surgeons was improving as well. This is shown by an increased knowledge of foreign languages: the Dutch translations of the five books of Le Dran were made by five different surgeons.[29]

Furthermore, qualified surgeons increasingly proceeded to their university doctorates, so that they attained an equal footing with physicians. Well-known examples are Cornelis Solingen, Govert Bidloo, Johannes Rau, Jan Sermes, Johannes de Gorter, Gerard Greeve and Anton Schrage. The acquisition of a university degree did not usually imply that they gave up their surgical practice nor indeed their barber's shops. Even if they had become affluent most surgeons kept their shops as a steady addition to their income. The majority of surgeons, however, still depended entirely on barbering, their surgical practice being restricted to bloodletting and the treatment of simple wounds. The earnings from such a practice were modest. Shaving was done for an annual fee of four guilders or less. Regular dressing of a wound earned the surgeon eight pence (stuivers) a day, and a bloodletting from fifty cents to a guilder.[30]

With the exception of Amsterdam, the average annual income in fifteen Dutch cities in 1742 amounted to 850 guilders.[31] Research of the assessment register of that year, conducted by Leonie van Nierop, showed that of the 269 guildsmen in Amsterdam — which at the time had some 200 000 inhabitants — sixteen were estimated as having an annual income of 2000 guilders.[32] In this they exceeded the income of about half of the doctores medicinae and equalled the annual income of a lawyer.

According to Van Nierop's study three surgeons — Ulhoorn, Plaatman and Adriaan Verduin Jr — had an annual income of between 4500 and 9000 guilders. Each possessed a house in the country and all three kept horses and carriages. When the streets were difficult because of snow, Verduin travelled by private horse-sleigh. A few surgeons owned a horse and a gig, these having estimated incomes between 2500 and 3500 guilders.[33] However, as appears from contemporary pamphlets and lampoons, such ostentation by a surgeon was disapproved of (cf. Fig. 63).

In the *Hollandsche Spectator* Justus van Effen complained in 1756 about the despicable urge among surgeons to live beyond the station in life in which God had placed them. In his article he reviles surgeons, known to him, 'who on Sundays are dressed like gentlemen and who, after the latest fashion, address one another in public by the title of Sir (mijnheer) and whose wives style themselves as Madam (juffrouw)'.[34]

Between the extremes of social affluence, there existed a group that managed fairly well with just a barber's shop and a surgical practice which they traversed on foot. The above- mentioned Abraham Titsingh makes a good example. As town surgeon he earned, on top of the income from his practice, a fixed annual salary of 175 guilders plus 25 guilders for expenses. He furthermore held the position of

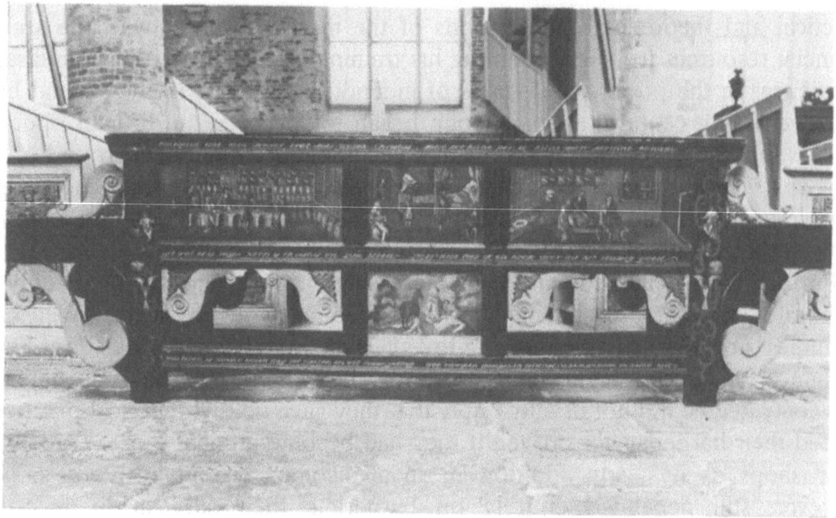

Fig. 59. Painted bier used by the surgeons and pharmacists of the small Frisian town of Workum. From left to right a pharmacy, a sick room and a trepanation scene which is evidently inspired by the vignette on the title page of *Medecynboec ende chyrurgie* by Joh de Vigo (Dordrecht 1614). In the lower middle the Good Samaritan.

surgeon to the admiralty, as well as to three orphanages and the old women's home. The tax collector assessed him for 1500 to 2000 guilders.[35] This income allowed him to live in a canal house on the Nieuwe Keizersgracht and upon his death in 1776 he was given, if not a splendid, at least a first-class funeral.[36]

One might well expect that the income of surgeons in the countryside was of more modest proportions than that of their city colleagues. The few available data confirm that suspicion. The diary and ledger of Philippe-Xavier Ceulemans (1733—88), which he kept from 1758 to 1788 for his practice in the village of Broechem — nowadays the municipality of Ranst in the province of Antwerp — reveal that his annual income was a little lower than that of a farm labourer, who usually earned about 260 guilders a year.[37] Naturally, the cost of living in the countryside was lower than that in the city. In the village of Durgerdam, a little north of Amsterdam, two surgeons appear to have earned a decent living with a population of 500 to 600. From the legacy of one of them, who bequeathed a house and some money to a total value of 1410 guilders, it would appear that he was moderately well off.[38] Both surgeons and physicians sometimes had other sources of income besides their practice.[39]

Relationship with Physicians

Notwithstanding the great professional prestige and evident affluence of a number of surgeons, the general public still saw a big difference in status between physicians and surgeons, 'who neither in knowledge nor good manners came up to the character of the physicians'.[40] Indeed, it was not unusual for physicians to be descended from well-respected, although not commonly the foremost families — or to be related to them by marriage — whereas surgeons generally were of a lower middle class descent. Physicians had been given a good education but their academic training was no guarantee of quality. The spectator-type periodical *De Philantroop* (The Philanthropist) complained that professors conferred the title of Doctor on the most stupid lads and roughest rakes with the same laudations with which they addressed the most well-behaved young gentlemen. For a few ducats it was possible to have one's dissertation written by so-called 'dispuutmakers' (disputation writers).[41] The number of physicians was still much smaller than the number of surgeons, so that they could rest assured of an ample income. Van Nierop's study reveals that in 1742 there were 58 Christian — that is non-Jewish — physicians in Amsterdam, of whom 27 had a yearly income of 2000 guilders or more.

As a counterpart to the surgeon with a doctor's degree in medicine, there appear from the middle of the seventeenth century physicians with an interest in surgery (cf. p. 128), which interest was no longer exclusively evidenced by writing books on surgical topics or prefaces to such books. Some physicians, such as the later professors of medicine Hieronymus David Gaub and Matthias van Geuns, even went to Paris to study anatomy, surgery and obstetrics. Others, like Cornelis Trioen in Leyden — the son of a surgeon who had taken a degree as doctor of medicine — were to specialize in surgery after graduating in medicine, sometimes combined with obstetrics. In Amsterdam Dr. Jan David Schlichting (1703—65) was sued in 1747 by the surgeons' guild because not only did he practise surgery but he also held a collegium anatomico-chirurgicum at his home. The defendant was acquitted, for a doctorate in medicine gave a person the right to a comprehensive practice; the only requirement was that the physician, on establishing himself, had to produce his degree certificate to the local Collegium medicum.[42] In the 'Voorreden' (preface) of his book *Traumatologia nov'antiqua* Schlichting called on physicians to take a greater interest in the practice of surgery: 'no city government, and even less a common trade or guild can impose rules on him'.[43] Surgery is 'much easier to know and to practise' than medicine, he argued, 'because it can be understood and known by means of one's sight and senses and requiring less powers of judgment'.[44] He advised surgeons not to be satisfied with the little they had learned and not to believe and adopt everything they had seen their teachers do, to study anatomy and to leave barbering to others.

Since the municipal lecturers in anatomy and surgery were traditionally always medicinae doctores, it is striking that some of them, for example Paulus de Wind in Middelburg, practised surgery and obstetrics without having taken the master surgeon's degree. This they probably did on the strength of the practice which they had acquired in Paris. It is noteworthy that Boerhaave did not hesitate to conduct minor operations himself when it suited his convenience.[45] In this he made a contribution to the eventual promotion of surgery as a decent profession for university men.

On the other hand it also happened that surgeons concerned themselves with the practice of medicine. This they did legally in villages and small towns without physicians, but sometimes also illegally in towns which had a physician. In 1742 Johannes de Gorter, professor in Harderwijk, argued for better relations between the two groups.

All this is evidence of the gradual start of a process that would lead to the ever increasing interweaving of these two related professions.

5.3.5.2. A Further Consideration of Surgery in a Few Dutch Cities and in the Countryside

After these general observations it is appropriate to cast a glance at a few individual Dutch cities and some of their prominent surgeons. Particularly in the first half of the eighteenth century Leyden and Amsterdam were still centres of European renown. On a smaller scale, The Hague, Rotterdam, and Middelburg were towns which also enjoyed a good reputation.

Leyden

Surgery at the university. Leyden owed its position to the quality of its university education in medicine under the great Boerhaave, which drew students from all over Europe, and even from America. Nevertheless, Boerhaave does not have a great significance for the history of surgery, even though in his *Aphorisms*, a work which was tremendously successful and which went through no less than 20 Latin editions outside Holland, he had something to say on the subject of wounds, bruises, dislocations, fractures, inflammations, abscesses and fistulae.[46]

Surgery, which did not appear as such on the university timetable until after 1700, continued to occupy an insignificant position in the Leyden curriculum until the end of the eighteenth century. Classes in this subject were taught by professors of anatomy. The lessons were of a wholly theoretical nature, and there were no practical exercises. Traditionally, however, courses on anatomy also included surgical aspects.[47]

While at the beginning of the century the professors Bidloo and Rau had gained great experience in surgery, their successors were primarily anatomists. During the professorates of Bernhard Siegfried Albinus (1721—1745), his younger brother Fredericus Bernardus Albinus (1747—70) and Eduard Sandifort (1771—1813) anatomy in Leyden flourished.[48] Dissection techniques reached a very high level of sophistication, illustrated by superb books and atlases. The casual collections of curiosities of the seventeenth century were substituted by systematic collections of specimens for teaching purposes. Particularly after the publication in 1761 of Morgagni's famous book *De sedibus et causis morborum*, interest in pathological anatomy grew in Leyden: it is probably no coincidence that it was in this town where a new reprint of this book appeared in 1778. The *Observationes anatomico-pathologicae*, a work in four volumes by Eduard Sandifort with magnificent illustrations, in scientific respects ranks a good second to that of Morgagni. A number of these observations concern surgical pathology (Fig. 60).

In 1791 Meinard Simon du Pui (1754—1834) was appointed professor extra-ordinarius chirurgiae practicae et artis obstetriciae. For the purpose of clinical instruction six beds were assigned to him in the ancient St. Caecilia Hospital, which can be seen as the first differentiation in the field of academic clinical tuition. In St. Caecilia Du Pui gave, as Petrus Camper had in Groningen, a 'Collegium causale chirurgicum', a regular clinical demonstration of outpatients. For the benefit of the pupils of surgeons he conducted classes in anatomy and

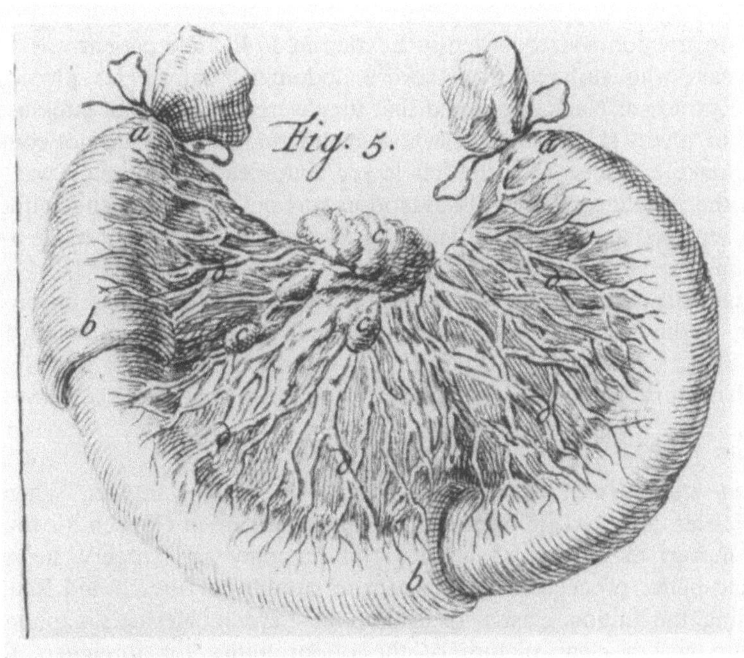

Fig. 60. A case of double intussusception, observed by Eduard Sandifort.

surgery in the Dutch language. Du Pui himself had acquired his practical knowledge in London — where he stayed for a year with the eminent surgeons John Hunter, Percivall Pott and Lowder — and subsequently in Paris, with Moreau, Pelletan, Louis and Desault. He had received practical training in obstetrics from the obstetrician Baudelocque in the Hospice de la Maternité.

Surgery in the guild. Existing in the shadow of the university, the Leyden surgeons' guild never came to full bloom.[49] The professors of medicine, who since the early years of the seventeenth century presided over the guild (see p. 109), among them Boerhaave in 1720, made little effort to improve the quality of the surgeons. The accounts that have been preserved show that, between 1669 and 1714, the opportunity to conduct anatomical dissections in the surgeons' hall (Fig. 42) was taken only six times. The unordered collection of curiosities was insignificant compared to those of the guilds in cities like Amsterdam, Rotterdam, Enkhuizen or The Hague: it was utterly useless for purposes of education. The guild did not have a library. The Leyden surgeon Alexander Balthazaar (1731—post 1793), who took his M.D. at the age of 53, describes his colleagues with great contempt in his *Heelkundige waarnemingen, inzonderheid van zwaare en moeielijke gevallen* (Surgical observations, in particular of serious and difficult cases) of which a second edition appeared in 1779; he accuses them of gross incompetence. At that time he had worked in Leyden for about 25 years and had witnessed a great deal of malpractice. He attributed this to poor training: surgeons did not profit from the flourishing of academic anatomy. Yet the first successful case of laparotomy for intestinal obstruction was recorded in Leyden in 1742. The patient was a woman of fifty years who suffered from severe abdominal pains. Her physician, the celebrated professor Nuck, suspected that they were caused by an intussusception. He called in 'a very skilful surgeon' whose name unfortunately has not come down to us, to make an incision in the left lower abdomen. The surgeon was then to draw out the intestines. The intussusception was quickly found and reduced, the intestines replaced and tbe abdominal wound sutured. The patient made a smooth recovery and lived for another twenty years.[50]

Although is is clear that there were a number of competent surgeons in Leyden — among whom was the well-known surgeon and obstetrician Jacobus Denijs (1681—1741), a distinguished lithotomist — it is beyond doubt that during the eighteenth century Amsterdam continued to be the centre of Dutch surgery.

Amsterdam

Amsterdam surgery seen through the eyes of a German student. When young Lorenz Heister, after having been a student of medicine in Giessen for four years, in 1706 moved to Leyden to improve his anatomy and surgery, he was told that he had better proceed to Amsterdam to study with Ruysch and Rau instead of attending the tuition classes of Bidloo in Leyden. Heister's experiences in Amsterdam give a clear picture of the opportunities for foreigners to study medical subjects in that city at the beginning of the century.[51] In spite of his advanced age the great Ruysch was still active. Together with Caspar Commelin he appears to have given practical lectures in botany in the beautiful Hortus medicus. At the time a knowledge of medicinal plants was still important for surgeons who, if necessary, had to compound their own ointments and wound potions. In the Theatrum anatomicum Ruysch gave public lectures on anatomy throughout the summer, making use of his famous specimens. Heister also attended the private collegia anatomico-chirurgica given by Ruysch and Rau.

Ruysch gave his private lessons largely through the medium of anatomical specimens, but if desired his students could conduct anatomical dissections themselves on human cadavers in the Binnengasthuis hospital.

The fee asked by the town surgeon Rau was considerable:[52] when Heister and a few others, including his compatriot Erndl and the Englishman Wickam enrolled with him, he charged no less than 100 'rijksdaalders' (250 guilders) each, half of which was to be paid in advance. Rau turned out to be a very unpleasant person who did not quite meet his commitments and who was unpleasantly vociferous when his pupils complained. Neither does Rau appear to have been a kind person from statements of other people. Nevertheless he was an outstanding anatomist and an excellent operator, very proficient in lithotomy.

Other prominent surgeons also offered students the opportunity to attend their operations (Fig. 61). Heister especially remembered those of Verduin (cf. p. 209) — whose name is also spelt Verduyn — and Verduin's son-in-law Gomarus van Bortel (1660—1724), a lithotomist of renown, and those of Adriaan Koenerdingh (1650—1710), who in speech and in print disagreed with Verduin's amputation method. From the list of the operations which Heister was able to attend in 1706 and 1707 there emerges a picture of what contemporary surgery involved:

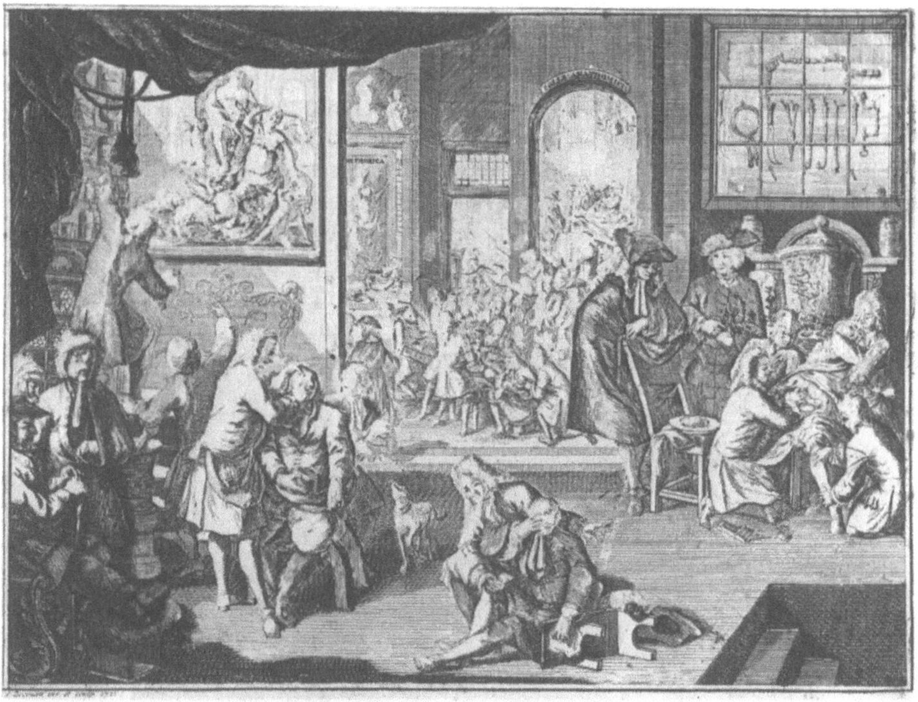

Fig. 61. Vignette of the Amsterdam surgeons' almanacs for 1731 and 1732, representing different aspects of surgical practice. From left to right: patients with sore extremities; the preparation of a medicament; an eye-operation; the drawing of a tooth; cutting for the stone. At the back a leg amputation and a patient being transported in a wicker stretcher. The wall painting on the left represents Aesculapius together with his daughter Hygeia, who is chasing the demons of disease. In the cupboard on the right, divers surgical instruments including a cutting clamp for mastectomy. On the floor behind the lithotomist a characteristic portable instrument case.

lithotomy, herniotomy, couching of cataracts, treatment of lacrimal fistulae, of symblepharon and other eye diseases, excision of cancer of the mouth and of the breast, removal of polyps and other growths, cutting the tongue-string, abdominal paracentesis for ascites, opening a 'dichtgegroeid achterste' (closed buttock: imperforate anus?). laying open of an anal fistula, incision of a festering finger, application of issues (small artificial ulcers) and setons (see p. 354 n. 44), treatment of wounds, ulcers, fractures and dislocations. Some of the operations mentioned belong to the 'grande chirurgie' of those days, but practised by only a few. Heister did not state the number of operations he witnessed. He did observe, however, that in Holland, as in his home country, good surgeons were much in the minority. During the summers of 1707 and 1709 he was eager to gain practical experience in the Dutch army, and took the opportunity on the bloody Belgian battlefields during the War of the Spanish Succession. Another, later well-known surgeon who used this war to acquire practical proficiency was Hendrik Ulhoorn (1687–1746).[53]

In the autumn of 1709 the war in the Southern Netherlands went into its winter recess, and Heister returned to Amsterdam with the intention of permanently establishing himself there. After taking his M.D. in Harderwijk he began a Collegium anatomico-chirurgicum in Amsterdam. His first course was attended by no fewer than ten French students, presumably expatriate Huguenots. In 1710 he was, however, appointed professor of anatomy and surgery at the university of Altdorf, near Nuremberg, and so he returned to his native country. The fruits of Heister's studies in Amsterdam were published in his *Compendium anatomicum* in 1717. This went through several editions, two in Amsterdam, and was for a long time the most popular book on anatomy at the West-European universities. His *Chirurgie* appeared one year later, originally in German but 'at the request of his Dutch friends', he soon had it rendered into Latin. It also appeared, with an extensive commentary, in a Dutch translation by the abovementioned Ulhoorn

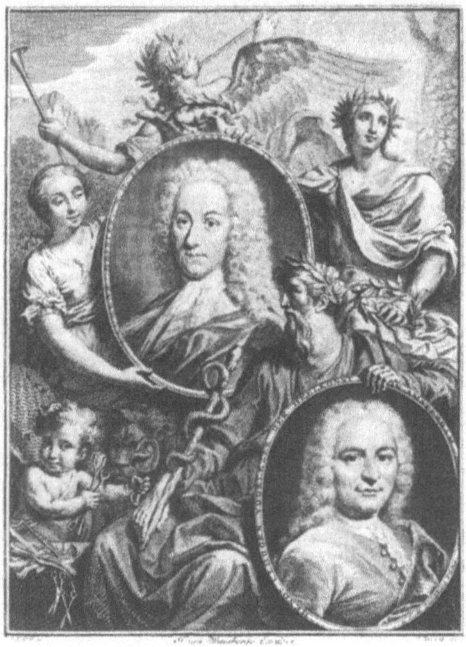

Fig. 62. Frontispiece of Ulhoorn's Dutch translation of Heister's *Chirurgie*. Heister's portrait is being held by Fame personified, Ulhoorn's effigy by Aesculapius. In the left lower corner a few qualities becoming a surgeon: courage (lion), prudence (serpent looking at itself in a mirror), diligence (bees), together with instruments held by the putto who also displays prudence.

(Fig. 62).[54] As both of them were contemporaries on the battlefields of Tournai and Malplaquet, it is quite possible that they knew each other personally, although there is no evidence for this. Heister's book, which also existed in an abbreviated version, was very popular all over Europe.[55]

Corruption in the Amsterdam guild. The Amsterdam corporation of surgeons did not remain free of the corruption prevalent in the eighteenth century.[56] This led in 1731 to the dismissal of the majority of the wardens when an investigating committee set up by the town corporation found them guilty of various types of malpractice. On the strength of sham examinations at high fees, they had admitted to the guild such people as barbers and Jews, excluded by the prevailing ordinance. The examination fees, as well as the entrance fees for the public dissections, found their way into the pockets of the wardens, who failed in their obligations to succour and support their sick colleagues and surgeons' widows; the collection of the taxation money of the wigmakers was farmed out to the guild's manservant and there was inadequate bookkeeping.

This scandal caused a great stir. A deluge of diatribes appeared for and against the dismissed wardens, sometimes with arresting titles like *De Clysteerspuit werksaam op de Amsterdamsche snykamer* (The clyster in operation on the Amsterdam dissection room); *Het kegel-spel, gespeelt op de Amsterdamsche snykamer* (Bowling, played in the Amsterdam dissection room). The controversy was sparked off by Abraham Titsingh, shortly after he was elected warden (Fig. 63).

Titsingh was one of the most colourful figures in the surgery of that time. Prior to establishing himself in his native Amsterdam he was for many years a ship's

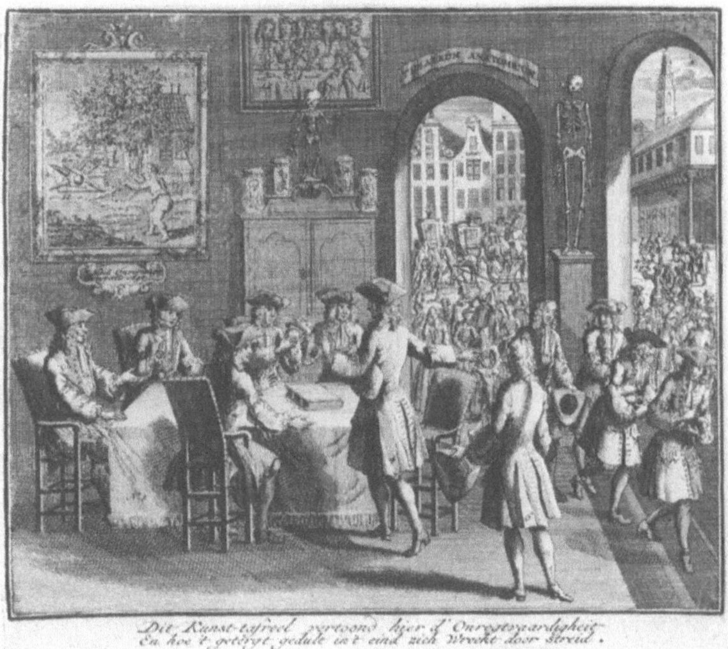

Fig. 63. Cartoon showing the characters of the corrupt wardens of the Amsterdam surgeons' guild in 1732. Five corrupt officers are seated at the table. Good Titsingh ('Brave Titsingh', no. 4), is refusing money offered to him as his share in the wrongfully collected examination and entrance fees, while pointing at wardens who are making for home with the money, stolen from the guild. Under the left archway, widows are wailing out their misery ('die om heur nooddruft schreeuwen'). In the background horses and carriages and a horse-sleigh owned by wealthy surgeons, now for sale. Beyond the right archway, the prison deserved by the corrupt wardens. The meaning of the painting on the wall, representing the bowling over of skittles, is unmistakeable.

surgeon, just like Solingen and Rau.[57] He had a good reputation, marked by his appointment as town surgeon and his attachment to various orphanages. He never received any teaching appointment, but he did give a private Collegium anatomico-chirurgicum. Basically he was a kind-hearted, honest man, but with a talent for antagonizing people by his sharp tongue and his arrogant, high-handed behaviour. He was a man of little education which later he did his utmost to remedy by self tuition. His numerous books show that he never quite succeeded in compensating for his early defective schooling. His vindictive nature is revealed in the frequent and unrelenting grudges he bore against persons and institutions. His enemies numbered Ulhoorn amongst them, a man who used to be his friend, but with whom he fell out on account of the proposal to send young surgeons to Paris in 1728 (see p. 157). Ulhoorn supported this idea, and with the rest was subjected to his ire. Nevertheless, Titsingh was inspired by a sincere desire to purge the guild of the abuses that had crept into it and to restore Amsterdam surgery to its former glory.

As dean of the new council he succeeded in restoring order (Fig. 64). The barbers who had been admitted illegally were given the opportunity to take a regular master-surgeon's examination. If they failed they were expelled on the reimbursement of their admission fees. The Jews were removed unconditionally.

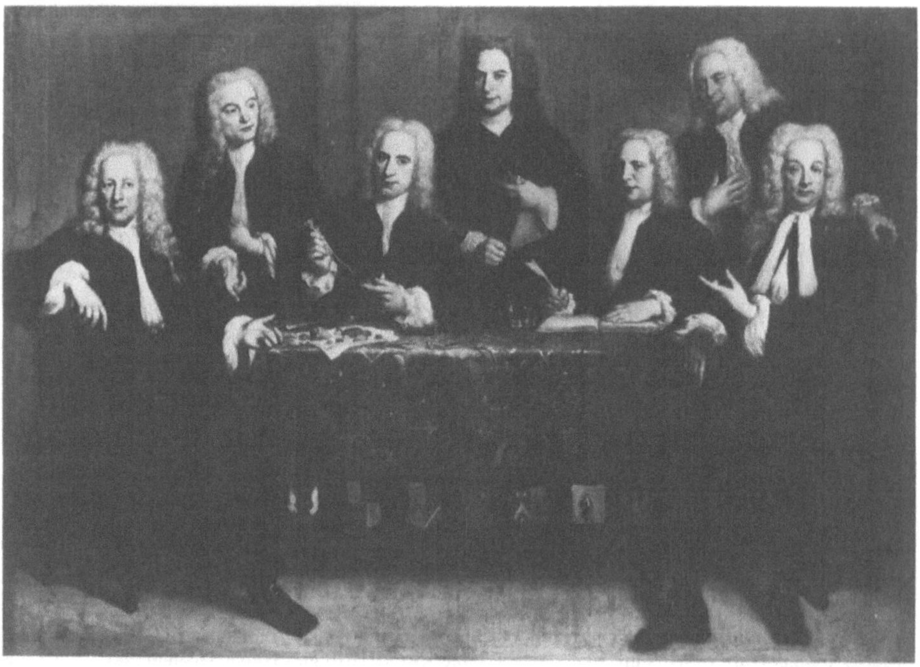

Fig. 64. The wardens of the Amsterdam Surgeons' Guild. The central figure is Abraham Titsingh. The officer sitting at his right side is the lithotomist H. Meyer, holding a lithotomy staff. On the table are seen other instruments as well as a collection of bladder stones. The other wardens are N. Craanmeester or perhaps P. Plaatman, L. Coster, A. Graver, J. Bekker and J. Lahrman.

Emancipation of obstetrics. In 1746 a new conflict arose in Amsterdam, this time between the surgeons led by Titsingh and the physicians of the Collegium medicum under professor Willem Roëll (1700—75), successor to Ruysch as instructor of anatomy. At stake was the right of surgeons to practise obstetrics. For centuries obstetrics had mainly been a matter between women. In the course of the eighteenth century, however, the male midwife ('vroedmeester') became of increasing importance. Male midwives were surgeons with a special interest in obstetrics, and they had often received further training in this subject abroad. Initially their task was confined to performing embryotomy when the child had died during labour before delivery. Increasingly, they became involved with assisted deliveries until, very gradually and hesitatingly, the caesarean section began to be performed on living women.

In the Netherlands instrumental delivery was introduced by the Amsterdam surgeon Hendrik van Roonhuyze with his use of the obstetric lever; he probably bought the instrument while travelling in England, from D. Chamberlen who, together with his sons, ran a successful obstetric practice in London. Roonhuyze tried to keep the shape and use of the lever a secret, which he sold to only a few, who in their turn resold it to only few, so that but a small number of obstetricians became familiar with it. Possessing 'the Roonhuyze secret' greatly enhanced one's status.[58]

In 1746 a prominent Amsterdam surgeon made an obstetric mistake with fatal consequences. For the Collegium medicum this was an excuse to advise the city council to prohibit the practice of obstetrics to all surgeons, with the exception of three 'Roonhuysians'. Titsingh, who was not among the three, appealed to the burgomasters, arguing that obstetrics was traditionally a part of surgery and should remain as it was. The city council, however, ruled that only those who had passed the relevant examination with the professor anatomicus and the inspectors of the Collegium medicum, were allowed to call themselves obstetricians. Probably as a consequence of Titsingh's zeal it was decided in 1749 that the obstetrician's examinations would be held — less disgracefully — by the professor anatomiae, the dean and the 'proefmeester' of the guild (see p. 109) and by two members of the Collegium medicum. Thus the obstetrician was granted official status as a specialized surgeon.

In 1749 Abraham Titsingh retired as dean of the Amsterdam guild and although he published several books, gradually faded into the background.

The Hague

Since 1591 The Hague had boasted its own surgeon's guild, named after Saints Cosmas and Damian. In 1629 it obtained a small two-storey building at the foot of the tower of the Jacob's Kerk, on the top floor of which an anatomical theatre was built. Among the professors who taught anatomy and surgery here, a few were of international renown, although this rested primarily on their anatomical writings: Anton Nuck,[59] Govert Bidloo (1649—1713)[60] and Thomas Schwencke (1694—1767).[61] Some of the other deserving figures from The Hague — Solingen, Cornelis Stalpart vander Wiel (1620—1702) — have already been mentioned on pages 132 and 134.

Utrecht

In both medicine and surgery, Utrecht was markedly overshadowed by Leyden and Amsterdam during the entire period of the Dutch Republic. Soon after the foundation of the university in 1636 the administration of the theatrum anatomicum, which moved house several times, was transferred from the surgeons' guild to the medical faculty. As in Leyden, the surgeons and their apprentices were admitted to the university courses on anatomy, and in both Utrecht and Leyden these courses were not very rewarding because of the students' insufficient command of Latin. Not until 1708 did they succeed in their requests for a course to be given in the 'Low German language'. The professor of anatomy at that time was Rudolf Leusden, M.D. (1671—1764), a skillful surgeon who until 1710 also served as the city lithotomist. He possessed a beautiful anatomical and surgical cabinet, which was much admired by Heister.[62] He produced only a few written works.

Harderwijk

At the time when Johannes de Gorter (1689—1762) was professor of medicine (1726—54) at the small Guelders university of Harderwijk, the doctorate of which was reputedly very easy, there was a period of modest prosperity. De Gorter seems to have been a good teacher who attracted many Dutch and foreign students. By the age of nineteen he was a master-surgeon and three years later he took his M.D. at Leyden. Being the only professor of medicine at Harderwijk, he taught all medical disciplines. From the outset De Gorter also gave extramural lessons — in Dutch — to surgical apprentices, on the subjects of anatomy and surgery. In 1751 he was given permission to teach surgery in the Dutch language at the university, too. In 1754 he accepted an invitation to go to St. Petersburg as court physician to the czarina. After four years, however, he returned to his native country and established himself in Wijk bij Duurstede.

He was the author of a number of much-used textbooks. One of these, *Compendium medicinae in usum exercitationum domesticarum digestum*, which in 1731 and 1737 was published in two volumes in Leyden, was translated into Japanese in 1792. Significant works for the history of surgery are *De gezuiverde heelkonst ter onderwijzinge van den leerenden en konstoeffenenden heelmeester t'zamengesteld* (The purged art of surgery compiled for the instruction of the student of surgery and of the practising surgeon) of 1731 and an adaptation of it, *Chirurgia repurgata, ab auctore recensita* of 1742. The latter work was not only published in Latin in Leyden and Vienna, but also in Dutch and Italian by three different publishers before 1785. It appeared in Spanish in Madrid, but curiously enough, never in German or French. The Dutch translation went through four editions. In the preface, addressed to 'the judicious reader' (Aan den bescheiden lezer) De Gorter explained that he wrote his book in his native language because 'the Netherlands are laden with thousands of surgeons and inquisitive souls all of whom have no command of the Latin language but are still in need of tuition'. He considered it objectionable that, as often happened, writers chose Latin in order to prevent 'the common people from entering into their secrets'. Such a practice was prompted by a thirst for power or money. An author must always have the intention 'to communicate what he knows to others'.[63] He had given his book the title 'Purged art of surgery' because in it he left out all unnecessary discourses. He had also omitted anatomical observations because there were already enough anatomy books in the Dutch language.

The *Gezuiverde heelkonst* is divided into nine books: the traditional pentateuch was thus abandoned. The first book gives a brief survey of general anatomy and general pathology. In pathology, he appears to follow his teacher Boerhaave. The ratio between the sizes of the particles which constitute the fluids and the diameters of the various tubes and small vessels through which the fluids are transported is of great significance for good health or illness. A further mechanistic line of reasoning is revealed in the view that a change in the shape of the particles of the fluid, which makes them sharp and pointed, is the cause of the pain which one feels with certain complaints.[64]

The classical four humours are still taught, but their significance is now primarily seen in the psychosomatic constitutional types. These 'temperaments' are related to each individual humour. Each one of the four temperaments is characterised by a specific bodily and moral build of the bearer, by peculiarities in his vital functions and his reactions to drugs. Finally they predispose a person for certain types of diseases: the sanguine temperament for inflammations or hot fevers, the bilious for erysipelas, the phlegmatic for oedema and for scirrhus, and the melancholic for scirrhus and cancer. To this extent the Galenic principles are still evident.

The following books deal successively with the bones and their defects (fractures and dislocations), the arteries, the veins, the brain and the nerves, more superficial disorders including wounds, glands, herniae and ulcers. The discussion of the subject-matter is largely practical: short descriptions of the organs and tissues in which the afflictions occur, and a short explanation of the pathology in its various manifestations.

The indications for the treatment to be adopted and its practical description — in the case of operations even step by step — are short and succinct, but pre-eminently clear and efficient.

At the end of each chapter there are a number of questions on its subject-matter, together with the correct answers, so that the reader can test his knowledge. Because of the deliberate absence of authors' names and source references and its compact form, this manual is in fact more or less a compendium. After the 442 pages of the actual manual there are another 200 or so pages with prescriptions for 359 different salves, powders, lotions, poultices, and so on. Numbers in the text refer to the prescriptions at the end of the book which allows the text to run on uninterruptedly, thereby gaining in clarity. The book concludes with an extensive index of subjects, which also serves as a vocabulary.

In the discussion of practical surgery in the next chapter of this book, De Gorter's *Gezuiverde heelkonst* will be referred to in more detail.

Middelburg, Goes, Zierikzee

Middelburg, which was cut off from Flanders as a result of the rebellion against

Philip II, had in the meantime developed into a flourishing mercantile town, being an important homebase of the East and West Indian Companies. Other Zeeland towns too, had attained great prosperity.

Around the middle of the seventeenth century the Middelburg hospital became instrumental in the training of surgeons because, as has already been mentioned on page 117, anatomical dissections were performed here.

The 'Collegium Anatomico-chirurgicum Medioburgense', a committee appointed by the city government and consisting of two surgeons and three physicians, more or less acted as a governing body for the local training course in anatomy and surgery.[65] In the eighteenth century the city lectureship was held for a period of more than forty years by father and son Helvetius, and during the second half of the eighteenth century by three members of the De Wind family in succession. All Middelburg lecturers held doctorate degrees in medicine from the university of Leyden.

The most important representative of the Middelburg lecturers was Paulus de Wind (1714—71). Prior to taking his doctoral degree he had studied in Paris. In his native town he held the posts of town surgeon, lithotomist, obstetrician and physician. In 1750, the year in which he became lecturer, he was also appointed surgeon and lithotomist of the province of Zeeland. These appointments were not just empty distinctions: De Wind practised surgery and obstetrics himself, and he also possessed the Roonhuysian secret. He was an eminent lithotomist who on one occasion had been summoned to Amsterdam to relieve the son of a colleague of bladder stones.[66] Neither did he hesitate to venture on other major operations. He performed a mastectomy on his own wife who suffered from cancer, unfortunately without being able to cure her.

In other Zeeland towns too, lectureships were instituted, although at a much later period.[67] In Goes in 1769 the town obstetrician Adriaan Huisman was raised to the rank of 'Anatomiae, chirurgiae et artis obstetricandi lector'. This appointment was probably a personal one, as a reward for his unselfish zeal in examining midwives. Only the instruction of midwives is mentioned in his educational tasks: surgeons were not included. After his death in 1785 the city of Goes did not appoint a successor.

In Zierikzee the city government had urged the trustees of the hospital as early as 1672 to 'provide for a suitable accomodation for anatomy', but there are no indications that the recommendation was adopted. It was not until 1768 that a lecturer in anatomy, surgery and obstetrics was appointed in the person of Jacques Rocquette (c. 1744—post 1800). Rocquette obtained his doctorate in Leyden several months after his appointment, with a surgical thesis called *De bubonocele in hernia inguinali.* Prior to his appointment in Zierikzee he had spent three years in France; in Rouen, no doubt with Le Cat, and in Paris with 'the first personal physician to the king'. The latter must have been Germain-Pichaut de la Martinière (1696—1783), a surgeon instrumental in effecting the emancipation of Parisian surgery by withdrawing it from the tutelage of the Medical Faculty.

Groningen

The university of Groningen, founded in 1614, had a medical faculty from the outset. On several occasions in the seventeenth and eighteenth centuries, however, Groningen did not have a professor of medicine. The Groningen faculty distinguished itself from those of Leyden and Utrecht by its instruction in the vernacular as early as the eighteenth century.

Anatomy languished in a very sorry state. It was only rarely that a human cadaver became available for public dissection. Anatomical collections were virtually non-existent. The dissecting room, which was furnished in a room adjacent to the Broerkerk in 1654, remained in use until 1829. The only time when the training in surgery received any impetus was when Wouter van Doeveren (1730—83) and Petrus Camper (1722—89) were connected with the faculty.

Van Doeveren had undertaken a study tour to Paris before taking his doctorate in Leyden. In Paris he attended the tuition classes of several surgeons, amongst whom were S.-F. Morand, De la Faye, Garengeot, Louis and Andouillé. Under Andouillé he had attended an operation course using the cadaver, which included lithotomy, and with the well-known obstetrician André Levret (1703—80) a course in the practice of obstetric manoeuvres using an obstetric mannikin. Not yet twenty-four years of age, he was appointed professor of anatomy, surgery and obstetrics in 1754.[68] It was not until Van Doeveren's appointment that the teaching of anatomy was taken seriously in Groningen: the new professor did not even hesitate to commit grave-robbery in order to obtain material. In 1756 Van Doeveren introduced academic training in obstetrics at Groningen. On the appointment of Camper in 1763, Van Doeveren had to surrender anatomy and surgery to his new colleague. In 1770 he left Groningen for Leyden.

Petrus Camper distinguished himself not only in the fields of anatomy, surgery and obstetrics, but also in those of zoology, physical anthropology, comparative anatomy and botany. He was undoubtedly the most versatile scholar which Holland produced during the age of Enlightenment: Goethe once called him 'ein Meteor von Geist, Wissenschaft, Talent und Tätigkeit'.[69] On top of that he was also a gifted draughtsman and was fluent in French, English, Italian and Latin, with a good reading knowledge of Greek. In 1746 he concluded his medical studies in Leyden with two doctorates on one and the same day, in philosophy — that is to say natural sciences — and medicine respectively. Both theses were written on the subject of the eye: the optics of vision and the physiology of various parts of that organ. During his studies he became greatly interested in obstetrics. He himself practised in this branch of medicine under Cornelis Trioen, M. D., a surgeon and obstetrician of Leyden as well as a lecturer and examiner of midwives (cf. p. 157). In 1748 Camper travelled to London primarily to attend a course in obstetrics under William Smellie. During this visit — Camper was in England altogether three times — he was introduced to other well-known British physicians, including William Hunter, Sir John Pringle and Sir Hans Sloane.[70] From London Camper went to Paris to take lessons with the famous surgeon Louis and the zoologist De Buffon. Under Louis he attended an operation course of three months in the Salpêtrière hospital, during the hot summer of 1749, about which his French host would later write:

I had been installed in Paris for more than five years at the head of the Salpêtrière, a division of the

Hôpital Général, where there were more than eight thousand persons. I had cadavers at my disposal at all times. The season of the year was never an obstacle to the demonstration of surgical operations, because, after very long conferences in which we discussed the need for an operation and the rules to be followed in different circumstances, we executed the procedure itself, often in less than a minute.[71]

In 1750 Camper accepted a chair in philosophy, anatomy and surgery at the university of Franeker in Friesland. In 1755 he was appointed to Amsterdam, where in the same year — perhaps in order to entice him — the city lectureship in anatomy and surgery was elevated to a chair in both subjects at the Atheneum illustre. In his inaugural speech, entitled *De anatomes usu in omnibus scientiis*, which only survives in manuscript, he argued, even before Morgagni, for the use of anatomy in establishing connections between the signs and the localisation and nature of diseases.[72]

As a result of Camper's joint appointment, his lectures at the Theatrum anatomicum were open to both surgeons and their apprentices as well as to medical students. On the payment of an extra fee he allowed his students to practise the performance of surgical operations as well as anatomical dissections on human cadavers.[73] He may have been inspired in this by the private school of anatomy of William Hunter (1718—83), which he had visited in London.[74]

After six years he left Amsterdam to settle on his wife's estate in Friesland. Here he prepared the edition of his *Demonstrationum anatomico-pathologicarum libri duo*, which Louis, with some overstatement, described as 'l'oeuvre le plus remarquable d'anatomie et de chirurgie de ce siècle'.

In 1763 Camper could not resist the call from Groningen, where he accepted the chair of anatomy, surgery, obstetrics, physiology, botany, and materia medica. It was during his Groningen years that Camper developed his major activities. With reference to his lectures the so-called 'collegium causale chirurgicum' should be mentioned, which he introduced into the Groningen curriculum in 1764. This course consisted of demonstrations on outpatients, but it is not known where it was held. Camper explained that for the benefit of his students he treated several external diseases in their presence. 'I also supplied the sufferers with medicaments, bandages, trusses, boots, iron corsets, etc. etc. giving the external medicaments free of charge to all those who came to this lecture. Each student paid four guilders if he had paid the entire lecture fee, or eight guilders, when he was dispensed from paying a tuition fee because he had attended the lecture-course three times already; I used to supply the deficiency out of my own pocket'. He continued this outpatient clinic until shortly before his departure from Groningen. About 500 patients are described in the registers that are extant.[75] After his voluntary resignation in 1773 he became more and more involved in politics, as a member of the Council of State in The Hague and an ardent Orangist. He travelled abroad on several occasions, once to Belgium, twice to Paris where in 1777 he gave lectures before the Académie de Chirurgie and the Académie des Sciences, to Germany where he was received by Frederick the Great, and to England for a third time.[76]

Petrus Camper is part of the audience in a rather caricaturist drawing by the English draughtsman Thomas Rowlandson. This drawing represents the dissecting room of the anatomy school of William Hunter in Great Windmill Street (Fig. 65).[77]

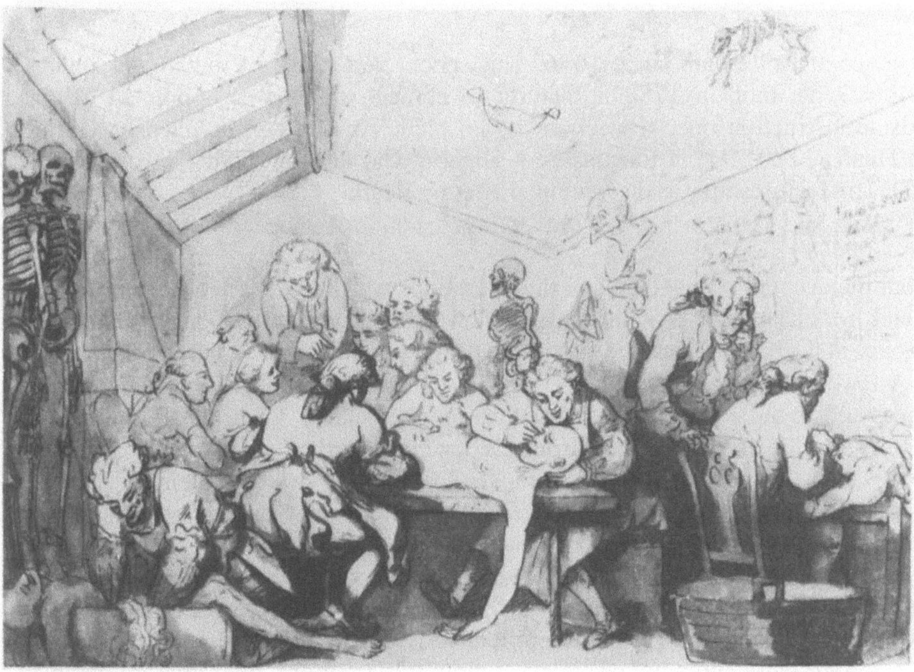

Fig. 65. Dissection room in William Hunter's School for Anatomy in Great Windmill Street, London. Mr. Hunter, wearing spectacles, is teaching from a somewhat elevated position at the back. The third student on his left, shown in profile, is believed to be Petrus Camper.

Camper published extensively, and some of his publications will be briefly discussed below.

The Groningen guild did not distinguish itself throughout the history of the Dutch Republic. Neither did the town ever appoint lecturers for the training of surgeons.

Rotterdam

The municipal lectureship in anatomy and surgery in Rotterdam was held from 1708 to 1790 by three members of the Vink family — all Leyden graduates. The first one, Willem Vink (c. 1680—1763), put together an extensive collection of anatomical specimens and 'curiosities' which for many years was the pride of the Rotterdam anatomical theatre. He was, moreover, the author of an illustrated textbook of anatomy.

In 1717 the apprenticeship period was extended to six years, whereas the examination for master-surgeon, apart from the traditional practical and theoretical parts, now came to include a clinical test in the hospital and the defense of a number of propounded theses.[27] Willem was succeeded by his nephew Pieter (1713—73), with whom we have already become acquainted because of his French sympathies (see p. 157). Apart from his translation of De la Faye's comments on Denis, Pieter deserves credit for establishing a co-operative lending pool for surgical instruments (see p. 254). His son Hendrik, who succeeded him in 1765, received the title of honorary professor at the Illustrious School which had been in existence at Rotterdam since 1636. This school was never of much consequence for medicine until, in 1788, a lecturer of clinical survey was appointed to give bedside instruction once a week in the hospital. This office was filled by Gerard ten Haaff (1720—91), a former army-surgeon who later in his life was promoted M.D. This lectureship was discontinued after his death.

The Country

From the account on page 167 of the operations which Lorenz Heister was able to attend in Amsterdam in 1706 and 1707, we gained an impression of what a city practice at the beginning of the eighteenth century could imply.

A few surviving account books afford a glimpse of surgical practice in smaller places and in the country. The diary covering the years 1758 to 1788 (see p. 162) kept by the surgeon Ceulemans from the Southern Netherlands town of Broechem shows that 25 per cent of his practice dealt with the treatment of injuries. Fractures, with about 12 per cent, were clearly important, and those of the collar bone and the lower leg were most prevalent. The actual number of fractures which this surgeon treated in the course of some twenty-six years however, is not more than 82. It is striking that he performed the caesarean section eight times, although it is not clear whether the patients were already dead or alive. The practice of this one country-surgeon may well have amounted to more than that of many a surgeon established in a city.

The surgeon Anthony Egberts (17?—1778), who practised in the North Holland village of Durgerdam, was mainly active in the treatment of wounds, ulcerations, including abscesses and ulcers, and swellings, but he also extracted teeth. In the course of forty-four years he only incidentally treated fractures of the lower leg, the ankle, the patella, the clavicule and only once a femoral shaft fracture in a child. In the absence of a resident physician in Durgerdam, he also practised medicine.[78]

5.3.5.3. Surgery in the Latter Days of the Republic

The Professional Level

In the evaluation of the level of practical surgery in any period, the results will differ as one focuses either on its prominent exponents or on the rank and file. As the latter group has always been the larger of the two, it would undoubtedly have been foremost in the critical eye of the public. This of course holds for every profession.

Complaints about the low professional level of surgeons could be heard in a variety of keys throughout the eighteenth century. Not only in medical publications, but also in the critical lay press: in the spectatorial magazines which are so characteristic of the Enlightenment. These magazines, by the way, also heavily criticized the manner in which many physicians chose to perform their duties.

The number of surgeons who attempted major operations must have been very small. In his preface to the *Aanmerkingen op de chirurgicaale operatien van den heere Dionis*, which he had translated (see p. 157), Pieter Vink complained in 1740, that many operations described in that book were hardly, if ever performed in Holland. Petrus Camper regretted in a speech made in Amsterdam on 15 March 1759: 'In this populous city, how seldom are there ever operations of any import? Not even four times a year is a lithotomy performed, and even then there are foreigners among those performing the operations. Not as much as once every four years is an arm or a leg amputated! Not as many as six times is a breast amputated with the likely prospect of success! Cutting strangulated herniae ('verstropte breuken') is not often performed either'.[79] At that time Amsterdam had a population of around 200 000 people.

In Paris, which had about 560 000 inhabitants, conditions were not all that different. Of the 300 members of the guild of Saint-Côme in 1743, there were only five who practised 'grande chirurgie'. The rest made a living out of minor surgery, but because there was not enough for all, and only a few kept barber's shops, the surgeons in Paris more and more took up the practice of medicine.[80]

Critical Observations of two Professors

Near the end of the century two professors chose the condition of Dutch surgery as the subject of a lecture. The first one was delivered by professor Bonn in Amsterdam in 1793 on the occasion of a prize distribution, the second one in 1797 by professor Mulder on accepting the chair of anatomy, surgery and obstetrics in Franeker. In both cases the speech was delivered in Dutch instead of the customary Latin.

Andreas Bonn (1738—1818) was descended from a wealthy family. He obtained his doctorate in Leyden in 1763 with an anatomical thesis, entitled *De continuationibus membranorum*, with which he entered the new field of histology. After having studied anatomy and surgery for a year in Paris, he settled in his native town, where he was appointed professor of anatomy and surgery in 1771.

In his speech of 1793 at the prize distribution, entitled 'On the present state of surgery and obstetrics in our native country',[81] Bonn lamented that other nations had entirely overshadowed the Netherlands in the fields of surgery and obstetrics. Whilst the flow of foreign publications was eagerly received, deserving compatriots on the other hand were hardly appreciated. The low standard of education was largely to blame for the relatively inferior position of Dutch surgery. Whoever was not fortunate enough to have a surgeon for a father and so receive a thorough training in the profession, had to learn surgery much in the way one learned a craft, with the barber's shop acting as his workplace. A young surgeon was extremely fortunate if his master was one of those skilled surgeons of which there were a number in the Netherlands. These, either as town surgeons or attached to charitable institutions and parish poor-relief boards, had the capacity to enable their pupils to acquire practical experience under their guidance and supervision. In other countries, where there were no, or at any rate fewer such charitable institutions, the hospitals were the nurseries of surgery. In Holland too, several surgeons who were attached to city hospitals would allow pupils of other surgeons to attend special operations, but, as with the public demonstrations in anatomy and surgery, which were given by dedicated masters, they failed to arouse the interest of the young, or eclipse the bad examples of some surgeons unworthy of the name.

Foreign colleges of surgery — Bonn probably had the Collège de Chirurgie of Paris in mind — attracted both young physicians desiring to qualify as surgeons as well as prospective surgeons wanting access to knowledge unavailable in the Netherlands. Bonn approved of a recent proposal made in Germany, to establish special schools for country surgeons and obstetricians.[82]

Johannes Mulder (1769—1810) came from a prominent Franeker family. He studied medicine in Leyden, but interrupted his studies for a year in order to observe medical practice in the large teaching hospitals in London. He became an honorary member of the Medical Society of Guy's Hospital. Back in Leyden, he took his degree as doctor of medicine. His thesis on the history of the obstetric forceps and lever was translated into German.

In his inaugural lecture Mulder analyzed the reasons underlying the negligible contribution of the Dutch to the improvement and expansion of surgery and obstetrics. He pointed to lithotomy, amputation and artificial deliveries as examples of surgical operations in the development of which the Dutch had taken no part.[83] He then went on to consider three issues.

1. Are the Dutch at all temperamentally suited to practise surgery and obstetrics;
2. Is there sufficient opportunity in the Netherlands to receive a thorough training in these subjects;
3. Are those who may call themselves surgeons and obstetricians sufficiently protected and are inexperienced practitioners adequately barred by the government from practising the profession?

On the basis of Celsus' well-known statement about the requirements of a good surgeon in courage, firmness, composure, and friendliness, Mulder came to the conclusion that Dutch surgeons certainly qualify.

Thorough instruction meant that the future surgeon should be trained in anatomy, physiology and also pathology by study of the cadavers of those who died from disease. Furthermore he ought to receive tuition in pharmacology and, of course, in operative surgery with its indications, and in bandaging. The last two were to be practised diligently on cadavers. Finally the student must attend upon his master when he was treating his patients.

In order to learn the practice of surgery as efficiently as possible, the student should visit hospitals made suitable for that purpose. This was equally necessary in obstetrics, which is really a part of surgery, though usually practised independently. Unfortunately there did not exist in Holland any opportunity to receive such a training in surgery or obstetrics. Subjects which could be of importance to future surgeons and obstetricians were taught in Latin at the universities, as a result of which they were not understood by these students. Here and there lecturers provided tuition using the vernacular, but there were no training colleges for surgeons and obstetricians as such. Although there were surgeons, obstetricians and midwives in the Netherlands who were in no sense inferior to their foreign colleagues, their number was far exceeded by incompetent practitioners.

The question finally whether the government took sufficient measures against quacks, was again answered by Mulder in the negative, although there did exist a few laws which prohibited the unqualified practice of surgery.

suited to practise surgery and obstetrics, but it was both the lack of regular training and adequate monitoring of the required skills which were obstacles in the way of developing these professions.

Mulder concluded his inaugural lecture with an appeal to the citizens' representatives — for we are now two years into the Batavian Republic — to take appropriate measures to eliminate the abuses described by him. He included the abolition of Latin and the establishment of university hospitals as two important measures which he felt ought to be taken.

A year after this inaugural lecture Mulder caused a sensation by performing the first successful hip disarticulation on a patient (see p. 214). In 1801 he went to Groningen, where, in the small university hospital already founded in that city in 1797, he established departments for surgery and obstetrics. He died of infection from a puncture of the antrum Highmori which he had performed on himself.

Measures to Arrest the Decline of Surgery

New anatomical theatres. On the whole there was a general recognition of the fact that national surgery had fallen into a rather poor state. It was also recognized that its cause lay in the inadequate method and standards of training. There were attempts at improvement: for instance in Rotterdam where, in 1759, a fine new anatomical theatre was built for Pieter Vink who, as a fervent advocate of French surgery, introduced in his lessons the latest surgical notions.[84] As late as 1770 Alkmaar built its first surgical theatre, while in 1799 there appeared a similar facility in Haarlem, the last old-style theatre to be built in the Netherlands. It may have already been constructed in 1788, the year when Meinard Simon du Pui, later to become professor of practical surgery in Leyden, was appointed city lecturer in anatomy, surgery and obstetrics in Alkmaar. On the occasion of this appointment Du Pui was given the title of professor.[85] However laudable such attempts at the improvement of the standards of education may have been, they were nevertheless not very effective. The guild system as such remained intact and with it the traditional apprenticeship system as the basis of surgical training. It was therefore difficult for new ideas to take root. This state of affairs was the more oppressive as in the second half of the eighteenth century a major change in the structure of surgery began to take place, a change from practical art towards applied science. This change was represented in Great Britain in the person of John Hunter, in Germany by Richter and in France by the work of the Academy of Surgery.

Society for the Advancement of Surgery. A society with the specific aim of promoting surgery was founded in Amsterdam in 1790. It was born out of an informal society ('weekelijks kunstkweekend gezelschap') in which the better surgeons in weekly meetings had been attempting for the previous twenty years to increase their knowledge and experience through an exchange of views. The driving force and chairman of the new society was Andreas Bonn, while David van Gesscher for years acted as its secretary.

David van Gesscher (1735—1810) was also born and bred in Amsterdam. A student of Camper, he was a skillful surgeon with a large practice, while he also acted as surgeon of St. Pieter's Hospital or Binnengasthuis. Although he had received no university training, he was a cultured, widely-read man, who knew French, German and Latin. He published a great number of articles in the transactions of the Dutch scientific societies, and appears to have been a member of all four of them. He was also the author of no less than thirteen books and monographs, four of which — on amputations, chronic swellings, the surgery of Hippocrates and spina bifida respectively — also appeared abroad in a German translation, his most important publication is *Hedendaagse oeffenende heelkunde* which appeared in three voluminous parts between 1781 and 1786. The influence of the French surgeon Louis — Camper's Paris preceptor — is unmistakable.

In the memorial which Bonn and Van Gesscher addressed to the burgomasters of the city for the endorsement of the new society, they wrote that it hoped 'if possible to raise the fame of Dutch surgery, which had often caught foreign attention because of its more simple directions and treatment, to a level which would sometime enable it to equal the College of Surgery in Paris'.[86] This aim was to be pursued by arousing in surgeons an ardour for scientific work. The society proposed to stimulate this interest by organizing competitions, a common practice in those days. Gold medals worth 30 ducats were to be offered to the prize winners. The *Verhandelingen van het Genootschap* (Transactions of the Society) which were to be published annually, would offer scope for the publication of important communications whereas the *Prijsverhandelingen* (Prize Transactions) would contain the prize-winning essays. In all this the 'Académie royale de Chirurgie' clearly set the example.

That the founders were serious about the high academic level of the society is illustrated by the fact that only five Amsterdam surgeons were among the early members. As the society was to bear a national character, professors, lecturers and other prominent surgeons from all over the country were invited to join. Many accepted the invitation, and the society began its activities with 36 members.[87] Already in 1791 the first competition was awarded with gold. The contributors had been invited to discuss 'the nature and the causes, symptoms and effects of 'kropgezwellen' (scrophulae) in the neck and elsewhere, a common affliction in our country'. The prize-winner was Willem Leurs, surgeon-major in the Personal Guard of His Serene Highness, the Lord Prince of Orange and Nassau, etc.

Abolition of the Surgeons' Guilds

Three years after the peaceful revolution of 1795, as a result of which the Republic of the United Provinces was transformed into the Batavian Republic, a joint constitution was effected after considerable political upheaval and French military intervention. In article 53 of this first ever national constitution the guilds amongst other relics of the Middle Ages, were abolished. Nor did this come as a surprise to those corporations.

The Amsterdam surgeons' guild had been active in reviewing the regulations, with the particular aim of improving educational standards. David van Gesscher, who repeatedly acted as warden and dean of the guild in those troublesome years, made supreme efforts to that end. But all to no purpose. At the end of February 1798 the municipal government of Amsterdam simultaneously abolished the surgeons' guild — which in the eighteenth century liked to call itself 'Collegium Chirurgicum' — and the Collegium medicum.[88] They were substituted by a 'Committee of Medical Supervision for Amsterdam and its jurisdiction' (Commissie van Geneeskundig Toeverzigt), composed of physicians, surgeons and pharmacists, with roughly the same powers of the earlier guild administration and Collegium medicum put together. The possessions of the guild were transferred to the city authorities, with the exception of the Surgeons' Widows Fund. That Fund gained its independence and still exists today. The days prior to the suppression of the corporations must have been full of excitement, but the minute books of the Amsterdam guild have left no traces of it. There is even no mention of the municipal council ruling on the abolition. The last minute entered into this book, dated 16 February 1798, records the permission granted to the widow of J. Harting to practise as a tooth-drawer. Earlier minutes give evidence of the political emancipation of the Jews, one of the effects of the Batavian revolution which led to their admission to the surgeons' corporation.

Van Gesscher sat on the new committee. Bonn could not reconcile himself to the new state of affairs and resigned as professor of anatomy of the Athenaeum, which included the office of instructor in that subject to the surgeons. He was succeeded by Gerard Vrolik (1775—1859), who in spite of his youth already held the chair of botany at the Athenaeum. He now was appointed professor of anatomy, physiology and obstetrics. In order better to perform the last mentioned teaching commitment he was granted a few beds in the Binnengasthuis hospital, which made Vrolik the first Dutch professor to have an obstetric clinic.

The daily surgical routine was hardly affected by the Batavian revolution. One of the first questions the Amsterdam Committee of Medical Supervision was confronted with concerned the desirability of a separation of barbering from the practice of surgery. It initially decided in the affirmative, but on further consideration it concluded 'for various weighty reasons' to leave things as they were. In Franeker the separation had already been effected by that time.

5.3.5.4. The Netherlands as French Vassal State and Part of the Napoleonic Empire

Political and Social Aspects

The Batavian Republic, a product of the ideals of the Enlightenment, was in fact a French vassal state. Bound to France in an offensive and defensive pact, the Republic soon entered into war with England, which led to massive losses in merchant ships seized by the British. This war also cost the Republic nearly all her colonies. The Peace of Amiens of 1802 was only short-lived, and hostilities were resumed in 1803. Once again the colonies which had only just been returned were lost to Great Britain, which after the victory of Trafalgar held unchallenged supremacy over the seas.

In domestic politics too, the overriding influence of France made itself clearly felt. The various constitutions which succeeded each other from 1798 on, were invariably modelled on those of France, in which country they were the products of the gradual development from a democratic republic to a despotic empire. While in 1804 the French Empire was born, this country in 1806 substituted the Batavian Republic by the 'Kingdom of Holland', with a brother of the French emperor Napoleon as its crowned head.

This kingdom, however, was granted only a short life. The Dutch king was less willing to be kept in French leading-reins than his powerful brother in Paris had wished. In 1810 he abdicated, whereupon Napoleon annexed the Netherlands as part of the French empire. The 'Continental System', which Napoleon had introduced with the intention of isolating England economically, was now also strictly followed in Holland. This system implied that all trade between England and the continental countries dominated by France, was prohibited. Since trade was vital for the Dutch, the introduction of this system had disastrous effects on their economy. Conscription — new to the Netherland, which formerly had always employed mercenaries — drafting young men into the army by a system of drawing lots, censorship of the press and vigorous police supervision, excited great discontent.

Against these disadvantages, however, there were also a number of salutary government measures, including the introduction of the Registry of Births, Marriages and Deaths and the French legal codes, products of the organizational genius of Napoleon. An injuction was furthermore issued forbidding intramural burials in churches, and cowpox vaccination was introduced. The legal codes remained in force in several countries for some time after Napoleon's downfall. The *Code Pénal*, with occasional modifications, remained in use in the Netherlands until 1886. This code has been of importance for medicine because it penalized the violation of professional secrecy by physicians, surgeons, pharmacists and midwives.

Training in Surgery after the Suppression of the Guilds

For surgery the twenty years of political subservience to France involved a period of stagnation if not deteriotation. Plans seem to have been made during the period of the Batavian Republic for the foundation of surgical schools, which were to provide training on a more methodical basis than had been possible in the traditional master-apprentice relationship with its occasional padding of lectures and demonstrations at the Theatrum anatomicum, but these plans failed to materialize. Everything therefore remained more or less the same, with the only difference that from 1801 onward, the examinations were held by the Departmental Committees of Medical Administration (Departementale Commissies van Geneeskundig Bestuur), introduced that year, instead of by the wardens of the defunct surgeons' corporations. Before the newly-fledged surgeon was admitted to practice, he was required to take an oath before this Committee, inspired by that of Hippocrates.[89]

When David van Gesscher was appointed lecturer in theoretical surgery (beschouwende heelkunde) after professor Bonn's resignation, he wrote three compendia 'for the use of his audience'. Student-surgeons had therefore access to a certain amount of official material. The pathology which Van Gesscher set out in his *Schets der heelkundige ziektekunde* (Outline of surgical pathology) (1803), involves an amalgamation of elements taken from late eighteenth century patho-physiological doctrines — not discussed in this book — in which a great deal of prominence was given to such notions as 'stimulus' and 'counter-stimulus' and to vitalism. The sthenic and asthenic diseases of Hoffmann are also included. It is important to note that Van Gesscher counts 'contact with infectants' (smetstoffen) among the external causes of surgical diseases in particular.[90] He does not commit himself on the nature of these infectants, however. It is to be doubted whether Van Gesscher's modest textbooks ever gained great popularity as it seems that no-one ever referred to them.

The demonstrations at the anatomical theatres did not amount to much during the first decades of the nineteenth century. Around the turn of the century student surgeons in Rotterdam lodged a complaint with the Minister of National Education against their anatomy reader, Johannes Ripping, M.D., because he would only very occasionally acquit himself of his teaching commitments. The Rotterdam theatre looked neglected when Dr. Eduard Meiszner, a physician from Töplitz, once visited the premises.[91] It was not in use, and trousers were left to dry on the dissecting table. The glass cases held a collection of the most heterogenous objects, including some sorry injection specimens and mouldy abortions along with stuffed birds and curiosities such as the shoe of the Giant Farmer of Lekkerkerk, a Moor's penis and the hairy hand of a 'savage man'. Both quantitatively and qualitatively this conglomeration must have been but a weak reflection of the original large collection, of which the printed catalogue of 1740 contains 328 items taking up sixteen pages, not counting the minerals.

The Medical State Settlement of 1804

The continuation in the interim of training in surgery along traditional lines did not imply that the government in The Hague was blind to the necessity of creating some measure of order in educational standards and health care. Far from it, because in 1804 this government effected an important medical settlement, the first one ever introduced in this country. This settlement was long-lived: until Thorbecke's laws of 1865 the practice of medicine in the Netherlands was largely based on it. The Medical State Settlement (Geneeskundige Staatsregeling) of 1804 continued to distinguish between two different classes of practitioners of medicine. The first category, those with a university education, now contained three sub-divisions: doctors of medicine, doctors of surgery and doctors of obstetrics. For each of these three qualifications the taking of a separate doctoral degree was required, and while it was possible to obtain more than one degree, the doctorate in medicine was prerequisite. The doctoral degrees in surgery and obstetrics were based on theses and could be taken a few days up to some months after the medical degree was obtained. They did not carry practical qualifications.

The second category which the Settlement of 1804 distinguished, was that of the surgeons. This was subdivided into city surgeons, country surgeons and obstetricians (stadsheelmeesters, plattelands-heelmeesters en vroedmeesters). Government control of health care in its several aspects was entrusted respectively to the Departmental Committees of Medical Enquiry and Supervision (Departementale Commissies van Geneeskundig Onderzoek en Toevoorzigt) — formerly the Departmental Committees of Medical Administration — and the City or Local Committees of Medical Supervision.

The Departmental Committees were charged with checking of the qualifications of those wishing to establish themselves in their provinces, organization of the extra-mural examinations, supervision of medical practice and with fighting of epidemics. Until French laws were enforced after the annexation in 1810, doctors of surgery too, had to have taken an examination with the Committee of Medical Enquiry in the department in which they wished to set up a surgical practice.[92] The Local Committees were required to supervise the observance of general and local ordinances and medical tuition, insofar as it took place in the vernacular. They also had to take measures in case of epidemics, and to supply the Departmental Committees with all necessary information. The members of the Departmental Committees were appointed by the central government. Local Committees had to be instituted by the municipality in places with at least four practising physicians.

Incorporated into France

After the annexation of Holland into Napoleon's French Empire in 1810, the Amsterdam Athenaeum and the Utrecht university were degraded to 'écoles secondaires', while both Franeker and Harderwijk, in 1811 and 1812 respectively, were entirely suppressed. Only Leyden and Groningen retained their university status by being appointed 'Académies de l'Université Impériale'.

Even in those difficult times there were in Holland a few eminent professors, especially Bleuland in Utrecht and Brugmans in Leyden. Jan Bleuland (1756—1838) taught anatomy, physiology and obstetrics to medical students, and to surgical apprentices and midwives surgery and obstetrics using the vernacular. He was personal physician to king Louis Napoleon. In the troublesome years 1811—1815, when the former university lead a poor existence, he did his utmost to preserve educational standards. Together with his very proficient collaborator Petrus Koning, he put together an anatomical collection of more than 2000 specimens. This collection was later acquired by the government for the Anatomical Museum in Utrecht, part of which is still on display. Bleuland wrote several superbly illustrated anatomical works.[93]

Justinus Sebaldus Brugmans, M.D. (1763—1819) was professor of botany at Leyden from 1786, in 1787 adding natural history, and from 1800 onward including chemistry. He was greatly interested in wound treatment and distinguished himself as Inspector General of the army medical service, which post he filled from 1795 as well as his professorship. More about him on pages 276 and 290.

Practical Surgery in the Seventeenth and Eigtheenth Centuries

6.1. GENERAL INTRODUCTION

In the two preceding chapters we have presented a social history of surgery in the seventeenth and eighteenth centuries, particularly although not exclusively concerned with the Netherlands. These were illustrated with representive features of works by the surgical authors whom we discussed.

In the present chapter we shall again consider the seventeenth and eighteenth centuries, but this time the intention is to give a more coherent impression of a few representative aspects of surgical practice within that period. Our survey of current texts will include soft part injuries and their treatment, bone and joint surgery including fractures and dislocations, orthopaedics and amputations, head injuries, vascular surgery, tumours, herniae, bladder stone and resuscitation.

6.2. SOFT PART INJURIES

6.2.1. *Introduction*

Before the introduction of antisepsis, treatment of traumatic lesions was the chief part of the surgeon's occupation. This subject therefore continued to command much interest as appears for instance from numerous and at times quite extensive articles in the *Mémoires de l'Académie de Chirurgie*. The wars which the Republic fought on land and sea are reflected in the case histories one finds in the Dutch medical literature: war wounds or the later results of them are by no means rare.

6.2.2. *The Natural Healing Processes*

In 1735, De Gorter described the normal healing process as follows:

1. little by little the edges separate further;
2. the haemorrhage comes to a standstill because the cut vessels withdraw and the extravasated blood forms a clot which fills up the cavity;
3. after one day some red fluid is being produced;

4. the edges become red and painful, swell and curl up, this is accompanied with thirst, some fever and a feeling of heat;
5. on the third or fourth day pus appears while redness, warmth and swelling diminish;
6. starting at the bottom the wound is now gradually being filled with flesh having a sky-blue or white, soft, even border;
7. the wound is covered by skin.[1]

Towards the end of the century John Hunter in his *A treatise on the blood* etc., one of the classics in this field, stressed the importance of the haemorrhagic clot filling the wound cavity in the first instance. Herein small vessels come into being, while the red components of the clot in course of time are being resorbed. What remains is 'plastic lymph' which brings about healing by first intention. Pus appears only when the edges remain separated for too long a time. The significance of Hunter's work was appreciated only in the nineteenth century.[2]

6.2.3. *Treatment of Fresh Wounds*

6.2.3.1. Haemostasis

It was as yet far from clear how nature herself brings about haemostasis which was the reason why Solingen performed the animal experiments referred to on page 104. In this context, Jean-Louis Petit emphasized the formation of a lymphatic plug or clot by which the damaged blood vessel would first be closed and subsequently healed.[3] This contention gave rise to quite some discussion. Some held that the formation of a thrombus was not possible at normal body temperature and that such plugs would only come into being after dealth. Others ascribed spontaneous haemostasis to pressure on the vessel exercised by extravasated blood amassed in the perivascular tissues. There also was a difference of opinion on the question of whether the formation of a thrombus was a necessary preliminary stage in the healing process of the vessel.

There was no unanimity either on the best way of checking bleeding by artificial means. The methods preferably used way into the eighteenth century were compression — strongly recommended by Petit as support of natural thrombus formation — thermocautery with redhot irons and styptic medicines (Fig. 66).

Pressure could be applied in several ways. Usually compression bandages were being employed after the wound-cavity had been filled up with lint and pledgets — of which more hereafter — dipped in some astringent. There existed furthermore all sorts of apparatus with which it was possible accurately to apply pressure on particular arteries. More than once records mention continued digital pressure. An interesting example occurs in Roonhuyze. He once stopped an obstinate arterial haemorrhage of the frenulum penis, resulting from an erosion of chancre treated with red precipitate, by digital compression maintained for eight days. For this he had hired two journeymen tailors who were used to sitting cross-legged, relieving each other every three or four hours.[4]

Irons used for haemostasis in the eighteenth century no longer had the big, round, flat head with which a large area of tissue could be scorched, but a much smaller, olive-shaped one suitable for accurate burning of individual blood vessels.

Agents arresting the flow of blood, styptics or astringents, were given in quantity, often as complex powders. Many of their constituents we came to know when looking into Antiquity and the Middle Ages, but doubts with regard to the efficacy of medicaments like finely chopped hare's fur or usnea: moss that had grown on a human skull, was increasing.[5] Such wound powders were applied either on tents — turunda, turon, steekwiek — or on pledgets — pulvibus, plumaceola, platte wiek — which had first been dipped into white of egg. A tent consisted of a somewhat cylindrical tuft of linen threads of about equal length, placed lengthwise to each other, halfway along their length bound together with a thread. By this thread, which was left long to be carried out at the wound, the turunda could be removed. A turunda particularly for arresting haemorrhage could also consist of a bit of bovista or alum or blue vitriol wrapped into fine cotton attached to a thread. A pledget likewise consisted of teased-out linen but now arranged as a flat piece of lint.

The vascular ligature was by no means in general use in the early eighteenth century. It was feared that the thread might slip off or might cut the vessel wall. Indeed, secondary haemorrhage caused by an infected thread would not have been a rare occurrence at a time when purulent wounds were the rule rather than the exception. If it was employed at all, it was usually done by undersewing. This of course entailed the risk that adjacent nerves were strangulated as well, immediately resulting in severe pains. The two ends of the thread were always carried out at the wound to facilitate its removal once it had answered its purpose.

Only after it became understood that the risk of ligation is less if done directly around the vessel without including any of the surrounding tissues, did the ligature come more and more into use; although it was of course only antisepsis which made it a really safe procedure. Towards the end of the eighteenth century ligation was generally accepted as method of choice (Fig. 67). Its use obviated the need of bulky pressure-bandages.

6.2.3.2. Depuration

A second step in the treatment of fresh wounds was 'depuratio', the removal of any foreign bodies, bone fragments, tattered tissue. When the foreign body lay dangerously near to a blood vessel or a nerve, or when the wounded was in a bad state, its extraction should wait until purulence had developed. According to De Gorter, depuration could best be done with the fingers.[6] Van de Voorde, however, still used forceps and other instruments such as were depicted by Dalla Croce, Guillemeau or Scultetus. The 'arcubalista' — described by Guy de Chauliac amongst others (Fig. 13) — had meanwhile fallen into oblivion because it sometimes happened that the foreign body to be removed was stuck that fast that in the release of the bow the bone was torn to pieces.[7]

6.2.3.3. Wound Closure

In pre-antiseptic times surgeons were very reluctant to use needle and thread in the closure of wounds, they rather had recourse to strips of adhesive plaster or

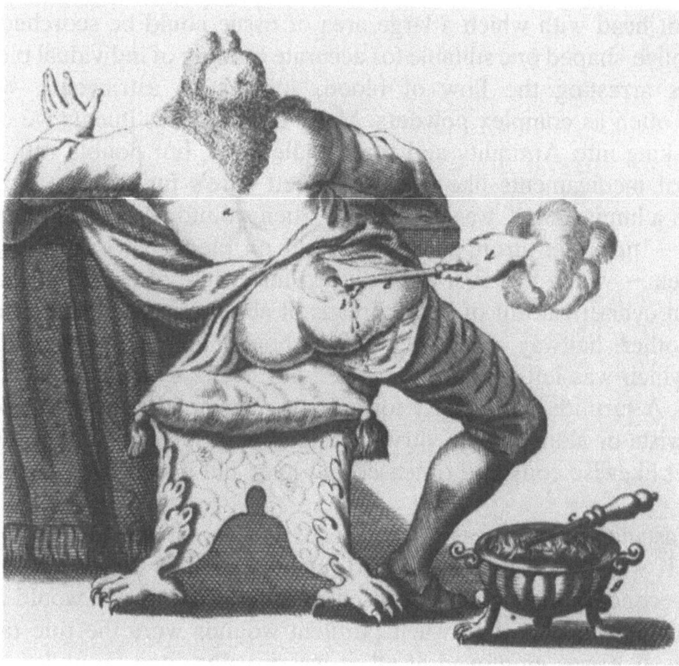

Fig. 66. The red-hot iron, also useful in the treatment of abscesses.

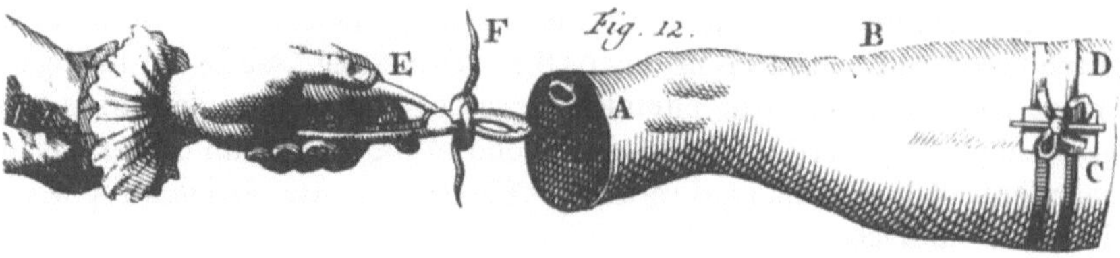

Fig. 67. Ligating blood vessels after amputation.

bandages like a two-headed roller bandage soaked in vinegar to approximate the wound edges. But in some wounds bloody suture could not be avoided. The different ways to do so were the traditional methods dating from the days of Galen and Albucasis and used and described by the mediaeval surgeons.[8] The most current method was the simple interrupted suture, starting in the middle of the wound, Van de Voorde informs us. In the treatment of facial wounds in particular the dry suture was still popular. Thus it appears that the technique of wound suture had not changed at all through the ages.

6.2.3.4. External Medicaments

Surgical textbooks abound with recipes for all sorts of medicaments which may be used in the treatment of wounds. On the sutured wound Van de Voorde applied a medicament which was believed to strenghthen the inborn heat, thereupon compresses which just like the bandages which had to fix them, were wetted with white wine or brandy, for these two fluids possessed fortifying and drying properties.[9] De Gorter first applied a 'balsamus vulnerarius' containing turpentine, then a digestive and finally a cloth wetted with vinegar and water.[10] Heister was amongst those who avoided stitches whenever possible. He much preferred to cover the wound with desiccant agents like brandy, honey, oil of turpentine, oil of St. John's wort, Peruvian balsam, camphorated spirits. In this way he hoped to prevent the formation of bad pus.[11] The application of poultices of all sorts of herbs, flowers or worts boiled in water or milk, or of linseed meal, was likewise a very common method of wound treatment.

It was only in the second half of the eighteenth century that some surgeons started to raise their voices against the prevailing use of bringing greasy or powdered substances into the wound and plugging it with lint whereby the efflux of 'acrimonious humours' was prevented. The Amsterdam M.D.—surgeon Schlichting, for instance, whose *Traumatologia nov'antiqua* (1748) has already been mentioned on page 163, was one of them.[12] Jacob van der Haar (1717—99), a well-known surgeon at 's-Hertogenbosch held that:

> Surgeons who make use of many cumbersome, costly balsams, ointments, plasters, waters, poultices etc. and put therein their confidence, show that they have no notion of the healing power of nature and are at the same time unsuited for preventing accidental impediments of nature or for removing them, if already present.[13]

This tendency could be observed in all countries. Frequent probing of fresh wounds also began to incur disapprobation but the reader might remember that as early as the fourteenth century Henri de Mondeville already had raised his voice against this practice.

6.2.3.5. Should Suppuration be Promoted?

There was still a difference of opinion on the ancient question whether the healing of wounds should necessarily be accompanied by the formation of pus. Heister was of the opinion that the appearance of pus was a normal phase in the process of wound healing, that is of creamy, non-offensive pus, which was to be looked upon as 'a very good wound balsam' and absolutely necessary for the healing. But this opinion was in the seventeenth century no longer shared by all. Matthaeus Gottfried Purmann (1649—1711),an outstanding German military surgeon of the period, related that at first he adhered to the traditional opinion that no wounds could be cured without suppuration and that medicines had to be directed accordingly. But after some campaigns in which he followed the old custom, he saw reason enough to leave it off. 'I soon found it true that wounds might be constantly and perfectly cured without suppuration'.[14] Van de Voorde too, rejected 'the promotion of suppuration in simple wounds, as so many surgeons did with so much zeal'. The formation of pus delays healing, can give rise to complications and is painful to the patient. 'He who keeps the outside air out of the wound and thus prevents the raw flesh from being adulterated, will very easily bring a wound to cure without "digestion" (purulence)'. he declared.[15] The dogma of the nefarious influence of atmospheric air was upheld by many. It was therefore of prime importance to cover up any wound as soon as possible.[16] But Petrus Camper, in a prize essay of 1775, denied any direct influence of the air on surgical diseases whatsoever. Air charged with the exhalation of a great number of people only acted injuriously on patients by affecting their constitution. He therefore stressed the importance of good ventilation in hospitals and on board ships.[17]

6.2.3.6. Lacerated Wounds

Ever since the days of Hippocrates there was a consensus that in lacerated wounds and wounds with a great loss of substance suppuration had definitely to be promoted to consume the contused parts. For this, surgeons had the disposal of several so-called digestive ointments. There were mild and strong digestives. An example of the first category is the 'unguentum digestivum' as prescribed by Barbette. It consisted of olive oil, yellow wax, incense, mastix, egg yolk and unsalted butter.[18] A strongly acting digestive had styrax as chief component, it was indicated in wounds and ulcers with unhealthy suppuration.

6.2.3.7. Bandaging

The art of bandaging, today almost extinguished, was in full bloom at the period under consideration. This not only held true for the treatment of traumatic and operative wounds, but of course also in the management of fractures and dislocations. Applying bandages was an essential part of the craft of surgery. Based on principles already laid down in Antiquity, this art attained at the time a level such as was probably never reached before or after. There were special manuals available. Well-known was the one by Jacques de Marque — *Traité des bandages de chirurgie* (1618). The number of bandages with their possible variations described in contemporary surgical textbooks is quite enormous: Heister for instance, presented no less than twenty-one illustrations of different head-bandages alone.

6.2.3.8. Supplementary Treatment

In the further treatment Van de Voorde recommended the observation of the 'non-naturals', the environmental factors affecting health and disease.[19] The diet had to be frugal, he stated, in line with Hippocrates. Cooling and exsiccating drinks should prevent wound complications and 'abundant humours' should be evacuated. The latter requirement explains why revulsive bloodletting — on the principles laid down by Galen and summarized on page 18 — still had a place in the treatment of wounds. Solingen performed venesection when there was 'a great orgasm in the blood'. He moreover prescribed opiates for internal use for sedation of that unfortunate condition.[20] The ancient custom of supplementing local wound treatment by bleeding and purging survived for quite a while particularly in Great Britain and France.[21]

6.2.4. *Treatment of War Wounds*

Because of the many wars, battle wounds occupied a large place in traumatology. Military and naval surgeons were not the only ones to occupy themselves with such lesions, civil surgeons too sometimes became involved since it was still customary to evacuate the wounded to hospitals in nearby or even faraway towns.[22] When after the naval battle near the Dogger Bank in 1781 the Dutch fleet had returned to the roadstead of Texel, 102 of the 404 wounded sailors were shipped to Amsterdam where they were admitted to the 'Binnengasthuis' hospital. During and after this engagement between the Dutch and the British, 24 major amputations were performed at sea by four Dutch surgeons. Only four of these patients did not survive, the cause of death being tetanus. For haemostasis, ligatures were used. Since the amputations were carried out in great haste, the ligatures in most cases included the accompanying nerves. From this Van Gesscher gathered, that tying the nerves was not as dangerous as he formerly had thought although it was just possible that the four cases of lockjaw had to be imputed to this occurrence. According to the preserved hospital records, the injuries for which the sailors were taken to Amsterdam mainly consisted of fractures, wounds from bullets and flying wood and severe burns. One man, hit by a cannonball, had a devastating injury of the upper jaw and face (Fig. 68). He survived for sixteen years.[23] No details were given on the treatment of any of these cases but we may presume that this would not have deviated from the methods in common use. Amputations occupied an important place in the treatment of the war wounded: we will enter into that on page 215.

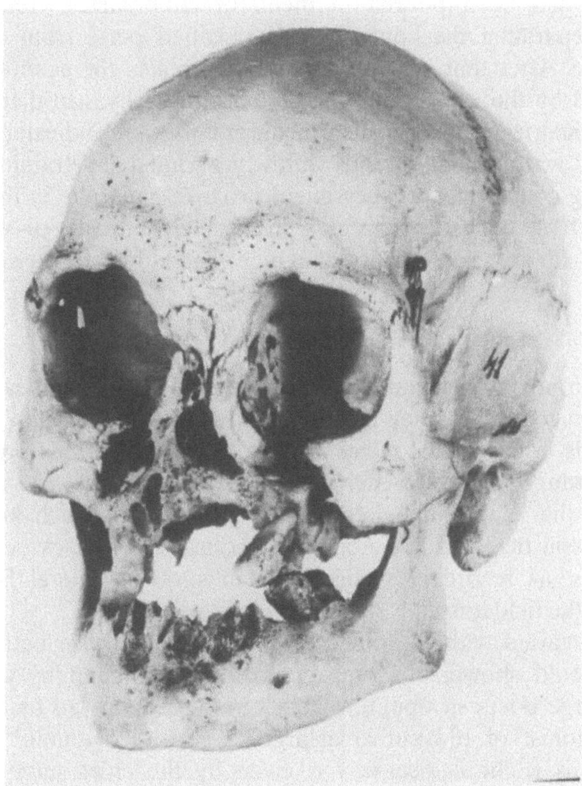

Fig. 68. Pyramidal or central middle third facial fracture (Le Fort type II), sustained by Able Seaman Frans Marcus at the naval battle near the Dogger Bank.

The danger of battlefield wounds of the soft parts when they did not immediately cause death and when no important blood vessels were directly involved, lay in life-threatening inflammation; in the case of gunshot wounds or stab wounds, favoured by the fact that any pus could not easily escape through the narrow wound canal. Heister recommended starting treatment by extracting any foreign bodies like bullets, shell-splinters, pieces of clothing, broken off bayonet tips. If such objects remain behind, there is a great risk of non-closure of the wound or fistulization. If needs be the wound should be enlarged to get hold of them. De Gorter and Van de Voorde were less aggressive: if it were not quite possible to remove a bullet it should be left in peace. John Hunter, in his *Treatise on the blood*, took a similar view. In the firm belief that the body is a perfect machine possessing within itself the innate power of repair, he was opposed to the prevailing practice immediately to open all gunshot wounds. Particularly those made by bullets entering with low velocity were well able to heal by first intention.[24] Surgeons no longer believed in shot wounds being poisonous but soldiers apparently did. When injured in the field, they used to suck each other's wounds in an attempt at removing any penetrated poison. There even existed professional 'suckers' who followed the armies to offer their lip-service for a consideration.[25] According to Heister, fresh battle wounds should first be dressed with lint soaked in brandy after brandy had been poured in them. In later stages, treatment should be directed at separating the contused and putrified parts from the healthy using digestive salve. After that separation had taken place, the generation of new flesh was promoted by the use of appropriate balsams or by 'eau d'arquebuscade'.[26] In the stage of cicatrization exsiccating medicaments were indicated. Van de Voorde recommended washing war wounds with white wine and refraining from the use of pus-generating compounds as they might provoke gangrene in the contused parts. Heister fought established gangrene with caustic ointments or waters, with 'aqua phagedaenica' for instance, composed of lime water and mercury sublimate.

6.2.5. *Tetanus*

Ever since Hippocrates, tetanus has been described by countless surgical authors all through the centuries, when mostly as a case history. Tetanus, as a complication of war wounds in particular, seems to have become a serious problem only in the eighteenth century (Fig. 69). After the battle of Prague in 1757 and of Liegnitz in 1760 during the War of the League of Augsburg in which king Frederick the Great of Prussia defeated the Austrians, thousands of cases occurred even after minor injuries, as recorded by the Prussian surgeon-general Bilguer. The poor ventilation in the field hospitals was largely held responsible.

Treatment varied with the different authors from warm baths or quite to the contrary by cold showers or the application of ice and by amputation. Some prescribed large doses of opium, others wine and Peruvian bark. Bilguer himself was a protagonist of preventive enlargement of the wound.[27] A good clinical account of this frightful disease was given by the chief surgeon of Napoleon's armies, the famous Larrey (see p. 216). As mode of treatment he favoured amputation.[28]

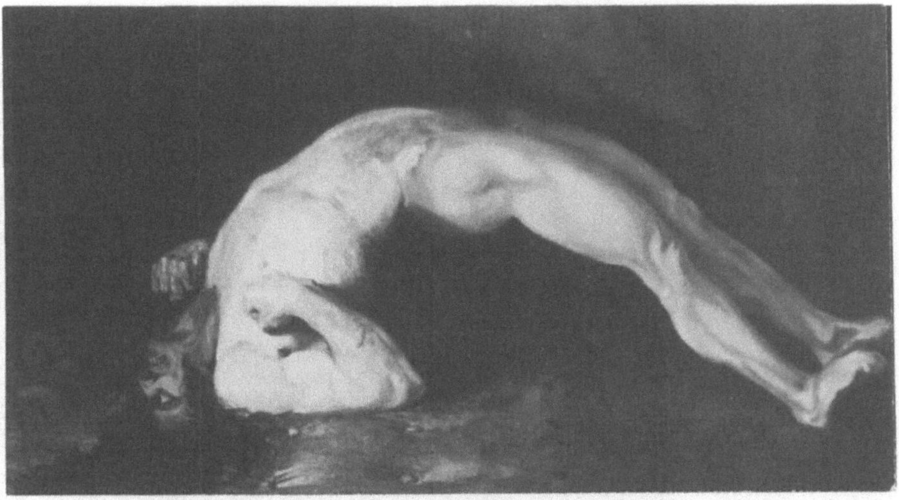

Fig. 69. Tetanic spasm in a wounded soldier. Composite picture form three cases of tetanus among soldiers wounded in the Battle of Corunna (Spain) in 1809.

For a discussion of the hospital gangrene which seems to have presented itself for the first time in the eighteenth century and of a few other wound diseases — septicaemia, pyaemia and erysipelas — the reader is referred to page 289.

6.3. BONE AND JOINT SURGERY

6.3.1. *Osteology*

Throughout the eighteenth century, great interest was manifested in osteology. That interest not only concerned anatomy, but also and in particular pathology. The science of diseases of the bones and joints occupied a special place in public and private instruction and there appeared a host of publications on the subject. By diseases of the bones were understood fractures and luxations as well as osteomyelitis, dry caries, osteomalacia and exostosis. Many a surgeon cherished a private collection of remarkable bones.

A well-known collection of this kind in Holland belonged to Jacob Hovius (1710—86) in Amsterdam. A catalogue of these specimens was prepared by Andreas Bonn.[29] The collection still exists and is well worth seeing. It is being kept in a large cupboard with Hovius' portrait on top in the Department of Anatomy of the University of Amsterdam (Fig. 70).

6.3.2. *Fractures*

6.3.2.1. Some Standard Textbooks

In the first half of the eighteenth century the treatment of fractures relied mainly on French texts. Amongst these, those by Duverney and Petit occupied a

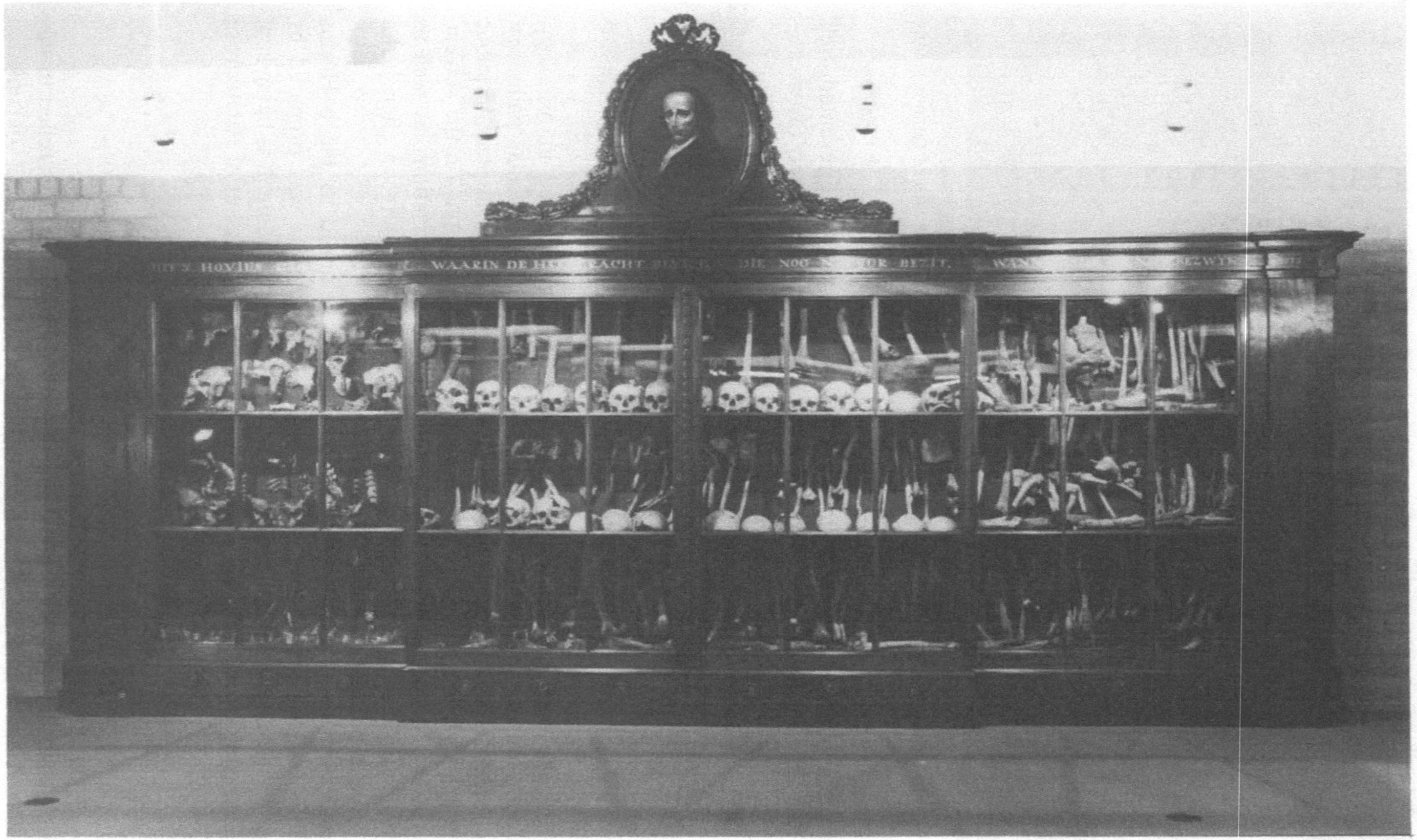

Fig. 70. Osteology collection of Dr. Jacob Hovius. Hovius, who was physician to the Amsterdam Buitengasthuis, presented this beautiful collection to the surgeons' guild in 1773. The caption on the cornice reads: 'Dit's Hovius geschenk waarin de heelkracht blijkt die nog natuur bezit, wanneer de kunst bezwijkt' (This is Hovius' present which gives evidence of the healing power nature possesses even when the art fails).

prominent place: both surgeons have already been referred to on page 155. They were both excellent teachers who also drew pupils from Holland. Duverney was one of the best anatomists of his days. His *Traité des maladies des os* appeared only posthumously in 1751, and five years later also in a Dutch translation.

A Dutch adaptation of Petit's well-known *l'Art de guérir les maladies des os*, first published in 1705, appeared in 1736 and once again in 1751. In his preface, the translator Hoogvliet cited Boerhaave as saying: 'As to the diseases of bones, the celebrated Petit in Paris outdistances all, his treatise stands unrivalled up till now'.

In the second half of the century it was especially English publications that in many languages dominated the field: Percivall Pott's *Some few general remarks on fractures and dislocations* (1765) taking the lead. On the continent Pott had a dedicated follower in the French surgeon Pierre Lassus (1741—1807). In 1771, Lassus translated Pott's textbook into French, a Dutch edition after the French saw the light of day in the following year in Ghent. Towards the end of the century Pierre-Joseph Desault (see p. 152) gave the lead in France. He brought surgical bedside teaching to a level never attained before.

6.3.2.2. Principles of Fracture Treatment[30]

The relevant sections in textbooks of the time usually start with an enumeration of the different possible types of fractures. There was difference of opinion on the actual existence of some varieties: Petit for that matter expressed his disbelief in fissured fractures. He moreover denied the existence of longitudinal fractures of which Benjamin Bell entertained a conviction. Epiphysial separations, both of the spontaneous kind seen in cases of scurvy which was a quite common disease as well as the traumatic variety, were first described by Georg Christian Reichel in Leipzig in 1759.[31] The life-threatening complications of the compound fracture, inflammation and suppuration, were blamed as before on the nefarious influence of the external air. Percivall Pott explained the happy outcome of an open leg fracture he once sustained himself by the circumstance that after reduction of the protruding bone fragment the wound of the skin no longer communicated with the fracture site so that no outside air could reach it.[32]

Any necessary reduction should be carried out as soon as possible. It should only be delayed in cases of severe swelling caused by contusion of the soft parts: then a decrease of the swelling should first be striven for by means of bloodletting and evacuation of the bowels. Reduction had to be accomplished by use of the hands, mechanical aids ('konstwerktuigen') were passing into disuse.[33] There was, however, disagreement on the question whether the extension required for the correction of the fracture should have to act on the distal end of the broken bone or beyond the adjacent joint.

Percivall Pott had reached the highly important conclusion that the displacement of the fragments is mainly due to tension and retraction of the muscles and that such forces may be eliminated by placing the injured extremity in such a position that the muscles are relaxed. Then reduction can be more easily done and displacement is less apt to recur.[34] Pott advised against the old Hippocratic method still generally adhered to in his day of reducing a broken limb by extension in a straight position.

Fixation was achieved by folded linen, wedge-shaped pads for filling empty spaces, bandages and splints. Splints were to be had in a wide assortment varying from rolled compresses to preformed cardboard. Cardboard was a widely used material at the time. For certain fractures special types of fixation devices were available. The old guttered splints of straw, wood or tinplate were still in use but mainly for transportation.

In 1768 the French military surgeon Hughues Ravaton whose years of birth and death do not seem to be known, introduced a tin boot, suspended on four rings, for keeping a broken leg in a hanging position. This suspended splint allowed the treatment of compound fractures when semiflexion seemed desirable to maintain reduction, but the wound required regular attendance.[35]

Suspension in combination with traction likewise dates from the late eighteenth century. According to Richter, its inventor probably was an otherwise unknown surgeon by the name of Posch in Vienna. In 1774 he constructed a suspension bed on which the leg was placed with bent knee, while over the ankle extension-straps were applied which could be tightened by means of a windlass.[36] This apparatus was widely used for quite a while.

At about the same time several other surgeons brought out different apparatuses for applying continuous traction on the lower extremity. It soon became clear, however, that such extension splints caused pain and that the bandages used to fixate them had all the time to be tightened with the consequence that the broken bone was granted insufficient rest. Compound fractures formed in principle an indication for amputation although conservative treatment, whether or not including the sawing off of any projecting bone ends of removing loose fragments, at times yielded satisfactory results.

An acceptable fracture bandage should not comprise roller bandages completely enveloping the extremity but should be such that it could be loosened or tightened without disturbing the fracture site. In the opinion of many, Scultetus' many-tailed bandage — 'boek-band' in Dutch — still answered that condition best (Fig. 71).

The importance attached to the proper use of bandages in the treatment of fractures and dislocations is apparent from the publication of special manuals like the one written in 1688 by Laurent Verduc, *La manière de guérir les fractures et les luxations par le moyen des bandages* of which a Dutch translation appeared in 1691. One had an eye for important details. Thus a sponge was placed under the heel of an immobilized leg for the prevention of a pressure sore. The development of talipes equinus was counteracted by a bandage or a foot board keeping the foot at a right angle to the leg and by the use of a cradle (Fig. 72).

These are some of the more important principles as they can be distilled from textbooks. It should be remembered, however, that in case of a fracture or dislocation people by no means always called in a qualified surgeon. Many had recourse to lay bonesetters as was pointed out on page 128.

6.3.2.3. Fracture Treatment in Practice

In this paragraph we will pay heed to those fractures which from the late

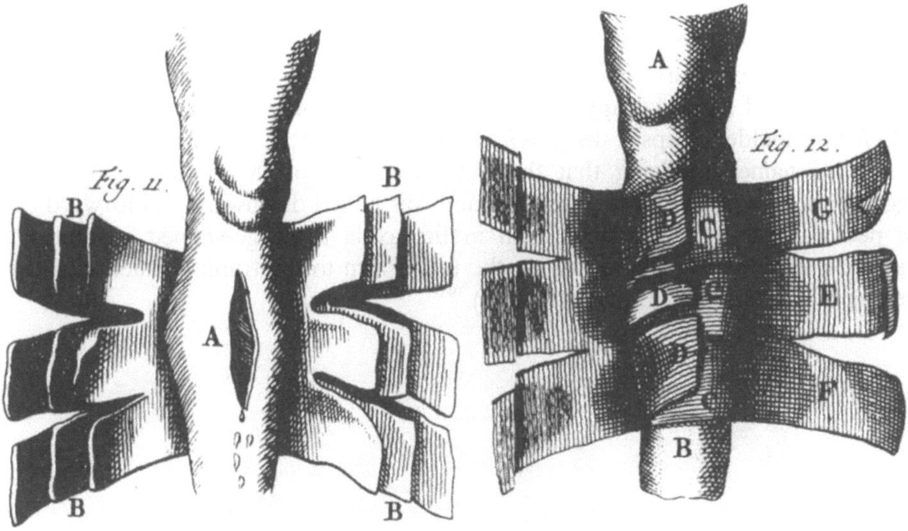

Fig. 71. Scultetus' multi-tailed bandage ('boekband').

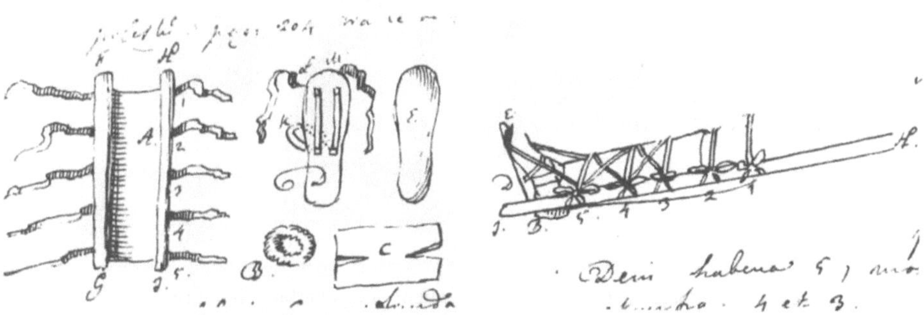

Fig. 72. Petrus Camper's bandage for a leg fracture, as drawn by himself, 1751.

seventeenth century onwards were receiving more attention than before or were being treated in some novel way. In doing so we will observe the traditional sequence 'a capite ad calcem' which continued to apply in the textbooks. Fractures of the skull are the subject of a separate consideration lower down in this chapter.

When William III of Orange towards the end of his life broke his *collarbone* as a result of a fall from his horse, it was immediately treated by the king's personal surgeon Ronjat who applied a bandage and an arm sling. When after a little while Govert Bidloo, the court physician well-known for his fine anatomical atlas, entered the scene, he of course disapproved strongly of the measures taken by the surgeon although the royal patient stated that he felt quite comfortable. A new bandage was applied incorporating a small splint and compresses. In the two weeks the monarch still had to live before he died from pulmonary tuberculosis and oedema which had bothered him for years, he hardly complained of his fracture.[37] Heister just bound such patients to a large wooden or iron cross. Some seventy years later, Pierre Brasdor (1721—97), professor of anatomy and surgery in Paris, devised a special apparatus to treat this fracture, consisting of a corset with firm shoulder-straps.[38] In 1787 Desault introduced the bandage that still carries his name. Realizing that the outer fragment of the broken collarbone sagged under the weight of the shoulder and was pulled downward and forward by the pectoral muscles, he placed high in the axilla a wedge-shaped cushion to neutralize these forces. By bandaging the upper arm to the trunk he succeeded in keeping the axilla-pad in its place (Fig. 73).[39]

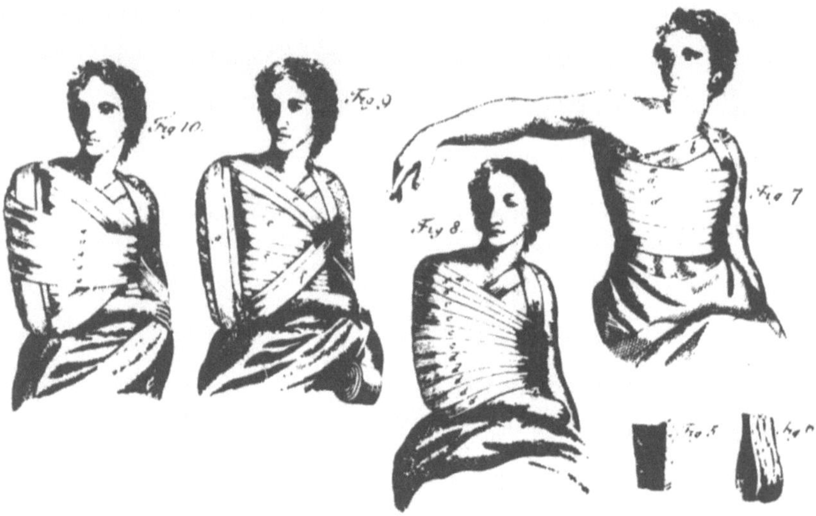

Fig. 73. Desault's bandage for the treatment of a collarbone fracture.

Fractures of the *scapula*, of which several types were already being recognized, were treated with appropriate bandages. In the treatment of the *upper arm* fractures which entirely followed the well-established rules, we first hear of the binding together of the two fragments with a wire loop. This cerclage was carried out using copper wire in about 1770 by Sicie and Lapujade, surgeons at Toulouse. There were no details given nor do we know any particulars of the bold operators.[40]

As to the *forearm* fractures no definite change in treatment occurred. Petrus Camper paid some attention to the fracture of the *olecranon* process in his *Dissertatio de patellae fractura et olecrani* which with fine illustrations by his own hand, came out posthumously in 1789. He believed the function of the olecranon to be almost analogous to that of the patella. Fractures of this part of the ulna therefore should be treated like those of the kneecap: one should not aim at a complete union but treat the swelling with rest, fomentations and bandaging. Afterwards one may allow movements starting cautiously. Others were treating this fracture with a fortnight bedrest with the extended arm lying somewhat higher on a cushion.[41]

Van Gesscher when discussing the fractures of the *spine* remarked that only those of the spinous processes can be directly diagnosed. Those of the vertebral bodies are only indirectly recognizable from signs of paralysis and incontinence which they may provoke.[42] In this respect no progress at all seems to have been made since Albucasis.

There was on the other hand much ado about the fracture of the *neck of the femur*, as has been pointed out on page 142. In 1680, the Amsterdam surgeon Gerrit Borst once again called attention to this little-known fracture in 1681.[43] He claimed to be able to make the diagnosis at first sight on account of shortening with external rotation and emaciation of the leg, with pain at the knee. Duverney also gave a description of the fracture of the femoral neck but the French claim that he was its discoverer, was already contested by Titsingh.[44]

The clinical signs of a recently sustained collum femoris fracture were further specified by Petit.[45] Prior to the introduction of radiodiagnostics in 1895 — and even for a number of years afterwards — this fracture often confronted clinicians with great diagnostic difficulties. This also held true for treatment. Most surgeons in the period under consideration simply applied splints whereas others merely prescribed bedrest since the fracture was considered incurable. Van Gesscher did not share that opinion. He claimed to be able to bring about cures with preservation of function by his favoured method. This entailed reduction carried out with the patient lying supine by slow and gentle traction at the heel, and at the same time giving the foot 'a half inward rotation'. To maintain the reduction, Van Gesscher used a bandage consisting of a double folded sheet around the hips, circular compresses around the greater trochanters and around the ankles, and firmly bandaging the injured extremity to the sound one which acted as a splint.[46]

Fractures of the *shaft of the femur* were not rare — perhaps even the most frequent Van Gesscher thought. To explain this remarkable phenomenon — the femur is indeed the largest bone of the entire skeleton — he referred to a theory advanced by William Porterfield, an Edinburgh physician living in the middle of the eighteenth century. Porterfield held that the fragility of bone would be the greater the more it contained 'solid substance'.[47] Treatment of fractures of the shaft of the thigh-bone underwent a fundamental change since Pott had demonstrated the importance of muscle action for the displacement. No longer was the leg splinted while in a state of extension, but in a flexed position. Pott himself preferred to bandage the upper leg after reduction with Scultetus' many-tailed bandage or to provide it with a guttered splint. Thereupon he placed the entire leg in a flexed position laterally on two cushions which could be turned forward and fastened over the limb. This position, however, was difficult to maintain: the double inclined plane devised by Charles White (1728—1813) in Manchester served the purpose more adequately.[48]

There existed differences of opinion on the curability of *patellar* fractures. Camper was particularly interested in this injury. Apart from his own treatise of 1789, mentioned above, he had one of his students defend a thesis on it as early as 1754. In his own work Camper describes the functional part played by the patella in bringing the knee into extension. When the knee is suddenly bent too vigorously or too rapidly, a transverse fracture may occur whereas direct trauma results in fragmentation or in a longitudinal fracture. The first of these two mechanisms can also induce a rupture of the common tendon of the quadriceps muscle or of the patellar ligament. Of the three possible types of fracture of the kneecap, comminution is the most difficult to recognize. The prognosis of the transverse fracture is bad in the view of Camper which differs here from that of some of his contemporaries. Relying on eleven cases, he concluded that this type of fracture never heals by bony consolidation but merely by a sinewy union. Such a tendinous repair nevertheless does to a certain extent restore the function of the knee owing to the distal bone fragment taking over the role of the formerly intact patella. A longitudinal fracture always heals without a problem, but a comminution in which often the joint is also involved, frequently ends up in ankylosis. Rupture of the common tendon likewise results in some residual weakness of the knee. On the prognosis of the ruptured ligamentum patellae Camper did not make any comment. His treatment of the transverse fracture was the same as one finds in Heister: a bandage of the extended knee that presses the two fragments together by turns running alternatively over and under the cap (Fig. 74). Mobilisation is allowed after two days, at first on crutches. The comminuted fracture requires a fixating bandage and prolonged rest.[49]

As of old, *leg* fractures were being treated by reduction and splinting. Van de Voorde's description of how he proceeded in such cases may well serve as an illustration of how this was done in practice (cf. p. 140). An interesting case of cerclage treatment took place in Antwerp in 1796. A certain Guilihelmus Sluyds had sustained a compound fracture of the lower leg in which in spite of reduction and splinting the displacement recurred time and again. Frans van Montfort, the attending surgeon, then wondered if there would be no other means to achieve his aim. 'Then it appeared to me to be a good idea to pass a gold wire around only the bone fragments by way of undersewing which after having been twisted would permit the unhappy patient to keep his leg'. Montfort carried this plan into execution and indeed did pass a gold wire around the oblique tibial fracture. The loop was removed after 33 days; the patient made an uneventful recovery.[50]

Fractures about the *ankle* are met with repeatedly in eighteenth-century case histories: they were no longer regarded as dislocations. The Utrecht professor Johannes Munniks (1652—1711) presented two instances of compound fracture-dislocations. In the first case, relating to a farmer, conservative treatment was initially adopted, but when the protruding bone started to taint, the leg was then taken off below the knee. This had taken place years before, but the man 'with a wooden leg still strolls the land of the living'. In a second similar case of a young woman, brought about by jumping from a gig, amputation was performed straight away. The patient bore it stout-heartedly. The postoperative course was at first quite satisfactory, until opisthotonus developed from which she died, 'the wound until the very end so to say smiling upon us'.[51]

Percivall Pott gave a classic description of a fracture-dislocation at the ankle, in which the foot is displaced outwards with tearing of the collateral ligaments which connect the distal end of the tibia with the talus and calcaneus and breaking of the fibula above the lateral malleolus.[52] This fracture continues to be known in the English-speaking world as 'Pott's fracture'. Fractures of the *calcaneus* apparently

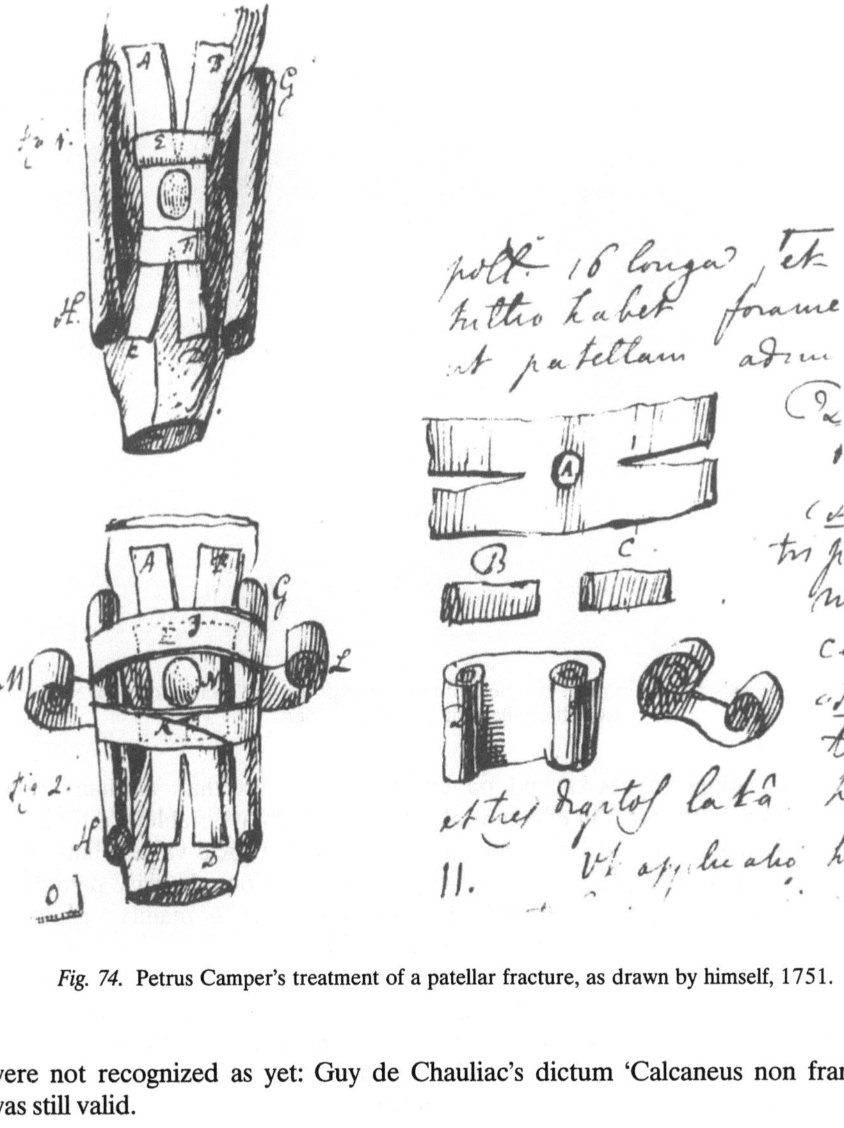

Fig. 74. Petrus Camper's treatment of a patellar fracture, as drawn by himself, 1751.

were not recognized as yet: Guy de Chauliac's dictum 'Calcaneus non frangitur' was still valid.

6.3.2.4. Results of Fracture Treatment; Osteoclasis

We are not too well acquainted with the outcome of fracture treatment prior to about the middle of the nineteenth century. Only a few authors troubled to mention — incidentally — any results. The many crippled who moved through the streets with crooked, shortened or otherwise deformed legs provide the evidence why our expectations cannot be oversanguine,[53] although the responsibility for that particular feature of the street scene may in an unknown measure be shared by the lay bonesetters. In fractures of the thigh bone in particular, healing with shortening would hardly have been avoidable (Fig. 75). Specimens in osteologic collections as

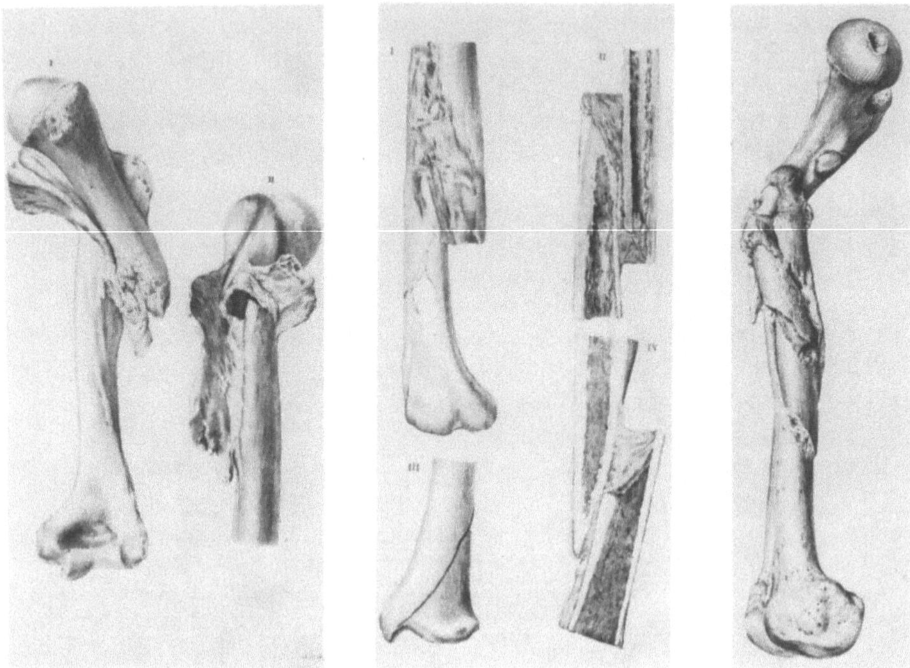

Fig. 75. Some results of 18th century treatment of femoral shaft fracture, as illustrated by specimens from the collection of Andreas Bonn.

well as illustrations in books and papers indeed suggest that, at many other locations as well, healing sometimes took place in an unfavourable position. But the relatively few preserved bones have of course no statistical value whatsoever: they may well have been kept for their very crookedness or otherwise pathologic condition. Once in a while an intrepid surgeon tried in a case of manifest malunion to achieve a more satisfactory result by refracturing and resetting the crooked bone as Celsus had already recommended. An example of this is provided by Gerard ten Haaff, reader in clinical surgery at the Illustrious School in Rotterdam. In 1775 he described a case of a sixteen-week old fracture of the shaft of the femur in a fourteen-years old boy which had healed with a severe anterior angulation and considerable shortening. Ten Haaff first tried to soften the callus by the application of mercury ointment and poultices for a week. Then he broke the leg by having two stalwart men applying strong traction and countertraction and straightened it by direct pressure using his full body weight. The result was quite to the patient's satisfaction.[54]

6.3.2.5. The Process of Repair

In the eighteenth century interest grew in the healing process of broken bones after Antonius de Heide, as described on page 104, in 1684 had been the first in modern history to approach this problem by way of animal experimentation. His conclusion was that callus is a real bone substance.

There were divergent opinions on how callus is formed. In Paris Henri-Louis du Hamel du Monceau (1700—82) believed that he had shown on the strength of experiments with madder (Rubia tinctorum), that bone receives its nourishment exclusively from the periosteum and that the formation of callus likewise proceeds from this structure. This would appear from an increased vascularization and swelling of the periosteum at the fracture site.[55]

Peter Detlef in Göttingen, who likewise fed his animals with the red-coloured madder, arrived in 1753 at a different conclusion. In his view repair began with the forming of a gelatin-like matter into which tiny blood vessels entered issuing from the bone. This vascularized mass would gradually turn into callus.[56] Petrus Camper too, occupied himself with the problem. In 1765 he sent to the Royal Society in Edinburgh an essay under the title: *Observationes novae circa callum ossium fractorum*. In this he stated that young callus initially is of cartilaginous character and later changes into a solid, organic matter of the same colour, substance and composition as any other bone. Callus is deposited as internal and as external callus, effected by slow ossification of a mucous matter exuded by the vessels of the periosteum or by the bone fibrillae. No external means whatsoever are able to promote callus formation.[57] Twenty years later, still another view was propounded by Andreas Bonn. He made callus grow from the fracture ends as young, vascular and tender flesh, like granulations in wounds and ulcers. This flesh not only established a connection between the fracture fragments, but also covered the sawn surfaces of amputation and grew out from the dura mater and the cut bone after trepanation of the skull. This young callus could undergo hypertrophy just like granulation. It never became cartilaginous and in ossifying it became more compact than ordinary bone, almost like ivory. 'Modus quo haec omnia fiant, incognitus est', he concluded.[58] At the end of the century John Hunter in his already repeatedly cited book, developed a theory which by and large was identical with the one he had drafted in regard to the healing of soft part injuries.

6.3.3. *Dislocations*

Until way into the eighteenth century the reduction of dislocations was considered mainly to be a matter of force (Fig. 76). This too was very often done by unqualified bonesetters. Petit reminded his contemporaries of the precept of the Ancients, that the head had to be brought back along the same path by which it had left the socket, therefore through the rent in the capsule. The question whether a dislocation is ever and always accompanied by tearing of the joint integuments, was, however, still unsettled. Pott condemned the use of traction apparatus in the treatment of dislocations as well. As in the reduction of fractures, the muscles had to be relaxed as much as possible by an appropriate positioning of the limb. The reduction of displacement of the femoral head for instance had to be undertaken with a flexed hip. Pott distinguished four different types of dislocation of this bone. Petit knew of three varieties at the shoulder. He described no less than nine different ways of reduction. After correction, the extremity was given rest for some weeks.[59] In 1791, Van Gesscher described a typical case of 'pulled elbow' in a child. To achieve a maximal relaxation, some surgeons recommended preliminary

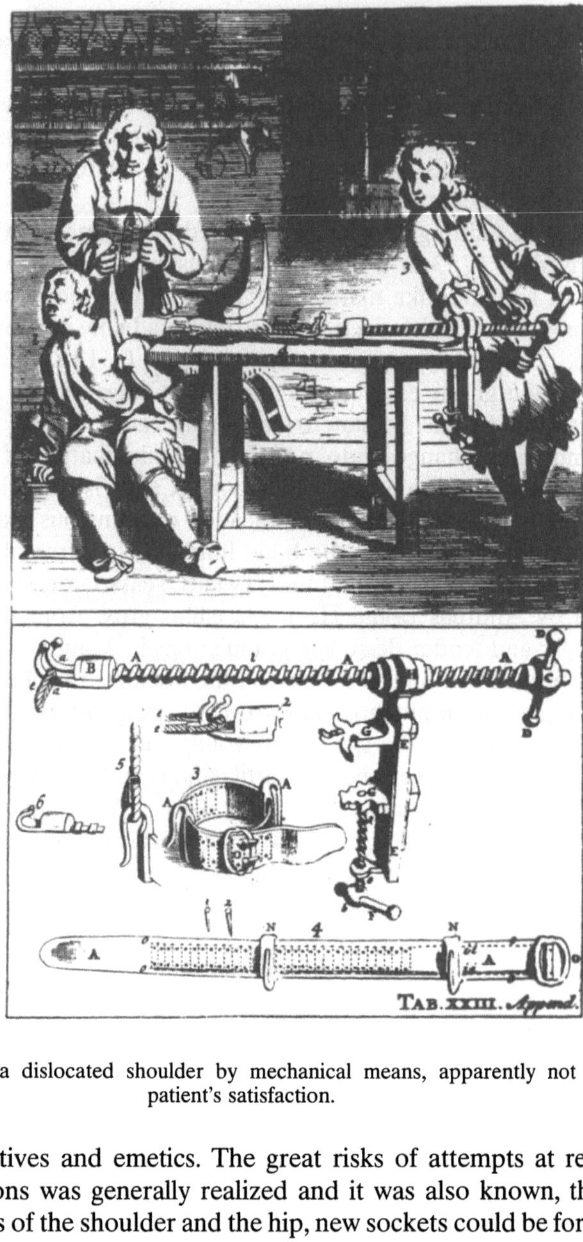

Fig. 76. Reduction of a dislocated shoulder by mechanical means, apparently not quite to the patient's satisfaction.

venesections, purgatives and emetics. The great risks of attempts at reduction of inveterate dislocations was generally realized and it was also known, that in non-reduced dislocations of the shoulder and the hip, new sockets could be formed.

6.3.4. *Orthopaedics*

The word orthopaedics was coined by Nicolas Andry (1658—1742), dean of the Paris medical faculty. He explained its meaning in the very title of the book that he published in 1742 on the subject: *L'orthopédie ou l'art de prévenir et de corriger dans les enfants, les difformités du corps*. This does not mean that this branch of medicine only originated in the middle of the eighteenth century. Iron corsets to correct scoliosis were described and depicted already by Paré and in the works of his slightly senior contemporary Arceo one finds a way of treating clubfoot with special splints and shoes. Other Renaissance authors too, wrote on clubfoot and deformities of the spine.[60]

From the older days the treatment of both kind of defects appears to have rested with 'specialists' who, although not always physicians or surgeons, had an extensive practical experience in this particular field. These early practitioners have left only few traces. In the second half of the seventeenth century, however, there were a few in Holland who enjoyed an international reputation. Thus the brothers Nicholas and Peter Schot ran a crookedness clinic in Utrecht which was visited by patients from all over North Europe. They were very experienced makers of iron and copper and other orthopaedic appliances to cure crooked limbs. The local blacksmiths' guild protested against their setting up a practice in Utrecht, arguing that their activities infringed on their monopoly, but the civic authorities shielded them and even granted Nicholas freedom from taxes for all the wine and beer consumed in his household.[61]

In the Brabant village of Oirschot Arnoldus Fey (1633—79) had a similar renown. He started his career as a tailor and began to make trusses as a side line. He styled himself a surgeon but it is doubtful whether he ever did pass any examination. The Grand Pensionary Johan de Witt sent his three daughters to Fey for the cure of their crooked spines.[62]

A third no less picturesque figure in this field was Hendrik van Deventer (1651—1724), trained as a goldsmith. He acquired his knowledge of medicine and surgery in practice. At the age of forty-three he took his M.D. in Groningen. He achieved much fame for his method of treatment of bones distorted by rickets and was once even called to the Royal Court in Copenhagen. Later in life he had a prosperous practice in the village of Voorburg near The Hague. Here he seems to have operated some sort of orthopaedic institute but no details are recorded. His book on diseases of the bone appeared posthumously in 1739.[63] Van Deventer was moreover a prominent obstetrician whose books on midwifery were translated into German, French, English and Latin.

Numerous other authors described ever more sophisticated corsets and traction apparatus. Amongst these was an apparatus of Van Gesscher, who for the first time applied the principle of elastic pressure on the protruding ribs at the convex side of the scoliosis.[64]

In the eighteenth century, orthopaedics unequivocally became a branch of medicine. Challenged by some of his former pupils who contended that original themes were exhausted, Petrus Camper published in 1781 a monograph on the best shoe, illustrated with drawings by his own hand. By way of introduction to the real theme, he gave an anatomical description of the foot and its static conditions on standing and on walking. On the strength of these data he reasoned which conditions a good shoe had to comply with. In the last chapter he discussed the foot ailments which may result from wearing faulty footgear. This article also appeared as a treatise in French and German, English editions saw the light of day even as late as 1861 and 1871.[65] For a more complete history of orthopaedics the reader is referred to the excellent book of Bruno Valentin.[66]

6.3.5. *Amputations*

6.3.5.1. Indications

Gangrene and serious injuries were as in earlier times the main reasons for removing larger or smaller parts of the extremities (Fig. 77). The physician Jan van Beverwyck stated that he had the legs of several soldiers amputated in the hospital of Dordrecht for gangrene caused by exposure to cold while standing on guard. In some patients the toes or even a whole foot had already fallen off spontaneously.[67] Less frequently, the operation was also performed for incurable osteomyelitis, uncontrollable haemorrhage, certain deformities, tumours and life-threatening aneurysms.

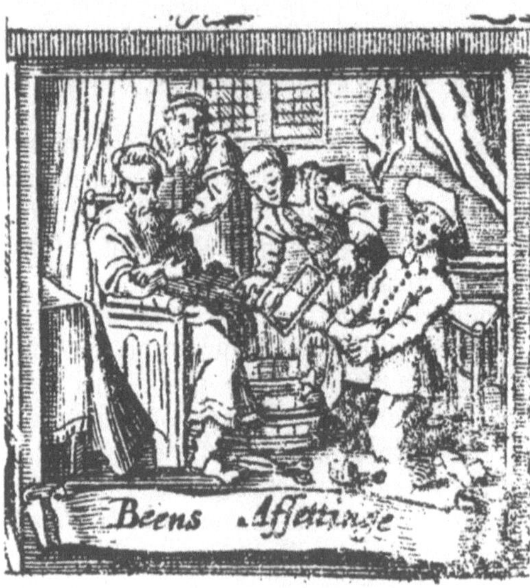

Fig. 77. Leg amputation, c. 1660.

6.3.5.2. Technique

Minor Amputations

Until the end of the seventeenth century there was hardly any change in operative technique for either major or minor amputations. There was some difference of opinion on the admissibility of the operation of Botallo, consisting of chopping off fingers or toes or even the hand with a chisel on a wooden block. Van de Voorde and Solingen rejected this procedure whereas others like Schouten, De Gorter and Roonhuyze continued to practise it. The following case is a fine illustration of how the latter would proceed in such a case. The foot of a woman suffering from a 'decayed' great toe was put with the sole on a wooden block and while the surgeon was pretending to be still making additional preparations, he unexpectedly delivered the mallet stroke (Fig. 78). The toe sprung at him but the woman

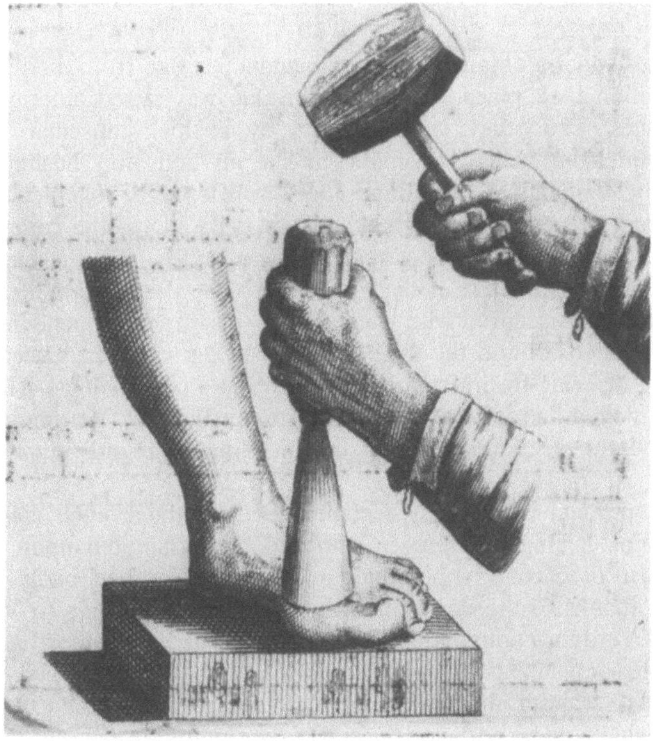

Fig. 78. Amputation of a toe according to Botallo, as depicted by Scultetus, c. 1672.

declared not to have felt any pain thanks to the deceit. The severed toe weighed 4½ ounces. After four years, the patient remained alive and in good health.[68]

Major Amputations

The method which is still to be found even in the last (1671) edition of Van Beverwyck's much-read *Heelkonste* is entirely that of Paré. The Middelburg surgeon Van de Voorde in teaching his students, likewise proceeded along traditional lines. His method only differs from Paré's in that he applied two ropes — one over and one under the knee — instead of one, and that he preferred the actual cautery to ligatures. Haemostasis should be complete 'lest the soul flows out together with the blood'. Van de Voorde did not share the apparently still prevailing view, handed down from the days of Hippocrates, that allowing a wound to bleed for some time would prevent inflammation. Infected blood moves through the veins and cannot flow out because of the valves, whereas arterial blood is 'pure', he argued.[69]

Towards the end of the seventeenth century, in 1696, the Amsterdam surgeon Pieter Adriaansz Verduyn or Verduin (1636—96) introduced a new technique for the amputation. This consisted in first making a transverse stab wound through the soft parts on the posterior aspect of the lower leg at the proposed level of the amputation, from which he obliquely cut down on the heel through skin and muscles. In this way he obtained a musculocutaneous flap from the calf. Then the actual amputation took place, whereafter the flap was raised anteriorly over the sectioned bones. Thus they were covered by a thick muscular layer which prevented them from being 'corrupted' by the air and after healing the stump would be of better quality. The wound edges were brought together and covered with bovista and the stump was tightly bandaged. To add to the compression and to prevent seepage of blood, a pig's bladder was pulled over the bandage like a cap, as was common practice at the time. Over this, Verduin applied a concave, metal disk which was secured with leather strips by way of suspenders to a broad leather belt fastened around the thigh. The upper leg was then placed in a metal guttered splint tapering from the knee downward at a certain angle. The distal end was provided with a flat disk to support the stump (Fig. 79). Verduin claimed that by his method the need for securing the bleeding from individual vessels was obviated.[70]

Verduin's approach was highly recommended by the French master-surgeon Joseph Vergniol, a Hugenot refugee who had been operated upon by Verduin himself because of chronic suppuration of his leg. This had badly affected his health which, thanks to the amputation, he regained. According to Vergniol, the advantages of Verduin's amputation were that no recurring haemorrhage was to be feared, that the movements of the knee joint were better preserved, that wound dressing was less painful and that in the end the prosthesis could be of a lighter type since weight could be borne on the end of the stump.[71]

Verduin's publication attracted considerable attention. It not only appeared in Dutch and Latin, but also in German and — in Vergniol's translation — in French. Frederik Ruysch recommended a technique which was only slightly different from that of Verduins.[72] The method also met with opposition, for instance by Solingen, but in particular by Verduin's fellow citizen Adriaan Koenerding, surgeon to the hospital. Preparing the oblique flap would be too painful and the wound would take a long time to heal whereas the arteries would easily dilate in an unnatural fashion.[73] Heister and Sharp raised the objection that the turned over position of the flap might result in its mortification. Verduin's method was very advantageous in the eyes of De la Faye, but it would not always be possible to obtain a satisfactory flap, in particular in cases of extensive gangrene.[74] Koenerding moreover pointed out that Verduin's mode of proceeding was not original: according to the Plymouth naval surgeon James Yonge it was first conceived by C.D. Lowdham of Exeter.[75] Verduin himself wrote with regard to this that, at the time when he was entertaining the thought of covering the stump with a thick, single flap, he was visited in Amsterdam by one of his former pupils who had established himself in London, where he had married an Englishwoman. This man told him that he had once heard from his wife that her grandfather, in his time a well-known surgeon in London, had once performed an amputation in this manner. The informant did not think that the operation had ever been repeated in England.[76]

By the writings in favour and against, however, the prime importance of a good covering of the amputation stump was brought out clearly. De Gorter in his *Gezuiverde heelkonst* (1735) paid due regard to this principle as appears from his

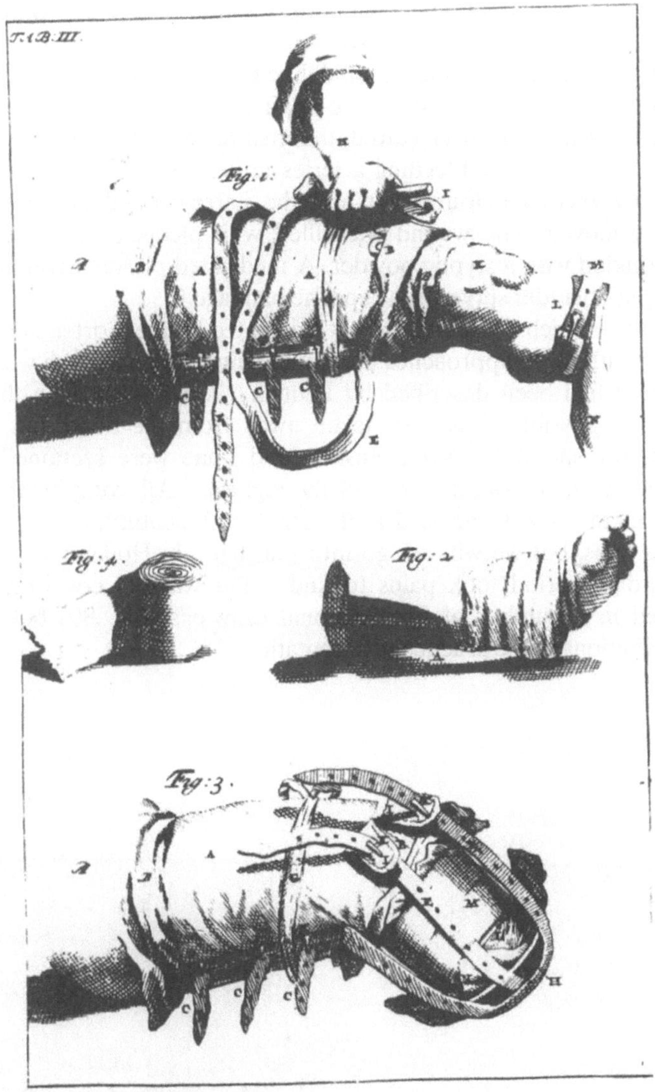

Fig. 79. Leg amputation by Verduin's method. I: The tourniquet around the upper leg, the leg having already been sawn off, leaving a muscle and skin flap posteriorly. II: The amputation specimen. III: Pressure bandage on the stump, kept in its place by a metal disk.

instructions for carrying out amputations of the leg. For the prevention of serious arterial haemorrhage he first fixed compresses in the bend of the knee and high on the thigh with bandages. Then he wrapped stiff paper around the upper leg over which he applied a solid linen bandage which served as a tourniquet when a short stick was pushed under its windings and twisted. The skin of the leg was to be pulled up as high as possible and a narrow linen bandage was firmly tied around the limb a few fingers above the scheduled amputation site: this was meant to produce some degree of numbness. Using a curved knife the surgeon should cut the muscles in one circular sweep to the bones. With a double-edged knife the soft parts between the bones were severed. An assistant then had to pull up the muscles as high as possible using a solid linen or leather strip which was split lengthways so that one half of it could be applied in front of the bones, the other behind. After the bones had been sawed, the muscles were lowered, the tourniquet loosened somewhat and any bleeding arteries undersewn. When haemostasis was satisfactorily achieved, the tourniquet and the narrow band just above the cut surface were removed. The wound was filled with pledgets moistened with egg white and sprinkled with a styptic powder. A medicated plaster covered it all up.[77] Once again a pig's bladder served as a capeline bandage.

This method — which was certainly not originated by De Gorter since we find it in many other authors — approaches the double circular procedure which became standard after it had been described by Petit in 1736. It rested on the principle that as much as possible should be taken away from the bone, but as little as possible from the soft parts. Skin, muscles and bone were sectioned at several levels, the skin at the lowest, the bone at the highest.[78] Allowing for this principle several more methods were devised in the eighteenth century, amongst which the use of double flaps, but we will not go into that here. In Holland, Petrus Camper in his Amsterdam period took pains to find better ways of covering the stump. These resulted in a number of fine sectional drawings (Fig. 80) but not in any original contributions to the practice of amputation.[79]

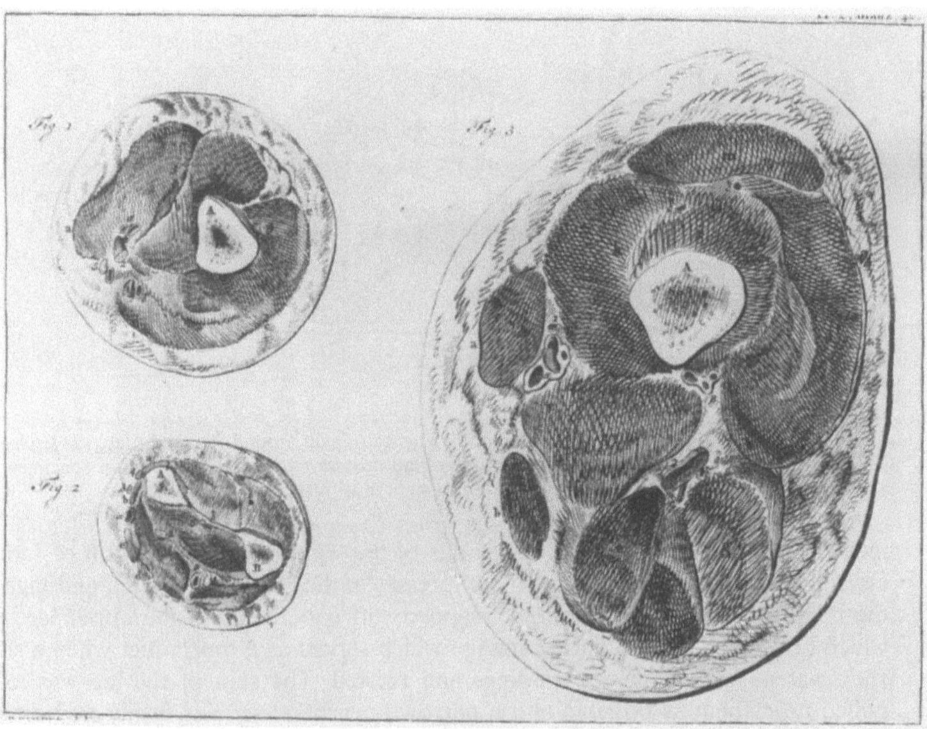

Fig. 80. Sectional drawings of an arm and an upper leg by Petrus Camper.

While a consensus was gradually being reached on the principles of amputation, there was still a difference of opinion on details of its practical execution. One of these regarded the important issue of controlling the bleeding. As in the treatment of accidental wounds, the ligature was by no means in general use in surgical operations. Van de Voorde and Solingen were amongst those who preferred to use the red-hot iron. Van de Voorde because ligating a blood vessel was time-consuming and dangerous since the thread might cut through the vessel wall. Solingen pointed out that the severed vessel often retracted into the muscles and was thereafter difficult to secure. In the first half of the eighteenth century, even in the Hôtel-Dieu in Paris the actual cautery was the only method in use.[80]

An adherent of the ligature was Van Beverwyck but then he was a physician who probably did not do practical surgery. De Gorter made use of needle and thread, undersewing the bleeding vessels percutaneously in the way described by Paré and Guillemau. Dionis, like Heister, rejected the cautery and preferred to tie the vessels.[81] In cases of secondary haemorrhage, manual or digital compression exerted by apprentices in turn was sometimes resorted to. To be able to lay the ligature with greater certainty around the vessel, the artery forceps invented by Paré, was constantly becoming more refined. William Bromfeild, when surgeon to St. George's Hospital in London, devised a special tenaculum, a slender sharp-pointed hook, not unlike Deschamp's needle, for the purpose of drawing the cut vessel out. This prevented the nerve being included in the ligature, which was extremely painful.[82]

Another mechanical means of stopping haemorrhage was external pressure applied by tight bandaging, by special devices like Verduin's apparatus or by hand as just mentioned. To this should be added Petit's screw tourniquet by which it was possible to exert aimed pressure.

A fourth method, favoured by many, was the application of styptics often combined with a compression bandage. Solingen may be cited as using firm tents made of compressed bovista or pledgets dipped into egg white and then into a styptic powder which he applied directly on the bleeding vessel.[83] De Gorter used small pieces of vitriol in muslin which he put on the vessel stump when haemostasis was not optimal: this had a cauterizing effect. Theden recommended his 'eau d'arquebusade'.[26]

The operation wound was usually closed by keeping the edges together by means of a firm bandage. The majority of surgeons, moreover, used strips of adhesive plaster. Only a few, like Van de Voorde in Holland and Sharp in England, applied sutures like Paré had recommended. As the eighteenth century advanced, healing by first intention was more and more striven after. This trend was originated by British surgeons, and on the continent Richter was a champion of 'speedy union'.[84]

There was also some disagreement on the optimal level for amputating a leg. According to Paré four fingers below the knee would be the site of election because a long leg-stump might be troublesome to the patient.[85] Garengeot on the other hand held that a long stump would not trouble the amputee so much at all. Pierre Dionis advanced as a rough-and-ready rule that the upper leg should be taken off 'as low as possible above the knee, the leg as high as possible under the knee, whereas the forearm should be left as long as possible'.[86]

Amputation of the thigh. In the surgical literature of the seventeenth and eighteenth centuries hardly any mention is made of thigh amputations. In textbooks of the time amputation of the leg apparently served as a paradigm for major amputations in general. Amputation through the femur was considered a most dangerous intervention because of the rich vascularization and the great mass of muscles. Besides, the patient's life might be endangered by the considerable suppuration which would result from such a formidable wound.[87]

From what has been said above it follows that nevertheless thigh amputations were actually being performed, be it only rarely. In 1740, the Rotterdam surgeon Johan van Wyck reported on such an operation which had taken place in Paris: the patient died from a secondary haemorrhage.[88]

Amputations through the joints. Amputation at a joint was already recommended by Celsus. Paré, Fabry of Hilden and their contemporaries sometimes resorted to this procedure in removing a leg or forearm. Disarticulation of the humerus at the shoulder joint was introduced in the eighteenth century by French surgeons, in particular by Morand the elder, Henri-François le Dran, Garengeot, De la Faye. Later in the century the famous Desault and Raphael-Bienvenu Sabatier risked doing it. In England, Samuel Sharp and Edward Alanson (1747—1823) published on the subject. Initially, a circular incision was used but after 1740 the joint was generally approached by the flap incision as described by De la Faye. The different modifications suggested in the eighteenth century, mainly considered the way the axillary artery should be taken up. Amputation through the shoulder joint was usually undertaken for dry caries and comminution, whether or not sustained in warfare.

There was much ado about hip disarticulation in Paris before this operation finally was put for the first time into practice in Dronrijp in Friesland. In 1739, the Dane Hans Frederik Wohlert (1703—79) and the Swiss Puthod published papers in the *Mémoires de l'Académie des Sciences* in Paris stating that experiments on the cadaver had demonstrated the feasibility of the operation.[89] At Morand's proposition, the Academy of Surgery in 1759 offered a prize for the best essay on its indications and technique. No less than forty-four entries were submitted, thirty of which accepted the practicability. The prize was won by a naval surgeon by the name of Barbet. He recommended this type of amputation in cases of comminuted fracture or dry caries of the head and neck of the femur, of aneurysm and gangrene. Barbet included the history of a fourteen-years old boy who in the Hôtel-Dieu at Orleans had a spontaneous hip disarticulation, brought about by extensive gangrene caused by ergotism.[90]

It seems that hip disarticulation was first performed in Holland by Johannes Mulder (see p. 179), professor of anatomy, surgery and obstetrics at Franeker. This was done with a happy outcome in an eighteen-years old girl in the village of Dronrijp on July 21, 1798, for reasons unspecified. A very short report of this operation appeared in a newspaper[91] but Mulder himself unfortunately never published the case. Twenty-six years later, his son Claas Mulder in a letter to the editor of the same paper reported that the woman was alive and well. She had borne five children. Indoors, she moved freely, hopping on one leg, being able to carry a pail of water or to climb a ladder.[92]

Joint excision. The resection of joints undoubtedly belonged to the top performances of eighteenth century surgery. A pioneer in this field was Charles White of Manchester, who in 1768 excised the head of the humerus in a boy of fourteen years for osteomyelitis. The result was satisfactory.[93] His compatriot Henry Park (1744—1831), surgeon to The Royal Infirmary in Liverpool and a former pupil of Pott and Le Cat, did, in 1783, a similar thing with regard to a knee and an elbow.[94] In Holland this operation does not seem to have been practised at the time.

Amputation as treatment of compound fractures. In the eighteenth century the question whether or not compound fractures with major laceration required immediate amputation, gave rise to the first international dispute of any dimension.[95] On the authority of French military surgeons amputation had become the standard treatment of such fractures once the fear of intra-operative haemorrhage had largely been dissipated by the introduction of the screw tourniquet. It was generally believed that sacrificing the limb before wound complications ensued would enhance the chance of survival. Dionis remarked that young military surgeons were most eager to perform operations and that they measured their exploits in a campaign by the number of arms and legs they had amputated.[96]

Matters were first taking a turn during the Austrian War of Succession (1740—48) in which Dutch, British and Austrian forces were opposing the French armies of Louis XV. It was after the bloody battle of Fontenoy on May 11, 1745, that Pierre-Joseph Boucher (1715—93) observed in the Hôpital St.-Sauveur in Lille which was packed with wounded, that two-thirds of those who underwent amputations because of shot fractures, mostly of the legs, had died, whereas out of 165 of such cases treated without amputation not a single one had taken a lethal course. 'Les grand accidents ne demandent pas toujours les grandes opérations'.[97]

In 1757 the ever-alert Royal Academy of Surgery in Paris offered a prize for the best answer to the question on how, given the inevitability of amputation, cases which required immediate operation might be distinguished from those which allowed postponement. The prize was won by Jean-Louis Faure, a regimental surgeon who on the strength of numbers, concluded that in the war now at an end the retarded operations were in the majority crowned with success, whereas the outcome was quite the opposite in those cases where amputation had been prompt.[98] His argument, founded as it was on numeration, is the first instance — primitive as it may be — of the use of statistics in surgery to establish the value of any form of treatment.

A prominent protagonist of conservative treatment was the Swiss Johann Ulrich Bilguer, surgeon-general in the Prussian army of Frederick the Great. The thesis with which he graduated in medicine in 1761, right in the middle of the Seven Years' War (1756—63), embodied his vast experience with shot fractures obtained in numerous engagements. It was translated into German, French, Spanish, English and Dutch. In this he expressed his view that amputation was only warranted in cases when the blood supply of the limb was arrested by injury of the main artery, or when gangrene had set in. His treatment consisted in generous enlargement of the wounds of entry and exit saving nerves and bloodvessels, extirpation of loose splinters and foreign bodies, digital reduction of the main bone fragments and sawing off any sharp protrusions. The wound was then filled with lint, covered with compresses and a circular bandage, which for several days was kept moist with spirit or wine. Afterwards he applied digestives and softening poultices. The limb was brought in extension between rigid supports or in a straw guttered splint. This course had to be continued even when suppuration was aggravating or maggots had invaded the wound. Bilguer, too, presented numbers to sustain his claim.[99]

Bilguer's communication made no small stir all over Europe. He was attacked by Saveur-François Morand, chief military surgeon of the French army, and by Germain-Pichaut de la Martinière, president of the Académie de Chirurgie. They both argued that Bilguer's way of treatment by incision, being nothing less than anatomical dissection, was far more painful than amputation.[100]

Some English surgeons too, were up in arms. Outstanding amongst them was Percivall Pott. Pott felt that in every instance of compound fracture, the surgeon should carefully weigh the risk of conservative treatment against the hazards of operation. His *Remarks on the necessity . . . of amputation*, published in 1762, was in substance an attack on the one-sided views of the Prussian surgeon.[101]

Yet another antagonist of Bilguer's method was David van Gesscher in Amsterdam. In a monograph of 1771 on the possibility and necessity of amputations in several surgical disabilities, he went fully into Bilguer's standpoint. He conceded that amputation was a hazarduous operation, but the hazards lay not primarily in the intervention as such, but in attending circumstances. These were:

1. a poor condition of the patient;
2. injudicious methods of operation, in particular dividing the limb in a single plane;
3. prolonged exposure to the 'infected air' of a hospital;
4. after-treatment of the stump with caustics and greasy ointments, as French surgeons in particular were wont to do.

Surgeons who operated with the necessary attention did not have reason to complain of their results. Van Gesscher quoted the results of Donald Monro (1727—1802) who in the Royal Infirmery of Edinburgh had amputated 14 big limbs without one single death. Van Gesscher finally reported on eight amputations performed 'during the last few years' in Amsterdam. Six of these patients survived.[102]

Like most other writers on the subject, Van Gesscher failed to clearly distinguish between the conditions of warfare and those in civil life. In wars of movement in particular, when field hospitals and sanitary personnel necessary to carry out any form of conservative treatment were largely absent, the only chance of survival for men who had sustained a serious fracture lay in amputation. Their useless limbs removed, they were in a better position to seek their way to some sort of shelter. This explains why even some thirty and forty years later, during the Napoleonic wars, army surgeons still performed amputations on the battlefield in large numbers. It is said that in the Russian campaign Dominique-Jean Larrey (1766—1842) performed with his own hands about 200 amputations within 24 hours during and after the battle of Borodino near the river Moskwa. This he did under the open sky of the Russian winter. The outcome of this heroic treatment never became known in detail.[103] It may have been better, however, than similar operations carried out in contemporary hospitals with their 'infected air'.

During naval engagements too, conditions precluded a careful preoperative examination and weighing up of the most appropriate course of treatment. Every so often the state of the amputation stump left much to be desired. Thus the Amsterdam surgeon Ulhoorn perforce had to reoperate upon Colonel Jan van Loon, whose leg he had amputated some years before. The bone had been sawed off obliquely. After this had been remedied by a reamputation which the patient endured 'with incomparable composure, not uttering a single word of complaint', a wooden leg could comfortably be fitted. With this the worthy officer lived in the best of health for another twenty-five years.[104]

Camper left a few sketches of unsatisfactory stumps which he saw in his Groningen clinic in 1765 and 1766: the centre of the scar was thin and adherent to the bone.[105]

Artificial limbs had been devised in the preceding ages by Paré, Fabricius Hildanus, Solingen and numerous other surgeons. In the eighteenth century, prosthetics largely benefitted by the high level reached by toolmakers all over Europe, not least in Holland.

6.4. HEAD INJURIES

Ever since Hippocrates, injuries of the head have occupied a prominent place in the textbooks of surgery. In the seventeenth century, there even appeared separate monographs on the subject, like the one by the Haarlem surgeon Wouter Schouten (1638—1704) in 1694. This work appeared one year later in German.[106] Hippocrates' famous treatise remained a basic text even in the early nineteenth century.

In the surgical literature of the seventeenth and eighteenth centuries we find good clinical descriptions of brain concussion which may or may not accompany fractures of the skull bones, of wounds of the scalp and face, and of what we now know to be fractures of the cranial fossae. The phenomenon of contralateral hemiplegia first recognized by Galen, was well-known.[107] Dionis distinguished no less than twelve types of fracture.[108] There was still some discussion on the existence of fractures by contrecoup, as described by Hippocrates and Celsus. Stalpart vander Wiel believed that skull bones could separate by mere fright: such cases required firm bandaging.[109]

6.4.1. *Pathology*

The serious consequences of skull fractures were generally imputed to blood or some other fluid running between cranium and meninges, or between dura mater and pia mater, resulting in compression of the brain. The extravasated blood could be converted into pus and infect the surrounding parts.[110]

In the middle of the seventeenth century, Job van Meekeren became interested in the phenomenon, first observed by Paré, that grave head injuries were often followed by suppuration of the liver. He entered into correspondence about it with the Rotterdam physician Nicolaas Zas (1610—63) and with his fellow citizen Paul Barbette. Zas oversimplified the matter by attributing the liver abscess to a direct injury of that organ, caused by that very accident, but was also prepared to accept the interpretation of Pigray who ascribed the formation of pus in the liver to 'sympathy'. Barbette on his part explained the phenomenon quite rationally by means of the blood circulation. Both explanations were published by Van Meekeren in his book.[111]

6.4.2. *Signs and Symptoms*

According to De Gorter, the presence of 'extravasation' could be gleaned from the type of the external violence and the localisation of the injury. Moreover from concomitant signs and symptoms such as bilious vomiting, loss of hearing, feeling, smell and taste, dizziness, falling to the ground, somnolence, snoring respiration, paralysis, convulsion, ravings, apoplexia, blood leaking from the eyes, the nose or the mouth, loss of speech, swelling of the face, swollen and red eyes. The site of the lesion could be determined from the history, from the swelling and redness of the scalp, from the movements of the hand that all the time reaches for the same spot, from any paralysis or convulsion. Many authors adhered to the old advice of incising an unbroken skin to ascertain the existence of any fracture.[112]

6.4.3. *Prognosis*

Dionis, like Ambroise Paré long before him, stressed the difficulty of forming a correct prognosis in injuries of the head. It was generally realized that extensive fractures are not necessarily followed by any bad sequelae whereas simple contusions may prove fatal.

6.4.4. *Therapy*

Conservative treatment aimed at the resolution of any accumulation of intracranial fluid by means of appropriate medication and by bleedings and purgings. Should this be of no avail, one should use the trepan.[113] Van de Voorde insisted that any respectable surgeon should possess at least five trepans with crowns of different sizes. Those crowns are best, that not only have sharp teeth on the underedge, but are provided with sharp edged teeth which descend from the upper edge in such a manner that the diameter of the crown diminishes from above downward. This prevents its all too easily slipping through on rotation.[114] In accordance with Hippocrates trephining should in the view of most authors up till the middle of the eighteenth century be resorted to in cases of contusion and when any crevice was too narrow to allow the blood that might have accumulated between the cerebral cranium and the meninges to escape freely. This indication was of a preventive character. Contrary to Hippocrates who proscribed all use of instruments in fractures attended with depression of bone fragments, depressed fractures were by most surgeons of this era accepted as an indication for operation. Percivall Pott in particular insisted that in every case of fracture with depression, the skull should be opened either to raise the fragment to its natural position, or to remove it entirely.[115] Dionis, who considered unconsciousness after a blow on the head as sufficient reason to interfere, advised operation without delay in any cases of doubt.[116] Van de Voorde adhered to the Hippocratic instructions and recommended the use of the trepan within the first three days.

The operation itself is described in detail by a great many authors. According to Dionis, the surgeon should as a preoperative measure have his hair bound together at the back of his head to prevent it from falling in front of his eyes on stooping. He should take off his wig should he wear one, and replace it by a cap which would not interfere with his work. De Gorter ordered the head of the patient to be put on a pillow under which a board was pushed and his ears to be stuffed with wax so that he would hear less of the frightening noise of the burring. The tripod screw-elevator for raising depressed skull fragments introduced by Hans von Gersdorff, was still in use with Pott, among others. Wouter Schouten referred to that instrument only to denounce it as being more difficult, more dangerous and less certain than the trepan.[117] Schouten claimed to have performed trephination many times, without ever having lost a patient.[118] De Gorter enumerated the places where the trepan may not be applied: the suturae, the temporal bone, the frontal sinus, wherever big blood vessels are running, below the occiput, on a loose bone fragment, on a bump or an indentation of the skull.

In the seventeenth century, an accomplished surgeon did not shrink from using the trepan (Fig. 81). As early as 1552 an Amsterdam city ordinance explicitly mentioned trephination upon a dead man's skull together with bleeding as the only practical parts of the master's examination.[119] The physician Nicolaas Tulp, who usually left the practice of surgery to the surgeons, sometimes did that operation himself.[120] In the opinion of Tulp's younger contemporary, the surgeon Hendrik

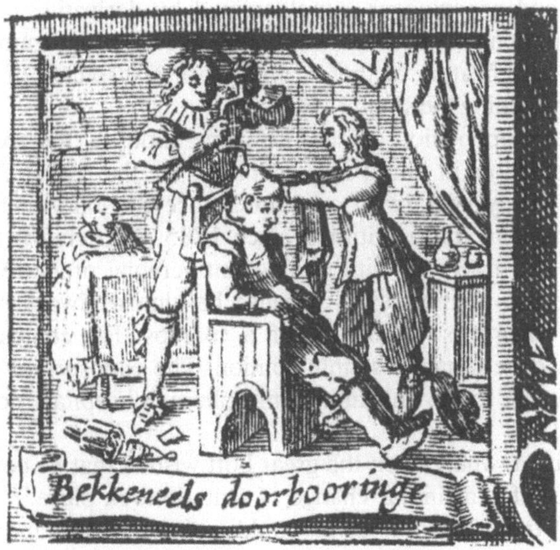

Fig. 81. Trephination of the skull, c. 1660. On the floor an opened instrument case.

van Roonhuyze, the trepan was often used too freely. Multiple operations in one and the same patient have been reported more than once. Thus Adriaan van den Spiegel, whom we have met already as an anatomist (see p. 366, n. 128). is said to have made seven burr holes in one of his patients.[121] Dionis recorded the case of a twelve-year old girl in whom, together with Mareschal, he had performed the operation twelve times.[122] It was Hendrick Chadborn, an otherwise rather unknown surgeon from Nijmegen, however, who bore away the laurels by trephining Philip of Nassau, a grandson of prince William I of Orange, no fewer than twenty-two times. The count had sustained multiple fractures when falling from his horse against a pole in the village of Wychen near Nijmegen. The outcome was quite satisfactory, the patient 'could afterwards drink three persons down on the straw'.[123] The result of the operation was not everywhere equally favourable. According to Dionis, in Avignon and Rome all patients recovered. In Paris the results were fair, in its suburbs better than in the city. In the Hôtel-Dieu, however, nearly all patients succumbed 'owing to the infected air which injures the dura mater and causes it to putrefy'.[124]

6.4.5. *Developments in the Late Eighteenth Century*

The developments which took place in the second half of the eighteenth century had mainly a bearing on indications for operation. It became clear that the results of indiscriminate trephination were not all that could be wished for. Amongst the Prussian army surgeons who, like Bilguer, trephined with a will, enthusiasm waned after Schmucker had reported that during the War of the League of Augsburg he had lost his first twelve patients, all light ambulant cases, after he had treated them with the trepan. He now reserved instrumental interference for cases of manifest fracture. In all other instances he confined himself to cold compresses wetted with sal-ammoniac and winevinegar, supplemented by derivative measures by way of bleeding and purging.[125] Richter whose works were also published in Holland, regarded only putrefication of the dura mater or a suspicion of that condition as a justification for opening the skull.

In France, too, opposition arose. This came about by the great mortality which followed trephination in the Paris hospitals. In the Hôtel-Dieu the operation therefore was hardly performed any more since the early eighties. Desault, who had been attached to that institution since 1785, restricted it to the most urgent cases of depressed fractures with signs of intracranial pressure. But even here he abandoned the use of the trepan because he almost always reached his aim by removing the fragments by means of a forceps. He contested the view that trephining would be a harmless intervention. The exposure of the bone defect to the air, in particular to the unhealthy atmosphere in hospitals, could be nothing but dangerous.[126]

In Great Britain, where even the great Pott wished that he could say that he was frequently successful, a similar change of attitude took place.[127] We may therefore summarize that trepanation, until the middle of the century more or less a routine intervention, often loosely aimed at the prevention of untoward consequences, at the end of it had become a curative operation which was only performed for urgent symptoms of which the evacuation of an actual extradural clot was the most important one.

For the rest, the history of trepanation in the eighteenth century is characterized by a gradual perfecting of the necessary instruments. The exquisitely made trepanation sets of that era in their elegant wooden cases with velvet lining are easily amongst the most beautiful surgical tools ever produced.

6.5. VASCULAR SURGERY

6.5.1. *Aneurysms*

6.5.1.1. Varieties and their Cause

It is easy to understand that the frequent venesections of former times more than once gave rise to complications. Immediate bleeding to death as represented in Figure 82 will indeed have been a rare occurrence, but the formation of a potentially dangerous traumatic aneurysm as a result of the erroneous incision of an artery was by no means an exception.

Aneurysms appear to have offered a serious surgical problem ever since Antiquity.[128] They seem, however, to have become even more so in the seventeenth and particularly in the eighteenth century if we may rely on the great number of publications on that subject then appearing. Not all of these publications referred to traumatic or false aneurysms, already in Hellenistic times physicians and surgeons were well aware of the existence of a spontaneous variety. Aneurysms caused by inexpert bloodletting understandably mainly occurred at the bend of the arm and on the foot, whereas endogenous or true aneurysms manifested themselves most frequently in the popliteal artery and in the thoracic aorta. A causal relation between spontaneous aneurysms and venereal disease was suspected by Giovanni Maria Lancisi (1654—1720), physician to pope Clement XI. In his work *De aneurysmatibus* that appeared posthumously in 1745, he explicitly imputed to venereal disease a case of popliteal aneurysm in a ‘running footman who was . . . proficient in the wrestling school of Venus, age thirty-three’.[129]

6.5.1.2. Treatment

False aneurysms were treated from the older days by pressure dressings. Since the seventeenth century, numerous mechanical contrivances for compressing the affected blood vessels were brought forward. Serious cases of false aneurysms and all true ones required operation, although many surgeons applied continuous pressure even in instances of the latter type. The increasing experience gained in arresting haemorrhages by means of ligation contributed to more surgeons daring to engage in operative treatment. The principle of the operation as laid down in Antiquity — ligation of the artery either or not followed by removal of the tumour by emptying or excising the sac — was still valid, but there were diversities in its actual performance. Dominique Anel, for instance, confined himself to ligating the artery just above the pulsating swelling, whereas Pierre Brasdor in a case of popliteal aneurysm placed the ligature far higher up at the origin of the superficial

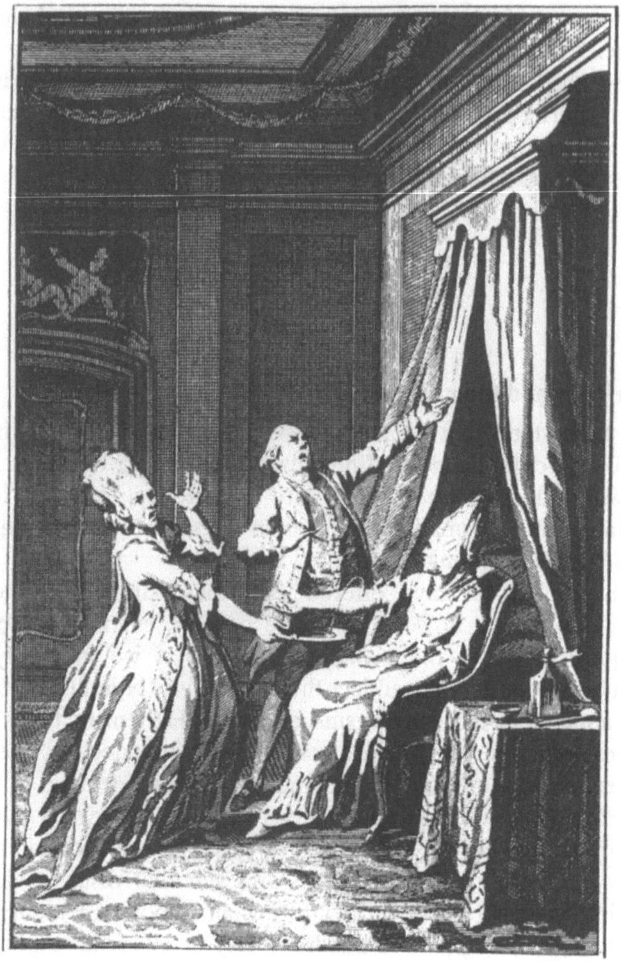

Fig. 82. Bloodletting with a fatal outcome.

femoral artery.[130] The principle of high ligation of the proximal artery was also endorsed by John Hunter, who appreciated that in endogenous aneurysm the pathological brittleness of the vessel wall was by no means confined to the dilated segment, but extended for some distance along the proximal and distal vessels.[131] To facilitate ligation, aneurysm-needles such as the well-known instrument of Deschamps (1797) were competitively invented. The ends of the ligatures were carried out of the wound, they were allowed to come out spontaneously during the process of healing. Heister uttered the warning that in the absence of a second big arterial branch, ligation might bring about gangrene requiring amputation.[132] Primary amputation of the affected limb was sometimes carried out in life-threatening cases,[133] but it seems that such a heroic approach usually had a fatal outcome. Aneurysms of the thoracic aorta — those of the abdominal aorta were apparently still unknown — were of course outside the reach of surgery. They were treated by repeated venesections and a very strict regimen as recommended by professor Antonio Maria Valsalva (1666—1723) at Bologna, the teacher of Morgagni.[134] They were of course always fatal. One such case was described by Eduard Sandifort in 1765. The patient was a 54-year old carpenter, with an enormous vascular swelling which had almost completely corroded the second up to the fourth rib inclusive at the front together with part of the sternum (Fig. 83). The man died from haemorrhage one and a half years after the tumour first became visible.[135]

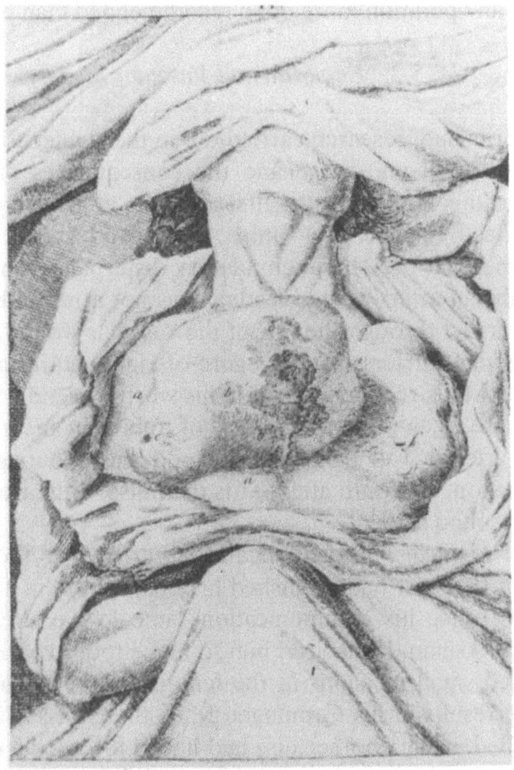

Fig. 83. Aneurysm of the thoracic aorta which penetrated the thoracic wall, 1765.

An Amsterdam Case History

Frederik Ruysch gave a dramatic account of the treatment of a traumatic aneurysm of the cubital artery in a Mr. Panhuysen from Dordrecht. At first external pressure was tried, but after a while the tumour burst, upon which the blood vigorously spurted out. By applying bovista and a pressure bandage, the haemorrhage was for the time being mastered but for a more definitive treatment there seemed to be nothing left but amputation. Yet an attempt was made to save the extremity. A closely fitting iron ring was laid around the upper arm by way of a tourniquet. The skin over the swelling, which had already become gangrenous, was incised and a large subcutaneous clot cleared away. Thereupon, in four jets, the blood started to spout again. After undersewing of the artery over and under the swelling the haemorrhage stopped. The wound was then filled up with bovista and astringent powder. A bandage was applied and an assistant was instructed to maintain continuous manual pressure on it for ten hours. In the end the patient recovered while retaining his arm. This operation was performed by Verduin in the presence of Ruysch and his good friend Abraham Cyprianus, to whom we will return below. In his commentary Ruysch stated that during the past twenty years he had not witnessed any surgeon undertaking this type of operation on an artery of that magnitude: it was an operation more often recommended than practised.[136]

6.5.2. *Experimental Vascular Surgery*

Much of the experimental research carried out in the eighteenth century considered the ways of arresting haemorrhage and the consequences of the ligation of big arteries. But we also come across the first attempts at arresting haemorrhage from partially cut arteries by means of a suture. It occurred to Mr. Lambert, surgeon at Newcastle-on-Tyne, that peripheral circulatory disturbances might be prevented in cases of a partially cut artery when bleeding was not arrested by means of ligation, but by a suture carried through the lips of the vascular wound. He had come upon the idea by observing farriers using a figure-of-eight suture in the neck of horses after bloodletting. At his recommendation, his worthy friend Mr. Hallowel, put this idea into clinical use when in treating a case of traumatic aneurysm he encountered a wound in the arterial wall from which blood was spouting. The haemorrhage indeed came to a stop. A month afterwards the pulse in the treated arm was nearly as strong as at the sound side.[137]

The periodical *Medical observations and inquiries by a Society of Physicians in London*, in which Lambert had published his observation in 1762, apparently had a wide circulation since his communication came to the attention of the Zwolle surgeon Conradus Asman. It inspired him to make four experiments in three dogs, in which he closed small incisions in the femoral artery in the aforesaid manner. He described the results in his Groningen M.D. thesis in 1773. In one animal the operation had failed, while another dog had licked the needle out after a few days, which had resulted in haemorrhage. The one remaining dog — having had two operations — was sacrificed by hanging after about two months. Both femoral arteries appeared to be markedly constricted at the site of the suture. Air, blown into the iliac artery, did not pass the constriction. It was observed, however, that the air passed readily via distended collaterals, but the significance of this was apparently overlooked. His experiments led Asman to the conclusion that at best Lambert's technique had the same result as ligation, but entailed a risk of secondary haemorrhage.[138] It is illustrative of the contemporary lack of critical acumen that Asman's conclusions have long been regarded even by surgical authorities like Velpeau in France, as definite proof of the futility of lumen-preserving arterial suture.

6.6. TUMOUR SURGERY

6.6.1. *Facial Tumours*

The removal of tumours from the head and neck belonged to the feats of seventeenth-century surgery. This appears from the fact that such operations were minutely described and illustrated in contemporary texts. Verduin recorded no fewer than three such cases in the addendum from his hand to the Amsterdam reissue of 1748 of the popular *Armamentarium chirurgiae* by Johannes Scultetus. The frontispiece, by an unknown artist, of the new edition calls direct attention to this particular operation (Fig. 84). Whereas earlier frontispieces of the *Wapenhuis* show a recumbent patient surrounded by surgeons — probably a case of a fractured upper leg being set — the central figure in this one is a patient in whom a huge tumour is about to be removed from the face, an operation which does not occur in the original Scultetus. The patient is restrained by two apprentices. His head is bound to the back of the operating chair which is separately depicted on the left. A physician standing behind the patient gives a piece of advice to the surgeon. Seventeenth century frontispieces often aim to confer a more general idea

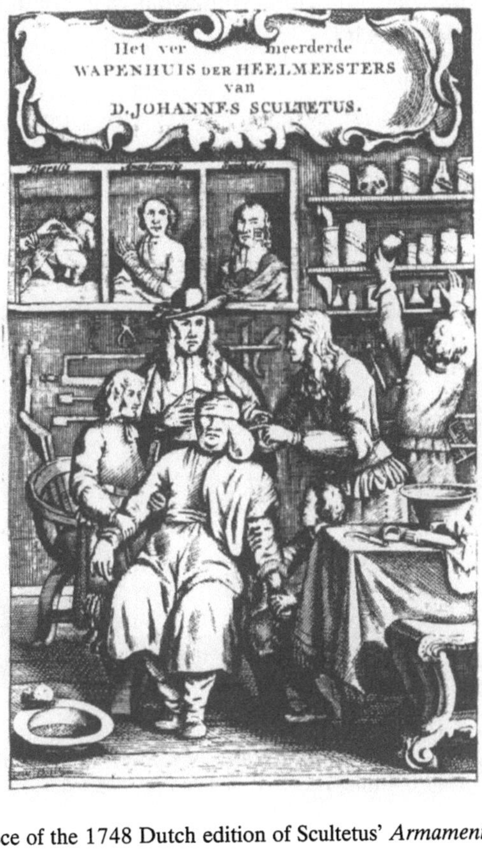

Fig. 84. Frontispiece of the 1748 Dutch edition of Scultetus' *Armamentarium chirurgicum.*

to the central representation by the use of allegories. Here the comprehensive notion is: 'surgery'. At the wall in the background some kind of a tryptich is seen hanging in which surgical therapy is symbolized by the three features of *diaeresis* – division or separation, here somewhat mischievously represented by the uncovered bottom of a child – *anapleurosis*, which means healing, illustrated by a splinted forearm and *synthesis*, represented by a wound in the face, closed by a dry suture (see p. 356, n. 22).

The first two cases published by Verduin, were in fact cured by his stepfather Jacob Cornelisz van Dalen (1608–63), a Mennonite minister who was known to be a particular skilfull operator (Fig. 38). The third patient was treated many years later by himself.[139] In all cases the operation was preceded by a detailed medical consultation in which well-known physicians and surgeons took part. In the first two cases, the tumour was removed by applying first a solid ligature around its base for some days. When it became apparent that the swelling did not proceed from the masseter muscle nor from the jaw, it was cut from its bed with a sharp curved knife (Fig. 85). Verduin in his own case first applied a caustic in the groove produced by the ligature in order to promote the formation of a scab that would diminish the danger of haemorrhage. All three cases ended well even when excision was not always easy because of hard areas in the swelling. The first patient was the only one to come out of it with a somewhat wry mouth. History is silent on how these patients fared in the end.

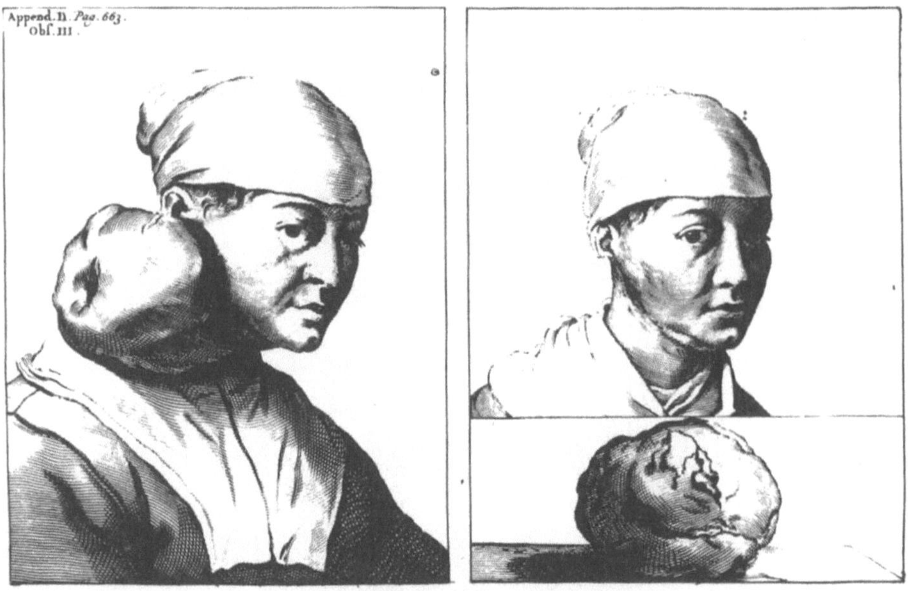

Fig. 85. Anna, daughter of Jacob, from the Holstein village of Scherenbyl, aged 17, presenting a solid, cartilaginous tumour under her right ear, which had grown to the depicted size in four years. On its removal severe arterial bleeding occurred which was stopped using bovista. The specimen weighed more than 3 pounds. The wound healed well. With mouth somewhat awry, the patient cheerfully went home (1656).

Van Roonhuyze too, once described and illustrated a similar case.[140] It seems, however, that Heister was the first to undertake it.[141] None of these authors expressed himself on the origin of such tumours, they presumably issued from the parotid gland which was first described by Caspar Bauhinus in 1605.

6.6.2. *Breast Cancer*

6.6.2.1. Pathophysiological Concepts

In the seventeenth and eigtheenth centuries, Galen's atrabiliary doctrine regarding the genesis of cancer was far from forgotten. Van de Voorde was amongst those who stuck to it (see p. 139). Influenced by rising iatrochemistry, however, several other theories appeared in which new categories like lymph, acid, acrimony, corrosion and coagulation played parts of varying importance. Lymph as a basic substance of malignant growth was accepted by François de le Boë Sylvius, for one. This Leyden professor of medicine held that a peculiar acrimony would cause the lymph to turn into cancerous matter (see p. 100). Others, like the Halle professor Hoffmann, imputed cancer to coagulation of lymph.

Cancer was still mainly thought of as a disease of the female breast. The Galenic distinction between scirrhus and carcinoma remained in force. Scirrhus was thought by the vast majority of medical people to have its immediate origin in stagnation and coagulation of body fluids, be it black bile, lymph, milk or blood. Coagulation could have a local cause, such as a fall or a blow. There was no unanimity, however, as to how scirrhus, once established, could merge into cancer.[142]

6.6.2.2. Metastasis

In the seventeenth century medical literature, ever and anon mention is made of enlarged and hardened glands in the homolateral axilla. The cause of such enlargements was thought to be the same as the one underlying the lump in the breast. Contemporary autopsy reports with an unequivocal description of visceral dissemination seem to be lacking. No definite explanation of the death caused by cancer was given either; there was some vague notion of a poison secreted by the afflicted parts. As time progressed, belief in the existence of a particular cancer poison grew stronger.

In the treatises on the nature and therapy of cancer which abound in eighteenth century literature, we find the first clear evidence of the concept of metastasis. As early as 1735, De Gorter wrote on 'cancereuse stoffe' (cancerous matter) that, after entering into the circulating blood, may make 'een metastasis van de eene glandule op de andere': a metastasis from one glandule to another.[143] Whether the notion of haematogenic metastasis was introduced here for the first time, I cannot say. Quite a few eighteenth century medical writers, however, appear to be familiar with 'remote' deposits clearly to be distinguished from direct spread.

The theory of lymphatic dissemination was greatly promoted by the admirable anatomic studies on the lymphatics by William Hewson (1739—74) in London and Paolo Mascagni (1752—1815) in Siena. Their work did much to clarify the lymph drainage system of the breast. Camper associated the only too common experience of local recurrence after mastectomy with the lymph nodes he had discovered alongside the internal mammary vessels.[144]

6.6.2.3. Contagiousness

A question that would remain unsettled until well into the nineteenth century, concerned the possible contagiousness of cancer, especially of the ulcerating type. The well-known Amsterdam physician and anatomist Tulp cited the case of an elderly lady suffering from open breast cancer, who was believed to have conveyed the disease to her housemaid.[145] The misfortune of these women served for a long time as positive evidence all over Europe.

6.6.2.4. Conservative Treatment

A great deal of attention was paid to conservative methods. 'Resolving' poultices and plasters were prescribed in great variety for external use in closed cancer and numerous ointments and powders for ulcerating stages. Internal treatment consisted of all sorts of diets (cf. p. 139), laxative medicines and, of course, bloodletting. Non-operative treatment was the rule in early cases. The Leyden professor of medicine Antonius Nuck and the well-known M.D.—surgeon and anatomist Govert Bidloo were amongst those who denied that any benefit whatsoever could be derived from drugs in the treatment of cancer. Yet belladonna and cicuta were much used in the late eighteenth century.[146]

6.6.2.5. Operative Treatment

Most surgical and medical authors appear to favour operative treatment. They enumerate, however, quite a number of contraindications. There was difference of opinion on the question whether ulcerated cancer was a case for operation. Van de Voorde was amongst those who held that ulceration amounted to a spontaneous and natural excretion of black bile and should therefore be left alone.

Straightforward ablation without closure of the wound appears to have been the favoured method. The patient was placed in a semi-recumbent position, the arm at the diseased side elevated to tighten the pectoral muscle (Fig. 86).[147] The breast was cut off in one sweeping movement with a big razor. Hot irons or styptic drugs together with a compression bandage were used to stop haemorrhage. Such an operation took only a few minutes. To have a firm grip on the breast during the operation, many surgeons introduced one or two solid traction threads through its base. Others used a big two-pronged cutting fork to lift the breast from the thoracic wall. Ulhoorn designed a cutting clamp which might remind the modern reader of a huge cigar cutter (Fig. 61). Diderot's and d'Alembert's famous *Encyclopédie*, that monument of the Enlightenment, rejected the use of any of these aids.[148]

Van Horne advised against operation in the presence of axillary enlargements, but some surgeons were prepared to take the swollen glands along. The first to be reported to have done so, was Fabry of Hilden. This he did with his forefinger, entering the axilla through a separate incision.[149]

Jean-Louis Petit, in his textbook which appeared posthumously in 1774, described a more extensive mode of mastectomy with excision of the pectoral

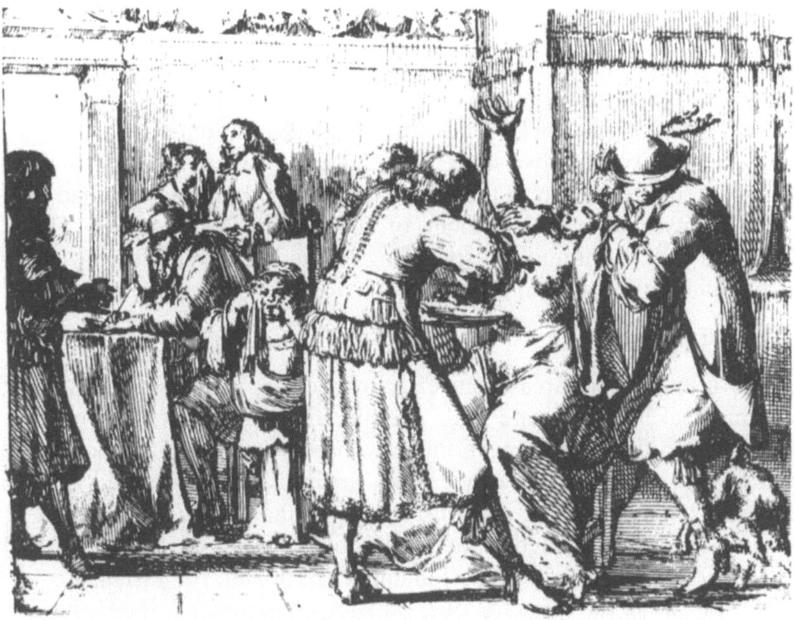

Fig. 86. Mastectomy in the 17th century.

fascia and removal of axillary nodes. In the same year Bernard Peyrilhe (1735–1804) recommended removing the pectoral muscle as well. So it appears that the principles of what later would become known as Halsted's operation, were already formulated in the second half of the eighteenth century.

6.6.2.6. Frequency of Operation

Numbers and figures hardly had any place in medical thinking before later in the eighteenth century. So we have to be content with statements like Van Horne's to the effect that breast amputation was a common intervention. Bidloo recalled that he had performed the operation twenty times in 1679 alone. He did not give any particulars. The French surgeon Henri le Dran (c. 1656–1720) claimed to have carried out 'a great number' of mastectomies, 'many' with success.[150]

There are a few statements suggesting that breast amputation was less frequently performed in the second half of the eighteenth century. Thus, in 1747, Ulhoorn remarked that in his day the notion was dawning that there was no point in operating on even small tumours, when cancerous matter had already spread to the body, as was evident from additional swellings at a distance. Thirty years ago, Ulhoorn added, this basic rule was not yet understood and surgeons 'cut off everything they saw'.[151] In 1757, Camper expressed his regret that in a densely populated town like Amsterdam — which at the time had some 200 000 inhabitants — 'not six times a year a breast was amputated with a reasonable chance of cure'.[152] In a small monograph in which he resisted the therapeutic use of cicuta in breast cancer, Jacob van der Haar at 's-Hertogenbosch stated in passing that he had a wide experience with mastectomy, but he did not go into details.[153]

6.6.2.7. Follow-up of Patients

Reliable postoperative survival rates are also lacking for this period, although there was a continued follow-up of at least some patients who had been operated upon or otherwise treated by Bidloo, Le Dran, Lambergen and Camper.

Bidloo's patient lived for five more years, despite having an ulcerating wound. Her physician wrote to Bidloo to the effect that during these years he had cut away wound excrescenses to a total weight of more than 400 pounds! There was hardness in the axilla continuously spreading to the back.[154] Follow-up reports of this kind are quite rare.

6.6.2.8. Quackery

Through the ages cancer, breast cancer in particular, provided a wide field for quacks. In medical literature one finds occasionally bits of information regarding their activities. Van de Voorde mentioned a widow from Workum who had a great reputation for curing ulcerating cancer with an infusion of pounded ash bark in milk, and with an ointment of mutton-fat, turpentine, yellow wax, salted butter, olive oil and verdigris. Remedies of graduated doctors were just as doubtful, however. The Amsterdam physician Johannes Hartmann, for instance, was cited by Van de Voorde as the inventor of a powder consisting of dragon-herb, white arsenic and chimney-soot.[155]

A certain reputation in the treatment of breast cancer was enjoyed by the nuns of a convent near the German town of Rees. These holy women sent beguines abroad to hand out a secret remedy which most probably consisted of a mixture of pounded crawfish and garlic, sewn in linen bags for external application.[156] Since the beguines — who were also active in Amsterdam — declared each small lump to be cancer but refrained from treating bad cases, they could boast of a high recovery rate.

6.7. HERNIA

6.7.1. *Incidence*

Herniae must have been of frequent occurrence since they figure largely in all surgical textbooks of the seventeenth and particularly the eighteenth century. In 1761, Petrus Camper described the gravity and incidence of this ailment in the following words.

> Amongst the infirmities of our body there are none, which in my opinion give more reason for grave concern, and therefore require more accurate investigation than the ruptures. For amongst aged men one finds very many indeed who show a descending hernia of the intestine only, or combined with the omentum, with a water- or fleshy hernia, or keep it in with a truss. Not rarely this inconvenience disrupts the groins on both sides, preventing the labourer from gaining his livelihood and the rich man from enjoying his abundance. Women, although less in number, groan under the same pains so far as the nature of their parts allows it. Even first-born children are not exempt, but may bring their ruptures with them into the world. So widespread is this pitiable ailment![157]

The same author stated elsewhere more precisely that in Holland one in five was cursed with the infirmity. This would be more than in many other European countries.[158]

The Amsterdam surgeon Monnikhoff to whom we will have occasion to return presently, was in 1775 the first to publish important statistics — 1230 cases in 1000 patients — of ruptures. These he must have observed over a period of 45 years. From which it appears that herniae in the umbilical region particularly befall obese persons, men less frequently than women, mostly next to the navel, occasionally above it. Inguinal herniae on the other hand are more often found in the male sex either on one or on both sides, on the left less than on the right and this in a ratio of one to two. Monnikhoff imputed the preponderance of the right side to the more frequent use of the right arm. Femoral herniae are only seen in adults, particularly in thin individuals. Herniae occur in particular in inhabitants of moist and boggy regions and may be hereditary in certain families.[159]

6.7.2. *Pathology*

6.7.2.1. Indirect Inguinal Hernia

About 1672 the naturalist Jan Swammerdam and the physician Justus Schrader dissected together a male cadaver in the Amsterdam hospital 'Binnengasthuis'. On the site from which inguinal herniae issue forth, they found a protrusion of the peritoneum which extended into the scrotum. When Swammerdam by means of a small tube blew air into the dimple marking its point of origin, the elongation assumed a pouchlike appearance. This ran alongside the spermatic cord in such a way that it became indented by that structure without being in any open communication with it.[160] Boerhaave, in his biography of Swammerdam, called this 'the precious discovery of the true nature of herniae'.[161] Yet this discovery, published by Schrader in 1674, did not settle the ancient dispute whether the inguinal hernia results from a stretching or a rupture of the peritoneum. Twenty-five years later, in 1701, Jean Méry (1645—1722), first surgeon of the Hôtel-Dieu in Paris, reconsidered the subject in a fundamental disquisition. He emphatically denied that the peritoneum would be ruptured in cases of hernia and stated that inguinal and scrotal herniae were surrounded by a dilated extension of the peritoneum.[162] This publication marks an epoch in which much anatomical research was conducted into the origin of herniae. Michel-Louis Reneaulme de la Garanne (1676—1739), dean of the Paris medical faculty, was prepared to accept a tearing of the peritoneum in those herniae which suddenly come into being, although he admitted never to have seen such a tear for himself. Reneaulme designated as the main cause of herniation the pressure of the abdominal muscles and the midriff on the viscera and the presence of a weak, stretchable spot in the abdominal wall, for instance where structures penetrate. In the latter instance, the orifice is not an open ring, but rather a slit through which the peritoneum protrudes like a sheath alongside the spermatic vessels leaving the trunk. Such places are gradually being dilated by increases in intra-abdominal pressure — jumping, dancing, walking, playing wind instruments — or by the weight of the intestines. When the bowels are filled with inspissated faeces they may slip through the weak spot either gradually or all of a sudden.[163]

Reneaulme who, by framing this theory, made the first important attempt at a scientific explanation of the causative mechanism of hernia, was well aware of the existence of the processus vaginalis peritonei of which, he wrote, Swammerdam was the discoverer. To this *vitium conformationis* he imputed the frequent occurrence of inguinal herniae in children.

Some ten years later De Garengeot formulated a similar hypothesis. He described the inguinal canal as consisting of three separate splits in the muscles which are lying behind one another mutually overlapping and thus closing the canal. On the tightening of the muscles they come to lie more directly in line. Garengeot gave an accurate description of this action of the transverse and oblique abdominal muscles. Femoral herniae would be caused by a similar mechanism. He did not mention rupture of the peritoneum anymore but neither did he seem to regard the open processus vaginalis peritonei as a predisposing factor.[164]

In 1747, Antonio Benevoli (1685—1756), surgeon at the Hospital S. Maria Nuova at Florence, raised objections to the theories of Reneaulme and Garengeot. In his opinion the presence of open, flaccid rings was not sufficient to explain the protrusion of the intestines. For this a pathological relaxation of the mesentery was first and foremost required.[165] In 1756 Percivall Pott wrote a treatise on the anatomy of the inguinal canal and the femoral ring. In his classical study, which included the first description of congenital hernia, he also gave a thorough account of the different possible modes of incarceration and the methods of surgical treatment.[166] The French surgeon Georges Arnaud de Ronsil (d. 1774), who practised successfully in London, was the first to distinguish between an irreducible and a strangulated hernia.[167]

Just splendid are the accurate drawings that Camper made of autopsy cases he examined in the 'Binnengasthuis' during his years in Amsterdam (Fig. 87). These were published in 1801 by the well-known German anatomist Samuel Thomas Soemerring (1755—1830) in Frankfurt-on-Main. Professor Richter in Göttingen who through his *Abhandlung von den Brüchen* (1777—79) which was translated into several languages including Dutch, may be regarded as one of the prominent authorities in the field, held the view that an 'unnatural relaxation' of the peritoneum and all other structures that keep the intestines in their place was an important factor. Intestines and abdominal wall continuously act counter to each other. The intestines filled with elastic air strive after expansion and enlargement of the abdominal cavity whereas the parietal muscles try to limit their dimensions. If this equilibrium is being disturbed to the detriment of the abdominal wall, then this may weaken, either entirely as in pregnancy or dropsy, or only at a particular site. Herniae result from the latter condition.[168]

The significance Benevoli and to some extent Richter attached to a lengthening of the mesentery was denied by Antonio Scarpa. His book *Sull'ernie* which appeared in 1809, is one of the classics in the history of herniology: it has been translated into many other languages but apparently not into Dutch. Scarpa stressed that the mesentery did not so much serve the purpose of attaching the intestines as of their nutrition. Any lengthening was not the cause, but the result of sliding down into a hernia. He shared Richter's conclusion, that its real cause lay in a disturbance of the equilibrium between pressure and counter-pressure which at

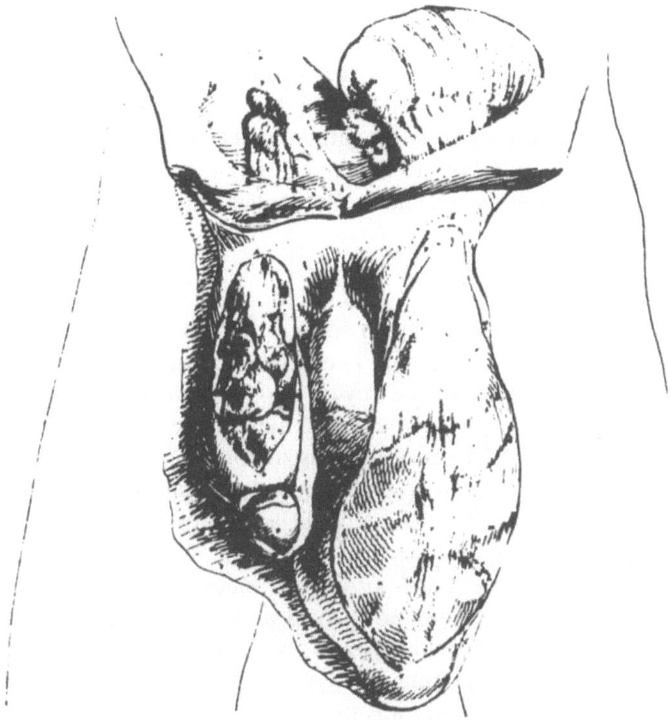

Fig. 87. Bilateral scrotal hernia: at the left side an omental hernia, at the right side an intestinal hernia. Drawing by Petrus Camper.

weak spots in the abdominal wall would result in hernia. In this treatise, Scarpa also gave an accurate description of the sliding hernia which was probably first observed by Pierre Franco.[169]

6.7.2.2. Congenital Hernia

Many authors investigated the problem of congenital hernia focussing attention on the significance of the patent processus vaginalis. Camper who, on the authority of Winslow and Douglas, initially had assumed that the peritoneum snugly encloses the spermatical cord, found so many newly born in his autopsy-material, boys in particular, with patent processus, that he came to accept this as a normal anatomical structure at that tender age — a remnant of testicular descent — which would gradually close around testis and cord. The failure of closure of the processus would give rise to an inguinal hernia in the newly born. Just like Monnikhoff, Camper attached some aetiological importance to the damp climate in this country. Infantile hernia was so frequent, he wrote, that most of the time the parents did not bother to call in the aid of a doctor or surgeon, but left its cure to 'old women'. Such ruptures usually heal after they have been bandaged for a year or perhaps slightly more. Their closure is brought about by alterations in intra-abdominal pressure which occur during growing. This explains why a patent processus vaginalis is rarely observed in adults. Herniae in adults are usually not a consequence of persistence of such elongations of the abdominal peritoneum. In adult cases the peritoneum can locally extend to a sac, arising at the site where a tiny scar is reminiscent of the former exit of the processus vaginalis. The Hague surgeon Dringenberg 'famous for his attainments and excellent dexterity in operations for herniae' pointed out to Camper in 1754, that such a hernial sac does not pass within the processus vaginalis, but outside and next to the spermatic cord.[170]

6.7.2.3. Strangulated Hernia

In the eighteenth-century literature much attention was paid to strangulation as the most dangerous complication of hernia. The extensive articles on herniology in for instance the *Mémoires de l'Académie royale de Chirurgie* while presenting much case material stress the aetiology and therapy of incarcerated hernia.

It was generally felt that the cause of constriction had to be looked for in the orifice. But according to some, an abnormal narrowing and hardening of the neck of the sac could be the cause as well as could an occlusion of the intestinal loop lying in the sac by faeces or by gas.

Richter distinguished three types of incarceration: a variety caused by an accumulation of faeces, an inflammatory form and a spastic form. Strangulation brought about by faecal occlusion would be slow developing, whereas the distinctive feature of the inflammatory type would be pain and fever. The inflammation could be the cause but was more often the result of the incarceration. Spastic strangulation is characterized by remissions and by its responding to spasmolytic agents. Its primary cause would be bilious defilement and intestinal worms. The seat of the cramp was the external oblique muscle which by contraction of its fibres would bring about a narrowing of the sinewy external ring of the inguinal canal.[171] Scarpa pointed out that a descended loop of intestine makes an oblique angle with the rest of the intestinal tract which by becoming still more acute may easily close the passage.

6.7.2.4. Direct Inguinal Hernia

Heister, when dissecting the dead body of a rope-dancer, once found an inguinal hernia which arose form 'a newly made opening next to the annulus, not far from the linea alba'.[172] This might be the first recorded instance of a direct inguinal hernia but it was only at the beginning of the nineteenth century that the internal—direct and external—indirect types of inguinal herniae, having their origin medial or lateral to the deep epigastric artery, came to be clearly differentiated.[173]

6.7.2.5. Other Types

In 1655 Barbette in Amsterdam was probably the first to describe an abdominal hernia 'below and beside the umbilicus, way above the groin', which may well have been a semilunar hernia. A swelling in the location, he wrote, may be taken for an abscess by ignorant surgeons and consequently be incised. Barbette also called attention to a type of herniation in the back which could have been the lumbar hernia more fully described by Jean-Louis Petit in 1774, and a rupture in the groin in such a way that the descending intestinal loop is not driven into the scrotum, but finds its way between the skin and muscles to the thigh. The latter condition may well have been a femoral hernia.[174]

6.7.3. *Clinical Features*

The clinical features of the several types of hernia are well described in the literature of the period. Yet it sometimes did occur, as Barbette had feared, that a surgeon took a swelling for an abscess and acted accordingly. Ulhoorn relates the case of an English student at Leyden who fell victim to such a diagnostic error. A certain surgeon cut into the swelling after Ulhoorn's father, a surgeon whose previous good services had been rewarded by this student with mere ingratitude, refused to attend upon him any more. 'Owing to which, to end this case briefly, that English extortioner in little time moved out of the world'.[175]

6.7.4. *Treatment*

6.7.4.1. Non-Strangulated Hernia

Conservative Treatment

Writing in the second half of the sixteenth century, the Dutch physician Pieter van Foreest stated that surgeons shrank from herniotomy leaving that intervention to empirics.[176] More than a hundred years later, matters had not changed. The Paris surgeon Pierre Dionis expressed opposition of the operation since in men it still implied at the time the removal of the testis. This he deemed to be at variance with divine and human laws. He was prepared, however, to make an exception in the case of a religious who has little use for 'his balls' anyway. 'He would derive two benefits from it: the first being that he would no longer be bothered by those parts, the second that he would be relieved from a difficult ailment'. The efficacy of the operation Dionis did not contest.[177]

In Holland too, the treatment of this condition, if it was treated at all, was conservative in principle. It seems that Dutch surgeons were even more conservative than their colleagues in some other countries. Particularly in Germany and Switzerland, herniae were cut liberally and rashly. This was what Solingen had heard from physicians and surgeons who had visited those regions and also from apprentices of German extraction as well as from one having lived in Germany with a rupture master and afterwards serving with him: they attested to that in most boastful words.[178]

The Rotterdam praelector Pieter Vink whom we heard once before running down his Dutch fellows for their little inclination to operate (see p. 178), wrote in 1740: '. . . herniotomies, how little are they heard of in most places? I know of important and populous towns in which it is not remembered that such an operation was ever carried out . . .'.[179] In general, the ruptured were provided with a truss.

Trusses and their makers. Dionis narrates that there were several people in Paris who applied themselves exclusively to the treatment of herniae with trusses. These 'rupture masters' were members of the surgeons' guild of Saint-Côme, to which company they were admitted after having presented a 'masterpiece' — presumably a truss framed by themselves — as evidence of their skill. Some of these artisans were so proficient, that most surgeons obtained their trusses from them. In the country, where 'rupture masters' were absent, surgeons had to make their own trusses.

In Holland trusses were made by the master-surgeons themselves, or on their prescription by artisans. Even prominent surgeons like Ulhoorn and Camper did not think it beneath their dignity to forge their trusses with their own hands. When Camper was professor at Franeker (1751—55) he thought the readymade trusses which he had sent to him from Amsterdam to be of inferior quality. This induced him to make a serious study of the conditions a properly made truss would have to fulfill. His investigation resulted in a few articles which did not only appear in Dutch, but also in French like the one in the *Mémoires de l'Académie de Chirurgie* of 1774 with diagrammatic representations. Camper's knowledge of trusses was not merely theoretical: ever since his disappointment from Amsterdam he made these resilient steel objects himself. He held the opinion that surgeons should not only know how to measure these bandages, but also be able to construct them. In his 'collegium causale chirurgicum' in Groningen he once a year used to make in the presence of his students a truss from the very beginning, including forgeing and hardening of the steel bow. At last he acquired such a skill in this art that allegedly it almost never happened that his devices failed to hold an inguinal or femoral hernia in place. Since many military men were suffering from ruptures, Camper made a plea for fitting them with excellent and cheap trusses 'for the good of the country'. Military tailors should make allowances for a truss in making breeches.[180]

Ulhoorn recalled the case of a wealthy miser whose hernial orifice permitted the introduction of the tips of all his fingers brought together. The truss Ulhoorn made for him was quite effective so that the man could live on in comfort, albeit with a heavy heart because of the fee.[181]

Ready-made trusses could be obtained from pharmacies and even renowned makers of physical instruments like Van Musschenbroek in Leyden fabricated such devices.[182] Eighteenth-century newspapers displayed advertisements in which these useful expedients were offered for sale. As truss-making improved, the empiric herniotomists slowly retired to the shade, whereas a new occupational group arose, that of the bandagists. They did not limit their activities to the making of trusses, but also measured ruptured persons without qualified control. The surgeons of course regarded such activities with disfavour as may be inferred from scornful remarks in contemporary textbooks.

Some of the bigger towns employed surgeons as 'town rupture masters' (stadsbreukmeesters) who on a part-time basis had to care for the town's poor.

Operative Treatment

Itinerant operators for hernia. All through the seventeenth century, herniotomy was mainly performed by travelling empirics. Pierre Dionis had little liking for them. Some of them must have been able operators since they managed to perform the castration which formed part of their cure in a cleverly inconspicuous way.

Dionis knew of an empiric who brought his dog along for the purpose. This animal 'lay in wait under the bed or the table near its master for that delicacy the master treated him to as soon as he had taken it out, without the bystanders noticing it. They would have sworn that the patient had kept all his parts'.[183]

In the Netherlands too, specialized empirics were active in this field as late as in the early part of the eighteenth century. Herniotomy seems to have been the last part of operative surgery in which empirics were active. Since they usually had a roaming existence, they left few traces in the guilds' or towns' archives apart from notes on a temporary admittance for a fee to be paid to the surgeons' guild or from a rare handbill preserved by chance. In 1700, Gerard Gorus described them as quacks who 'proceeding from the dregs of the people . . . lay their hands on this holy art, pillage the patients and in the manner that assassins and privileged executioners with impunity play with human lives, leading innumerable people to ruin'.[184]

It is, however, a different question whether this qualification held true for all those who applied themselves to herniotomy. lithotomy and the couching of cataract, difficult operations the average surgeon preferred to leave alone. For before such 'operators' were allowed to practise, they had to submit proofs of their competence, usually in the form of written testimonials, to the satisfaction of the Collegium medicum and the wardens of the surgeons' guild.

Among the travelling empirics there were several foreigners, Germans mostly, who had received a sound surgical training in their country of origin but for some reason or other had not managed to establish themselves there in practice.

Johann Francken (16?—17?). A case in point is the 'German master' Johann Hermann Francken from Brunswick who had acquired much experience on battlefields in North Italy before coming to Holland in 1694. Since in his surgical writings he gave many particulars of his chequered career, we are in the position to form some idea of the life and work of at least one representative of this curious group of practitioners who in their time played such an important rôle.

Francken initially behaved entirely like an itinerant quack who in his boastful handbills promised to cure blindness and bladder stone as well as intestinal hernia. After many wanderings he established himself in the small Frisian town of Workum where, according to a testimony by the city government, he successfully operated on several people for the stone, for hernia and cataract. In 1729 in the same town he passed the examination for master-surgeon, after which he was appointed town surgeon in Amersfoort. All would have been well, were it not that he could not refrain from advertising himself in handbills. In these he also boasted of his knowledge of uroscopy, an art which was no longer part of official medicine but lingered on in quackery. Because of quarrels with the surgeons' guild he left his office after three years. He then succeeded in getting a similar position in Utrecht. Twice — in 1717 and 1731 — Francken also practised in the environs of Amsterdam where by his own account he performed 208 herniotomies, 4 lithotomies and 36 eye operations. In case records in his book, Francken also relates some interesting hernia cases. In Ylst in Friesland, for instance, he once operated upon a certain Pals Palsen for an unusually voluminous rupture, almost as big as a distended calf's bladder. On the fifth day after the operation the patient, instead of using the bedpan as he was instructed to do, sat himself on a chamber pot on the floor, straining so fiercely, that the tied peritoneum burst open and his intestines were shot out over the floor which was covered with sawdust, sand and other dirt. Master Francken, who was summoned in great haste, washed the prolapsed intestines with warm milk and pushed them back into the abdomen. Since he did not have any instruments with him, he could not resuture the defect. He then made a quick decision: he shelled the testis out of the scrotum, pushed it through the orifice into the abdominal cavity and tied a string around the neck of the scrotum. The patient regained his health.[185]

Operative techniques. In 1724, Francken still practised the age-old 'punctum aureum', the ligation of the hernial sac with a gold thread (cf p. 58). This method had meanwhile become obsolete, which is why the Collegium medicum in Amsterdam did not allow him to practise in that city. But in his book, which appeared in 1733, he described his mode of working as follows: exposure of the sac and pulling it outwards as far as possible without opening it, pushing back its contents into the abdominal cavity and ligating it as short as possible. Should the sac contain a tag of omentum, then it was opened and the omentum drawn out as much as possible and tied off. When after a number of days the ligated tag had fallen off, the omentum stump was to be pushed back and the sac tied up behind it.[186]

This method was in keeping with the general trend at the time to preserve the testicle. To this end some surgeons tried to provoke an inflammatory obliteration of the internal ring of the inguinal canal by the use of a tight truss with a hard pad, others aimed at obliterating the sac by etching with sulphuric acid.

The Académie de Chirurgie strongly raised its voice against the latter method after the famous mathematician Charles-Marie de la Condamine fell victim to it.[187] Richter condemned all such methods. A really radical cure of hernia should consist of closure of the sac, followed by narrowing of the external orifice. 'Of all surgical operations there is perhaps none which is more painful to the patient and requires so much knowledge, judgement, attentiveness and presence of mind as herniotomy', Van Gesscher noted as late as 1781.[188] He hardly ever thought the operation to be indicated. Gesscher himself performed it only twice in his practise of twenty-five years standing. Besides, the outcome did not always give reason for rejoicing.

Surgeon-herniotomists. Only few established surgeons ventured on herniotomy in non-obstructed cases. The enormous size many herniae had assumed in the course of time would surely not have encouraged any operative approach (Fig. 88). Van Meekeren presents the case of an able seaman whose hernia on standing reached to below the knees while the abdomen had almost disappeared, yet who was second to none in striking the topsail.[189] Thus it is understandable that those surgeons who dared to undertake operative correction, asked substantial fees. Rochus van Dyck, town lithotomist and herniotomist in Amsterdam since 1642, asked for 125 guilders in advance and another 125 guilders after the cure. Any

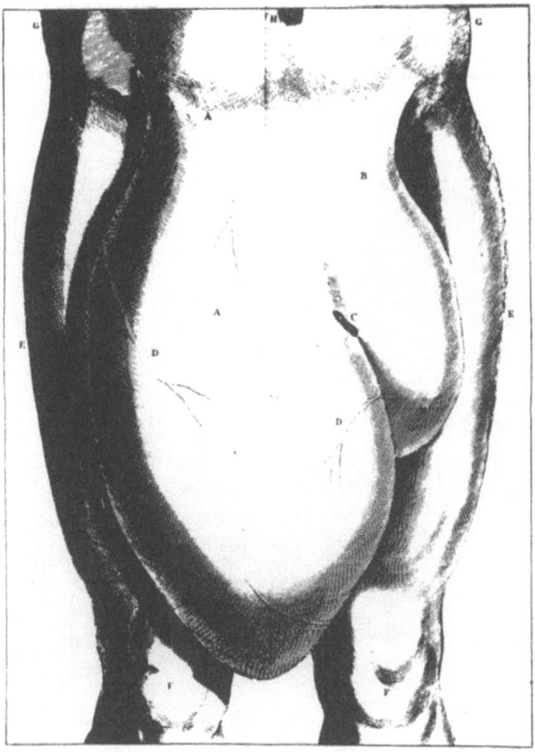

Fig. 88. The bilateral intestinal hernia of Anthoni Helt in Amsterdam which was successfully operated upon by Mr. Joannes Steiger in 1730, while sparing the testis. The wound healed in 7 weeks.

recurrence within two years, however, would be treated free of charge.[190] 'All hernia operations are attended with danger to the life of the patient and take place at the cost of his purse', Monnikhoff remarked some hundred years later.

After about the middle of the eighteenth century, itinerant empirics are no longer heard of and herniotomy came to the responsibility of properly trained surgeons although by no means of all. Even an outstanding anatomist like Camper seems to have performed this operation but once in his life.[191] The availability of good trusses largely obviated the necessity of the operation.

6.7.4.2. Strangulated Hernia

The treatment of strangulated hernia consisted first and foremost of reposition. This was first aimed at in an indirect way. Copious bleeding until the patient was on the verge of fainting, might bring about a salutary relaxation causing the hernia to slide back. Or one could apply a clyster to void the large intestine and lay relaxing poultices on the swelling. Heister sometimes had good results with a tobacco smoke clyster. Other surgeons expected more of a local treatment with astringents or with cold, in the form of wet compresses, snow or the sudden pouring of ice-cold water. If all this was of no avail, the hernia should be reduced manually with the greatest possible carefulness. Some surgeons carried this out in a lukewarm bath. When reduction failed, there remained no choice but to operate (Fig. 89).

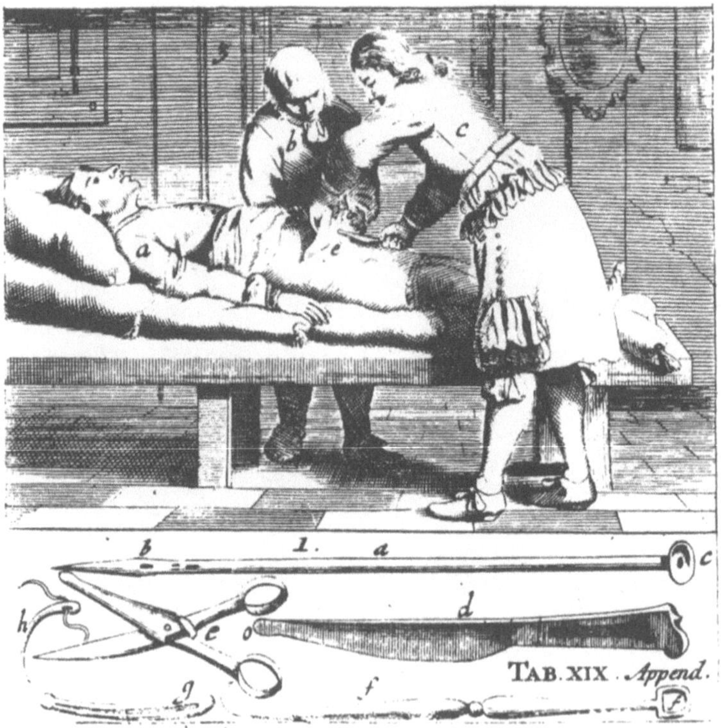

Fig. 89. Herniotomy.

The operation consisted — in case of an inguinal hernia — of enlargement of the outer inguinal ring and reposition of the contents of the sac. A case history which the M.D.—surgeon Abraham Cyprianus (c. 1660—1718) published in 1700 shows how this was done. His patient was a labourer of fifty years of age with a large, strangulated scrotal hernia causing faecal vomiting. Cyprianus first incised 'the scrotum and the stretched abdominal membrane' exposing the strangulated loop of large intestine. Then he notched on his finger 'the coverings and the muscles of the lower abdomen which constitute the ring through which the elongated peritoneum together with the intestines had slipped into the scrotum'. In this case reposition through the enlarged orifice was at first impeded by attachments of the colon to the elongated peritoneum that had to be severed by knife. The inguinal ring and other divided parts were sutured. In spite of his advanced age the patient had a smooth recovery. Cyprianus was most disappointed to find that the hernia later recurred although the scar had become so firmly attached to the pubic bone, that there had seemed to be little danger of relapse. This gave him a rather pessimistic outlook on herniotomy in general.[192] Other surgeons used a grooved director instead of their forefinger to protect the intestine while notching the ring. Incarceration of a femoral hernia required the incision of the lacunar ligament, first described in 1793 by the Spanish surgeon Don Antonio de Gimbernat (1734—1816).

Such enlargement operations entailed the risk of cutting into a nearby blood vessel: the epigastric artery in case of an inguinal hernia or an aberrant obturator artery — Hesselbach's 'corona mortis' (1819) — in case of a femoral hernia. Opinions differed as regards the best direction to incise the orifice: upward and inward, or upward and outward. Lethal haemorrhage did, however, sometimes occur in either way, which would not particularly have stimulated surgeons to take up the knife.[193] This may explain the procrastination and even omission one frequently encounters in case histories of the time, although textbooks urged that operation to be carried out as soon as possible to forestall mortification of the trapped intestinal loop.

Tulp recorded the case of an incarcerated scrotal hernia with faecal vomiting which even on the thirteenth day was successfully reduced by the surgeon Cornelis Sasbout.[194] Operation was apparently not considered at all. As late as 1759, Camper recorded that in Amsterdam 'cutting of tangled ruptures' was very rarely done.[195]

Following the case of a patient who, after attempts at taxis had failed, died on the fourth day of his hernia becoming strangulated, Job van Meekeren recommended replacing the contents of the sac via a small laparotomy immediately above the swelling. He derived the details of the operation which he himself had never put into practice, from Pigray's *Epitome*.[196] The Leyden physician Frederik Dekkers (1644—1720) described a case in which the proposed laparotomy really was performed, but the patient did not survive.[197]

An important question concerned the hernia which had already become gangrenous. Sometimes nature herself performed a cure as in the case of the town midwife Engel Tyssen. Mrs. Tyssen was a very obese person about forty years of age. She had an umbilical hernia the size of a child's head, which one day became strangulated causing her much pain. She was released from her agony when the swelling perforated with the passage of much pus and faeces. Being a 'particularly courageous woman', she soon dressed the wound herself. The opening grew gradually smaller until in the end a defect the size of a bean remained. Through this she passed her daily motions: nothing came anymore per anum, not even flatulence. Three years after her mishap the woman was in the best of health, having delivered in the meantime 394 children.[198]

Inspired by similar cases Méry, Heister, Garengeot and still others created a gun barrel enterostomy in the herniotomy wound after resection of the affected intestinal segment. There were even attempts at joining the two intestinal segments. In 1730 Ramdohr, surgeon to the duke of Wolffenbuttel, after excision of the gangrenous loop, succeeded in restoring the continuity by inserting one of the cut ends into the other. He then fixed the two components of this invagination with a single suture catching the intestinal wall at either side. When after a year this patient died from pleurisy, Ramdohr had the opportunity to do a post mortem examination and to remove the anastomosed segment. He presented the specimen to Heister.[199]

6.7.5. *Legacy Monnikhoff*

In the foregoing we have already referred more than once to the Amsterdam surgeon Johannes Monnikhoff (1707—82). This man, after becoming a master-surgeon, confined himself entirely to the treatment of hernia. In 1752 he was appointed 'town rupture master' in his place of residence. Two years previously he had published a book on the subject, a second edition of which appeared posthumously in 1792. At the beginning of this section on hernia we have already presented the most important items from his work.

Shortly before his death, Monnikhoff instituted a fund for the promotion of surgical sciences, herniology in particular. Out of the interest from this capital, consisting of 22 000 guilders, gold medals had to be paid for to present to the winners, Dutch or foreign, of a yearly contest held by the curators. The prize-answers, twenty-seven in number, were published between 1797 and 1850 in fourteen octavo volumes. The last prize-winning essay came from the pen of J. M. Schrant: it is on benign and malignant tumours and gives an excellent survey of the existing knowledge on that subject in the middle of the last century. In 1852, the fund was suppressed by a judgment of the court because the curators had not honoured for three years their obligation of instituting a prize subject once a year. What remained of the capital was made available to the Monnikhoff heirs.[200]

6.8. BLADDER STONE

6.8.1. *Incidence*

Right up to the end of the eighteenth century bladder stones seem to have occurred very frequently all over West Europe. It is true that statistical evidence for the earlier ages is lacking — medical statistics came only in the early decades of the last century into more general use — but the numerous and extensive case reports together with pertinent statements by contemporary medical authors testify to that. According to Tolet, the disease was particularly prevalent among the lower classes and in small children, in the country more so than in the cities.

In the Netherlands in particular, bladder stones seem to have been of frequent occurrence. The Dordrecht physician Jan van Beverwyck, whose treatise on the stone is referred to on page 130, designated vesical calculus 'an evil very common in this country, and killing many people'.[201] This was confirmed by the English physician Thomas Muffett, who in 1655 in his *Health's Improvement* wrote that although his fellow countrymen had to bear their share of this inconvenience '... no people in the world are more subject to that disease (than the Dutch), as the number and excellency of stone-cutters in that country may plainly prove'.[202] About a hundred years later the Amsterdam surgeon Abraham Titsingh remarked that the ailment was very common especially in the province of Holland.

6.8.2. *Operative Treatment*

As was pointed out on page 59, there are indications that by the Middle Ages operative treatment had already been resorted to in the Netherlands. Pieter van Foreest, the most distinguished physician in this country in the sixteenth century, wrote however, that in his day surgeons generally shrank from operations such as herniotomy and cutting for the stone. Foreest mentioned a single Dutch lithotomist, a certain Willem van Dalen at Delft, but he does not seem to have thought much of him.[203]

In the seventeenth century this situation began to change as amongst other things appears from the interest for lithotomy displayed in medical literature. Van Beverwyck described two modes of operating in some detail, the Celsian cutting directly on the stone pushed forward by the surgeon's fingers and the Marian operation involving the use of a metal sound or staff. The suprapubic cystotomy advanced by Franco he only mentioned in passing, he was not aware of that operation ever having been put into practice. In his description of the operation with the staff he closely followed Paré although it is not quite clear whether he had a sectioning of the membranous urethra in view, or the lateral cystotomy which we came across in Franco (see p. 93). Being a physician, Van Beverwyck had never performed any of these operations himself, but he had attended many: in his opinion the first mentioned was the easiest, surest and best. In the middle of the century the Amsterdam physician Barbette wrote that in his place of residence there were such expert lithotomists as to outdo the famous French specialists in this field.[204] Other authors too drew comparisons which went in favour of the Dutch. In regard to bladder stone operations too, as Paris was apparently leading, we must fix our attention for a few moments on what went on in the French capital.

6.8.2.1. France

An important part in the emancipation of lithotomy was played by the Colot family in Paris. Laurent Colot, the first representative of this family, had learnt the 'greater operation' sometime in the middle of the sixteenth century from an itinerant Italian who himself had been introduced into the art by no less a person than Mariano Santo in Rome, who had first described it. This had procured him the appointment of operator for the stone at the Royal Court. Laurent Colot (who flourished in the middle of the sixteenth century) and his descendants performed this operation so successfully that from all over Europe sufferers from the stone travelled to Paris to have themselves treated by the Colots. In the Hôtel-Dieu until well into the seventeenth century lithotomy continued to be performed by descendants of that family.[205]

Since the second half of that century, when in Paris surgery in general was strongly rising, lithotomies regularly took place in the Hôtel-Dieu as well as in the Charité, a much smaller hospital exclusively for men managed by Franciscan friars. Pierre Dionis mentions in his *Cours d'opérations de chirurgie* (1707) as prominent lithotomists in the former institution Jacques Petit (1611—1708) and one Bonnet. Jean Méry (cf. p. 231), who was the first to give regular courses in anatomy and surgery at Hôtel-Dieu, likewise enjoyed a good reputation as a lithotomist. In the second half of the eighteenth century, when Paris had some 600 000 inhabitants, more than a hundred patients a year were cut for the stone at the Hôtel-Dieu, on a 'jour de grande taille' at times ten or even more one after another.

'Malheur au malade destiné à tomber entre les mains d'un chirurgien, lequel aura pu assister sans émotion à 7, 10, 12 opérations en moins d'une heure, qui aura gardé assez d'indifference et de sérénité pour tirer des derniers actes de ce spectacle de sang, de cris et de douleurs les mêmes instructions que des premiers ... Les jours de taille sont de véritables autodafés. Ce grand jour annoncé depuis quelque temps a rassemblé le plus grand nombre de spectateurs et il n'est sans doute pas ignoré de ceux qui doivent faire les honneurs de ce spectacle. Quel est l'état d'âme des malades qui attendent, entendent et voient les autre malades opérés dans leur lit?'.[206]

Lithotomy by now came to belong almost exclusively to the realm of regular surgery, albeit that surgeons who ventured on it were proportionately few. Charité-surgeons with a good reputation in that particular field were Claude Morel and Georges Mareschal but it was François Tolet (1647—1724) working in that same hospital, who brought the operation with the greater apparatus to its height, in its practical execution as well as in its didactic presentation. His *Traité de la lithotomie* which appeared in 1681, was a masterpiece of precision and clarity. It went through many editions in French and was translated into English, Dutch and German. Tolet marked the end of a period. He was the last of those lithotomists who like the Colots, only engaged in this one operation.

6.8.2.2. Lithotomy in the Netherlands in the Seventeenth Century

Thomas Muffett was right when he recorded in 1655 that the Netherlands also had many capable lithotomists. The main reason must have been the high prevalence of bladder stones: from the older day the high frequency of an ailment which requires special skill to treat it has favoured specialization. Just as in France, lithotomy gradually passed from the hands of the incisors into those of specialized surgeons: a line came to be drawn between qualified and non-qualified healers. At the end of the seventeenth century more than twenty surgeon-lithotomists were active in Amsterdam alone. Almost every charitable institution in that city had its own lithotomist.[207] Some of them could do the operation in four, six or ten minutes.[208] Camper related that in Amsterdam as elsewhere, spectators used to note carefully by their watches the time required for producing the stone.[209]

Supervision by the Civic Authorities

The great risks of lithotomy induced the town governments at a relatively early time to enact restrictions. Taking Amsterdam — which in so many aspects was leading — as an example: already in the guild's charter of 1552 which regulated the practice of surgery, the condition is found that masters who want to carry out that operation are only allowed to do so in the presence of the aldermen, with the examiner of the surgeons' guild who have 'to see through their work and to testify to their being worthy and capable of doing it or not'. In 1688 a penalty of 100 guilders was imposed for performing this operation without explicit permission of the burgomasters, which had to be obtained in each individual case. At that time the operation had to be watched by a doctor of medicine and two aldermen.[210] In order to obviate any unnecessary intervention, these three officials had by probing with a metal catheter to satisfy themselves that a stone was really present in the bladder. When in 1728 the professor of anatomy was added to the supervising body, as many as four persons were entitled to 'torture the patient prior to the actual operation', scorned Camper as late as 1777.[211]

Gradually the superintendence grew into a regular examination before the aldermen of the surgeons' guild, of anyone who wanted to be recognized as a qualified lithotomist.[212] Larger towns appointed a municipal stone-cutter. He was by now always a qualified surgeon. Most lithotomists had their little tricks which they jealously kept a secret. The trade was usually learned for a fee from someone already in business. The celebrated Rau, however, was largely a self-made man in this respect. He once confessed to Titsingh to having performed the operation for the first time at sea on a sailor when he was still a naval surgeon. This had happened at the instance of the commander 'for the patient bothered the crew by his moaning'. It is not recorded in what way the operation was done nor what the outcome was.[213]

In Amsterdam an account of operations for the stone performed in that city was kept in a special register. The register, referring to the years 1700—1821, has been preserved with the exception of the years 1704—1724.[214] In this book the names and ages of the patients are recorded, together with the name of the surgeon who had done the lithotomy, the postoperative course, the number of calculi found and their weight, sometimes also the duration of the operation. The methods used are only infrequently mentioned. The number of operations recorded is 363, 254 of which or 70 per cent in children under 14 years of age. The overall operative mortality was about 20 per cent. Nieuwenhuys remarked that during the eighteenth century there had been a steady decrease in the incidence of bladder stone. Whereas at the end of the seventeenth century more than twenty surgeon-lithotomists were active in Amsterdam, there was only one left in 1817.[207]

Two Well-Known Dutch Lithotomists of the Golden Age at Work

Rochus van Dyck. Celebrated lithotomists were sometimes invited to come and operate outside their place of abode. At the Public Record Office a dossier is kept relating to the lithotomy performed in 1653 on the eleven-year old Henrik Wolraet, count of Waldeck and Culemborg, in his residence at the latter city. Its contents give a good record of the course of events. The complaints of the young patient dated from the time that he was about six years of age. His personal physician at Waldeck, Matthias Ramelo, for a long time favoured a conservative treatment. But he changed his mind when written advice obtained from the medical faculty at Leyden and from a few prominent physicians at Amsterdam, amongst whom Nicolaas Tulp and Paulus Barbette, all recommended a surgical intervention. The operation was performed by Rochus van Dyck, town lithotomist and herniotomist at Amsterdam since 1642. Apart from an uncle of the patient and Dr. Ramelo, there were present Dr. Willem van der Straten, physician at the court of the stadtholder at The Hague, the doctors Tulp and Barbette, a Dr. Timan Gessel from Utrecht and a few more physicians who all for this occasion had travelled to Culemborg. After the presence of a stone was confirmed by rectal palpation and by the use of a sound, the surgeon went to work while the gathered physicians shouted words of advice at him. It took half an hour to extract a hard calculus with spines the size of a raspberry. The boy endured the intervention heroically. The dossier unfortunately gives no information on how the operation was done, but it seems that Van Dyck usually followed the Celsian method (Fig. 90).

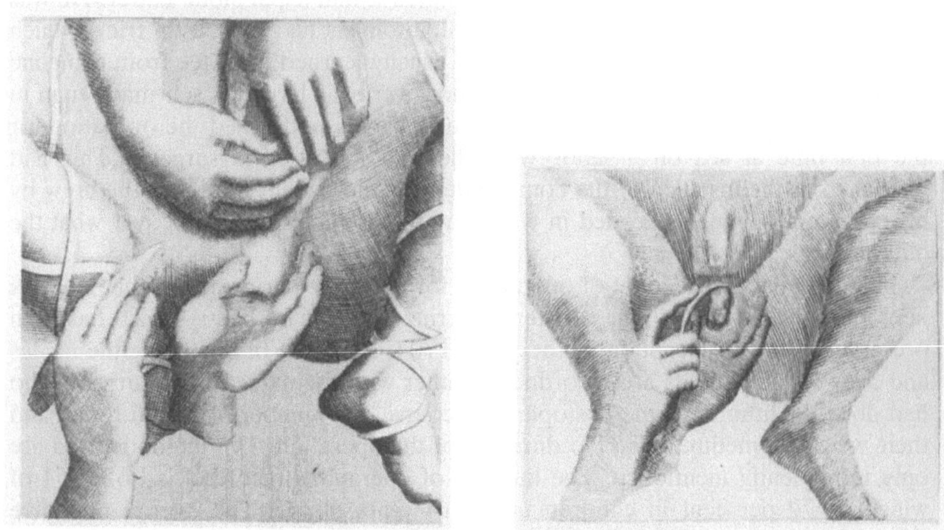

I II

Fig. 90. Lithotomy, according to Celsus, in a child, c. 1686.

The postoperative course was uneventful. The surgeon received 1000 florins as a fee, the physicians 250 florins each. The remaining expenditure contains a bill of 6 florins and 5 pence for a silver box with the young count's coats of arms for keeping the stone.[215]

Jacob Sasbout Souburg. Outside Amsterdam too, one could encounter surgeons who mastered this difficult operation. Solingen mentions in this connection the Dordrecht surgeon Jacob Sasbout Souburg who in October 1683 delivered the four-year old son of a minister of the Walloon Church from five bladder stones, using the apparatus minor. The child recovered within a month. It seems that Sasbout by preference used the operation of Celsus. That did imply some risks. It once happened that he cut right through the concretion which apparently had a soft consistence and then right through the rectal wall into his own digit.[216]

A Visiting Incisor: Frère Jacques de Beaulieu

Even towards the end of the seventeenth century it could happen that in spite of the existence of qualified surgeon-lithotomists a wandering stone cutter from abroad would make his appearance. A well-known example was the French pseudo-monk Jacques de Beaulieu who in 1699 and once again in 1704 paid a visit to the Low Lands. Frère Jacques, as he called himself, wore the habit of a Récollet — a Franciscan of the strict observance — with the distinction, however, that he was shod and wore a jaunty hat instead of a cowl. He had taken private vows of celibacy and poverty and therefore accepted hardly any remuneration from his patients. He had learned the operation from another empiric, called Pauloni. After having gathered experience in the French countryside he had made for Paris where his operations had been attended with small success. From Paris Frère Jacques moved onwards to a number of foreign countries including the Netherlands where he visited Amsterdam, Rotterdam, The Hague, Leyden, Zutphen and 's-Hertogenbosch. In all these towns he operated with permission of the civic authorities upon a few patients. The results of his first tour are not known but it is recorded that at his second appearance in Amsterdam five years later, he performed in the presence of surgeons and doctors many operations with favourable outcome. Through the years when travelling all over Europe, his results constantly improved, he is said to have operated on nearly five thousand patients with considerable success.

His technique was quite coarse. Without having prepared the patient in any way, he introduced a big steel staff having no groove into the bladder in such a way that its tip would be felt projecting against the pelvic floor at the left buttock. Then he plunged a long knife as if he were wielding a dagger into the left buttock, two fingers from the perineum in the direction of the tip of the staff, opening the body of the bladder near the neck. This was followed by the introduction of a conductor the exact shape of which he kept a secret. Guided by this instrument he searched for the stone with either his finger or a forceps. Having found the calculus he deftly extracted it saying: 'Jacques te taille, le bon Dieu te guérisse'. The summary after-treatment consisted of some oil and vinegar applied to the wound without any bandaging.[217]

This mode of action is strongly reminiscent of the second one of the four that were described by Pierre Franco. Since Frère Jacques as well as Franco had learned the art from travelling cutters for the stone, we may assume that the method was a current one in those circles. With the Celsian method, popular with these cutters as well, it has the direct approach of the body of the bladder in common.

6.8.2.3. Improvements of Lithotomy in the Eighteenth Century

Risks of the Traditional Operations

The time-honoured operation of Celsus fell largely into disrepute as the eighteenth century wore on. It was found that the neighbouring parts — the seminal ducts and vesicles — did by no means always escape unhurt. Even the urethra was in danger of being cut, being pushed forward as it was by the fingers in the rectum. There was, moreover, the possibility of deep extravasation, giving rise to inflammation, abscesses and fistulae. Tulp described a case of malignant degeneration of a urinary fistula in a middle-aged man, who as a child was cut for a stone. Once in a while a previous Celsian operation offered a distinct advantage in case of recurrence. An example of this is given by the case of Jan de Doot, an Amsterdam blacksmith who had already twice been cut before he was once again bothered by a bladder stone. In 1651 he cut himself several times in the perineum until he succeeded in getting hold of the stone and extracting it. As it is quite impossible that someone in this way could incise his own bladder, we must presume that this stone had already descended to the perineum as a result of inflammation of the bladder wall and the adjacent soft parts.[218]

The Marian operation by the greater apparatus or cutting on the staff was likewise the cause of much irreparable damage, if not death. The frequent occurrence of permanent urinary incontinence — 'pisbroeken' (piss breeches) the unhappy sufferers were called — appears from the aids devised to prevent 'leaking' such as copper receptacles to be hung between the legs fastened to the trunk, or apparatus which enabled a pad to be pressed onto the perineum as a substitution for the lost sphincter. Impotence might also ensue from this operation. Therefore other avenues had to be followed.

Lateral Cystotomy

One of the possible alternative courses was taken by Johannes Rau in Amsterdam, after he had discovered Frère Jacques' principle of lateral cystotomy at autopsy of patients who had not survived the latter's intervention.[219] Rau, like Frère Jacques, was not much inclined to expose his particular tricks, but he welcomed anyone as a spectator. When Lorenz Heister presented himself to follow Rau's course of anatomy and operative surgery, he was told straight away that he would hear nothing on lithotomy since Rau had to maintain himself mainly on that particular operation. One had only to look closely at how he did it but, Rau added, 'one can also read up Celsus'. With this somewhat cryptic reference he probably suggested that he, just like the ancient Roman, opened the bladder directly. Heister indeed used his eyes to good purpose and by an instrument maker 'In de Blauwe Klok' (In the Blue Bell) at Amsterdam he had Rau's instruments copied.[220] The most important one was a grooved staff which was thicker than the usual ones whilst the curved portion ended in a long, straight grooved beak. The description Heister gave of Rau's mode of operating may be completed by an eye-witness' account of Christian Heinrich Erndl, a German physician who spent five months in Amsterdam attending lectures by Rau (cf. p. 166): actually Heister and Erndl followed the same course.[221] Their combined reports are very much in agreement with Albinus' explanation some eighteen years later. Erndl was twice given the opportunity to watch his preceptor operating for the stone.[222] After the patient had been secured in the usual position, the grooved staff was introduced into the bladder. Using a wide-bladed lancet the blade of which was wrapped with a narrow band leaving only the point denuded over the distance of about a phalanx, Rau made an incision one inch to the left of the anus, where the tip of the staff could be felt through the pelvic floor. Aided by his intimate knowledge of anatomy, he carefully dissected by the side of the prostate, carrying the incision to the tip of the staff. Having reached the bladder wall, he inserted a concave conductor or gorget which was to guide the point of the lancet to the tip of the sound while incising the bladder wall. The actual incision was most probably done by placing the point of the knife in the groove of the staff while cutting forward. Once the bladder was opened, Rau replaced the knife by a dilator, like the gorget a concave, shallow, pointed instrument. Between gorget and dilator — Albinus spoke of male and female conductors — the wound in the neck of the bladder was dilated until it admitted the forceps by which the stone was extracted. One of the operations witnessed by Erndl was upon a Jewish boy of seven years of age who cried so hard, that during the intervention a rectal prolapse made itself visible. This was digitally replaced upon which the unperturbed surgeon brought the operation to a successful conclusion. In reliance upon a statement of Titsingh we may assume that Rau's method which its originator apparently did not for long manage to keep for himself, was standard ever since the beginning of the century in Amsterdam, as probably elsewhere in Holland.[223]

In 1713, the M.D.—surgeon Rau was appointed professor of medicine, anatomy and surgery at Leyden. In his inaugural address he prided himself on having performed no fewer than 1547 lithotomies (Fig. 91).[224] In his Leyden period he especially achieved merit by turning out beautiful anatomical preparations, some of which are still on display.

The lateral cystotomy according to Frère Jacques and Rau, inspired the perineal bladder puncture using a long hollow needle for emptying the bladder in case of urinary retention. This in its turn was conducive to a technical variant on lateral cystotomy in which a puncture needle introduced into the bladder previously filled with water, showed the way for the cutting instruments performing the actual cystotomy.

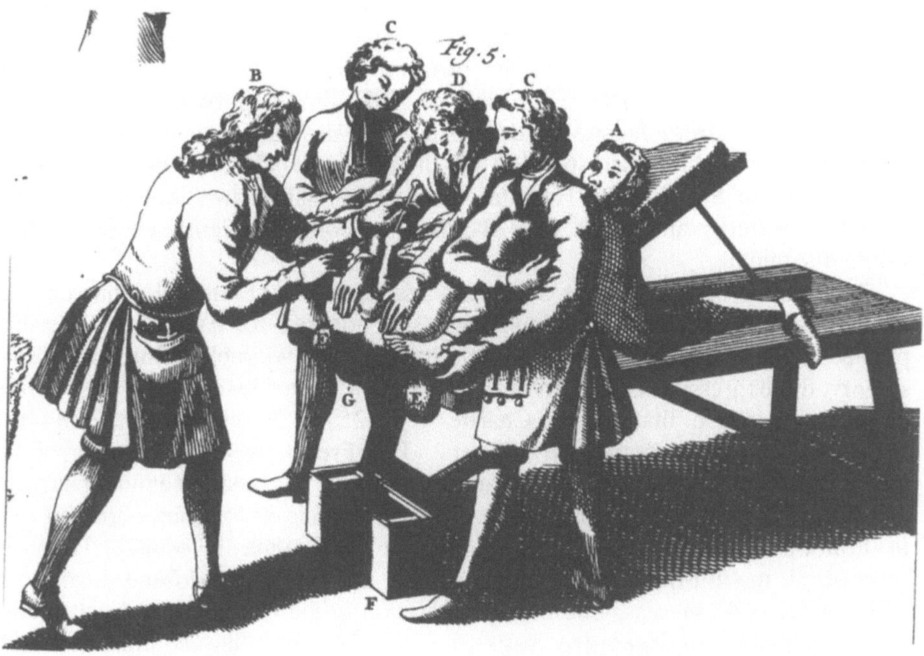

Fig. 91. Lateral cystotomy in the 18th century. The surgeon as usual has his instruments in a bag hung around his waist. A box of sand prevented the spattering of the blood as it streamed down.

Jacques Petit, Bonnet, John Douglas, Cheselden, Morand, Le Cat. Another escape from the Celsian and Marian operations was offered by the suprapubic approach as suggested by Franco in the sixteenth century. In Paris, this method seems to have been successfully applied by Petit and Bonnet, the Hôtel-Dieu lithotomists mentioned by Dionis. Some time later John Douglas (?—1759) in London adopted it after his brother, a skilled anatomist whose name has been given to the recto-uterine pouch, had shown that such an approach would be feasible. He was soon followed by William Cheselden, the leading surgeon in England in the first half of the eighteenth century. As a preliminary step, the bladder was filled with water. This operation was not without mishaps either. The peritoneum could be cut into or might burst, followed by extrusion of abdominal viscera. Sometimes the bladder itself burst from injecting too much water. A regular inconvenience was that wound healing was retarded by urine continually welling up from the bladder. Its great advantage was that no incontinence of urine was to be feared.

Cheselden lost no more patients than one in seven, whereas in 'the old way' — the traditional Marian operation — it appeared from a calculation of more than 800 cases, made by Morand in France, almost two in five died. Yet, hearing of the great successes of Rau, Cheselden turned for a while to lateral lithotomy but lost four patients out of ten from inflammation caused by extravasation of urine. He now returned to the operation by the greater apparatus with the difference, however, that he cut upon the staff beyond the bulb of the urethra and carried the incision from below upwards through the prostate into the bladder. The resulting opening was large enough to allow the extraction of stones of any size. Since in this operation the left lateral lobe of the prostate was cut, Cheselden called it 'the lateral way'. This is somewhat confusing, since the direct approach by the bladder as practised by Frère Jacques and by Rau was also known as 'sectio lateralis'. Cheselden was highly successful with his prostatotomy. Of 213 patients operated on 'publicly' in St. Thomas' Hospital, only twenty laid down their lives.[225] His operative dexterity and speed were dazzling, he could frequently extract a stone within one minute.

The rumour of Cheselden's successes also spread in France. In that country the cutting by the greater apparatus was still adhered to. Even the Rotterdam praelector Pieter Vink, who on the whole had a very favourable opinion of French surgery, did express his disapproval in this respect. As evidence of the poor results in Paris, he stated that in the Charité in 1725 of 20 cut patients only five recovered 'and thereabout (in) all years'. The French were well aware of the unfavourable situation and in 1729 Sauveur-François Morand, an eminent surgeon attached to the Charité, by instruction of the Académie des Sciences crossed over to London to study Cheselden's method at St. Thomas' Hospital. There he received all the information he could wish for. On his return Morand introduced, with considerable success, Cheselden's operation in the Charité, thereby attracting a great number of interested surgeons from all over the continent.[226] This contributed to Cheselden's method becoming standard for more than a century.

In the course of the eighteenth century many instruments were invented or being improved to render prostatotomy an easier and safer procedure. A well-known example is the 'lithotome caché', a slightly curved sound with a groove in which a knife was concealed. This knife was hinged to the rod and could be unfolded. By introducing the instrument with its concealed blade and then withdrawing it with the blade protruding a nice cut could be made in the prostate. Other urethrotomes and cystotomes were invented by Le Cat in Rouen, a first-rate lithotomist who just like Cheselden commonly needed less than a minute to produce the stone. He did not exactly shun publicity. From time to time he had lists published in the regional newspapers of his most recent lithotomy patients together with the exact time he had needed in every case.[227] Camper held him in high esteem.

Sermes, Francken, Denijs. The suprapubic lithotomy revived by Douglas and Cheselden achieved some following in Holland. In 1726, the M.D.—lithotomist Jan Sermes (1686—post 1731) in Amsterdam — a former student of Duverney in Paris — gave a detailed description of this method, comparing its advantages and disadvantages with that of Rau: these were apparently the two modes to choose from. The Celsian operation with the lesser apparatus 'rightly fell into disuse long ago' — Sermes was expressing himself a bit too strongly here — and cutting by the greater apparatus left many patients, women as well as men, with lasting incontinence. His conclusion was, that any lithotomist should be able to carry out the lateral operation according to Rau, as well as the suprapubic operation. He agreed with Heister, that the latter one should be the method of choice.[228] This he maintained in spite of the circumstance that he had lost a child three days after the operation in which, when performing a suprapubic lithotomy, he had accidentally cut the peritoneum which had resulted in a protrusion of the intestines. This disaster happened the very first time he did this type of operation. It stirred up such a commotion that Sermes, although otherwise having a good reputation as an anatomist and surgeon, had finally to leave the town.

Yet the suprapubic method continued to have a supporter in the person of Johann Francken, whom we have met already as a herniotomist. He developed a rather spectacular procedure. The patient was stretched face downward on a ladder which at a horizontal level was fixed to poles of a man's height (Fig. 92). The operator took his stand under the patient and brought in a metal catheter in such a way that its tip could be felt over the pubic bone. Over this landmark he laid the incision which should be no longer than a finger's breadth. Then he hooked a leaden weight on each side of the incision. As a next step the catheter was withdrawn and the wound in the bladder sufficiently enlarged to let out any concretions which might even fall down spontaneously at the surgeon's feet.[229]

About 25 years later, the Leyden town surgeon and lithotomist Jacob Denijs, a former ship's surgeon and introduced into the art of lithotomy by Rau himself, recorded that the method of Douglas was not much heard of anymore. The filling of the bladder with water and the tying of the penis to prevent its pouring out, was very painful and took so much time that an experienced lithotomist could easily have finished the whole operation within it. The method of Rau should therefore

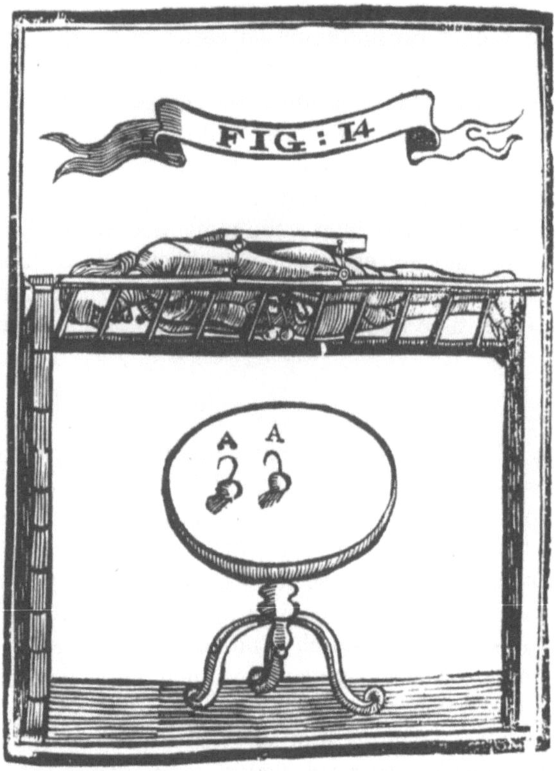

Fig. 92. Position and fixation of a patient for a suprapubic lithotomy, according to Francken. On the table, the weights to be hooked in the wound margins to keep the wound open.

be preferred by far over any other. This he stated on the strength of experience, gained in eight or ten Dutch towns 'in the presence of many learned men'. During the eleven years that he had practised that operation, he had lost only four patients.[230] Denijs did not state, however, the total number of people treated by him in that period. The suprapubic operation was never quite relinquished, however. In Paris, Joseph Souberbielle (1754—1846) is said to have performed it over twelve hundred times.[231]

Operation in Two Stages

Petrus Camper, although not practising the operation of lithotomy himself, was all in favour of an operation in two stages as had been advocated long before by Franco. Its advantages had been pointed out to him by his friend Antoine Louis whom he visited in Paris in 1777. Louis used to limit the first intervention to a lateral incision in the neck of the bladder. The second stage consisted of extracting the stone after five or six days when it appeared of its own accord in the suppurating wound. Its extraction then went quite painlessly.[209]

Needy patients were usually operated upon in the hospital. In 1820 Nieuwenhuys mentioned the existence of a special lithotomy-room in the 'Binnengasthuis' in Amsterdam, but it is not known, when it was fitted up as such (Fig. 93).[232] Anyone who could afford it, had himself treated at home or in a room rented at an inn. The frontispiece of Tolet's book allows us to cast a glance into what may be a private bedroom at the moment when someone is going to be relieved of his bladder stone (Fig. 94). The patient is placed with fastened legs in the lithotomy position, restrained by a few men. An assistant is holding with his right hand the free end of the staff introduced into the bladder. The surgeon, kneeling down, is just making the incision. Amongst those present we observe to the left a gentleman wearing a tabard: he is surely the doctor of medicine who, as prescribed by law, had to be present whenever a grave operation was being performed. On a round table behind the doctor the instruments are lying in readiness: metal sounds in a basin with oil, lithotomy knives and a pair of forceps. In the background the bed stands ready to receive the patient, while a servant is bringing a warming-pan. Beside and beyond the door a few onlookers can hardly conceal their anxiousness. To the right, his hat in his hand, stands a protestant minister: a surgical operation was usually immediately preceded by a prayer. Praying did not always come out well, as Francken remembered:

It happened in the year 1716 that I had to cut a boy of fifteen at Hoog Soeren on The Veluwe; that boy was so well disposed that he stripped with zeal; seeing no instrument or bandage whatever on the table or in my hands — many operators kept these in an abdominal bag to conceal them from the patients — he climbed bravely on the table; just when I was going to get hold of him after my own fashion, I heard the minister from Apeldoorn, called Van Bommel (who was present) say: 'Master, if you allow me, I would say a prayer'; I let him do it. This same clergyman in his prayer used the following expression: 'That if this patient should come to die under the hands of the master, O Lord, then have mercy on his soul'. No sooner had he uttered these words, than the boy jumped from the table before anybody could prevent him, burst through the people, and rushing from the house, climbed to the top of a haystack. He had to be fetched back with force by several strong men; and the operation was harder for me than any before or after. Since then no clergyman has been allowed, nor will any clergyman or whoever he may be, ever again be allowed to pray aloud, where I am going to operate.[233]

6.8.3. *Chemical Composition of Bladder Stones*

It was generally known from older times that there are different kinds of calculi. Denijs for instance, distinguished two types: the one fast-growing, brittle and calcareous, the other slow-growing, hard, heavy and compact. When at the end of the eighteenth century chemistry developed rapidly, the composition of urinary calculi began to be better understood. The Swedish chemist Carl Wilhelm Scheele (1742—86) attributed the formation of all stones to uric acid, his compatriot Torbern Olof Bergman (1735—84) stated that many calculi contain calcium phosphate and some oxalic acid. In 1797 the British physician and chemist William Hyde Wollaston (1766—1828) added calcium oxalate, ammoniomagnesium phosphate and cystic oxide to the constituents already known. In 1799 Antoine-François Fourcroy (1755—1809) and Louis-Nicolas Vauquelin (1763—1829) established the presence of ammonium urate and silex in some urinary concretions.[234]

6.9. RESUSCITATION

The late eighteenth century witnessed the foundation of so-called 'humane

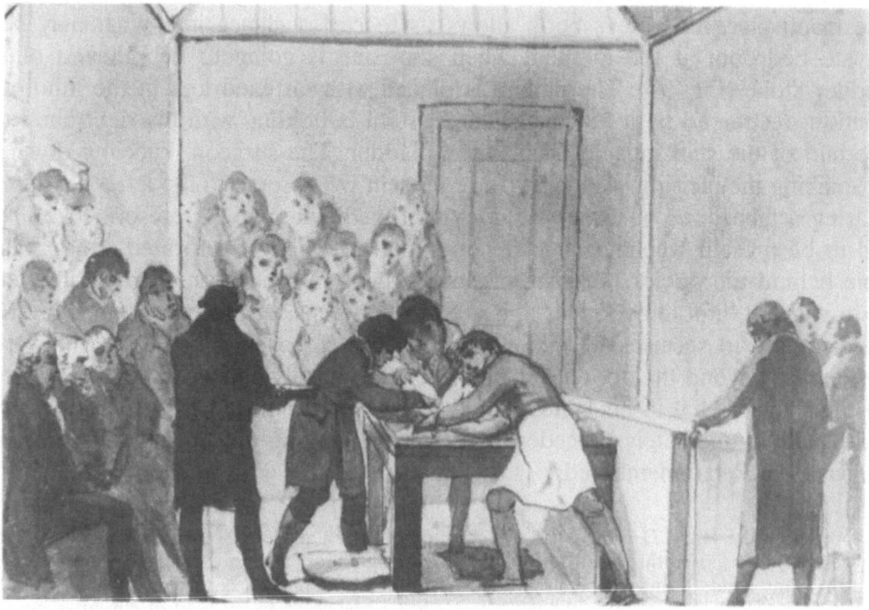

Fig. 93. Lithotomy performed by the town lithotomist Clemens van Demmeltraadt in 1807 or 1808, in the Binnengasthuis Hospital at Amsterdam.

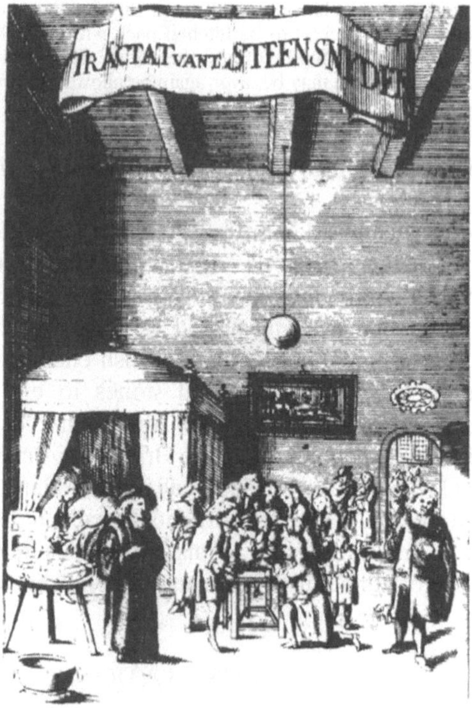

Fig. 94. Lithotomy in a private home, c. 1686.

societies' in numerous cities in Europe and even in North America. Such societies aimed at reviving unconscious drowned bodies: they proceeded from the social ideals of the Enlightenment.[235] The eldest is the 'Maatschappij tot Redding van Drenkelingen' which was founded in Amsterdam in 1767. In that town, which abounded in public-houses, quite a few people ended their days prematurely in its picturesque canals. The Amsterdam 'Maatschappij' tried to reach its goal by placing boxes with life-saving implements in ginshops on the waterfront, by the distribution of printed instructions and the offering of public rewards for successful attempts at resuscitation. The society performs the last two activities even today. Amongst those who in the eighteenth century were awarded a gold medal for recalling a drowned person to life was Johannes Mulder, whom we met already on page 179 as professor in Franeker. The means recommended by this society were warming up, rubbing, rolling, hanging upside down or rocking the apparently drowned, and furthermore by bleeding, the application of artificial respiration by mouth-to-mouth technique, the use of the tobacco smoke clyster. Tobacco smoke blown into the rectum was believed to have a powerful stimulating property (Fig. 95). This peculiar therapy was introduced into Holland in the second half of the seventeenth century on the recommendation of among others Frederik Dekkers,

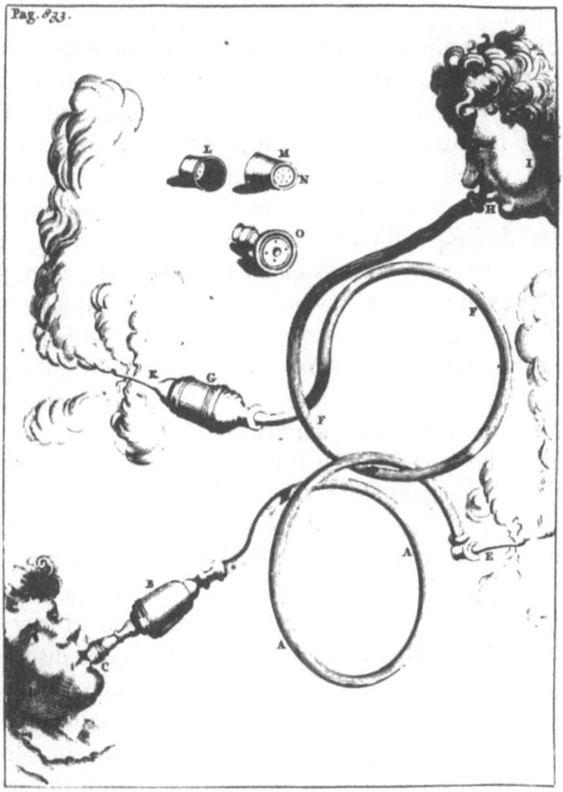

Fig. 95. Tobacco smoke clysters used for resuscitation and in the treatment of intussusception.

the Leyden physician who was also the first to describe albuminuria. The tobacco smoke clyster remained in use as a restorative until the middle of the nineteenth century.[236] It was also used in cases of obstruction of the intestines, sometimes, when intussusception was the cause, with good success. Supposedly Bauhin's valve impeded the passing of enema fluid, whereas tobacco fumes penetrated readily into the small intestine. By their 'stretching' and stimulating action they set the intestinal wall in motion.[237]

6.10. THE SURGEON'S TOOLS

Surgical instruments, preserved from Graeco-Roman antiquity, show that the basic tools used by surgeons through the ages, were largely contrived at the time when Western surgery was experiencing its first flourishing period.[238] Comparatively few authentic instruments dating from the Middle Ages have survived being largely made of iron or steel, which were less enduring than the bronze instruments of Antiquity. But drawings in mediaeval medical manuscripts suggest they had not much changed. A three-bladed vaginal speculum for example, which could be operated by means of a screw, was about equal to a similar instrument found in the ruins of Pompeii.

Guy de Chauliac classified instruments into those for cutting, burning, extraction, examination and suturing, apart from those for special interventions like trepanning or the laying open of fistulae. From a more detailed enumeration it appears that Guy used cutting instruments of several types; scissors and dilatation-scissors, cauteries, forceps, vulsella, needles for suturing, probes, spatulae, blunt and sharp hooks, instruments for bone surgery such as the trepan, chisel, elevatory and hammer, besides drains, catheters, specula etc.[239] In short, most of the basic instruments that we use today were available to the mediaeval surgeon.

In the sixteenth century a few new instruments were added amongst which were the grooved director and the artery forceps, both probably devised by Paré; whereas Paré's pupil Guillemeau improved the forceps by adding a spring between the handles to keep them closed. The scissors, formerly of the sheepshearing type, were replaced by the models now generally used.[240]

It appears from the woodcut illustrations in works like those by Dalla Croce, Paré, Fabricius ab Aquapendente or Fabricius Hildanus and from specimens handed down to us, that Renaissance instruments were in accord with the artistic taste of the time, richly ornamented as they were with flourishes and grotesques (Fig. 25). Typical were also the beautiful pointed portable instrument cases with their ambossed leather coverings, which surgeons used to carry fastened to their belts since the late Middle Ages (Fig. 46). Fabry of Hilden disclosed their contents: 1 small razor, 1 pair of scissors, 1 forceps, 2 spatulas, 2 probes, 2 lancets, 4 phlebotomes, 1 curved lancet for the incision of apostemes, 1 mouth-spatula, 1 small scoop, 1 small hook simple at one end, double at the other, 1 pointed and sharp instrument for the evulsion of teeth, 5 or 6 suturing needles in different sizes, 1 fenestrated canula to facilitate the passing of needle and thread through the wound margins, 1 small grindstone.[241] Fabry's personal instruments were made of silver, but when he went to war he took only iron and steel ones with him for fear that the soldiers, who as a rule did not have much respect for church silver, might also not leave him for long in undisturbed possession of his own precious instruments.

Cornelis Solingen did not fancy the ornate commercial instruments of his day. 'Those detestable instruments of Nuremberg mass-manufacturers' were difficult to clean, were easily attacked by rust at the least accessible spots and were made of inferior steel to keep down their price.[242] He therefore devised his own implements, devoid of any superfluous ornamentation, plain and easy to cleanse, and made of excellent steel. Folding plates in his works, with full size drawings in his own hand very clearly represent his ideas (Fig. 96 and 97). Some of Solingen's own instruments, which after his death passed into the possession of the University of Leyden, have been preserved.

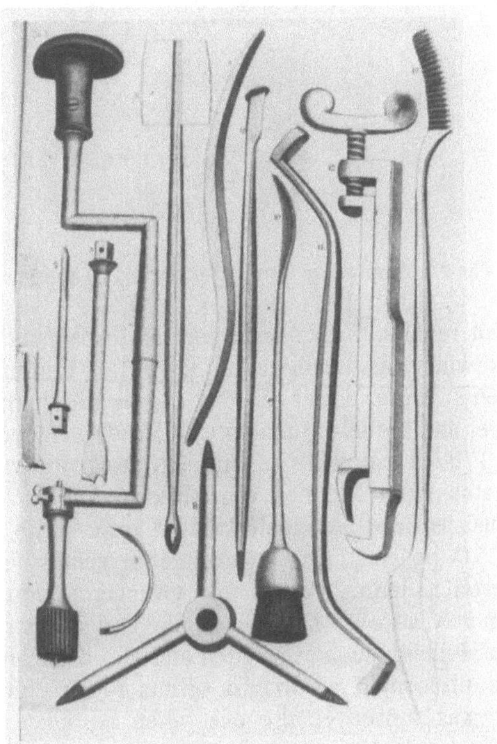

Fig. 96. Trepanation instruments devised by Solingen.

While it appears from Solingen's condemnatory words that German manufacturers were placing their products on the Dutch market, we know that ever since the seventeenth century specialized instrument makers were active in this country as well, whereas formerly surgical instruments were universally made by armourers. The archives of the Middelburg surgeons' guild, for instance, reveal that in 1658 this corporation obtained its instruments from Gisbrecht Servaesz at Rotterdam,

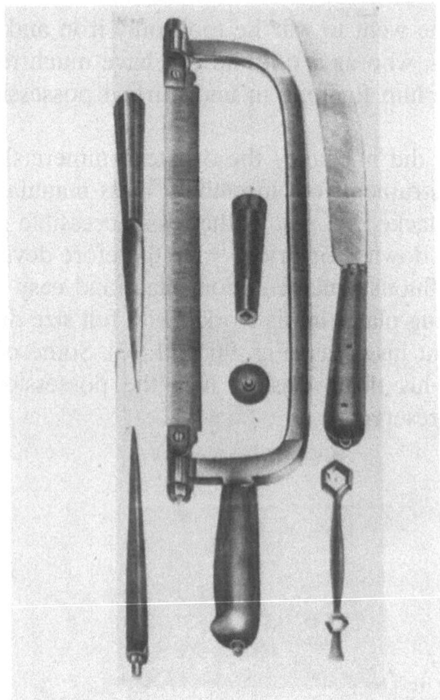

Fig. 97. Amputation instruments devised by Solingen.

who also carried out repairs.[243] In Amsterdam an instrument maker kept a shop 'In de Blauwe Klok' where, as mentioned on page 248, Rau and Heister had their lithotomy instruments made. Later in the eighteenth century, Van Gesscher recommended Pezzet and Gobels in that city.[244] Erndl included in his report of his visit to Leyden in 1707 a 'catalogus instrumentorum' of anatomical and surgical implements obtainable from Joannes van Musschenbroek: 'celeberrimus nostri temporis mechanicus', as Erndl designated him. A trepan with six burrs was priced at 7 guilders and 10 pence.[245] In the eighteenth century products of French artisans like Vigneron le jeune, Perron and Grangeret, 'coutelier de la Marine Royale' found their way all over Europe. A few British instrument makers, too, were well-known in Holland, such as Migden and Holmes from London: the latter particularly for his preformed cardboard splints for fractures of the leg. The eighteenth century was moreover the age when complete sets for particular operations in luxuriant velvet or plush cases were put on the market. Until the middle of the nineteenth century surgical instruments were made of carbon steel.

In the second half of the eighteenth century the introduction by Desault of gum-elastic catheters meant a valuable addition. It was not long before these useful objects could also be had elsewhere. In 1772, the Amsterdam merchant Bicker Raye in his diary analyzed by Van Nierop, noted the demise of Hermanus Mulder, a master carpenter who not only was an excellent maker of dentures, but also of flexible catheters so that one could easily tap one's own water in case of urinary retention.[246]

Inventories that have survived give a fair picture of the instruments kept by seventeenth and eighteenth century surgeons. Apart from the standard utensils of the barbers and pharmacists, their armamentarium usually was limited to knives, scissors, needles, tourniquets, forceps, dental extractors and similarly basic tools. Even well-to-do surgeons able to afford silver instruments did not usually possess anything like a trepan or even an amputation saw. Such pieces were borrowed from the instrument collection of the surgeons' guild, mentioned on page 111, or some independent co-operative lending pool for surgical instruments, which came into being in the second half of the eighteenth century. Some instrument pools continued to function even after the suppression of the guilds, only to disappear when, in the 1880s, surgery became more and more concentrated in hospitals.

CHAPTER 7

The Beginning of Modern Surgery

7.1. THE POLITICAL HISTORY OF THE NETHERLANDS IN THE NINETEENTH CENTURY

After Napoleon had suffered a decisive defeat at Leipzig in 1813 from the allied forces of Austria, Russia, Prussia and Sweden, freedom dawned on the areas which had been occupied by France. At its liberation the Netherlands took on the monarchial form of government, with the eldest son of stadtholder William V exiled to England as its sovereign. The territory of the new nation under king William I was larger than it had ever been in the time of the Republic, because the Congress of Vienna, on redrawing the map of Europe, had joined the South Netherlands to Holland. This unity did not last long. In 1830 dissatisfaction with the government of William I led to a revolt and the separation of the South, which then became the independent kingdom of Belgium.

The constitution of 1815, which granted parliament only limited power, allowed the first king to reign as an 'enlightened despot'. He worked hard to uplift the destitute situation in which he had found his new realm, putting forth every effort to promote trade and industry. The maintainance of an active army between 1831 and 1839 due to the state of war with Belgium had, however, resulted in a considerable increase in the national debt compared to 1815. When in 1840 William I left the throne, there was great poverty throughout the country.

In 1848, the aspirations of the bourgeoisie toward more influence on the government led to liberal revolts in Vienna and Berlin and to the February revolution in France which drove Louis Philippe from the throne. In the Netherlands these events brought about a constitutional reform which greatly increased the influence of the States General at some costs to the power of the king. The new constitution was mainly the work of the liberal statesman Jan Rudolf Thorbecke (1798—1872) who became prime minister twice between 1850 and 1872. His ministries were of great importance for the recovery of the economy thanks to measures stimulating trade, fishery, agriculture and industry. The colonies in the East Indies, which England had returned in 1816, yielded considerable profits. Thorbecke's significance in the modernization of medical education will be dealt with in chapter 9.3.

Political life between about 1850 and the outbreak of the First World War was characterized by the development of new political parties. The largest problems at that time concerned education and voting rights which we need not enter here.

A period of prosperity gradually evolved, although industrialization had brought with it a factory proletariate. For more than a century the country was not involved in war. The Prussian-Austrian war in 1866, which was in essence about the hegemony in Central Europe, the Franco-Prussian war of 1870—71, which resulted in a strong German empire, and even the First World War all bypassed the Dutch borders.

7.2. MEDICAL SCIENCE IN THE FIRST HALF OF THE NINETEENTH CENTURY

The nineteenth century was an extremely eventful era. In every field of Western society more changes took place than in all the previous twenty centuries put together. This is also largely true for science and technology. The development of new sources of power in the last century is often referred to as the second great revolution in the history of mankind.

As far as the pattern of illness was concerned, the whole of Europe was characterized by epidemics particularly of smallpox, scarlet fever, puerperal fever and other 'fevers', purulent ophthalmia and cholera. Among the endemic diseases tuberculosis and venereal disease took very prominent places. It was not until the last quarter of the century that the cause of these infectious diseases began to be better understood. The picture of European medicine, however, was far from homogenous in the first half of the century and displayed differences in countries like France, Great Britain and Germany.

7.2.1. *France*

During the French Revolution, the old educational system had been replaced with schools which no longer only gave tuition in either medicine or surgery, but in both subjects as different parts of one and the same medical science. This meant that in this country the traditional rift between doctors and surgeons had become much smaller. The Napoleonic wars had produced large numbers of practically orientated, energetic doctors. The clinicians who, in the first decades of the nineteenth century were in charge of the large Parisian clinics, including the ones of internal medicine, had for the greater part received their training in the practical school of war.[1] The prestige of French medicine remained unimpaired in spite of the downfall of the first empire.

The enormous amount of patient material enabled the Parisian clinicians to carry out autopsies on a grand scale. By correlating the patients' symptoms to the findings at autopsy as Morgagni had taught, a clinical medical science originated which was based on morbid anatomy. Pathological anatomy was no longer of interest to surgery only; internal medicine as well became more morphologically orientated.[2] At the beginning of the century Xavier Bichat (1771—1802) had introduced a refinement to anatomy and morbid anatomy by pointing out that organs were not homogeneous structures, but were composed of different tissues.[3]

This anatomical train of thought called for diagnostic methods which would enable accurate localization of morphological disorders. Percussion, which Leopold

Auenbrugger (1722—1809) from Vienna had demonstrated as early as 1761, was now given a firm place in physical examination through Napoleon's favourite physician, Jean-Nicolas Corvisart (1755—1821).[4] René-Théophile-Hyacinthe Laennec (1781—1826) invented the stethoscope in 1819, thus revolutionising the study of diseases of the thoracic organs.[5]

Attracted by this new form of clinical medicine, especially aimed at accurate diagnosis, foreign scholars once again thronged the French capital. Not solely for anatomy, surgery and obstetrics as was the case in the eighteenth century, but now also for the sake of internal medicine.

7.2.2. *Great Britain*

The French revolution had fewer consequences for medicine in Britain than in many other European countries. The traditional educational system was maintained far into the nineteenth century, with theoretical tuition at the universities and clinical instruction by various physicians at the hospitals. English medicine had traditionally paid close attention to anatomy and physiology as basic medical sciences. Private schools for anatomy, physiology, surgery and pharmacy continued their activities until 1824, when the Royal College of Surgeons of England decided not to accept certificates of attendance at such schools any longer: they thereafter gradually disappeared.[6]

7.2.3. *Germany*

In Germany, romanticism — a cultural movement determined by an idealistic philosophy pervaded by imagination and emotion — arose as a reaction to the rationalism of the Enlightenment. This trend of course manifested itself particularly in the fine arts, but also had an influence on medical science by calling more attention to the influence of the mind on somatic diseases. Idealism now came first. No longer was the learned scholar the beau ideal of doctors, but instead was replaced by the self-effacing physician, unremittingly devoting himself to his patients. This ideal contributed to the origin of the modern general practitioner, a medical man unknown in the earlier centuries. Medical practice was now to be based on intuitive art rather than science.

In the first three or four decades a second important tendency became manifest, particularly in German speaking countries, which directed itself to the natural philosophy of Schelling. This trend was based on the principle that nature, mind, organism and development all formed one unity. Nature and mind were not essentially different; nature was visible mind, mind was invisible nature. Nature was in a situation of constant development. There was no room for scientific experimentation in this manner of thought: nature can be constructed in the mind.[7]

Embryology and comparative anatomy, as typical 'developmental subjects' benefitted in particular from the natural philosophical line of thought. Haeckel's fundamental biogenetic law is a case in point.

Yet a third trend in German medicine was eclecticism keenly directed to practice, where Christoph Wilhelm Hufeland (1762—1836) from Berlin was the leading man. Hufeland was an extraordinarily prolific writer, his books and magazine articles were widely read in the Netherlands. It was particularly the latter variety of German medicine which acted as an example to Holland during the first half of the last century.

7.2.4. *The Netherlands*

After Holland had regained its independence in 1813, the old universities were restored and new state universities founded in Louvain, Ghent and Liège in the South, but education retained its typical eighteenth century catechetical character for some time to come. Even as late as 1848 the Dutch physiologist Jacobus Moleschott (1822—93), one of the advocates of scientific medicine, passed some very sharp criticism on the old-fashioned and inadequate tuition at Dutch universities. For most of the lecturers, Boerhaave and Gaubius had not lost any of their authority. Although the direct and indirect French dominance had lasted almost twenty years, medicine in this country had not become orientated towards that of France. True, scholars still enjoyed going on study tours to Paris, but for the time being the new French clinical medicine they became acquainted with was not transported to the Netherlands. The probable reason for this was that the university hospitals in Holland, because of their small scale, were entirely unsuitable for clinical tuition in the French style. It took until 1847 for auscultation and percussion to be absorbed into Dutch medical education.

As of old, medicine was practised by many different kinds of practitioners from very varied scientific and practical levels. The prime motive of the foundation of the Dutch Society of Medicine in 1849 was to achieve uniformity amongst practitioners through uniformity of education. This objective was not realized until 1865, when tuition became centralized at the universities (see p. 307). The Municipal and Provincial Committees for Medical Supervision, dating from the time of the Batavian Republic, continued to exist until the same year 1865 which in several aspects was a remarkable point of time in the history of Dutch medicine.

7.3. SURGERY IN THE FIRST HALF OF THE NINETEENTH CENTURY

In the first decennia, the interest of surgeons in all countries still circled around the questions which had occupied their attention from of old. The most important were trephination, lithotomy, exarticulation of the large joints, Caesarian section and the treatment of aneurysms, fractures, dislocations, herniae and tetanus.[8] Fundamental studies, such as John Hunter's on the nature of inflammations, were an exception: those surgeons who occupied themselves with research usually limited their efforts to refinements in operative techniques or the designing of more sophisticated instruments. This unimaginative trend was clearly visible in the journals of that time which for the most part were filled with inane and long-drawn-out case histories, with superficial treatises and — even then — with rarities. In the first forty to fifty years there were no indications that surgery would achieve its unprecedented heights towards the end of the century.

7.3.1. *France*

When shortly after the overthrow of Napoleon, Paris once again became the centre point of continental surgery, one of the leading surgeons was Alexis Boyer (1757—1833) at the Charité, formerly first surgeon to Napoleon. His *Traité des maladies chirurgicales*, which he published in eleven volumes between 1814 and 1826, was a masterpiece, such as had been unknown in the French literature since Paré. Simple in design, eminently practical and easy to comprehend, it served as a guideline for several generations of practitioners and students. Even so it was not entirely up to date, and as Malgaigne observed, it was more of an impressive conclusion to surgery in the eighteenth century as embodied in the Académie royale de Chirurgie.[9] Boyer believed that in his time surgery had reached its absolute zenith. 'La chirurgie', as he wrote in the preface, 'a fait de nos jours les plus grands progrès et semble avoir atteint le plus haut degré de perfection dont elle paraisse susceptible'.

Some of the foreigners, who once again travelled to Paris kept diaries or made reports which enable us to form an impression of the most important lecturers and operating surgeons of that time. In this way Hendrik Jan Logger (1789—1839), a Dutch physician who paid a working visit to the French capital in 1818[10] described how Boyer once conducted an operation on ulcerating cancer of the breast. Via two large half-moon shaped, horizontal incisions the entire breast was removed, after which various 'considerable indurations' had to be detached from the chest wall and axilla. For haemostasis, five ligatures were applied to the chest and one in the axilla. Between the various actions Boyer gave a detailed account of the whys and wherefores and perforce the patient had to wait in the meantime. Accordingly, the operation took about ten minutes. The very broad wound surface was covered with lint and the edges of the wound were approximated as much as possible by means of adhesive plaster. This was covered by a pressure bandage.

Foreign visitors, however, directed their steps in the first place towards the Hôtel-Dieu where Guillaume Dupuytren (1777—1835) had been working since 1803. Dupuytren, a student of Bichat, was the most famous French surgeon of the nineteenth century: he was a shrewd clinician and noted for his remarkable dexterity.[11] His most striking cases were lithotomies, particularly in children, using his 'lithotome caché'. An American student reported to his surgeon-father that Dupuytren could usually take out the stone in two minutes flat. An upper arm amputation took him six or eight minutes, dressing included. Dupuytren was the first to perform partial mandible resections. He was, moreover, a brilliant teacher who understood how to convince his audience that the art of surgery should be based on a solid knowledge of surgical pathology.[12] At the same time, however, he appears from private notes as a dominating man with a difficult character, charming at times but frequently discourteous or ever rude to students and patients alike. He left few scientific publications: his well known *Leçons orales de clinique chirurgicale* (1832) was committed to paper and edited by others.

The sometimes extensive diary annotations of the Dutchman Christiaan Bernhard Tilanus (1796—1883), who visited the Parisian hospitals with two friends in 1818, give a good interpretation of the manner in which Dupuytren conducted, for example, lithotomies, amputations, mandible resections, herniotomies in cases of strangulated inguinal, femoral and umbilical hernias and in which he treated fractures.[13]

Tilanus and his friends — J. C. Broers who subsequently became professor of surgery and obstetrics at Leyden and P. J. I. de Fremery who later became professor of chemistry at Utrecht — also visited Boyer in the Charité and Larrey in the 'Hôpital militaire de la Garde royale' in the rue du Gros-Caillou. Napoleon's former army surgeon still mainly occupied himself with trauma cases. The German Johann Ludwig Casper who visited Larrey in 1822, praised him for his skill in applying bandages but thought him a mediocre surgeon. Just like Logger before him, Casper observed that French patients could tolerate pain remarkably well.[14]

Important contemporaries of Dupuytren were Balthasar-Anthelme Richerand (1779—1840), engaged at the Hôpital St.-Louis, Philibert-Joseph Roux (1780—1854) at the Hôpital de la Charité and Jacques-Mathieu Delpech (1777—1832) in Montpellier. The former was the author of a *Nosographie chirurgicale* (1805—06), a very systematic and complete survey of the state of surgical science, with a classification of surgical diseases similar to those which were in use in natural history. This book ran through various editions before it was surpassed by Boyer's handbook. Roux, Boyer's son-in-law, made an important contribution toward the internationalization of surgery by arousing the interest of his fellow countrymen in the surgery on the other side of the English Channel. The book he wrote about his visit to London in 1814 is still well worth reading.[15] He introduced in his country the English method of wound treatment which aimed at healing by first intention if at all possible, of eligible traumatic and operative wounds. He also took up the English double-flap method applicable to amputations.[16] Delpech deserves to be remembered for his orthopaedic work in particular.

After Dupuytren's death in 1835, the number of foreign doctors visiting Paris sensibly decreased. Yet, there still were in that city excellent surgeons following Dupuytren. In the first place was Alfred-Armand Velpeau (1795—1867), whose work included an extensive book on operative surgery, *Nouveaux éléments de médecine opératoire* (1832), which acted as a guideline for many generations of surgeons. His *Traité des maladies du sein* (1854) placed him among the best oncologists of that period. Of his contemporaries we must mention Joseph-François Malgaigne (1806—65), an extremely productive writer whose many publications, especially *Traité des fractures et des luxations* (1847) were greatly appreciated. His studies on the history of surgery have kept their value until this day. Finally, Malgaigne should be credited with the introduction of the statistical method into surgery.[17] Auguste Vidal (1803—56) deserves to be mentioned here owing to his extensive *Traité de pathologie externe et de médecine opératoire*, the book which from 1839 superseded Boyer's. The German version of this work, adapted by his student Adolf von Bardeleben (1819—95), professor of surgery in Greifswald and later in Berlin, under the title *Lehrbuch der Chirurgie und der Operationslehre*, was one of the most popular textbooks in Germany during the last century.

We conclude our brief enumeration with Jean Civiale (1792—1867), who should be remembered for his invention in 1826 of the lithotriptor, an instrument for crushing stones inside the bladder, thus obviating the need for lithotomy.

7.3.2. *Great Britain*

The good name British surgery had acquired in the eighteenth century due to its thoroughness, sober-mindedness and great aptitude for surgical technique, was maintained in the following years. The school of Edinburgh still enjoyed an excellent reputation throughout Europe. Its most important representatives were John Bell (1763—1820) and his younger brother Charles (1774—1842). The latter established himself in London after reaching the age of thirty, where he took over the Great Windmill Street School of Anatomy, founded by William Hunter. Both Bells were first-rate draughtsmen who illustrated their own work. John was especially known for his *Anatomy of the human body* which first appeared in 1793 and his *Principles of surgery*, which was published in three parts between 1801 and 1808. Both books were reprinted repeatedly until way into the 1820s. He is considered as one of the founders of surgical anatomy. In London Robert Liston (1794—1847) at University College Hospital, was one of the most skilful surgeons of his time. 'A tall and powerfully-built man, he was possessed of such strength that he could amputate the thigh with the aid of one assistant, compressing the artery with his left hand and doing all the cutting and sawing with his right'.[18] He was the first surgeon in Europe to perform an operation under ether anaesthesia, and we will return to this on page 280.

However, the most popular of all London surgeons was one of John Hunter's students, Sir Astley Cooper (1768—1841) at Guy's and St. Thomas's Hospital.[19] His fame equalled Dupuytren's but contrary to his French peer, Cooper was a friendly and courteous man. He was an outstanding diagnostician and a bold and rapid, but elegant surgeon. Cooper owed his baronetcy to the successful removal of an inflamed wen from the scalp of king George IV. Like most of his contemporaries, he had a passion for anatomical dissections. His detailed knowledge of anatomy enabled him to carry out ligation operations on aneurysms of big vessels, such as the common carotid and external iliac arteries and once even on the abdominal aorta. However, in the latter case the patient only survived for forty hours after the operation. Cooper was a voluminous author. He published valuable monographs on the anatomy and surgical treatment of herniae, on diseases of the breast, joint injuries and diseases of the testis. The majority of his works were translated into German, some of them also into French and Dutch.

Human bodies for anatomical dissection were scarce in Great Britain at the time. By law only the corpses of executed criminals could be used and these were in short supply. 'Resurrectionists' were trying to meet both the demand of anatomy schools and private persons by robbing bodies from newly dug graves. The increasing scandal of the black market in human corpses, in which Cooper became involved, ultimately brought about the Anatomy Act of 1832, which legalized the dissection of human bodies on certain conditions.[20]

After Cooper's death Benjamin Collins Brodie (1783—1862), a surgeon to St.

George's Hospital who had been president of the Royal College of Surgeons of England for some time, became the acknowledged leader of the profession in Britain. His famous book *Pathological and surgical observations on diseases of the joints*, which first appeared in 1818, was translated into German, French and Dutch. A representative of surgery in Dublin, Abraham Colles (1773—1843) gained eponymous fame by recognizing the true nature of the traumatic condition of the wrist named after him.[21]

7.3.3. *The United States of America*[22]

In the first half of the last century a few surgeons from the USA, which had become independent in 1793, began to gain some reputation abroad. John Collins Warren (1778—1856), professor of anatomy and surgery at Harvard University was amongst them. He had studied in London, Edinburgh and Paris. It was in his operating theatre at the Massachusetts General Hospital in 1846 that general anaesthesia was used for the first time in a surgical operation. We will deal with this important occasion more fully below (see p. 279). Philip Syng Physick (1768—1837), sometimes referred to as 'the father of American surgery', held the chair of surgery at the University of Pennsylvania from 1805, the year it was established, until 1837. His numerous contributions to practical surgery were either published in *The American journal of the medical sciences* or became known through a popular textbook written by his nephew, which contained much of his experience. The surgeon who is best remembered from the early part of the history of American surgery is Ephraim McDowell (1771—1830) from Danville, Kentucky. In 1809 he was the first to perform a methodical excision of an ovary affected by tumour. An account of this operation appeared in a Philadelphian medical journal; but it was only after 1824, when the case was published in the *Edinburgh medical and surgical journal*, that it became generally known.[23] McDowell was a contemporary of Samuel D. Gross (1805—84) from Philadelphia, one of the most distinguished surgeons of his time. Gross was, moreover, a prolific author, whose *System of surgery* written in 1859, met with great success. It was translated into several continental European languages including Dutch.

In 1895 John S. Billings (1838—1913), when looking back on American surgery in the nineteenth century wrote at the end of his *History and literature of surgery* that American surgeons in that epoch had for the most part been 'practical men'. It was only within the last twenty years that the scientific problems of surgical pathology had become the subject of experimental study. He expressed the hope that the John Hunter or Joseph Lister of America was now busy with his preliminary work. Meanwhile American surgeons and physicians flocked to Europe — to Edinburg, London and Paris and towards the end of the century also to Vienna and Berlin — to acquaint themselves with the scientific progress which was still largely a European affair.

7.3.4. *Germany, Austria*

In the German-speaking countries surgery began to prosper at a later date than in most other parts of Europe, but when it began to gain a profile in the twenties and thirties it did so in several different places simultaneously. It sought to free itself from French influence, evident amongst other things, by the appearance of a large number of German translations of English publications. There was also no lack of original German handbooks and textbooks.

The schools especially of Würzburg, Göttingen, Vienna and Berlin were in the making.[24]

One of the descendants of Richter's school in Göttingen, already referred to (see p. 154), was Conrad Johann Martin Langenbeck (1776—1851), an extremely fast-working surgeon. The story goes that an older colleague from another university once visited Langenbeck to see him perform an upper leg amputation. While the patient was lying on the table and the surgeon took up the knife, the old gentleman turned away for a pinch of snuff. But, oh surprise! When he turned back he found that the operation was already over.[25]

Vienna owed its recovery mainly to Vincenz von Kern (1760—1829), who founded a school for surgery there in 1807, which produced professional experts. Six young surgeons at a time who had graduated with honours, were trained to master all operative procedures in a gratuitous two year course.[26] Of the men taught by Von Kern we will mention Max Joseph Chelius (1794—1876), professor of surgery at Heidelberg since 1817, on account of his *Handbuch der Chirurgie* of 1822, which underwent numerous reprints and translations. For almost forty years it was a very well-known textbook in many European countries: fuller reference to it will be made below (see p. 277).

On their way home from Paris, Tilanus and his two fellow-travellers paid short visits to several university towns in Germany, paying their respects to some professors including Chelius in Heidelberg and Langenbeck in Göttingen. They portray Chelius as an amiable man and an excellent lecturer. His 'Clinicum', complete with a good, well-lit operating theatre, was neat and clean. It had roomy and airy wards containing eight beds at the most. Unfortunately, the Göttingen pages of the diary are missing.

The surgical clinic in Berlin, dating back to the foundation of the university in 1810, had as its first professor-director Carl Ferdinand von Graefe (1787—1840), an excellent teacher and surgeon. He is regarded as the initiator of modern plastic surgery. His successor in the professorial chair, who likewise occupied himself with plastic surgery, was Johann Friedrich Dieffenbach (1792—1847), the author of a surgical textbook, also translated into Dutch.

7.3.5. *The Netherlands under its First King* (1813—40)

7.3.5.1. Medical Legislation

King William I maintained the enactments which the Batavian Republic had taken regarding medical tuition, the practice of medicine and public control and built on them further. In the Royal Decree on Higher Education of August 2, 1815, which aimed at reshaping university tuition following its deep depression under French control, the contents of medical education were defined more fully. As in all the other faculties, there were to be two academic degrees: candidatus and doctor.

With regard to the examination for the grade of candidatus the demands included 'an anatomical demonstration'. It is obvious that without practice no student would be able to meet this condition. So it is not surprising that the classical anatomical theatrum gradually transformed itself into an anatomical institute through the addition of a dissecting room for students.

The doctor's degree was gained by taking an examination in practical medicine and in the theory of surgery and obstetrics, followed by the writing of a thesis — 'specimen' — which had to be submitted in printed from and defended either or not in public. Following this the graduate had to take the oath of office before actually receiving the certificate of 'doctor medicinae' which entitled him to practise internal medicine throughout the country. Anyone wishing to acquire an additional degree as 'doctor chirurgiae', 'doctor artis obstetriciae' or 'doctor artis pharmaceuticae', had to submit to a supplementary examination. For surgery this consisted of a theoretical part as well as the execution of various set operations on a cadaver. The Royal Degree had further regulations relating to anatomical and other collections and to university hospitals. Each university had to be associated with a hospital for the purpose of practical tuition. But as the existing 'nosocomiums' were of rather modest size the legislator insisted on cooperation with local parish and town hospitals.

The Statute of 12 March 1818 with its accompanying enabling order 'to regulate that which applies to the execution of the various branches of medicine' maintained the old professional difference between university graduates and surgeons.[27] Section 11 and 12 stated that if anyone was in possession of diplomas entitling him to practise medicine as well as surgery, he was permitted to carry on a combined practice only in rural areas. However, the practice of surgery in combination with obstetrics was allowed everywhere throughout the land.

On this law special 'instructions' were superimposed for the separate professional groups. From section 13 for the regulations of surgeons it appears that in cases of strangulation, injury or other bodily harm which might have legal consequences, the surgeon was obliged to report such, immediately and without further request to the public prosecutor. This is contrary to the silence demanded by the oath of office which permits divulgence of such events only by order of the court. Nieuwenhuys correctly pointed out this contradiction. The requirement of taking an oath of office only confirmed an age-old custom. As was described above (see p. 114), ever since the sixteenth century the surgeon-to-be had to take an oath upon his promotion to master-surgeon and a similar tradition existed at the universities since at least the seventeenth century.

7.3.5.2. Surgical Apprenticeship

At first the kingdom omitted to regulate extramural surgical education. Just as before, the prospective surgeon was dependent on such private tuition as he was able to get. A neat picture of such a training course between 1814 and 1817 in Amsterdam was given by Pieter Klases Pel (1797—1878), country practitioner of medicine, surgery and obstetrics in Drachten.[28] His first tutor was apparently a barber-surgeon of the old type. He kept his pupil so fully occupied in shaving beards at his barber's shop that the young man was left with too little time to attend the lectures of Gerard Vrolik, professor of botany, anatomy and surgery at the Athenaeum Illustre. After some while Pel managed to become a living-in pupil of the surgeon Anthonie van der Hout (1782—1859), a young man with already a good reputation in surgery and obstetrics. For the price of 75 guilders quarterly, he had both board and lodging and admission to the lessons of his new master. The morning hours were spent at home in giving consultations for the poor who were members of the large sick fund ('ziekenbus') with which Van der Hout was associated, followed by visits to the local orphanage 'Burgerweeshuis' and to panel patients ('buspatiënten') in the city. In between there was usually time to observe instructive cases and operations at the nearby Binnengasthuis-hospital. After a midday meal at half past two, Pel had the rest of the day to himself, for studying or attending lectures. As he progressed he became more and more involved in teaching younger apprentices. The private tuition of Van der Hout was followed by about twelve young people. In his last year Pel, together with eight other advanced pupils, held a 'colloquium-medico-chirurgicum' evening once a week in which a particular topic was discussed. By 1817 he had reached the stage when he could take the medical, surgical and obstetrical examination before the Provincial Committee for Medical Supervision in Friesland, and in which he was successful.

Nieuwenhuys was probably thinking of, amongst others, Van der Hout, committee member of the Society for the Advancement of Medicine and Surgery, when he wrote in 1816: 'Much as it is learnt here without preparation and degraded by the association with lowly manual work, through scientific fellowship surgery has risen far above medicine in this city'.[29]

7.3.5.3. The Continued Existence of Barber-Surgeons

The maintenance of private training 'on the job' favoured the survival of the barber-surgeons. In spite of the numerical reduction which, according to Nieuwenhuys, the Amsterdam surgeons suffered in a period of some thirty years — 125 in 1816 against 261 in 1787 — there were still enough left to necessitate the reliance of quite a few of them on the return from their barbershops for a livelihood, even if the number of inhabitants had dropped from over 217 000 to about 180 000 during that time.[30] Conversely, there was a great shortage of practitioners in the countryside.[31]

Even in the 'twenties and 'thirties the genus barber-surgeon was not yet completely extinct. Jacob Vosmaer (1783—1824), professor of semiology and therapia generalis in Utrecht, created such a barber-surgeon as his central character in a series of delightful novels. This worthy person decided that his having a left shoulder somewhat higher than its counterpart was a consequence of his barber's activities.[32] The *Camera obscura* contains a letter by the Amsterdam surgeon Joris Krastem in which he complains that shaving oneself is rapidly becoming the fashion.[33] As late as the middle of the nineteenth century it was not unusual to see a signboard in a barber's shopfront exhibiting a painting of a muscular arm from which a fountain of blood was gushing rather like the spouting of a whale is depicted in old illustrations. Indeed, a high level of operative skill was not expected from these surgeons. An important part of their daily routine was bandaging the setons of those old ladies who held the firm belief that they should maintain a continual suppuration for the good of their health.[34] A municipal order from 1804 obliged the Amsterdam surgeons to 'always have the necessary instruments ready for resuscitating drowned people, as well as a tourniquet, threaded needles for ligating blood vessels, a male and female Cayenne catheter, and further every sort of appliance which might be necessary in emergencies, under penalty of a fine of 100 guilders.[35] Nor do lists of instruments which surgeons were required to have always ready for inspection, enacted in later years by the kingdom, suggest that these practitioners were expected to do much major surgery.[36]

7.3.5.4. Clinical Schools

Training schools for surgeons, which were already under discussion during the Batavian Republic, did not come into being until 1823, but it took five more years for them actually to open their doors.[37] They were founded in order to fulfil the need for medical assistance in rural areas, as stated in the appropriate Royal Decree from 1823. In a four year course, youngsters of at least sixteen years of age with some knowledge of Latin, who were capable of putting their thoughts to paper, were trained as either town surgeons or country surgeons ('heelmeester ten plattelande'), as obstetricians or — in a two year course — as pharmacists or midwives. Apprentice midwives needed only the ability to read and write. For the prospective surgeons or obstetricians the curriculum consisted of the subjects anatomy, physiology, pharmacognosy, chemistry, pharmaceutics, natural history, materies medica, pathology, therapy, surgery and obstetrics. The final examination was held by the Provincial Committee of Medical Supervision. A town surgeon's diploma enabled the owner to practise surgery — but surgery only — in the city. Country surgeons had also the right to practise internal medicine in the absence of medical doctors. The latter group can better be looked upon as general practitioners than as surgeons: they are comparable to the apothecaries in rural England at the time.

Clinical Schools were established in Amsterdam, Alkmaar, Haarlem, 's-Hertogenbosch, Hoorn, Middelburg and Rotterdam. These places were chosen because they had suitable hospitals. The cost fell on the appropriate municipalities. The schools in Rotterdam and Amsterdam experienced a certain amount of prosperity, as both managed to recruit a superior teaching staff.

In Rotterdam the school was partly established in the attic of the hall of the porters' guild in the Nieuwmarkt where surgical tuition had been taking place since the middle of the previous century, partly in a former barracks and partly in the old, rather unsuitable hospital for the purpose of clinical teaching. Many of the teachers — lecturers — from the Rotterdam school became professors at universities later in their careers.[38] Between 1836 and 1849 surgery was given by Frederik Willem Krieger (1805—81), an M.D. who had also acquired a doctor's degree in surgery and obstetrics. Before he graduated, Krieger had studied in Berlin for 2½ years. There he attended the lectures of Carl Ferdinand von Graefe at the university and probably those of Johann Nepomuk Rust (1775—1840) at the Charité Hospital. At the latter institute he can hardly have failed to see Dieffenbach in action. Opposition from the governors and surgeons at the hospital meant that Krieger in 1846 gladly left his Rotterdam chair for the far more prestigious one at Leyden. He entered upon office with a Latin oration on the contribution made by morbid anatomy to the recent progress of surgery.[39] His successor in Rotterdam, Machiel Polano (1813—78) adapted the *Lehrbuch der Chirurgie* by the Swiss Carl Emmert (1813—1903) in Bern for Dutch readers.[40] It can be stated in general that the lecturers at the Clinical Schools greatly contributed to the development of a medical literature in the vernacular, as tuition there unlike at the universities was given in Dutch.

In Amsterdam the school was housed in the ancient Binnengasthuis and it was not until 1839 that it took possession of its own residence in a mansion in the Kloveniersburgwal, adjoining the grounds of the hospital.[41] It acted in close cooperation with the Athenaeum Illustre: the teaching staff of the school were honorary professors at the Athenaeum. Their clinical lectures at the Binnengasthuis were also open to the medical students of the Athenaeum, while, conversely, the Athenaeum professors gave preclinical tuition to the pupils of the school. Lectures on anatomy, physiology and surgery took place in the old anatomical theatre. Assisting staff did not appear until 1843, yet there existed from the very beginning the system of resident students, chosen from the best in each year.

Among those who lectured at the school in Amsterdam we must especially mention Christiaan Bernard Tilanus (Fig. 98). We have already met him and his two friends earlier when they visited Paris and several German cities on their study tour (see p. 264). Tilanus was the first professor of surgery in the Netherlands to perform surgical operations in a hospital. Shortly after his appointment he had a new operating theatre built, which for its time was excellently equipped, with two isolated recovery rooms. It had previously been the general custom to perform operations on the ward, in the presence of other patients. Formerly even casual visitors were permitted to attend after paying an admission fee.

Tilanus was a cautious surgeon who, like most others of his generation, did not readily take up the knife. In his inaugural address he endorsed the view of Boyer that surgery was not susceptible to very much more advancement. For years he was the soul of medical-scientific life in the capital, among other things as chairman of the Society for the Advancement of Surgery. He was easily the leading Dutch surgeon of the last century[42] and produced quite a few papers. Two years after his death the Society for the Advancement of Surgery instituted a Tilanus medal in his memory. It is still being presented for special achievements in the field of surgery (Fig. 99).

For almost forty years, during the whole existence of the Amsterdam Clinical School, Tilanus lectured on surgery, and also for the first twenty years on obstetrics. We are well informed on the contents of his surgical lectures. He produced a concise *Schets der heelkunde* (Outline of surgery, 1835), as a syllabus of his lectures 'to spare himself and his audience the time-consuming dull dictations in his lessons'. The modest book runs to 193 pages. In 182 short paragraphs it deals with the pathology, the symptoms and treatment of surgical disorders without going into operative details. The text is succinct; literary references and illustrations are absent.

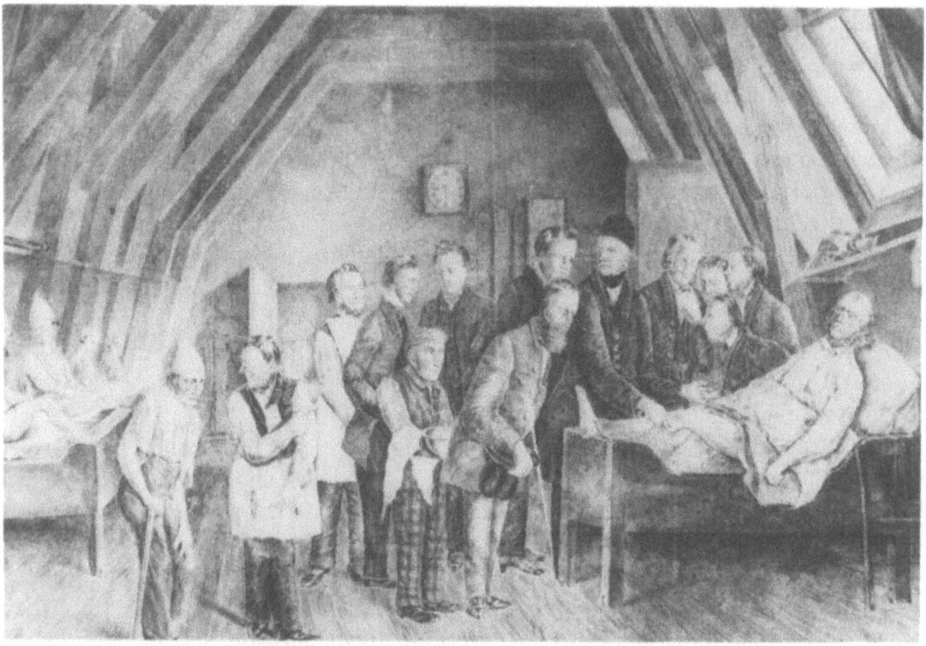

Fig. 98. Morning visit of Professor C. B. Tilanus, 1862.

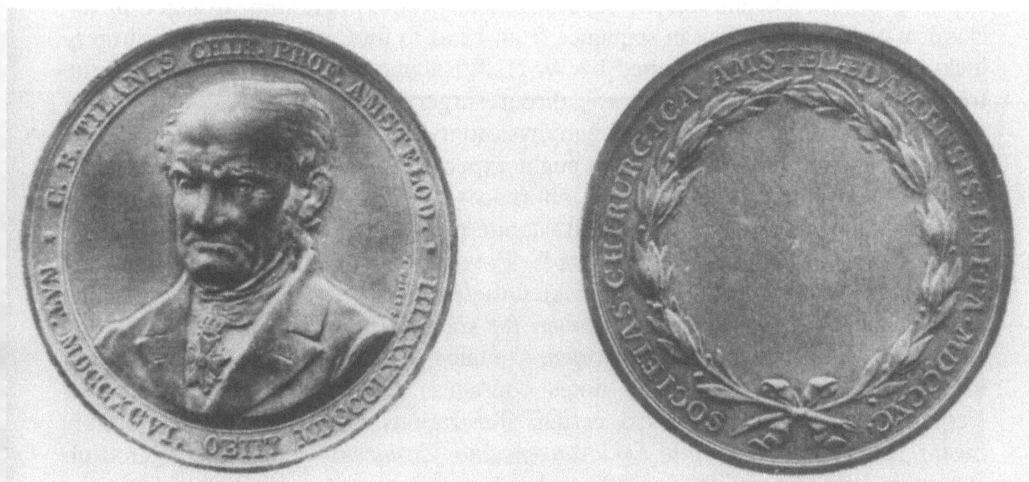

Fig. 99. Tilanus medal.

The subject matter is in two 'divisions'. The first deals with 'ailments of a dynamic origin', viz. inflammations, ulcers and abnormal growths. The second is about 'ailments of a mechanical origin and nature', embracing wounds, fractures, dislocations, orthopaedic and vascular abnormalities, as well as foreign bodies and spontaneous concretions: urinary, lacrimal, salivary and biliary stones.

In his study of inflammations — which is more extensively explained in a preserved handwritten student's notebook of 1834 than in the printed version — Tilanus shows himself to be a vitalist. Augmentation of the 'vital force' will lead to an increase in nerve sensibility — *dolor* — and a dilatation of the vasculary system which accounts for *rubor*. The circulation will be accelerated (!) which results in the red 'globules' being carried into vessels which normally only admit serum. This causes the fine serum vessels to become blocked, increasing the pressure in the supplying capillaries: these then also become dilated producing *calor*. Swelling — *tumor* — at first a direct effect of the vital forces, at a later stage develops from serum escaping into loose connective tissue.

Tilanus was not the only one who presented himself as a vitalist in the 1840s. Chelius, too, attributed the basic cause of inflammations to an increased activity of the life force.

As stated above, operative surgery was not included in Tilanus' lectures. A separate set of lecture notes made by one of his students, shows that this aspect of surgery — either as part of the official curriculum or in private courses— was taught by the city surgeon Gottfried Dietrich Schröder (1761—1835). Schröder was a German by birth who, as a doctor in the Prussian army, had studied at the well-known Berlin academy for military surgeons for three years. He established himself in Amsterdam in 1788 and became town surgeon shortly afterwards. Moreover, he was associated with the 'Buitengasthuis', the former plague hospital.[43]

Schröder's course of operative surgery fills 153 note-book pages.[44] Following a discussion about several elementary procedures such as suturing, bloodletting and applying setons, we find descriptions of more specific operations arranged in the classical order descending in sequence from head to foot, with ophthalmic surgery including keratonyxis, developed by W. H. J. Buchhorn at Halle in 1806 for the treatment of cataracts, ear-, nose-, throat surgery and in the obstetric section dealing with Caesarian section and symphysiotomy.

Pathology and diagnostics, as we might expect, are not brought up here. Unlike Tilanus, Schröder sometimes gives references to publications, but these always have a bearing on foreign literature. It is quite natural that as a German and having studied in Berlin, he should often cite C. F. von Graefe ('Graeve' is the name the student consistently wrote in his notes). Graefe's work from 1812, under the title quoted in full by Schröder as *Normen für die Ablösung grösserer Gliedmassen nach Erfahrungsgrundsätzen entworfen*, contains a description of an amputation using the funnel method. The notes contain a few rare diagrams. Schröder frequently makes references to certain illustrations in 'Bernstein': he possibly meant the *Kupfertafeln mit Erklärungen und Zusatzen* which Johann Gottlob Bernstein brought to light in 1802, a book of prints apparently available to the students.

It is noticeable that Schröder also referred to English publications, including an article by Sir Philip Crampton at Dublin in the *Medical-chirurgical Transactions* of 1816 on 'a new method of operating for the cure of external aneurism'. Schröder's operative surgery is still largely in the style of the eighteenth century, although some innovations are to be noted. For instance, he described a new approach to herniotomy, derived from Von Graefe, where the hernial sac, once opened and the contents replaced in the abdomen, was stuffed with wicks spread with a digestive. These needed to be replaced regularly until granulations appeared at the edges of the sac, then the wound could be closed. Obliteration of the hernial sac through accretion was apparently the set aim.

By means of an appendix or addendum at the end of the notes under the title 'The restoration of lost noses', an extract is given of a review in the *Konst- en Letterbode*, a magazine for the general public, of the work *An account of two successful operations of a lost nose, from the integuments of the forehead in the cases of two officers of H.M. army*, etc., which Joseph Constantine Carpue (1764—1846) at London brought out in 1813. This excerpt gives a fine historical survey of rhinoplasty in 13 pages, with two successful applications of the Indian method which Carpue, as the first European to do so, carried out in 1814 and 1815.

After a promising start, the Clinical Schools did not bring about the surgical improvements that had been hoped for. An important reason for this was that the examinations were held by the Provincial Committees and not by the school itself. Moreover, in order to fulfil the urgent need for surgeons in the war with Belgium, the compulsory attendance at a Clinical School, required for admission to the examination was dropped after a few years. Once again the situation developed where it was possible to prepare for the test via private tutoring. These schools were discontinued in 1866 (cf. p. 307).

The Binnengasthuis in Amsterdam, in which the Clinical School was established, also served as 'academic hospital' for the Athenaeum, when in 1876 it was raised to university status. This did not lead to the restoration of the operating theatre built by C. B. Tilanus in 1843. In 1893 it was described as a room of 7 by 8 metres, of which only half was open space. The rest was taken up by seating accommodation for 82 spectators (Fig. 108). The decaying floor allowed air and light to filter through from the first-aid room below. The attic, which formed the floor of the sleeping quarters of the man-servant, let dust and scrubbing water through. Everything in the theatre was always covered with a layer of dust. The stove in the corner had to be heavily stoked to heat the whole area, whilst nearby it was too hot to bear. The lift for the patients consisted of a large wooden crate which had to be noisily hoisted up from the ward below by means of a windlass.[45]

7.3.5.5. Military Doctors

Military doctors — already lauded by Homer — held an important position in the Netherlands in the nineteenth century. Their glorious past goes back as far as the seventeenth century,[46] but they distinguished themselves in particular during and shortly after the battle of Waterloo. The surgeon in charge of the Dutch medical service in the field was on that occasion Carl Georg Eduard Mergell (1781—1851), born in Germany, who had been serving in the Dutch forces since 1802. During the period of French rule he served in the Napoleonic army partaking in many campaigns. He had become good friends with the celebrated French army surgeon Larrey.[47] In the Belgian contingent we should mention Jozef Kluyskens (1771—1843) who had already served in the Austrian army as surgeon, before in 1794 coming under the command of the prince of Orange — later to become king William I — in the last catastrophic war between the old Republic and France.

After the battle of Waterloo, Kluyskens, who in his function of chief of the hospital service was responsible for more than 9000 wounded, conducted 300 amputations personally. In this respect he ceded nothing to Larrey.[48] Sebald Justinus Brugmans in particular met with much appreciation; we have already met him as professor at Leyden (cf. p. 186) and in the next chapter he will figure as one of the founders of antiseptic wound treatment (see p. 293). In his function of Inspector General he clearly showed his talent for organization when in the days following the battle of Waterloo, vast numbers of wounded were not only being conveyed to Brussels but also to dozens of villages and hamlets in the surrounding areas. For instance, between 16 June and 15 July, some 10 000 Prussians alone were taken to Brussels. By requisitioning buildings for miles around for use as emergency hospitals, mobilizing civilian doctors to supplement the military surgeons whose numbers could not cope with so many wounded at once, instigating measures for preventing the spread of hospital infections and spreading and evacuating the wounded as rapidly as possible, he was able to avoid the outbreak of epidemics.[49]

In 1817, the king converted the military hospitals at Louvain and Leyden into 'Great State Hospitals, for the Training of Medical Officers'. In 1822 both military schools were replaced by one central institute, the State Training College for Military Physicians in Utrecht. In the 1840's and fifties, this school grew into the best medical and surgical training centre in the Netherlands, known particularly for its clinical tuition which was made possible through its association with the Great State Hospital.[50] It could boast of many excellent teachers, including — to mention only one — the celebrated Franciscus Cornelis Donders (1818—89), himself a graduate of the school. As a physiologist Donders was one of the advocates of the modern natural science approach to medicine, and as an ophthalmologist he was one of the leading figures of his time.[51] Military physicians played a significant part in the development of scientific medicine in Holland, as intermediaries between academic and non-academic medicine as well as between medicine and surgery.[52] Unlike the civilian physicians who as a rule oriented themselves toward German medicine, army doctors were rather influenced by French medical ideas. In 1865 the school was transferred to Amsterdam and largely amalgamated with the Athenaeum Illustre there. It was closed in 1880, as a consequence of the statute, that all medical schooling in this country should be concentrated at the universities (cf. p. 307).

7.3.5.6. Textbooks of Surgery

Until about the middle of the century, the most important surgical textbooks available in this country besides the work of Tilanus, were mostly of foreign origin, especially German. The German influence on Dutch surgery was recognizable very early in the century; actually long before the Germans, inspired by a new natural scientific élan had taken a leading position in medicine and surgery. An explanation for this remarkable phenomenon could have been the nature of the German literature. This consisted primarily of those publications aimed at the practice of medicine and having little recourse to theory, which fitted well into the mentality prevailing in this country at the time. Another factor which may have contributed was the not inconsiderable percentage of Germans within the medical and surgical professions. Ever since the seventeenth century, increasing numbers of German doctors and surgeons had come to work here as university professors, as medical officers in the army and in the colonies, or as private practitioners.[53]

As a translator of German surgical works in the years following the French occupation, Anthonie van der Hout, (cf. p. 270) especially springs to mind. He took it upon himself to bring out Dutch editions of the textbook of surgery by Johann August Tittmann (1774—1840) in Dresden in 1816, the beautifully illustrated manual of bandaging by Johann Christian Stark (1769—1837), professor of surgery at Jena in 1817, and the handbook of surgical anatomy by Friedrich Christian Rosenthal (1780—1829), professor of anatomy and physiology at Greifswald in 1821. Tittmann's book ran through three Dutch editions, the last one appearing in 1827.

It was superseded by the celebrated *Handbuch der Chirurgie* by Chelius which was produced in Dutch in 1830, 1834 and 1853, translated by Gerardus Johannes Pool, a surgeon who had graduated in medicine in Germany, while Dieffenbach's operative surgery, by an unknown translator, appeared in 1846—1850. Taking a close look at Chelius' book, we find that the subject matter is arranged in an orderly and methodical fashion, with a concise and clear text. The author does not usually enter very deeply into the possible causes of surgical diseases, but does give a clear account of their diagnostic features and of their differential diagnoses. Regarding treatment he firstly gives an outline of the basic principles before explaining the practical therapeutical measures to be taken, with only the necessary details and no more. The book is largely aimed at surgical practice but regularly shows evidence that the author himself was a man of great theoretical knowledge and wide reading. The bibliography has maintained its value until today. References are provided in two ways. First in lists at the beginning of the book there appear in subject order history, textbooks and manuals, surgical science, instrumentation, dressings, miscellaneous and surgical journals: these being works of a general nature. Then he precedes each individual chapter with literary sources having special bearing on its particular subject; under some paragraphs further references, often from journals, are given with a short summary. Besides German, he also included much French and English literature: Chelius was clearly internationally orientated, which must have added to the popularity of his book. Dutch contributions are hardly referred to at all, which tells us something about the international regard of surgery in this country. Diseases of the eyes and ears, nose and throat, which still formed part of surgery at that time, are not considered and neither is obstetrics.[54]

Towards the middle of the century, British surgery came to be represented by no less a person than Sir Astley Cooper, who became widely known in Holland when Med., Chir. et Art. Obstetric. Dr. W. M. D. Junius translated his book *Principles and practice of surgery* in 1842. This translation, as well as a few more surgery books was done directly from the English. Up till then, English and French works had often been translated indirectly from German versions. Knowledge of the English language became somewhat more wide-spread than before, although most doctors and surgeons were still barely familiar with it.

7.3.5.7. Medical Journals

In the Netherlands the first medical journal — *Collectanea medicophysica* oft

Hollands Jaar-register — made its appearance in 1680: it survived for eight years. Since the 1720s several other journals existed for varying periods. The most successful periodical in the first half of the last century, was the *Practisch Tijdschrift voor de Geneeskunde in al haren omvang* (Practical journal of medicine in its entirety), established in 1822 and intended in particular for 'young doctors . . . and country surgeons' according to its subtitle. It contained a great many case histories, and besides epidemiology there were directions for the use of new medications — mercury preparations, prussic acid, iodine, cod-liver oil and even alkaloids — and especially abstracts from foreign journals. It is notable that original French or English publications were discussed in Dutch periodicals via abstracts in German journals. The fact that the *Practisch Tijdschrift* existed for 27 years thriving on this formula, proves that it fulfilled the requirements of the class of medical practitioners, to which the surgeons belonged.[38] Due to its mediocre level it can hardly have contributed to the advancement of surgery. On the other hand a higher scientific standard would probably have frightened off many of its potential readers. So long as the primary training of surgeons and obstetricians had not been elevated to a higher plane, very little continued education could be expected to originate from journals.

The *Nederlandsch Lancet*, founded in 1838, was likewise initially chiefly filled with abstracts and for the rest of its content with not very original contributions to surgery, ophthalmology and obstetrics. Its scientific level rose considerably after 1845, when it was edited, among others, by F. C. Donders and had received the subtitle 'Journal of the medical sciences to their full extent'. It took on the new natural scientific trend of medicine, which in those days had its focal point in Utrecht. The journal continued to exist until 1856.

7.4. NEW DEVELOPMENTS TOWARDS THE MIDDLE OF THE NINETEENTH CENTURY

7.4.1. *The Emergence of Scientific Materialism*

Towards the middle of the nineteenth century, fundamental changes took place in medical thinking. Aprioristic modes of thought, such as those which brought about various vitalistic and natural philosophical systems in the eighteenth century and the first decades of the following one, had to make room for scientific materialism under the influence of the developing natural sciences which in their turn were partly fired by the positivism of Auguste Comte. This French philosopher once again hammered home that only knowledge of the facts can be fruitful and that the researcher must stick strictly to observation. Experimentation was assigned a fundamental place, university departments changed into scientific institutes and staff apart from the professors entered upon the scene. Science and learning were no longer private affairs. The great German pathologist Rudolf Virchow (1821–1902), who was one of the most important apologists of the new trend, included animal experiments together with clinical observation and autopsies in his well-known cognitive triad. None of these components were new in themselves; it was the close connection into which Virchow had brought them which was new. Virchow further occupies an important place in the history of medicine on account of his doctrine of cellular pathology. The tissue cell, discovered in 1839 by Theodor Schwann in Berlin, was designated by him as the basic element of life. And as disease is nothing other than life under altered conditions, the cell is also the fundamental carrier of disease.

In the Netherlands Gerrit Jan Mulder's school of physiology in Utrecht played an important part in helping scientific materialism take shape here too. In a speech, entitled 'The material world, a means to higher development', held on the occasion of the opening of a new laboratory, Mulder said:

> Knowledge of matter and forces, and their interrelationship; ceaseless endeavours of the mind to become more familiar with these matters and forces; how to generate the latter and put them into operation: that, gentlemen, is what the science of Nature today considers her purpose.[55]

7.4.2. *The Introduction of Anaesthesia*

Two conditions which had traditionally imposed limitations on the scope of operative surgery were pain and wound complications, both of which had carried off many a patient. Until the nineteenth century surgeons were able to restrict the pain only by operating at breakneck speed with razor-sharp instruments. A typical ritual in the pre-anaesthetic operating theatres was the taking out of pocket watches by the audience the moment the operation was started (cf. p. 244). The invention of surgical anaesthesia was the first important American contribution to medicine — in fact one of the most important contributions of all time. Its history is too well-known to necessitate going into detail here.[56] A brief recollection will suffice: on the evening of the 10th of December 1844 a dentist in Hartford, Connecticut, observed that during a public demonstration with laughing-gas one of the experimental subjects fell while under the influence of that merry-making substance, without apparently hurting himself. This dentist, Horace Wells, took some of the gas himself the following day and had a tooth pulled out while intoxicated. The extraction was painless.

Wells obtained permission from Dr. John C. Warren, professor of surgery at the Massachusetts General Hospital in Boston, to demonstrate a painless extraction in the hospital lecture room. In the event, the demonstration was rather unconvincing, compelling Wells to beat a hasty retreat.

A colleague and former associate of Wells, William Morton, who had attended the unfortunate demonstration, started to experiment with ether: on himself, his family, his domestic animals, including the goldfishes: without any success, however. It was only after he had used a glass bottle with a spout, on the advice of the chemist Charles Jackson, that he was able to obtain satisfactory results. The method was subjected to a clinical test on October 16th 1846, in the same theatre at the Massachusetts General Hospital, where Horace Wells had failed. This time, however, the effect was indeed of general anaesthesia. Dr. Warren removed a tumour from under the jaw of the patient in dead silence, after which he spoke the memorable words: 'Gentlemen, this is no humbug!'. It was clear that a momentous discovery had been made and before long, heated arguments burst forth on the issue of priorities. We will not enter into that unpalatable story here, but prefer to retrace the way in which anaesthesia was accepted. A striking feature is the remarkable speed with which the invention became known all over the world after it had been made public in a paper published on November 18th 1846 by Dr. Henry Jacob Bigelow, one of the surgeons at the Massachusetts General Hospital.

The Cunard steamer Acadia, which sailed from Boston on the 3rd of December, carried a letter from Dr. Bigelow to his friend Dr. Francis Boott in London. On December 19th, Boott reported in the *Lancet* that 'a firmly fixed molar tooth was extracted in my study from Miss Lonsdale, by Mr. Robinson (a neighbouring dentist), in the presence of my wife, two of my daughters and myself, without the least sense of pain, or the movement of a muscle . . .' (Fig. 100). Subsequent trials all failed, however, apparently due to various shortcomings of the inhaler employed.

Robert Liston (cf. p. 266), was present at one of the attempts. He subsequently instructed his assistant William Squire, with the help of Peter Squire, a chemist, to contrive a better device. On December 21st, i.e. only two days after Dr. Boott's first trials, Liston operated on two etherized patients at University College Hospital, performing an evulsion of a great toenail in one case and an amputation of a thigh in the other. The news spread quickly over the country; the medical journals of 1847 contained numerous descriptions of inhalers, devised by just as many competitive inventors. The first operation to be performed under general anaesthetic in Holland took place on March 8, 1847 in the Hague, when the surgeon and obstetrician S. T. C. Schoevers in the presence of the medical doctors Mouton, Volgraff, Evers, Holtrop ad Blom Coster used ether for 'a surgical intervention' in a 22-year old girl by means of a simple device designed by the reader of chemistry F. P. Stutterheim.[57] Very shortly afterwards it was also introduced in Utrecht (Fig. 101) and Amsterdam. In the latter place, the attempt apparently went off less smoothly. The surgeon J. W. R. Tilanus (1823—1914), son of C. B. Tilanus, when referring to this memorable event many years later, was pointing to one corner of the theatre when he explained: 'That's where we began'. He then pointed to the opposite corner and finished his sentence by saying: 'We were there when we sutured the wound'.[58] Within a year, anaesthesia had travelled around the world (Fig. 102).

7.4.3. *Plaster Bandage*

An important invention by the Dutch military surgeon Antonius Mathijsen (1805—78) which took place in 1852, was the modern plaster bandage.[59] The principle of hardening dressings in the treatment of fractures was already very old. Hippocrates used a mixture of wheat flour and gum or incense powder for fractures of the nose and collarbone. Rhazes recommended chicken eggwhite, chalk and plaster for this purpose. In the Middle Ages and later white of egg bandages were commonly used (cf. p. 40). Larrey's 'bandage inamovible' consisted of compresses soaked in a mixture of eggwhite, lead subacetate and spirits of camphor. These were attached to the extremity with Scultetus' many tailed bandage (Fig. 71). For further reinforcement Larrey applied straw gutters before the whole was once again coated with the solution. Thus, a very solid dressing was

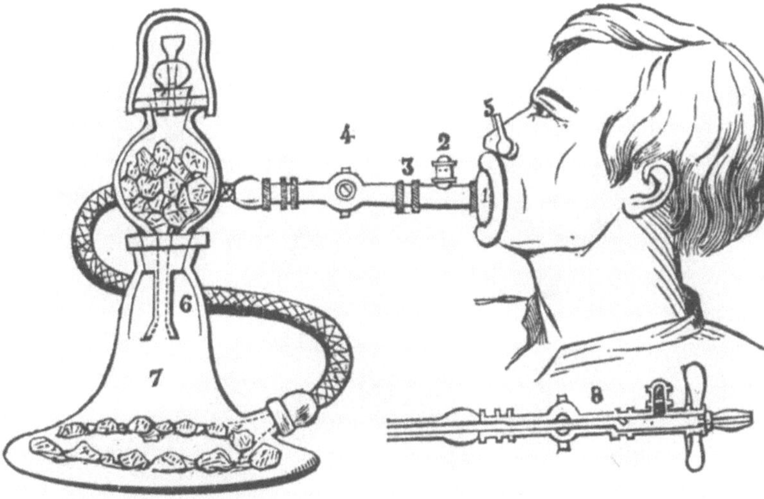

Fig. 100. Ether inhaler by Boott and Robinson, London, used on December 19th, 1846.

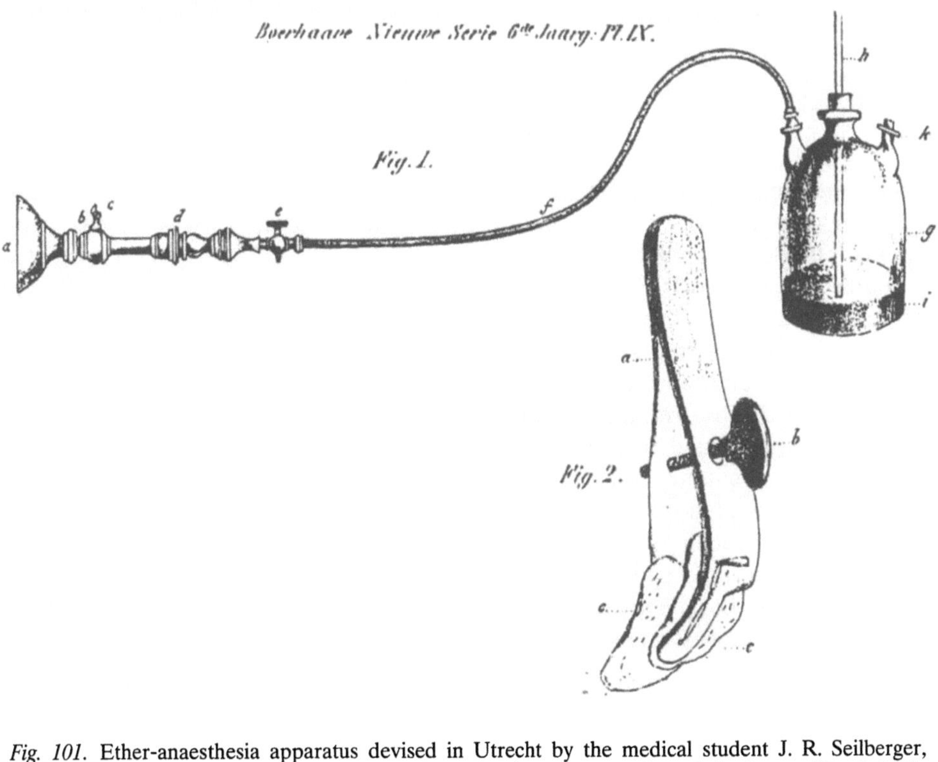

Fig. 101. Ether-anaesthesia apparatus devised in Utrecht by the medical student J. R. Seilberger, successfully used by the surgeon A. C. van Woerden in an amputation of the leg on March 16th, 1847. The clamp was used for pinching the patient's nose.

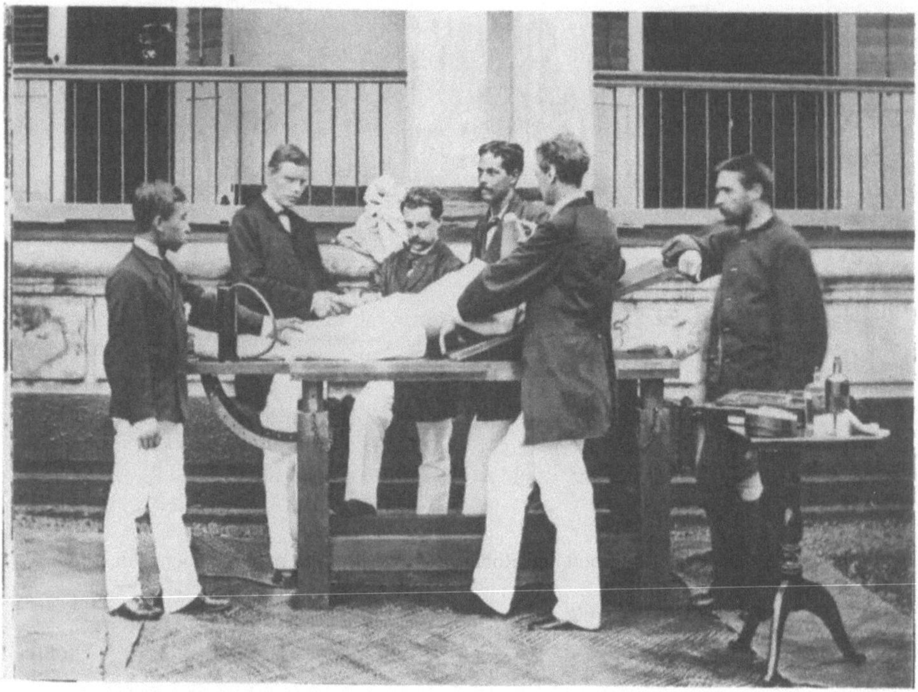

Fig. 102. Operation staged outdoors in the former Dutch East Indies. The operation was probably for an amputation of the right arm. No visible antiseptic precautions are being taken. The conical mask with which the chloroform anaesthesia was given, is clearly visible. Wooden operation table. Military Hospital at Batavia (?) in 1888.

produced, enabling the wounded man to be transported more easily, whilst obviating the necessity of constantly tightening the binders, as was the case with splints. The Belgian military surgeon Louis-Joseph Seutin (1793—1862) introduced a starch dressing in 1835. It consisted of many layers of linen and wet cardboard as splints, stuck together with starch. This dressing had the advantage that it was light to wear and even allowed the patient to move around, albeit without weight-bearing. However, it was rather complicated and it took several days to dry.

Plaster in liquid form applied directly to the extremity, was already being used for the immobilization of fractures by the Arabs. The first application of plaster reported in this country, took place in the nosocomium chirurgicum in Groningen in 1814. Petrus Hendrikz (1779—1843) who was associated with this institution by means of a teaching commitment in surgery, placed the broken extremity after reduction in a box splint, which he subsequently filled with liquid plaster. Mathijsen must be given the credit for hitting upon the idea of using bandages impregnated with plaster (Fig. 103).

7.4.4. *Surgery in the Netherlands in the middle of the century*

At about the middle of last century the existing medical journals, largely filled with case histories, no longer met the demands of the times. The readers now wished to

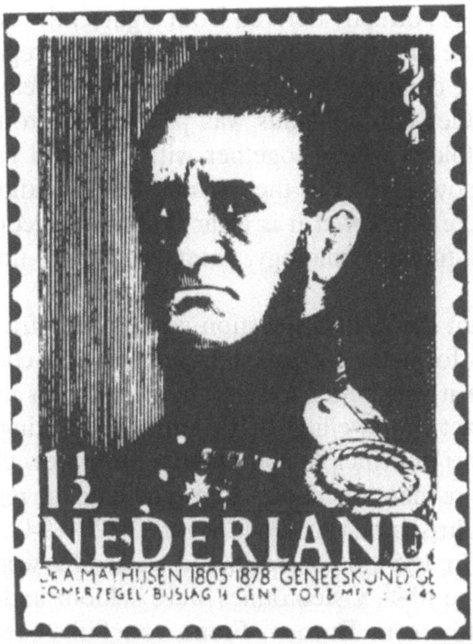

Fig. 103. Dr. A. Mathijsen, inventor of the plaster bandage.

be kept informed of new developments in their field and of social evolution associated with medicine. This desire was reflected in journals that came into being at the time. One of the more interesting new or renewed medical journals was the *Nederlandsch Weekblad voor Geneeskundigen* (Dutch weekly for physicians), which was published for six years from 1856. The information it offered its readers covered all aspects of medicine and was generally of good quality. That quality was safeguarded through the superior scientific level of its editors.

It breathed a positivistic spirit, departing from the idea that medicine should be a 'physical science', in which factual knowledge must be sought. In this it was in strong contrast with that of the good-old *Practisch Tijdschrift.* It is thanks to this formula, as well as to the frequency of issue, that the *Nederlandsch Weekblad* became the most important medium of its time for the publication of practical and experimental studies of Dutch surgery at its best.

Leafing through the volumes of the *Weekblad* it appears that the optimistic belief in progress chiefly concerned pathology and diagnostics.[60] Therapeutic possibilities were still in a sorry state. The introduction of anaesthesia, gratifying as it was for patients and surgeons alike, had not advanced operative surgery one single step further. Wound infection, which by shading off into pyaemia carried off patients within a few days, was still an oppressing problem. It is therefore understandable that most surgeons were disinclined to operate. In an extensive article containing a critical survey of surgical therapy C. B. Tilanus claimed an important gain had been made, when the various theoretical systems which had dominated medical thought during the decades at the turn of the century, had been abandoned in favour of 'the positive direction of medicine'. In his explanations of the action of pharmaceuticals he himself, nevertheless, made use of such concepts as ‘general nerve tuning’, directly derived from eighteenth-century neural pathology and ‘blood crasis of the sufferer’, a humoral pathological representation taken from Rokitansky’s blastema concept,[61] which Virchow had already haughtily dismissed in 1846.[62] On the other hand Tilanus was progressive in his appreciation of the new microscopic histology which, together with chemical research, should be the ‘foundation of our knowledge’. But then again he was traditional in his support of blood-letting. From the *Weekblad* it is clear that the surgeons particularly focused their attention on fractures, herniology, vascular surgery, urology and the surgical treatment of cancer.

The most important theoretical question asked about fractures was the manner in which callus was formed. As far as treatment was concerned there was an argument on whether it was better to wrap fresh fractures in cold, wet cloths for a few days to counteract the swelling or to apply supporting bandages right away. Fracture treatment was in principle conservative. Very few cases of open reduction of simple fractures were mentioned, and then each time the results were disastrous.

Professor Louis Christiaan van Goudoever (1820—94) at Utrecht did not let this discourage him. In 1851 he performed a successful wedge resection in a case of antecurvature of the tibia. Osteotomies were seldom undertaken at that time in this country or elsewhere in Europe. Franz von Pitha (1810—75), professor of surgery at the Medico-chirurgical Josephs Academy in Vienna, quipped in 1868 that for this operation ‘sich doch wohl selten die zwei nöthigen Männer finden werden’.[63] The invention of the plaster bandage naturally received all the attention. Amputation was still the treatment of choice for compound fractures. It gradually dawned on surgical thinking that the socalled ‘contusion of the foot’ was frequently a heel bone fracture.

Inguinal herniae still presented an important surgical problem. Standard treatment consisted, as before, of prescribing a truss. Caoutchouc, which had been invented in the meantime, made possible the design of better models. The inventiveness displayed here often demands admiration. Clinicians were also trying to find methods of obliterating the hernial sac. One idea was to inject this structure with tincture of iodine, another idea was to invert part of the skin of the scrotum into the inguinal canal on the top of a finger and fix it in that position with a few stitches by way of internal pad. Herniotomy was still only performed as an emergency operation in cases of strangulation. The death rate remained appallingly high. The clinical picture of ileus, often resulting from a strangulated hernia, was generally well-known. An excellent article by Nicolai Ivanovich Pirogov (1810—81), the greatest surgeon ever produced in Russia, on the pathogenesis and diagnostics of an abdominal obstruction, was extensively reviewed in the *Weekblad*. On the strength of post-mortem findings in patients who had died of this unfortunate condition Samuel Senior Coronel (1827—92), a general practitioner from Middelburg who later in his life was a pioneer in social medicine, once declared that operative treatment would have saved these cases. ‘And yet, however rational laparotomy might seem and as it were the only expedient, the operation will not easily find acceptance amongst our cautious Dutch surgeons’.

Vascular surgery was still mainly concerned with peripheral aneurysms. It was understood by then that atheromatous changes in the vessel walls were the direct cause of the dilatation. The classical therapy by ligation was accompanied by an operative death rate of 20—30% as appeared from reports at home and abroad. For this reason, foreign surgeons in particular diligently sought other methods for congealing the blood in the aneurysmal sac. A number of them can be found described in the *Weekblad*: galvanopuncture which was unsuccessful in this country; injection of sclerosing fluids as recommended by Pravaz,[64] or continued compression. The latter was no longer carried out on the aneurysm itself but on the proximal artery, using a specially designed device. Two of the eighteen aneurysm patients who were admitted to the Binnengasthuis in Amsterdam between 1829 and 1854, were cured by Tilanus using this method of treatment. One patient had responded well to the application of ice compresses, another to continued direct compression. In fourteen patients the femoral artery was ligated, eight times with success, whereas six patients died of secondary haemorrhage or 'purulent fever'.

There are not many reports on varicose veins in the *Weekblad*. Velpeau in Paris gave a survey of all the different forms of varicose vein treatments which had been invented over the years, including a new technique of injecting iron salts to produce sclerosation. On the basis of his own experience with 250 patients whom he had treated in all sorts of ways, he decided to abandon the treatment of this condition altogether.

In urology important developments were in progress. Lithotomy — a speciality of J. W. R. Tilanus — was gradually being replaced by lithotrity, crushing the stone with specially designed instruments. Due to the fact that bladder calculi were becoming increasingly rare, removal of stone was no longer the main urological operation. Urethral stricture, a late complication of the common infection of gonorrhoea, had meanwhile become the most prevalent urological problem.

The *Weekblad* also often contained thorough reports on cancer. The discussions included the question of whether a separate cancer cell existed, such as Hermann Lebert (1813—78), a leading German pathologist who worked in Paris for many years, had claimed. Microscopy was developing: although vital staining was not yet being used, various forms of cancer were being distinguished on their histological appearances. A second question was whether microscopy would ever make it possible to draft a division of cancer types, useful in clinical practice. A third point at issue was whether or not malignant processes were in principle curable at all. Yet another subject for discussion concerned the existence of a particular cancer diathesis. Statistics first became significant in the history of oncology as arguments for or against a given hypothesis. Two important contemporary contributions on oncology by Dutch authors, however, did not appear in the *Weekblad*. The first one was by Johannes Matthias Schrant (1823—64), perhaps the greatest Dutch pathologist of the last century. He was the author of a prize essay on benign and malignant tumours, in which he tried to define pathognomonic microscopic criteria (1851).[65] Following the example of Lebert, Schrant took soft medullary cancer to be the prototype of malignancy and looked for elements which might also be present in cancers of less malignant types. Noting the constant presence, more or less in abundance, of what he called 'free nuclei' in all his specimens, he concluded that such a profusion must be characteristic of the disease. After a critical review of the conservative methods of treatment still in use at that time, he strongly recommended early and wide surgical excision. Schrant had been working in Amsterdam before he was called to Leyden at the age of 39, as professor of internal medicine. Unfortunately, he died of typhoid fever two years later.

The second significant contribution was made in 1853 by Jacobus Ludovicus Coenraad Schroeder van der Kolk (1797—1862), professor of anatomy and physiology, later also of pathology, at the University of Utrecht. He found cancer cells in apparently healthy tissue some distance away from the primary tumour.[66] This finding gave support to the clinical maxim that cancer should be treated by wide excision, rather than by local extirpation. Schroeder van der Kolk's paper was cited with much appreciation by Virchow.[67]

Patients with breast cancer do not appear to have presented themselves in large numbers for operation. Professor C.B. Tilanus recorded only six such cases amongst 861 patients admitted to his clinic at the Amsterdam Binnengasthuis in 1853. All six were treated by excision: five were said to have been cured, one patient 'improved'. The annual report in which these favourable results were recorded was written shortly after the end of the year in which the operations had taken place, so the follow-up period can only have been a matter of months.[68] Professor Van Goudoever in Utrecht had even fewer cases to report: of the 241 patients admitted between 1849 and 1853, only two women suffered from breast cancer, both of whom underwent surgery.[69]

CHAPTER 8

Antisepsis: A Turning Point in Surgery

The introduction of antisepsis by Joseph Lister in 1867, as is generally known, made possible the healing of wounds without suppuration. In a very short time operative surgery advanced to unprecedented levels. It did in fact reveal an entirely new era. In order to visualize clearly the special meaning of this discovery let us first try to form an impression of the seriousness and scale of the problem of wound infection in the 100 years preceding Lister's breakthrough.

8.1. HOSPITAL SURGICAL DEPARTMENTS IN THE SIXTIES OF THE LAST CENTURY

The following account is derived from the memoires of a general practitioner who was a student in the surgery department of the University Hospital in Leyden between 1865 and 1866.[1] Since 1799 the hospital was housed in an old mansion in the Oude Vest, which is still standing. It comprised a medical and surgical department, an obstetric clinic, an operating theatre, a pharmacy and a mortuary, all under one roof. Infectious diseases were not isolated but lay among the other cases: a typhoid patient beside a terminal case of tuberculosis, venereal diseases among the amputations.

There was hardly any question of disinfection. The hands were washed occasionally with chlorinated water or spirit soap, when after the physical examination or dressing of an malodorous wound they had become unduly soiled. Semmelweis' discovery, which he had been publicizing since 1848, had no more permeated the surgery in this country than it had anywhere else in the world. In each department a student served as assistant to the professor. Residents in the modern sense of the word were not yet known. Frederik Willem Krieger, M.D., whom we have already met on page 271 as a lecturer at the Clinical School in Rotterdam, was professor of surgery at that time. It fell to the 'praetor' to supervise the two surgical wards and, among other things, to make sure that the patients did not smoke, a ticklish problem as the 'father of the sick' also enjoyed a good pipe. This functionary was a person of minimal education. Although a married man, he had to be present in the hospital day and night. He only had half a day off on Sunday afternoons, when his responsibilities were taken over for a few hours by one of the convalescents. The women's ward was entrusted to a 'mother of the sick', a former kitchen maid. This was all the nursing help available for the surgical department. In the absence of the professor, the praetor had to take over the outpatient clinic. He also had to assist at operations after having laid out the instruments that were taken unwashed from the cupboard and to provide a couple of buckets of pump-water for sponges and dressings.

It was the generally established custom in those days for the dressings to be prepared in the hospital itself by the convalescents and the chronic sick, including coughing consumptives and patients with leg ulcers, to help them while away their time. The dressing materials consisted of pledgets made from old linen which was teased out, 'English lint' — a type of brushed cotton — and swaddles torn from unbleached cotton. At operations the surgeon, his assistant and the spectators wore their oldest frock coats in view of the blood spatters. These coats had usually been worn at previous operations and were consequently crusted over with dried blood and matter. After use these status-bestowing garments were carefully put away in a closet in the theatre until the next time.

Scrubbing up — at least preoperatively — did not take place. After the operation the table and floor were washed down with wet sponges. Patients who had undergone major surgery such as an amputation or jaw resection stayed in bed in the theatre until another important intervention had to take place. Minor operations were carried out in the presence of the first patient when he was still in the theatre.

It was part of the praetor's duty to sit up with the post-operative cases for the first few nights and call the professor should secondary bleeding occur. The dressings were changed for the first time on the third day. Very occasionally the wound would heal by first intention, but in most cases it looked terrible and gave off a ghastly smell. Quite a few patients died of wound fever and wound diphteria. Nevertheless, 'comparatively many' were cured under such unfavourable conditions which is probably explainable by the circumstance that most of the operations were not very serious.

The situation was no better abroad.[2] An insipid, sweetish smell of matter, and not uncommonly even the stench of putrescence, hung about the surgical wards of the pre-antiseptic era. The German surgeon Ernst Küster (1839—192?) recorded that since the middle of the nineteenth century it was mixed with the odours of vegetable and chemical applications: camomile, camphor, and later carbolic acid.

The seriousness of the disease could be read in the face of the patient. Hectic flushing, glistening eyes and perspiring foreheads, the apprehensive look of a fever patient next to the pale, disinterested countenance of one ill with sepsis, moaning and mumbling in unfinished, half-intelligeable sentences. The bandages were stinking and soaked through with purulent matter, when even changing them several times a day could not prevent the effusion from soiling the adjacent parts of the body, the bedclothes and the mattress. Each change of dressing also meant a change of bedclothes and mattress. It was unavoidable that the patient was lifted from his bed for this purpose, which often drew screams of pain. Trained nurses were not yet available to perform these tasks. For many of the wounded, their being taken to hospital meant certain death. This picture of human misery, with its high mortality, the ever recurring disappointment of a successfully completed operation having a fatal outcome, demanded great dedication and strength of character from the surgeons in the pre-antiseptic era. Even about 1870 professor Polano, Krieger's successor, discouraged by disappointing experiences, apparently exclaimed: 'The government ought to forbid us to operate!'[3]

8.2. CLASSIFICATION OF WOUND DISEASES

Wound infections had already been described in the classical literature, but it was only in the first half of the nineteenth century that surgery began to make clear distinctions between the clinical varieties. According to Küster, at the time when antisepsis was being introduced, doctors were familiar with such deadly diseases as wound putrefaction or septicaemia otherwise known as sepsis, purulent fever or pyaemia, hospital gangrene or gangraena nosocomialis, lockjaw or tetanus, rose or erysipelas.[4]

In the second half of the nineteenth century, *septicaemia* was referred to as a condition in which the wound exudate took on a yellowish grey or dark brown, more or less bloody appearance, while emitting an obnoxious smell, sometimes like that of carrion. The edges of the wound became pinkish and swollen, though not particularly painful, in advanced cases rather insensible, probably due to the reduced state of consciousness. The symptoms developed gradually in the space of a few days. There was an increase in pulse rate before the local signs became apparent, accompanied by a remittent fever which reached a peak in the evening and increased day by day. The patient's countenance became dulled with glazed eyes.

Pyaemia usually occurred in cases with larger wounds, especially of the limbs. Contrary to septicaemia, pyaemia was of sudden onset with rigors followed by a rise in temperature, sometimes even as high as 41°C., while the wound was seemingly clean and covered by healthy granulations, exuding odourless matter. The fever fell after several hours with copious sweats. Many similar bouts of pyrexia followed. After the first few times the wound acquired a different aspect. The granulations became pale and flat, reduced in number and swollen with a glassy appearance. The exudate changed into a broth-like fluid usually with a slightly unpleasant smell. The wound was very painful. The most typical characteristic, however, was the formation of numerous abscesses in the internal organs and on the body surface elsewhere: they mostly followed the rigors. At the height of his suffering the wounded person wore an expression of fear and tension with the glistening eyes of a fever patient. Mixed forms of these two conditions existed and it was often impossible to make a sharp distinction between them.

Strangely enough, *hospital gangrene* does not seem to have been observed until the second half of the eighteenth century. It frequently occurred in the military hospitals of the armies which took part in the Seven Years' War (1756—63). Towards the end of the century gangraena nosocomialis was also prevalent in Dutch military hospitals, particularly in Leyden, Utrecht, Nijmegen, Alkmaar, Den Helder and Woerden. The French surgeon Claude Pouteau (1725—75) of Lyons gave a description of it, probably in 1760, claiming that nobody had written on the subject before.[5] Since we could not get hold of Pouteau's publication, we based our description of the disease primarily on the exemplary, nearly forgotten article of 1814 by the Leyden professor Sebald Justinus Brugmans, who also held the position of Inspector General in the Dutch Army Medical Service.[6] Brugmans reported having seen many such cases during a long succession of years (Fig. 104).

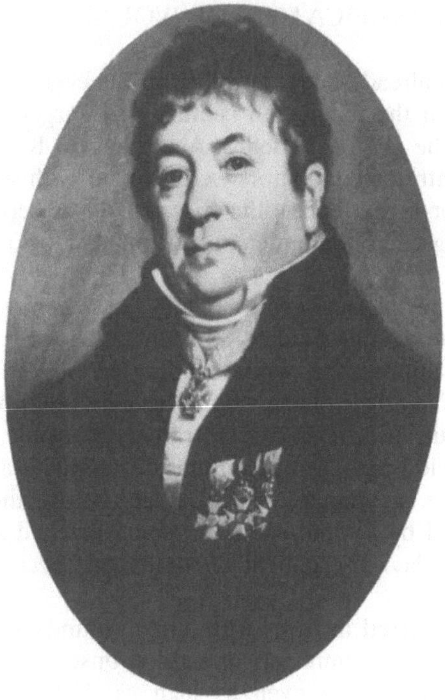

Fig. 104. Professor Sebald Justinus Brugmans.

After a short period of feeling unwell, sometimes for only a few hours, the patient became feverish. His wound which had thus far been producing healthy pus, rapidly changed its appearance. The edges swelled, showing dark red elevations. A short distance away from the wound a dark red ring appeared on the skin, more or less parallel with its contour and steadily widening. The surface of the wound itself began to mortify and necrotic areas sloughed off. Circumference and depth of the defect continuously extended. Connective tissue and muscles melted away, nerves and blood vessels offered the longest resistance. The wound bed changed into a putrid, grubby and discoloured pulp mass. Even bone could not escape the necrotic process. The pus became thin and ichorous, the wound exuded a very characteristic nauseating stench. The disease was usually fatal, although some patients survived; it tended to recur after an apparent recovery.

According to professor Delpech at Montpellier, the process could start in two ways: either through the formation of a white, adherent pseudomembrane which gradually became thicker, or through the formation of peculiar, pointed ulcers all over the surface of the wound which grew rapidly larger and finally coalesced.[7]

Autopsy reports were not present in the works of the contemporary authors which we consulted.

Hospital gangrene was especially prevalent in overcrowded hospitals, prisons and ships. It was highly contagious: the arrival of a patient suffering from the disease on an uncontaminated ward led irrevocably to a general outbreak within one day. In a French military hospital in Leyden the disease ran rampant among the patients on one of the downstairs wards, whereas those in the attic above were not affected. However, shortly after a hole had been sawed in the attic floor to improve ventilation, the wounded on the upper ward also became affected. Brugmans records that the first to be stricken were the ones lying closest to the opening.

Brugmans did not comment on the treatment of patients contaminated with the disease because his publication was primarily concerned with its aetiology. We learn from Delpech that the treatment in the early stages consisted of vinegar dressings, after the possible pseudomembrane had been peeled away. If the wound had already degenerated into the pulp mass mentioned above, the red-hot iron had to be used. It seems that good results were often achieved by the latter method.

There is no modern medical name for hospital gangrene and the microbiological pathogen has remained obscure. It disappeared so rapidly once antiseptic treatment had been introduced, that the still inadequate bacteriological techniques of the last century were unable to identify the infectant before the disease had become extinct. It was apparently last encountered in the Russo-Japanese war. Could it have been a form of wound diphtheria?[8]

In the case of *erysipelas*, which Küster included among the serious wound complications, distinction was made between a surgical form (proceeding fom a wound), and a medical (idiopathic) variant. The latter was thought to have been caused by 'biliary sharpness' of the blood. With the emergence of bacteriology it became clear, however, that erysipelas was an infectious disease, whereby the pathogen always made its entry via a wound. The portal of entry could be very small and due to the fact that the disease had an incubation period of 15—61 hours, it could already have healed up before the appearance of clinical symptoms. The signs and symptoms consisted of a general malaise, while a red swelling developed near the wound and quickly spread in all directions. The illness usually subsided within a few days, but could persist for several weeks. It became dangerous in prolonged cases and in combination with metastatic ulceration. Some few decades after the introduction of antiseptic wound treatment it too became very rare.

8.3. AETIOLOGY OF WOUND DISEASES

8.3.1. *Infection as Understood in the Pre-Microbiological Era*

From days of old a distinction was made between 'epidemic' and 'contagious' diseases. Epidemic diseases, such as the plague and hospital fever — the old name for exanthematous typhus — were caused by contaminated air.[9] The defilement of the air was thought to be due to 'miasmata', mysterious polluting agents which were suspended in it (cf. p. 138).

Conversely, contagious diseases spread via direct or indirect means from person to person, conveyed by unknown contagions which developed in the patient's body. It was not possible for miasmata to spread directly from person to person, but in some cases they could cause diseases which provoked the production of contagions.

Miasmata as well as contagions were infectious. Before the discovery of bacteria, infection of course was not held to be an invasion of the tissues of the body by pathogenetic microorganisms. Yet 'infection' had been a medical concept ever since late Antiquity. Temkin pointed out that the word, derived as it is from the Latin 'infectio', actually means staining or dyeing; staining something in the sense that it becomes tainted or corrupted. Infection is therefore basically a form of pollution. The same is true for the term 'contagion', which indicates pollution by direct contact. Infection, whether by miasms or contagions, would 'stain' the body with diseases, disease regarded as decay and putrescence. Indeed, putrescence became the pattern of pollution and the evil smell it propagated was taken as an indication and guide. The evil smell from sick persons and putrid wounds was supposed to transmit the infection just as the unpleasant odour did hovering over marshes and refuse.[10] Thus, putrid, foul-smelling wound conditions were traditionally thought of as being caused by polluted air. We have met this concept repeatedly in the foregoing pages, beginning with Albucasis, the Arabian surgeon who had such a great influence on Western surgery during the late Middle Ages and the Renaissance. As a consequence, wounds through the ages were packed with lint and covered by several layers of bandageing in an effort at excluding the air.

In what way precisely did air harm the wound? According to Heister, air caused the tiny blood vessels to contract and dry out, inhibiting the growth of flesh.[11] Benjamin Bell, who like Van de Voorde and Richter deemed it expedient to cover the wound with the shortest possible delay, considered the air dangerous 'qua talis'.[12] According to Le Cat, air would induce purulence in the blocked vessels, induration of the wound edges, ulceration and the movement of pus into the blood. Jean-Pierre David (1737—84) from Rouen, the son-in-law of Le Cat, had experience of a case where the initially healthy matter from a loin abscess had turned bad after incision, which change he attributed to the action of air.[13] However, other authors, including De Gorter, did not mention the possibly noxious influence of air on wound healing, which may indicate a rising skepticism.

The Académie royale de Chirurgie finally wanted to know the full facts of the matter and set up a prize competition in 1775. The entry which was awarded gold was by Petrus Camper. His conclusion was that there were no surgical diseases which were influenced directly in a positive or negative manner by air.[14] In particular, the British surgeons shared this opinion. John Bell wondered why air which was essential to life should be so harmful to wounds. Abernethy pointed out that the air in subcutaneous emphysema was usually harmless and that this was also true for air injected intraperitonally in animal experiments. John Hunter argued that the mucous membranes of the nose and urethra produced pus in cases of catarrh and gonorrhoea respectively, without being exposed to the air any more than usual.[15] It nevertheless took some more years before Vincenz von Kern from Vienna, a declared opponent of polypragmatism in wound treatment, introduced in 1810 the so-called 'open treatment' of wounds. This consisted of leaving the wound partly or wholly open and covering it only with a wet compress.[16] Because of the favourable results shown in terms of operative mortality, this method found partisans among German surgeons in particular, Billroth being amongst them.[17] It is not known whether open wound treatment was much practised in Holland.

Most surgeons however, continued to regard air as a menace. This attitude favoured the development of subcutaneous surgery in the 1770s. By making the incision in skin which had been moved laterally, the outside air was prevented from gaining access to the wound cavity once the skin had been returned to its original position (cf. p. 372, n. 82)

Towards the end of the eighteenth century the suspicion was raised by the French chemist Gay Lussac that oxygen, discovered simultaneously by Priestley and Scheele in 1774, was the harmful factor. This led to attempts to neutralize it, for instance with the aid of carbon dioxide. Jules-René Guérin (1801—86), especially famous for his orthopedic work, had a large apparatus installed on the ward at his Institute de la Muette in Passy in 1878 which made it possible to place all the wounds under bell beakers from which the air could be evacuated all at the same time. Etienne-Frédéric Bouisson (1813—84), professor of 'operative medicine' at Montpellier, considered stagnant air to be dangerous and therefore had a strong current of air blown over the wounds.[18]

On the ancient 'contagion' too, although still largely not understood, a more specific theory was being formed in the second half of the eighteenth century: it began to be regarded as a material contaminant ('smetstof'). David van Gesscher from Amsterdam was amongst those who used the word 'smetstoffe' in such a casual way at the beginning of the nineteenth century that we may surmise that it expressed a general notion. Let us now return to Brugmans to see how he tried to fathom out its nature.

8.3.2. *Brugmans on Hospital Gangrene*

The exceptional contagiousness of hospital gangrene was an indication for Brugmans that it was caused by 'a special infectant', a morbific matter, which was spread via direct contact with contaminated patients or objects and through the air. The disease was often limited to one ward of a hospital and therefore could not be due to changes in the composition of atmospheric air.[19] He sought the origin of the infectant in profusely putrefying wounds, in the emanations of certain ulcers, in rotting animal flesh and — probably remembering Pringle[9] — in 'enclosed air in which people live, without it being freshened'.

Using chemical means, Brugmans tried to gain an insight into the precise nature of the pathogenic agent. For this purpose he compared the night air of a ward which accommodated patients without suppurating wounds with that of a ward containing patients with hospital gangrene, using eudiometers. He concluded that there was more carbon dioxide and hydrogen sulphide in the night air where the gangrene patients were than in the 'healthy' air. When these gases had been precipitated out, the characteristic stench of hospital gangrene, however, still remained. This brought Brugmans to the conclusion that in the contaminated air yet another 'special principle must be present, which cannot be demonstrated by chemical means'. In a second series of experiments he showed that pieces of meat placed in contaminated air putrefied more quickly than in pure air. He drew the following conclusion: 'Thus this fine animal material, which gives rise to the peculiar smell of contaminated air, which has a general putrefying capacity and certainly, when present in the atmospheric air, can cause hospital gangrene, seems to be the actual infectant or at least the last and finest transport medium for the infectant'.[20]

In order to prevent the development and spread of such 'smetstoffe', Brugmans considered regular dressing changes and proper general hygiene to be of the utmost importance. Patients with hospital gangrene had to be nursed in isolation, were not to be approached by other wounded men and the nursing orderlies were not allowed to move from the former to the latter group. Dressings coming from these patients had to be burned; clothes, bedclothes and instruments had to be thoroughly cleaned. Surgeons had to be careful not to handle healthy wounds with fingers or instruments which had been in contact with 'impure ulcers'. The air in hospital rooms could be purified by using nitric acid fumes or concentrated hydrochloric acid gas.[21] By removing the stench of putrefaction such fumes would free the air from its nefarious constituent.

Brugmans' views on hospital gangrene in 1814 — including the significance of contaminated hands — bring to mind the observations made by Semmelweis in 1847 on puerperal fever. Neither Brugmans, nor at first Semmelweis, founded any school with the theory of a transmittable agent, in spite of the fact that through a German translation of Brugmans' paper his ideas did become known abroad. In both cases, the source of the deficiency probably lies in a passivity caused by the feeling of impotence against these specific hospital plagues.

8.3.3. *Gynaecological Contributions to the Notion of Contact Infection*

8.3.3.1. Oliver Wendell Holmes

In the second half of the eighteenth century a few English gynaecologists had already voiced the opinion that puerperal fever was a contagious disease and had emphasized the importance of cleanliness in connection with its prevention.[22]

In 1843 Oliver Wendell Holmes (1809—94), a general practitioner in Boston, was the first definitely to establish the contagiousness of puerperal fever.[23] He left the question about the particular mode of infection open: 'whether it be by the atmosphere the physician carries about him into the sick- chamber, or by the direct application of the virus to the absorbing surfaces with which his hand comes into contact'. Holmes urged that physicians who had been in contact with patients suffering from puerperal fever should wash themselves, put on clean clothes and refrain from obstetric work for at least 48 hours.

8.3.3.2. Ignaz Philipp Semmelweis

Holmes' advice met with little response and was not heard at all in Europe where, five years later, a young Hungarian obstetrician, Ignaz Philipp Semmelweis (1818—65), working at the General Hospital in Vienna, recognized that the examining fingers of the accoucheur should be inculpated as the most important transmitter of post partum infections.[24] He conceived the idea after a friend of his had cut his finger at the autopsy of a woman who had died of puerperal fever. The wound became inflamed and the man subsequently perished having shown similar septic signs to those of the diseased lying-in women. Just as a wound caused by a knife contaminated with ptomaine resulted in death from septicaemia, Semmelweis reasoned that the septicaemia which was fatal for so many new mothers resulted from infection with cadaveric poison. This infection would have been introduced into the uterus by the hands of students and assistants who, following the usual practice of the time, conducted their own autopsies on patients who had died on their ward. This reasoning implied that the cavity of the puerperal uterus was a wound and puerperal fever a septic wound disease. The accuracy of this conclusion was proved when the mortality rate due to puerperal fever dropped considerably when hand washing after autopsy was introduced.

8.3.3.3. Puerperal Fever in Amsterdam

Semmelweis' discovery that puerperal fever was a form of pyaemia resulting from direct contact was not accepted right away by everyone. Among those who expressed their adherence to his theory was C. B. Tilanus of Amsterdam.[25] However, when Semmelweis made his discovery public, Tilanus was no longer in charge of obstetrics at the Binnengasthuis, where since 1849, Dr. Leopold Lehmann (1817—80) had been head of the maternity ward. This obstetrician of German extraction was an excellent specialist with a keen scientific interest, but he never attached any credence to Semmelweis' discovery. Even when the favourable results of the introduction of Lister's antiseptic method had become manifest in the surgical department, he stubbornly left things in his own clinic as they were. Due to a serious outbreak of puerperal fever in 1871 and again in 1880—81, the Amsterdam maternity clinic had to be closed for several months. Lehmann died just before bacteriology started its advance. Shortly after his successor introduced antisepsis, puerperal fever was to become a thing of the past at the Binnengasthuis too.[26]

8.4. ANTISEPSIS AND ASEPSIS

The hypothesis of aerogenic infection persisted throughout the whole of the nineteenth century and even today has not entirely been rejected. The introduction of antisepsis by Lister was inspired by his endeavouring to eliminate the harmful influence of air, or rather of the 'floating particles' in it. He based his ideas on the fundamental research of the French chemist Louis Pasteur (1822—95).

8.4.1. *Louis Pasteur* (Fig. 105)

It was already recognized that alcoholic fermentation was caused by living

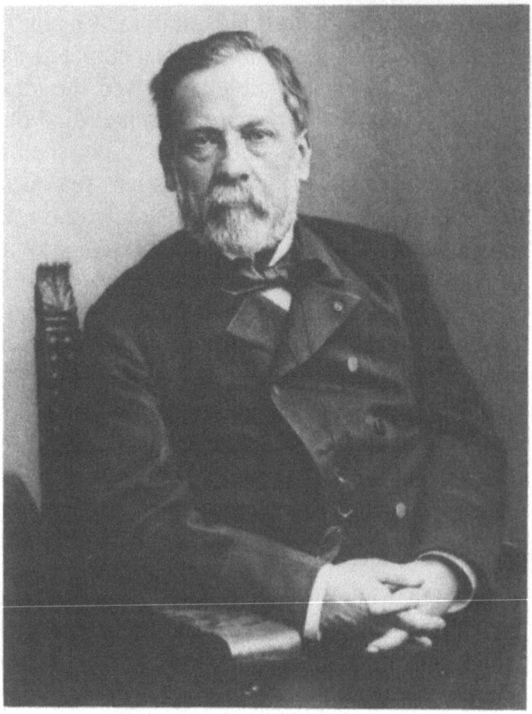

Fig. 105. Louis Pasteur.

micro-organisms, single-celled fungi, when Pasteur showed that unicellular micro-organisms were present in large numbers in sour milk and rancid butter, and that they were not present before putrefaction set in. The next question was whether these cells were the product or the cause of the rotting process. In the former case we would apparently be confronted with spontaneous generation, an Aristotelian biological principle which, remarkably enough, still appeared to have had supporters in the middle of the last century. In a series of ingenious experiments Pasteur proved that these micro-organisms did not originate from rotting material but were introduced from the outside air. If their entry is obstructed, no putrescence occurs.[27] If this work made the concept of spontaneous generation untenable, its consequences were no less important for practical surgery.

8.4.2. *Joseph Lister*

These were the conclusions drawn by Joseph Lister (1827—1912) when he was professor of surgery at Glasgow.[28] In accordance with contemporary belief, Lister at first had held that suppuration was brought about by the influence of the atmosphere as such.

> But when it had been shown by the researches of Pasteur that the septic property of the atmosphere depended, not on the oxygen . . . but on minute organisms suspended in it . . . it occurred to me that decomposition of the injured part might be avoided without excluding the air, by applying as a dressing some material capable of destroying the life of the floating particles'.

To materialize his concept, Lister had to find a suitable antiseptic agent, strong enough to kill 'the minute organisms' without being too noxious for the patient. For this he chose a strong solution of phenol, or carbolic acid as it was called then, since very satisfactory results had been reported from its use in deodorizing the sewage water in the city of Carlisle. As Temkin has pointed out, in the use of disinfectants or antiseptics physicians and surgeons have largely relied on their deodorizing action. Thus Semmelweis prescribed chlorinated lime for the disinfection of hands, guided by its deodorizing effect.[29] On the 12th of August 1866 Lister put his idea into practice. He treated an eleven-year old boy, admitted to the Glasgow Royal Infirmary with a compound fracture of his leg, by covering the wound with lint soaked in carbolic acid and splinting the fracture. The result was most satisfactory. After six weeks the wound had closed without having shown any signs of infection and the fracture had healed.

Lister's antiseptic method basically consisted of promoting healing under a scab without the formation of pus, by preventing 'floating particles' from having access to the wound by means of an occlusive bandage soaked in a fluid chemical compound. He devoted the rest of his life to the perfection of his system. It ultimately resulted in the disinfection of operative and accidental wounds, surgical instruments and the surgeon's hands, and for some time even the air using a spray soon nicknamed 'puffing Billy' (Fig. 106).

Professor Jan Egens van Iterson (1842—1901), successor to Polano at Leyden, visited Lister in 1881 at King's College Hospital in London, on the occasion of the

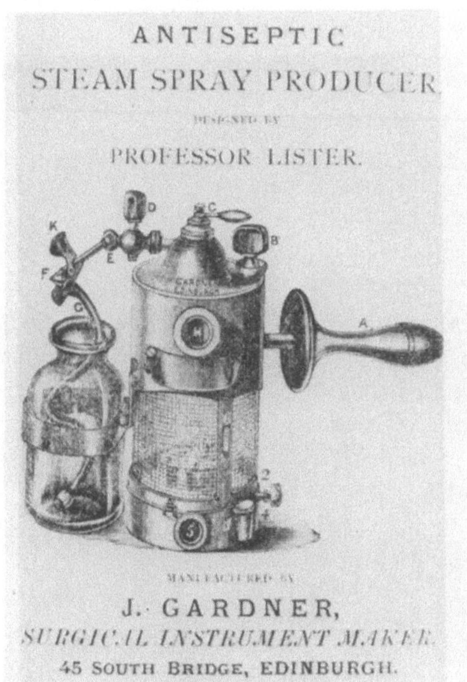

Fig. 106. Lister's carbolic acid spray.

International Medical Congress (Fig. 107). He made the following report of his visit:

When my curiosity had been sufficiently satisfied after touring London for a week, I felt great inclination towards visiting Lister's clinic. There are in King's College Hospital, where he is a surgeon, three wards containing altogether about thirty beds at his disposal. . . . Notwithstanding the intense heat, there was on each ward a fiercely burning fire in an open hearth. Lister felt that this was even more essential in the summer than in the winter for the sake of ventilation. It was not very pleasant. . . .

The carbolic spray was used while changing dressings, but only as long as the wound was *completely* uncovered; the area around the wound was cleansed with a piece of gauze soaked in 2½ per cent carbolic acid solution; the drainage tubes were washed in this solution and only inserted in the wound after the carbolic acid laden steam of the spray had been conducted through the lumen of the tubing. Lister particularly alerted us to this small precautionary detail. I cannot conceal that this measure very much attracted my attention, especially in comparison with the other things I saw and heard. Lister himself diligently took part in the changing of dressings. He and his assistants wore cloth frock coats; I did not see any washing of hands between one dressing and the next (there was blood in his nailfolds). . . . The bandages were applied very loosely. For instance in the case of a femoral amputation fairly high up which had been performed three days before, it seemed to me that it would be very easy to pass the fingers under the dressing to the wound itself.[30]

The science of bacteriology was only in its infancy when Lister introduced his method. Nothing definite was yet known of the micro-organisms that caused wound infections. Even so, the results of Lister's antisepsis were very rewarding: the incidence of wound diseases dropped to a fraction of what it had been before. Yet it took some time before the method was generally accepted. It was not until 1890 for instance, that the value of antiseptic procedures was recognized in America.[31]

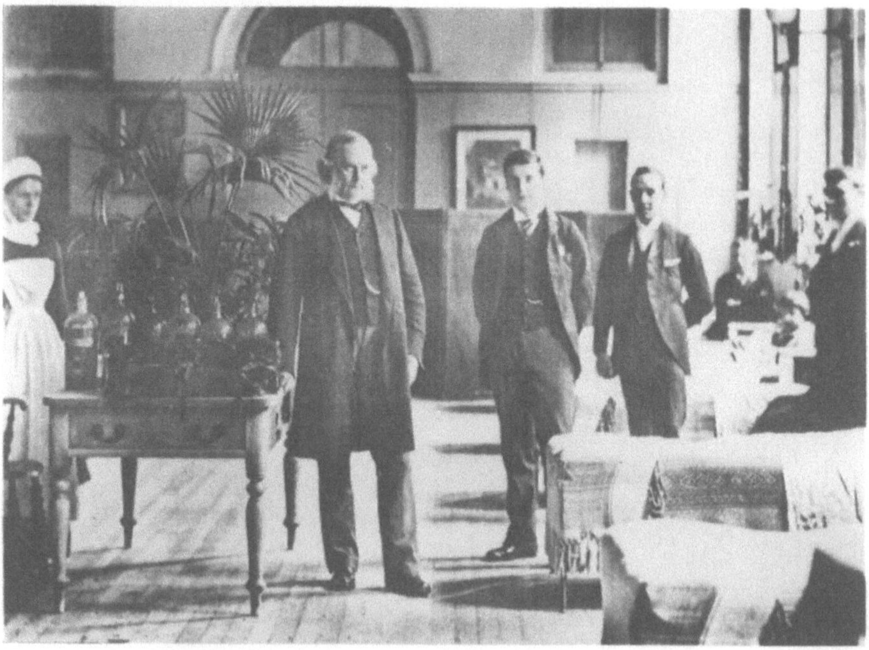

Fig. 107. Joseph Lister in a ward of King's College Hospital.

Lister's antisepsis has gradually evolved into the more modern system of asepsis, in which infection is prevented by physical sterilization — with heat — of all objects that may touch the wound. A system which is quite harmless for the patient and the surgeon, in comparison with antisepsis, which makes use of toxic chemical compounds.[32]

In contrast to Lister's original concept, primarily concerned with the prevention of airborn infections, the system of asepsis stresses the importance of transmission by direct contact. The latter was mainly developed in Germany in the eighties. It was initiated by Viktor von Bruns (1812—83) in Tübingen, who, in an article entitled 'Fort mit dem Spray!', took leave of the puffing machine.[33] In the period of transition from antisepsis to asepsis, sublimate (mercury bichloride) was used for some time as an antiseptic agent. But the smell of carbolic acid remained familiar in hospitals and sanatoria until the Second World War.

8.5. THE INTRODUCTION OF ANTISEPSIS IN THE NETHERLANDS

Neither Pasteur's research, nor Lister's wound treatment that it inspired, at first received much attention in the Netherlands. In the first few years following 1867, we find only a few short references to antisepsis in the *Nederlandsch Tijdschrift voor Geneeskunde*, mainly from German publications. Initially, these were rather unenthusiastic. In 1874, a review appeared in this magazine by the — then retired — Leyden professor Krieger, on the book by Billroth: *Untersuchungen über die Vegetationsformen von Coccobacteria septica und den Anteil, welchen sie an der Entstehen und Verbreitung der accidentellen Wundkrankheiten haben.* The Viennese professor wrote that he was not a follower of Lister's dressing method, but preferred to stick to irrigation treatment of open wounds.

Following a visit to Lister in Edinburgh, professor Carel Lambertus Wurfbain (1837—1904) of Amsterdam, successor of C. B. Tilanus, became the first to use antisepsis according to the rules in the Netherlands in 1874.[34] The results were very spectacular: 'Feared diseases such as erysipelas, suppuration, gangrene (the latter only at the Buiten Gasthuis) were either seldom seen any more or had completely disappeared', remembered J. W. R. Tilanus (Fig. 108).[35]

It appears that Tilanus jr. knew Lister personally fairly well. During the International Congress for Medical Science in Amsterdam in 1879, where Lister read a paper on wound treatment, they could often be seen walking arm in arm along the street. Antisepsis was generally accepted in Holland by this time and Lister received great acclaim at this congress.

It is hard to say when antisepsis was introduced in the Leyden clinic of professor Polano. From a doctoral thesis of 1875, which in fact is a report of that clinic for the academic year 1873—74, it appears that 'Lister's bandage' was already in use. This consisted of lint soaked in carbolic acid 1 per cent which was introduced into the wound. Sometimes the wound cavity was flushed with a carbolic acid solution. There is no reference, however, to any other antiseptic precautions being taken before or during operations. Yet the author stated:

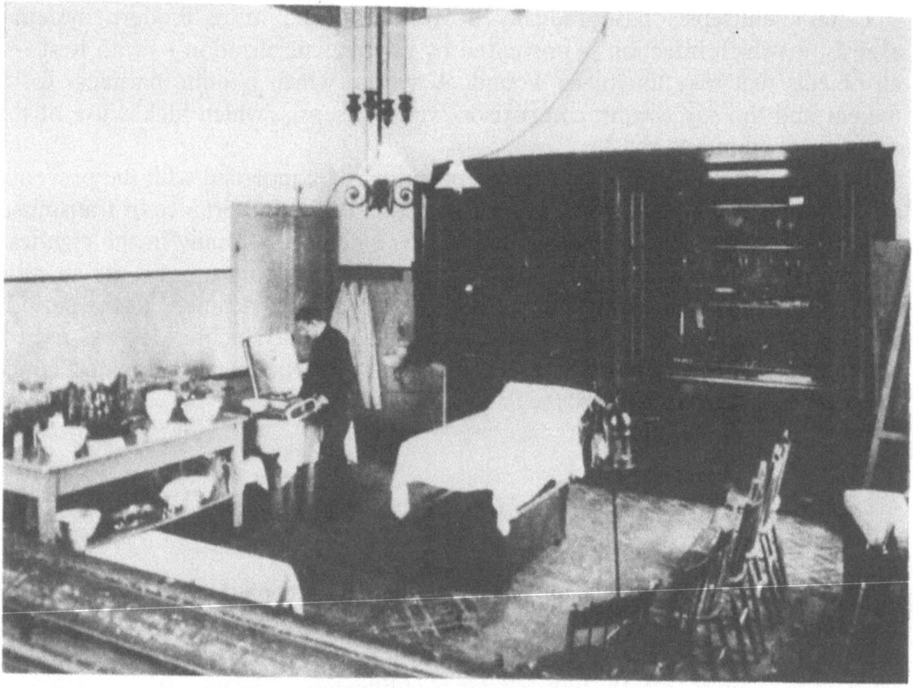

Fig. 108. Operating room Binnengasthuis Hospital Amsterdam, 1897. Lister's antiseptic steam spray apparatus was apparently still in use: it figures on a small occasional table.

'Lister's wound treatment is the best of all the presently known methods of treating wounds'.[36]

In Utrecht the new form of treatment was not initiated until 1876.[37] It is probable that Dr. Johannes Engberts van der Meulen (1848—1941), professor Van Goudoever's assistant, had a decisive influence here: prior to his being engaged at the university surgical clinic in 1874, he had spent a year abroad. In Berlin he had visited Bernard von Langenbeck (1810—87) at his clinic and perhaps heard the memorable lecture by Volkmann at the Third German Surgeons' Congress in April 1874, in which he gave an account of his favourable results using Lister's antiseptic method. He also went to visit Lister in Edinburgh.

The smell of carbolic reached the nostrils of those in Groningen even later. It took until 1878, the year in which Johann Rudolph Ranke (1849—87) was promoted professor. Born in Germany, Ranke was a student of Richard von Volkmann (1830—89) at Halle, one of the first of Lister's followers in that country.[38]

8.6. BACTERIOLOGY

Listerism was found to have a rational explanation when the organisms responsible for causing wound infection had been properly identified, so that it was no longer necessary to describe them merely as 'floating particles'. Bacteriology owes its development to various factors, the most important being the improvement of the microscope through the addition of the achromatic lens system, the introduction of artificial staining and the use of laboratory animals.

The most important pioneer of the new science — besides Louis Pasteur — was Robert Koch (1843—1910). Koch's significance in bacteriology lay not only in the micro-organisms he discovered, such as the spores of anthrax and the bacilli of tuberculosis and cholera, but also and especially in his research of a more fundamental nature (Fig. 109). He came up with proof that bacteria can cause

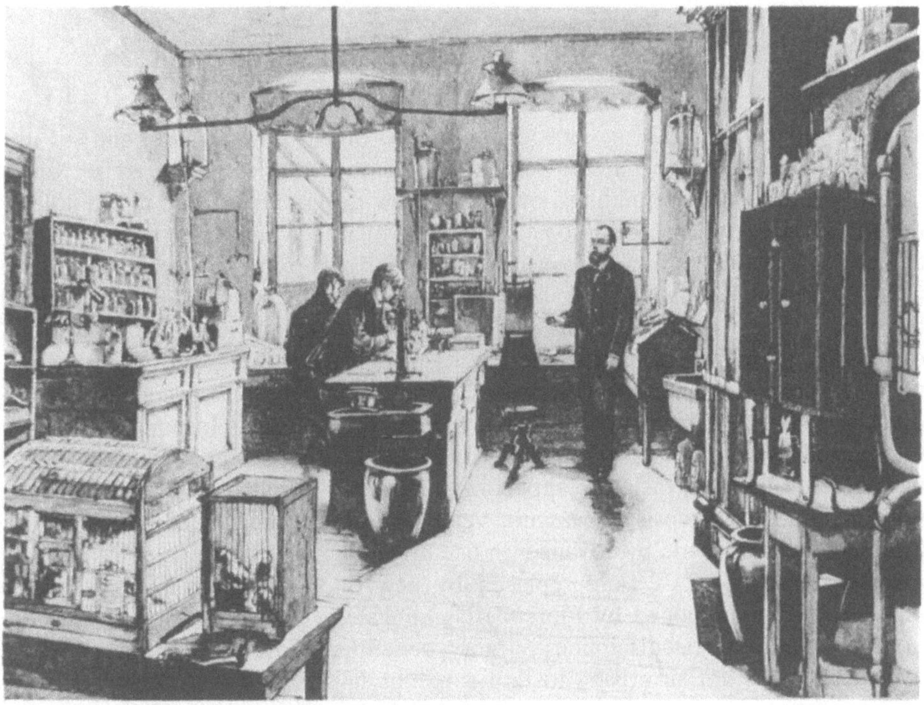

Fig. 109. Robert Koch in his laboratory.

disease and that each and all the various infectious diseases have their own specific pathogens. He also drew up the general conditions which have to be fulfilled before a particular bacteria can be considered as the causative organism. And finally, be was the founding father of bacteriological technique. His finding that instruments can be sterilized with the use of steam was of great relevance for surgery.

Once bacteriology had developed and standardized its methods, the pathogens of one infectious disease after another were found in quick succession. This meant that practical hygiene received a whole new footing. Among those who actively occupied themselves with bacteriological research in the last two decades of the nineteenth century we find quite a number of surgeons, for instance the Viennese professor Billroth to whom we will return on page 308. Staphylococcus pyogenes, the archenemy of surgeons, was discovered by Sir Alexander Ogston (1844—1929), surgeon at the Royal Infirmary in Aberdeen in 1881; streptococcus erysipelatis pyogenes by Friedrich Fehleisen (1854—1924), an assistant at the university surgical clinic in Berlin in 1882. Anton Julius Friedrich Rosenbach (1842—1923), surgical assistant in Göttingen, isolated streptococcus haemolyticus in 1884, classified staphylococcal bacteria into 'albus' or 'aureus' strains and described the development of acute osteomyelitis. Via the science of immunology, bacteriology had made it possible to prevent and cure infectious diseases using sera and vaccines.

8.7. NEW UNIVERSITY CLINICS

The university hospitals — nosocomiums — which towards the end of the eighteenth and at the beginning of the nineteenth centuries had been set up at random in pre-existing buildings, only had a few dozen beds. Since the middle of the last century larger institutions have been founded, far better suited for the demands of clinical tuition and specially built for that purpose. This happened in Groningen in 1852, in Utrecht in 1870 and in Leyden in 1873: they contained between 100 and 150 beds. The building of new hospitals at that time was not only inspired by the teaching commitments of university clinics but was part of a more general phenomenon synchronous with hospital systems gradually untying themselves from their function as care providers for the poor. Hospital buildings at that period, at home and abroad, were constructed on the so-called block plan and had therefore very barrack-like appearances. As they were planned just before the introduction of antisepsis, it was not very long before they failed to satisfy the hygienic demands made by advances in bacteriology. About the turn of the century most of these hospitals were replaced by new ones, often constructed on the pavilion plan championed by Florence Nightingale, which did fulfil such perceptions.[39] Of all clinical disciplines surgery benefitted most by a proper hospital hygiene, so it is not surprising to find surgeons in several countries at that time beginning to take an active interest in the design of hospitals. The university hospitals of Holland, around the turn of the century, were in their turn larger than their immediate predecessors.

8.8. MODERN NURSING

It is not a coincidence that nursing as a modern profession made its synchronous appearance with the developments in hospital construction which took place towards the end of the last century. With the new insight into the importance of hygiene gained from the achievements of bacteriology, new demands arose in the nursing of patients suffering from infectious diseases. The recent advances in operative surgery made possible by the antiseptic system asked for better care for those who had undergone major surgery.

At the time when antisepsis was introduced, there was nothing like an intelligent and competent nursing service in Holland. After the Reformation the religious orders which since the Middle Ages had applied themselves particularly to the care of the sick and the needy, had largely withdrawn from protestant soil: they had been replaced by poorly paid lay attendants, men and women, who did not satisfy even minimal requirements.

In 1844 a 'Society for Nursing' was established which aimed at offering suitable women a training course as sick-nurses. Once again religious congregations — now including Protestant deaconesses — took to nursing. The well-known *Notes on Nursing* (1859) by Florence Nightingale (1820—1910) which in 1862 also appeared in a Dutch translation, was instrumental in establishing the foundations of professional nursing (Fig. 110). The aspirations toward the emancipation of women which began to manifest itself in the second half of the century, contributed to the idea of nursing as a recognized profession with a fitting salary. Towards the end of the 1870s the first vocational training courses opened but it took some little time before the registered nurse became a common phenomenon. It was, for instance, only in 1892 that the first 'cultured nurse' ('beschaafde verpleegster') made her appearance in the university hospital at Utrecht.[40]

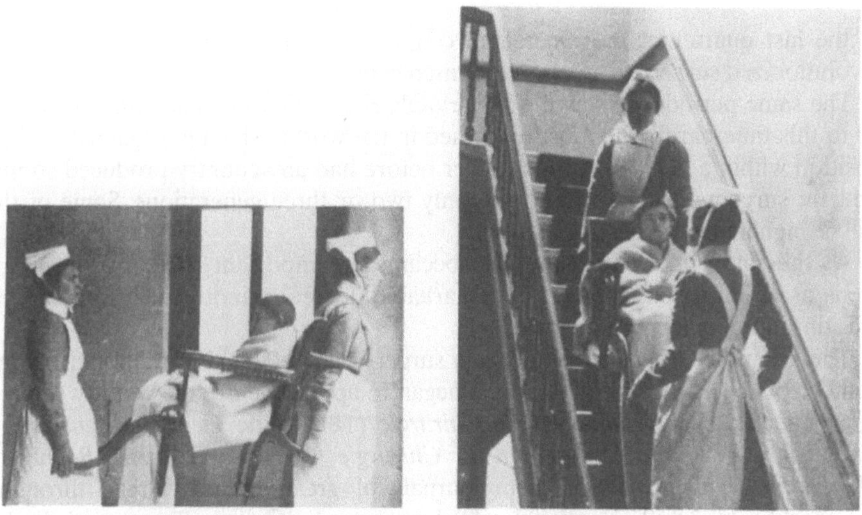

Fig. 110. Trained nurses ('beschaafde verpleegsters') at the beginning of this century.

Trained nurses who were exclusively or mainly employed in the operating theatre first appeared in the early years of the present century, and then only in the larger hospitals.

CHAPTER 9

The German Period in Dutch Surgery

9.1. THE SUPREMACY OF GERMAN–AUSTRIAN SURGERY

In the last quarter of the nineteenth century, anaesthesia, antisepsis and asepsis revolutionized surgery to an unprecedented extent.

The same period also saw the remarkable rise of German and Austrian surgery, up to this time hardly the most renowned in the world, which now gained a leading position within a very short time. Never before had any country produced so many brilliant surgeons within a period of only two or three generations. Some of them will be highlighted below.

At the same time, Germany also became an important name in the political arena as an imperialist power. Its remarkable degree of industrialization earned it the admiration of the whole world.

The scientific expansion of German surgery was reflected in the relatively large number of specialized journals which began to appear before the century went out: Langenbeck's *Archiv für klinische Chirurgie* (1861), the *Deutsche Zeitschrift für Chirurgie* (1872), the *Centralblatt für Chirurgie* (1874), and Bruns' *Beiträge zur klinischen Chirurgie*, all of them journals of great authority, read throughout the world.[1] In 1872, Bernhard von Langenbeck, Gustav Simon and Richard Volkmann founded the 'Deutsche Gesellschaft für Chirurgie', a society which greatly stimulated the growth of surgery in that country.

Asepsis was an important factor in the development of turning operative surgery, up to then a purely individualist trade, into a form of teamwork, requiring the observance of strict rules. The surgical university clinic, with its strict discipline and hierarchical structure, was developed especially in Germany, which in this respect set the example for other countries such as the United States and the Netherlands. The tight organization of surgical training and practice in the German and Austrian clinics must have contributed considerably to the supremacy of German surgery. This, to be sure, does not mean that no great surgeons were to be found in France or in the British Isles.

9.2. FOLLOWING THE GERMAN LEAD

Although a growing interest in German surgery had existed in our country as early as the late eighteenth century, as is evident by the appearance, already signalled above, of Dutch editions of German textbooks, this interest increased to such an extent in the second half of the nineteenth century, that one might well refer to a 'German period' in the history of Dutch surgery. Numerous Dutch surgeons worked in German clinics for shorter or longer periods, and after their return they introduced the organizational structure and working practice of those clinics in their own hospitals. German words found their way into the professional jargon; thus, 'Tupfer' was the commonly used name for a swab. German textbooks, in common use since the end of the previous century, no longer needed to be translated, as all Dutch physicians now had a good command of the German language. The annual congress of the Deutsche Gesellschaft für Chirurgie was visited by an ever-increasing number of Dutchmen. In fact, it was not only surgery which was heavily orientated towards Germany and Austria: the same was true for medical science as a whole, including the basic sciences and laboratory practice. This influence was to last until the Second World War. During all this time, chairs at Dutch universities were often held by Germans and Austrians, but Holland was by no means exceptional in this respect.

The appointment of Ranke to the chair at Groningen in 1878 meant an extension of the surgical school of Volkmann in the Netherlands; that of Adalbert Salzer (1858—93) at Utrecht in 1890 marked the appearance of the school of Billroth. Both found themselves in clearly outdated clinics, with little surgical activity. Operating theatres fell far short of requirements in the era of antisepsis. Nursing staff was traditionally made up of domestic servants with little or no training. When Ranke accepted the professorship, he found in his entire 57-bed clinic only one patient who had undergone an operation. In his ten years of work at Groningen, Ranke increased the number of operations to about 250 a year, including a relatively large number of amputations, joint resections and mastectomies.[2] At the Utrecht clinic, the first herniotomy for a non-strangulated hernia was performed in 1891. Appendectomy and major gastrointestinal surgery were soon to follow. The number of patients, outpatients as well as inpatients, increased rapidly. Salzer, however, apparently a man with a deep sense of responsibility, could not endure for long the heavy pressure under which he had to work in the primitive circumstances at Utrecht. In 1893, as he was staying in Dresden on his way to Austria, he took his own life.[3]

Salzer was succeeded at first by Anton von Eiselsberg (1860—1939), then by Albert Narath (1864—1924). Like Salzer, both were pupils of Billroth. Eiselsberg stayed in Utrecht for three years (1893—96), Narath for ten years (1896—1906). The three of them left an Austrian mark on the Utrecht clinic, which was to remain in evidence for a long time after they had left. At Amsterdam, the Swiss surgeon Otto Lanz (1865—1935), a pupil of Kocher of Bern, was appointed professor of surgery alongside Rotgans in 1902. Lanz was familiar with modern bacteriology, and it was at his clinic that antisepsis was replaced by asepsis. He should also be credited with the introduction of modern thyroid surgery in this country. However, he shied away from major abdominal surgery. Lanz was a tidy surgeon, who liked to leave fine scars: 'The surgeon's handwriting must be neat!' He was an inspired teacher, who spiced his lectures with anecdotes and references to current affairs. It is said of him that he never missed a lecture. He has been called 'the greatest antiquarian among surgeons, and the greatest surgeon among antiquarians'. This referred to his large collection of fine art and antiques.

The German influence was not only noticeable at Groningen, Utrecht and Amsterdam, but throughout the country.

On February 9, 1902, a Dutch surgical society was founded, following the example of the 'Deutsche Gesellschaft für Chirurgie'.[4] Its objective was to hold meetings at which papers and demonstrations 'concerning surgery in the widest sense of the word' could be presented. Founding members of the society were 36 surgeons, from all over the country, but predominantly from the West. First president was professor Rotgans of Amsterdam.[5] The old Athenaeum Illustre in that city had been raised to the status of university in 1876, and in 1900 Rotgans had been provided with a splendid, large operating theatre-*cum*-lecture room at the Binnengasthuis (Fig. 111). It was in this theatre that the first ordinary meeting of the society was held, and it was to return there many times afterwards.

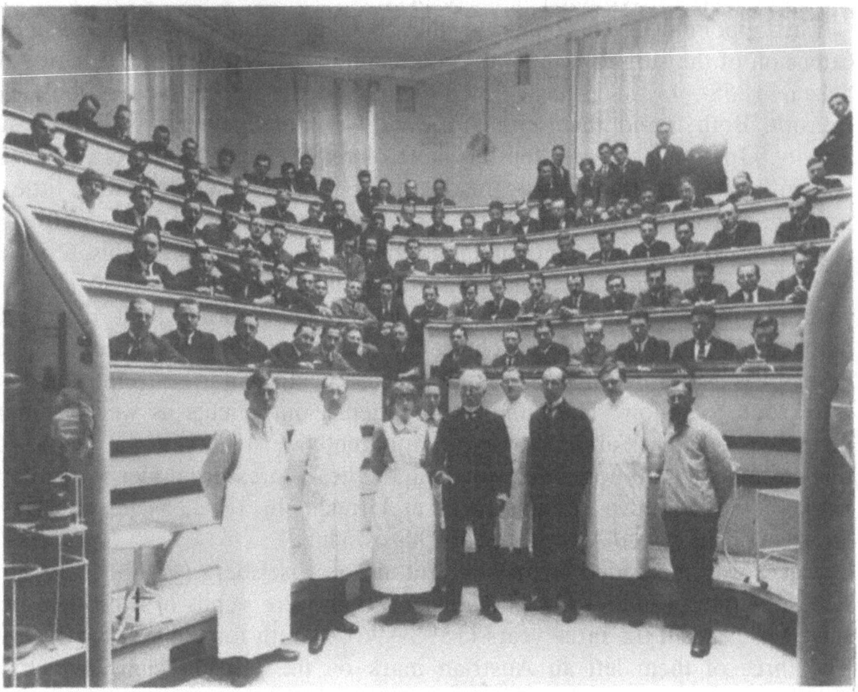

Fig. 111. Professor J. Rotgans in his new theatre cum lecture room. Binnengasthuis Hospital Amsterdam, 1901.

One may well ask why such a society was not founded earlier: not only Germany, but also France and England already possessed surgical associations. Various other scientific societies were in existence in this country, including the 'Amsterdamsch Genootschap tot Bevordering der Natuur-, Genees- en Heelkunde'

(Amsterdam Society for the Advancement of Physics, Medicine and Surgery, see p. 181). The question cannot be answered with certainty, perhaps surgeons felt that the local and national meetings of the Dutch Medical Association sufficiently met their needs. Moreover the number of Dutch physicians applying themselves exclusively to surgery was still limited in the last decades of the nineteenth century. Young Jan Schoemaker, however, who appears to have been foremost among the founder members, had visited Germany several times. In addition, Schoemaker, based from 1898 to 1902 at the provincial town of Nijmegen, must have felt the absence of stimulating contacts with colleagues there. His father, also a surgeon, had visited the meetings of the Deutsche Gesellschaft in his days: he even read a paper at one of them, in 1876. Schoemaker himself will be discussed in more detail on page 331.

9.3. THE GROWTH OF SURGERY AS A MODERN SPECIALITY IN THE NETHERLANDS[6]

One of the changes resulting from the laws on the practice of medicine (wetten betreffende de uitoefening der geneeskunde), drawn up by the liberal minister Thorbecke of Interior Affairs, and passed by Parliament in 1865, was that an end was put to the separate, non-academic professional training of surgeons, and hence in the long run to the difference in social and scientific status between physicians and surgeons. Those old-style surgeons still practising their trade were allowed to continue this practice. But this unity within the medical profession, which had been so ardently sought, was not to last for long. New developments in medicine, triggered by scientific materialism, rapidly led to a situation in which a physician could no longer know and practise the full range of medicine, surgery and obstetrics.

It was not long before a number of doctors began to specialize in one of the three major branches of medicine. In the beginning, there was no organized training for specialists in any of these three areas; candidates served an assistantship for a few years at a hospital in Holland or abroad. Abroad usually meant Germany. It then depended on the inclination and temperament of the individual doctor whether he would go on to practise surgery exclusively, as a 'professional surgeon', or whether he would perform surgical operations within the context of general medicine.[7] Thus Jan Schoemaker, the greatest Dutch surgeon of the period 1900—40, was for two years an assistant at the Elisabeth Gasthuis in Haarlem, under Benjamin Jan Kouwer (1861—1933), later professor of obstetrics and gynaecology at Utrecht, before settling as a surgeon and gynaecologist in Nijmegen, at the small but modern Wilhelmina Ziekenhuis. Until the Second World War and even afterwards, surgery was not rarely combined with gynaecology in a so-called 'double-specialty'. There were even skillful surgeons who had never held assistantships. It was only at the university hospitals and a few other, usually large hospitals, that one could find specialized surgeons around the turn of the century.[8] Until 1931, any physician had the right to practise surgery.

9.4. OPERATIVE SURGERY

We shall now outline — albeit very broadly — the revolutionary developments in operative surgery after the 1880's: no more than a few of the most important related names can be mentioned.

9.4.1. *Abdominal Surgery*

9.4.1.1. Gastrointestinal Surgery

Anaesthesia and asepsis enabled surgeons in the 1880s to open up the abdominal cavity in order to remove, partly or wholly, one diseased organ after the other: operative surgery was largely dominated by *extirpation.*

A major problem in gastrointestinal surgery — and one which, mutatis mutandis, crops up in connection with all tubular structures in the body — is finding a reliable method of closing a partial injury to the intestinal wall, or, in the case of a complete transection, even of reuniting the two ends of the intestine.

From ancient times onwards, until the end of the eighteenth century, one finds descriptions of four possible methods of repairing an incised or transected intestine: simple suture (Celsus, cf. p. 14); suturing over an endoprosthesis (Four Masters, cf. p. 40); bringing about an adhesion between the injured intestine and the inner lining of the abdominal wall (Palfijn, De La Peyronie, Le Dran, Bell); and, in the case of a completely transected intestine, invagination (Ramdohr, cf. p. 241).

The inverting suture, in which the intestinal wall is turned slightly inward on both sides of the injury, after which a suture is made between the two outer surfaces without entering the lumen of the organ, a method proposed in 1826 by Antoine Lembert (1802—51), eventually became the basis of modern gastro-intestinal surgery. It was performed — successfully — for the first time ten years later, by Dieffenbach at Berlin, after a resection of an injured segment of the small intestine. Almost all later suturing techniques were based on the same principle.

The development of gastrointestinal surgery owes a great deal to Theodor Billroth (1829—94) of Vienna, and his school.[9] In 1881, Billroth performed the first successful gastric resection, after experimental studies in dogs at his clinic, had shown it to be practicable. The operation amounted to not much more than a pylorectomy. The stomach was anastomosed with the duodenum using the method we now know as the Billroth I resection. It was also at his clinic that the anterior and posterior gastroenterostomies were developed; in 1885 a combination of pylorectomy and gastroenterostomy resulted in the operation now known as Billroth II, although it was described by his pupil Viktor von Hacker. The latter method is also named after Pólya.

Billroth was perhaps the most important representative of Austrian surgery at the end of the nineteenth century (Fig. 112). He was immensely creative, and had the gift of turning his wealth of ideas into surgical actions. In addition to his clinical activities, he also made a great name for himself as a pathologist and bacteriologist. Of his numerous pupils, many were to occupy important professorial

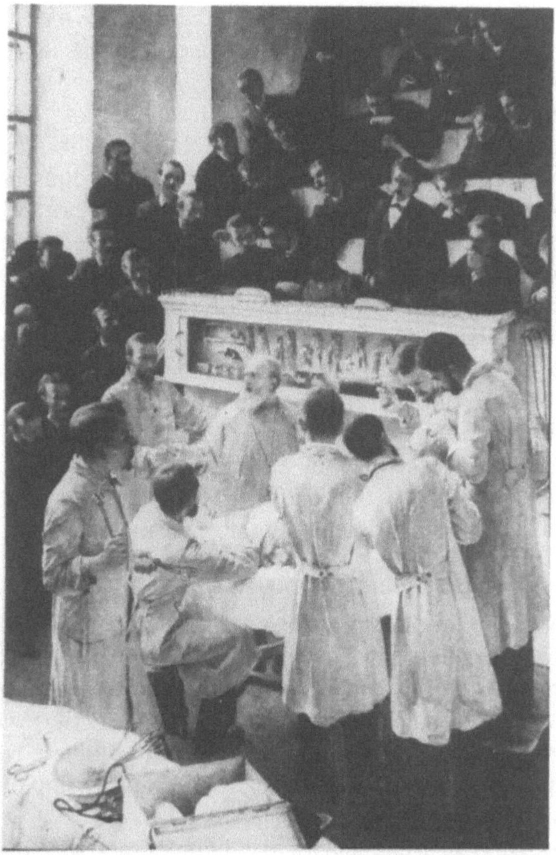

Fig. 112. Professor Billroth at the operation table, 1890. Among his assistants are two future Utrecht professors: Salzer (fourth from the right) and Von Eiselsberg (second from the right).

positions, both inside and outside German speaking countries including, as we have seen, the chair at Utrecht.

Gastric surgery in the Netherlands saw a relatively rapid development too. One year after Billroth had performed his first pyloric resection, Lambertus Theodorus van Kleef (1846—1928) successfully performed a similar operation at Maastricht. Where Carl Schlatter (1864—1934) of Zürich was the first to perform a complete gastric resection in 1897, professor Rotgans followed suit within a year at the Binnengasthuis at Amsterdam, where he performed the same operation, also successfully. Rotgans' patient was a 22-year old woman, who had been vomiting for seven years, and who on the day before the operation weighed no more than 23.7 kilogrammes. The stomach was removed in its entirety, in an operation lasting two hours and four minutes. The oesophagus had to be held as tightly as possible between the thumbs and forefingers of both hands of the assistant to prevent it from slipping upwards. The stomach was found to have been completely obstructed by a 'process of inflammation'. Eight months afterwards, the woman was found to be in good condition. Her digestion was normal, and she now weighed 37.4 kilogrammes.[10]

An important Dutch contribution to the treatment of peritonitis was gastric suction, introduced by Westerman in 1911.[11] Intestinal resections, among which particularly those of the large intestine were very hazardous because of the high degree of bacterial contamination of the contents, did not become widely used until the 1890s. As late as 1914, René Leriche included colectomy, as well as gastric resection, in 'la haute école du moment'.[12] Apart from a few successful colon resections performed in the pre-listerian era, the development of intestinal resection was also largely done by the Billroth school. At the end of the 1870s, colon resections for carcinoma were followed by resections of the small intestine because of necrosis resulting from strangulation: initially in that case the sutured segment was left temporarily outside the abdominal cavity. When in 1883 Vincenz Czerny (1842—1916) succeeded in extirpating the rectum using a combined abdominoperineal approach, the entire gastrointestinal tract, except for the oesophagus, had become accessible to operative treatment.

9.4.1.2. Surgery of the Gallbladder

At least as early as the fourteenth century, gallstones were found from time to time at autopsies, and Vesalius gave a clear description of them. In 1584, Johann Schenk von Grafenberg (1530—98), town physician at Freiburg in Breisgau, gave a clinical account of cholelithiasis in his famous *Observationum medicarum rararum, novarum, admirabilium et monstrosarum volumen*, regarded by Haeser as the most important collection of clinical observations since Hippocrates, and a book which saw some ten editions.[13]

Father of the surgical treatment of the biliary tract was Jean-Louis Petit, the French surgeon whom we have met several times before. In an interesting article, still worthy of perusal, which deals with acute distension of the gallbladder, Petit stated that this condition is usually brought about by stones impacted in the neck, just as acute distension of the urinary bladder may be engendered by calculus.[14] He explained how a dilated gallbladder could be differentiated from a liver abscess. The treatment of choice usually consisted of cholecystotomy, with a view of either evacuating any concretions present or diluting inspissated bile by injections of water, should this be found to be the cause of the occlusion. Some instructive case histories enliven the text. One of these concerns a man suffering from upper abdominal pains, who passed light stools and dark urine, while gradually taking on a saffron appearance. This may well be the first description of obstructive jaundice. In autopsies of patients who had suffered from gallbladder disease, Petit had found internal fistulae more than once.

In 1859 the German-born British physician Johann Ludwig Wilhelm Thudichum (1829—1901) proposed, where gallstones were suspected, to make a small abdominal incision above the lower edge of the liver, just large enough to allow the exploring forefinger into the peritoneal cavity. Should calculi be present, then the gallbladder was to be seized with a small hook, pulled out through the abdominal wound, and fixed there with a few stitches without being opened. After a week or so it could then be incised without the risk of fluid being spilled into the abdominal cavity. It was not until 1878 that this two-stage procedure was put into practice by several surgeons at about the same time.[15]

Carl Johann August Langenbuch (1846—1901), surgeon at the Lazarus Hospital in Berlin, was the first, in 1882, to remove the gallbladder of a patient suffering from severe colic.[16] He correctly assumed that gallstones were formed in a diseased gallbladder, so that cholecystectomy would be the only truly curative method of treatment. At first the operation met with opposition, from English-speaking countries in particular. But within a few years it was generally accepted as the procedure of choice for cholelithiasis. In 1915, Hans Kehr (1862—1916) at Berlin claimed to have performed personally more than 2600 cholecystectomies in 25 years. He greatly contributed to the operating technique, for instance by introducing the T-tube.

Meanwhile, in 1890, the Swiss surgeon Ludwig Georg Courvoisier (1843—1918) had demonstrated the feasibility of choledochotomy. The introduction of roentgenological cholecystography by Evarts Ambrose Graham (1883—1957) and Warren Henry Cole in 1924 meant a major diagnostic breakthrough. Although the first choledochoscope was constructed as early as 1923, this diagnostic tool only recently came into general use.

9.4.1.3. Appendectomy

The history of appendicitis, the most frequent acute abdominal disease in the Western World, started in the eighteenth and early nineteenth century, when a number of cases of acute inflammation with suppuration in the right iliac fossa were described.[17] Most physicians agreed with Morgagni that the inflammation originated in the retrocoecal connective tissue or in the psoas muscle. This view gave rise to the designation 'perityphlitis', probably coined by Gottfried Goldbeck in his academic thesis, submitted at Giessen in 1830. This unfortunate term, still widely in use in the early years of the present century, was largely responsible for keeping erroneous views alive.

The practical possibility of performing laparotomies, resulting from the introduction of anaesthesia and antisepsis, once more stimulated interest in the actual cause of inflammation in the right iliac fossa, and as a consequence of the growing number of abdominal operations in the 1880s, the true nature of the disease ultimately began to emerge clearly. The first to perform a successful appendectomy was probably Robert Lawson Tait (1845—99) at Edinburgh in 1880. His patient was a girl aged seventeen, suffering from a characteristic swelling in the right lower abdomen. After evacuation of the abscess, the appendix was encountered on its floor; it was inflamed and gangrenous. The surgeon therefore snipped it off, inverted the stump into the cavity of the caecum, and stitched the inverted peritoneal surfaces together with fine silk.

In the early 1880s, surgical intervention was still considered to be indicated only when the peri-appendicular abscess appeared. The disastrous consequences of this policy of procrastination were demonstrated in 1886 by Reginald Heber Fitz (1843—1913), a Harvard professor of pathology. He calculated that as many as 35 per cent of the patients treated by this conservative method died of acute peritonitis, and recommended removal of the appendix at an early stage. It was

Fitz who introduced the term 'appendicitis'. Before long, his advice was taken over by most American surgeons. Ever since, clinical diagnosis and surgical treatment have been developed predominantly in the United States; the names of Charles McBurney, John B. Murphy and Albert J. Ochsner in particular are linked with this evolution.

In Europe, however, most surgeons continued to take a conservative view, operating only when a mass had developed or after the acute signs had subsided. Although the British king Edward VII, who was operated upon in 1902 only after a painful swelling had appeared, made an uneventful recovery, his case greatly influenced the acceptance of early operation as the method of choice.

For years, appendicitis occupied an important place in the reports of the Dutch Surgical Society. In this country, too, operative intervention was only undertaken when the acute signs and symptoms had subsided after recurrent attacks with a favourable outcome. If an abscess developed, it was opened.

Among those who have occupied themselves with this problem in particular, the first name to be mentioned is that of Otto Lanz of Amsterdam. His achievements in the diagnostics and treatment of appendicitis include the indication of a spot on the lower right abdomen where the location of the appendix is to be sought on external examination, and advocating timely operation when most surgeons still preferred to await developments.[18]

Apart from the matter of the best time for an appendectomy, the Surgical Society also debated whether a chronic form of appendicitis existed or not.

9.4.1.4. Herniae

A milestone in the anatomical exploration of herniae was the book *Recherches sur les causes et l'anatomie des hernies abdominales* (1819) by Jules-Germain Cloquet (1790—1883). On the title page we find a quotation from Friedrich Hoffmann, printed as a motto: 'Ars medica tota in observationibus'.[19]

The introduction of antisepsis meant a fundamental change in hernia therapy as well. At the German Surgical Congress in 1878, Pauly of Posen reported the case of a female patient with an inguinal hernia dangling halfway down her thigh. Pauly dissected out the hernial sac, opened it to make sure it was empty, and ligated the neck of the sac with catgut. After extirpating the sac, he closed the hernial ring with a few catgut sutures. Despite the application of an antiseptic dressing, some suppuration occurred, but in the end the wound healed completely. The hernial sac, which could contain 700 grammes of water, was brought along by the lecturer as a rare trophy.[20] Thus the hernial sac extirpation proposed by Celsus eighteen centuries before, but rarely performed since then, was reintroduced.

From the 1870s onward, the closing of the hernial orifice was adopted as a new basic principle. At first, however, the results of the new 'radical operation' were far from satisfactory, as it showed a very high rate of recurrence. This was the reason why from 1889 onwards William S. Halsted (1852—1922), the famous professor at Johns Hopkins University, Baltimore, took the view that in indirect hernia, after resection of the hernial sac, a new internal abdominal ring should be constructed, which 'should fit the cord as snugly as possible'. In order to do this, Halsted cut through the aponeurosis of the external oblique muscle, the internal oblique and transversalis muscles and the transversalis fascia. The spermatic cord was isolated, the hernial sac excised after closure of the neck and the different layers which constituted the inguinal canal, were all in one sutured to Poupart's ligament, posterior to the cord. In this way the spermatic cord was made extra-aponeurotic and subcutaneous.[21]

At about the same time the Italian Eduardo Bassini (1844—1924) presented his epoch-making paper on hernia. As an ardent patriot young Bassini, after having completed his medical studies, took part as a common soldier in the Risorgimento, the war of liberation that eventually led to a united Italy. In a hand-to-hand combat during the siege of Rome in 1870, a papal Zouave dealt him a bayonet wound in the groin, and a fecal fistula developed, which took a long time to heal. It can hardly have been a mere coincidence that, ever after, he displayed a special concern precisely for the topographical anatomy of the inguinal region. Bassini was one of the first in Italy to introduce the antiseptic treatment of wounds. In 1882 he became a professor, first of surgical pathology and later of clinical surgery, at the ancient university of Padua. In his search for an anatomically reliable operation for inguinal hernia, Bassini proceeded from the observation that in large indirect hernias the internal ring is shifted in a medial direction, as a result of which the inguinal canal loses its diagonal course. After resection of the hernial sac, therefore, the inguinal canal must be reconstructed in such a way that it assumes its normal oblique direction again, for the inguinal canal closes as a result of the rear wall being pressed against the anterior wall by the intra-abdominal pressure. The method he used in trying to carry out this principle need not concern us here: 'Bassini's operation' is known far and wide. There have been no essential improvements in the surgical technique or the operative results after Bassini.

Bassini's operation became known outside Italy in 1890, when his pioneering paper *Nuovo metodo per la cura radicale dell' ernia inguinale* (1889) appeared in a German translation, published in the *Archiv für klinische Chirurgie*. Shortly afterwards, Bassini's method was accepted by surgeons all over the world, including those in the Netherlands.

It was especially with the hernia operation that Dutch operative surgery entered the era of antisepsis. The first modern hernia operation for a non-strangulated hernia was performed on February 11th, 1891, at Utrecht, where Salzer had been appointed professor the year before. Soon, more of these operations followed, and in 1900 Van der Minne in his dissertation was able to report on a postoperative study of 212 patients who had undergone an operation for inguinal hernia at Utrecht between the years of 1891 and 1900. All these operations had been performed by the professors themselves, an indication of the weight then attached to this operation. Among the methods used, Bassini's was greatly preferred. For all the antiseptic precautions taken, unmistakable wound infection was found to occur in 14.2 per cent of the cases.[22] Seven years later, professor Laméris calculated that the percentage of infections after an operation for inguinal hernia in the same clinic was 6 per cent.[23] Laméris, incidentally, for a long time held that in a direct inguinal hernia no operation was necessary, and that in the indirect operation torsion and resection of the hernial sac sufficed.

9.4.2. *Skull and Brain*

At the dawn of our understanding of cerebral localization, at about the middle of the last century, anaesthesia and asepsis seemed most promising for the further development of brain surgery, which up to that time had been largely limited to the evacuation of blood or pus.

A survey of the Surgeon General's Index Catalogue for the years 1886 to 1896 revealed the amazing fact that during the 10 years period immediately following the successful removal of a brain tumor by Horsley, more than 500 different general surgeons reported operations performed upon the brain! The fact that in the next 10 years, from 1896 to 1906, the number of surgeons reporting cases had fallen to less than 80 reflected discouragement and a beginning of return to sanity.[24]

The problems facing the early brain surgeons lay in the sphere of diagnosis, for which they had to rely entirely on the internist or the neurologist, as well as in that of the operation itself, in which haemostasis usually presented a major difficulty.

It is largely the achievement of the school of Harvey Cushing (1869—1939) at Baltimore, afterwards at Boston, that neurosurgery became an independent specialty. Cushing not only introduced numerous technical refinements — including the silver clip method of haemostasis — he was also a competent pathologist, who made many important contributions in the field of brain tumours. In the Netherlands, the modern neurological examination methods of ventriculography and encephalography were applied for the first time by Hendrik Jan Boevé (1884—1978), surgeon at Rotterdam. In order to acquire the necessary technique, Boevé spent some time with Cushing and with Walter Dandy (1886—1946) in 1916.

Before the time when neurosurgery had established itself as an independent specialty, the proceedings of the 'Nederlandsche Vereeniging voor Heelkunde' often reported on brain surgery performed by general surgeons. This included a case of drainage of a hydrocephalus through the vertebrae, forwards into the retroperitoneal fibrous tissue, performed in 1909; the extirpation of a ganglion Gasseri while leaving the motor radix intact, and of an acoustic nerve tumour in 1916; and the removal of a pituitary tumour after reflecting the nose upwards.

9.4.3. *Thoracic Surgery*[25]

While antisepsis and anaesthetics had made it possible to enter the abdominal and skull cavities, in opening the thoracic cavity there was still the problem how this could be done without the lung collapsing under atmospheric pressure. In 1904, young Ernst Ferdinand Sauerbruch (1875—1951), at that time assistant at the Breslau clinic of professor Johannes von Mikulicz, had designed a negative pressure chamber, which helped to solve this problem.[26] Yet the surgical treatment of pulmonary diseases — abscesses, caverns, echinococcus, neoplasms — had started some ten years before this. An important name in this connection is that of Théodore Tuffier (1857—1929), who worked at the Hôpital de la Cité du Midi in Paris. At the end of the century, Tuffier was able to quote from the literature 306 such cases, with a mortality rate of 29 per cent. Operations were undertaken most frequently in cases of echinococcus, abscesses and gangrene.

Tuffier himself successfully performed the first apex resection for tuberculosis.[27]

At about the same time, in 1895, Sir William MacEwen (1848—1924) undertook a pulmonary resection for tuberculosis at the Royal Infirmary at Glasgow. His patient was still alive in 1940.

During the entire nineteenth century and the first half of the twentieth, tuberculosis was very common. Therapy was basically conservative. Any surgical treatment of pulmonary tuberculosis was still largely indirect, consisting of drainage of empyemata and the collapsing of the cavernous lung. For the latter purpose, Carlo Forlanini (1847—1918) of Turin had introduced the artificial pneumothorax in 1888. Other methods serving the same aim were inversion thoracoplasty, a technique developed largely by Ludolph Brauer (1865—1951), Paul Leopold Friedrich (1864—1916), Sauerbruch and others, in which up to ten or eleven ribs are resected, pleuropneumolysis and — somewhat later — sectioning the phrenic nerve.[28] Thomas Mann's well-known novel *Der Zauberberg* (The magic mountain) gives a lively impression of diagnosis and therapy — both conservative and operative — of pulmonary tuberculosis in a Swiss sanatorium shortly before the First World War. Surgical treatment there consisted of costal resection, an operation in which, as lung specialist Behrens relates, formerly fifty per cent of the patients used to die on the operating table. But even now, he says, it sometimes happens that he can leave off early, 'mortis causa'.[29]

Direct operations in thoracic organs were very rarely reported before World War I, but they already included some cases of lobectomy. In Dutch pre-war literature, only a few reports on thoracic surgery can be found. Thus Westerman of Haarlem, a well-known figure during the first two decades of the century, sutured a wound of the heart in 1900, four years after Ludwig Rehn of Frankfurt-on-Main had successfully performed such an operation for the first time. Westerman's attempt failed, but in 1909 Schoemaker achieved a complete success with the same operation. In 1903 Westerman performed a low, intrathoracic, transpleural oesophageal resection for carcinoma, without the benefit of insufflation anaesthesia, although the patient was given oxygen. He made the anastomosis using Murphy's button. The patient appeared to have survived the operation in good condition, but died the same night in great respiratory distress. At autopsy the cause of death was found to be pneumothorax; the anastomosis was intact.[30]

Zaayer of Leyden, a man full of original ideas, whom we shall meet again in the next chapter, also moved into the field of thoracic surgery before the war. He constructed a simple insufflation apparatus for administering nitrous oxide anaesthesia, with the help of which he performed a thoracic wall resection in a case of recurrent breast cancer. Before applying insufflation anaesthesia to human beings, he had performed eight transpleural oesophageal operations in dogs: one intrathoracic resection and seven cardia resections. Five of the animals died, but in no case was their death caused by insufficiency of the suture. Zaayer had made the anastomosis in two layers by means of interrupted sutures. It was a surprise to him that this type of suture turned out to be usable, as Sauerbruch had rejected it in these cases.[31]

9.4.4. *Cancer of the Breast*

Around the middle of the last century there were important developments in the study of malignant tumours. With the aid of the microscope, researchers began to understand the epithelial origin of the carcinoma, and to distinguish various types on the basis of their histological characteristics. The old distinction between scirrhus and cancer was abandoned.

By the middle of the nineteenth century there was no standardized treatment of breast cancer. Some surgeons only removed the lump; others cut out the segment of the breast in which the tumour was situated, or began with excision of the central mass and removed successive portions of doubtful soundness afterwards; still others amputated the entire breast. In 1867, Charles Hewitt Moore (1821—70), surgeon at the Middlesex and St. Luke's Hospitals in London, urged that the breast should be taken away, along with the pectoral muscles and the axillary glands en bloc.[32]

The methods for the surgical treatment of mammary carcinoma proposed since the 1870s illustrate the gradual application of the requirements formulated by Moore. Partial or complete mastectomy, whether or not including removal of the pectoral fascia and enlarged axillary glands, was followed by complete mastectomy and axillary clearance, including removal of a smaller or larger part of the pectoral muscle. Finally, in 1890, Halsted of Baltimore conceived the radical mastectomy which was to become the standard method of surgical treatment of mammary cancer for the next three quarters of a century.

After the turn of the century, Dutch surgeons did not yield in their operative skills to their colleagues abroad. In 1910, Westerman reported on three very extensive operations in cases of recurrent breast cancer. In one instance he had exarticulated the arm and resected three ribs, covering the thoracic wall defect with a pedicle flap left over from the amputation. For the anaesthesia he had used Henle's insufflation apparatus. In two other patients he had performed a partial thoracic wall excision, and closed the defect with the remaining healthy mamma. The first patient was still alive and well after 1½ years, the other two died, one within a few months, the other after several weeks.[33] Today, all three cases would have been regarded as inoperable.

A development of the utmost importance was the introduction of the statistical method. The history of medical statistics goes back to the eighteenth century, but it was only after about 1830 that the medical profession began to appreciate statistics as a scientific tool. In 1878, Alexander von Winiwarter (1848—1917), who had just been appointed to the chair of surgery at Liège, published an important statistical study of cancer cases treated by his teacher, professor Billroth, at Vienna between 1867 and 1875. This study comprised 548 patients, including 170 instances of breast cancer. At the time of publication, 19 patients out of 143 who had undergone surgery (13.3 per cent) were still alive and were regarded as cured or had died from non-related diseases.[34] Similar statistics from other major German clinics followed. The most important conclusion from all of these publications was that mammary cancer was not always or inevitably incurable. Three-year survival rates rose from 6 per cent to slightly over 13 per cent around 1875, to from 16 per cent to 30 per cent at the turn of the century. During the same period, operative mortality fell from 20—30 per cent to almost nil.[35]

By the end of the nineteenth century, Johannes Adrianus Korteweg (1851—

1930), who held chairs successively at Groningen, Amsterdam and Leyden, gained a degree of international reputation for his statistical studies on breast cancer. In 1880, 1888, and again in 1903, he discussed the statistics published by a number of clinics abroad, combining them and drawing his own conclusions from the data collected. The fact that he relied solely on German sources is indicative of the strong influence of German science in the Netherlands at the time. Korteweg concluded from the data that early operation and axillary dissection, even in so-called simple cases, had indeed improved the overall results of surgery in terms of survival rates. When upon careful examination of the operative specimen the axillary fat was found to be free of nodal involvement, chances of survival were twice as high as when, even minute, metastases were detected.[36]

The limitations of cancer surgery were an inducement to look for others modes of therapy. After the discovery of X-rays in 1895 by Wilhelm Roentgen (1845—1923) of Würzburg, it was not long before their possible action on malignant tumours became the subject of research. Although the first results were not exactly encouraging, and especially finding the effective dose was a major problem, radiotherapy soon became the treatment of choice in inoperable cases.

Radiotherapy of cancer made its appearance in the Netherlands around 1903. In 1908, Van der Goot presented results of this new method of treatment, obtained over a five-year period in the Bronovo Hospital at The Hague. Whereas some types of malignancy reacted most favourably, and others showed varying degrees of success, no satisfactory response whatsoever had been obtained in his 13 cases of breast cancer, which had been treated with radiation only.[37] Five years later, postoperative irradiation appears to have become an accepted procedure.

9.4.5. *Surgery of the Thyroid*

Surgery of the neck was practically created in the last two or three decades of the nineteenth century. Tracheostomy, although practised every now and then from time immemorial, became a standardized operation, finding a wide application in diphtheria, which in the last century appears to have increased considerably.

Before Vesalius, who was the first to describe the thyroid gland, goitre was thought of as a new growth. Celsus, and after him Paul and the mediaeval surgeons, distinguished several types, based on such characteristics as consistency, vascularity and swelling. Lanfranc imputed the condition to particular qualities of the drinking water and to living in particular regions, 'in confinibus Alpium et planitium Lombardie' especially.[38] Surgical treatment, when considered at all, consisted of enucleation, excision, the application of caustics or the redhot iron, or the passing of a seton. Spongia usta, applied internally, was a widely used popular remedy.

The modern treatment of goitre was pioneered by the Swiss surgeon Theodor Kocher (1841—1917) of Bern, one of the most prominent among a generation that produced such an astonishing number of excellent surgeons.[39] Kocher, a pupil of Georg Albert Lücke (1829—94), was an enterprising and inventive surgeon, who wrote on a great variety of subjects, including hernia, fractures, and carcinoma of the rectum. He invented several instruments, of which the haemostat named after him is still in current use. It was for his work on goitre, however, that he received the Nobel Prize in 1909. As a result of his continuing refinements in surgical techniques, the mortality rate for thyroidectomy gradually dropped from 12.8 per cent in 1883 to less than 0.5 per cent. He is said to have personally performed the operation more than 2000 times. Respiratory distress, caused by the gigantic size of many of the goitres, was the prime indication for operation. Before long, however, it was found that total extirpation of the thyroid was followed by a condition characterized by a dry, non-pitting swelling of subcutaneous tissues and striking facial changes, in combination with mental inertia. This finding made it clear that the thyroid, the function of which was still unknown at the time, had an important physiological role to play. It was now also clear that similar congenital or juvenile cretinoid states, often encountered in Switzerland, likewise resulted from thyroid insufficiency.

Tetany, as another complication of thyroidectomy, was at first regarded as an acute form of postoperative myxoedema. It was only towards the end of the century that it was discovered that this condition resulted from the inadvertent removal of the tiny parathyroid glands, first described by the Swedish anatomist Ivar Victor Sandström (1852—89) in 1879. In 1913, professor Laméris at Utrecht was the first in the Netherlands to report tetany after strumectomy. The sequelae of injuring the recurrent laryngeal nerves had been known since Galen.

It was now also understood that the typical signs of exophthalmic goitre as described by Caleb Hillier Parry (1755—1822) of London, posthumously published in 1825, and by his fellowcitizen Robert James Graves (1796—1853) in 1835, as well as by Carl August von Basedow (1799—1854) of Merseburg, Germany, in 1840, were due to hyperfunction of the thyroid. In a large number of such cases, thyroidectomy appeared to bring about a cure. The problems connected with the surgical treatment of hyperthyroidism were largely solved by American surgeons, including George W. Crile. Iodine as a preoperative measure, introduced in 1922 by Harry Stanley Plummer (1874—1937) of the Mayo Clinic, greatly diminished the risks of surgery in such cases.

Thyroid surgery meant more than the development of methods by which yet another organ could be removed. It helped in acquiring a better understanding of the phenomenon of internal secretion. It also stimulated surgeons to take an interest in physiological problems.

As was pointed out on page 305, thyroid surgery in this country was introduced especially by Kocher's pupil Lanz. Various afflictions, including catatonia and angina pectoris, have been seen as grounds for total extirpation. During World War I, Brand in Holland examined 46 476 mobilized soldiers, and found that 2615 of them had an enlarged thyroid. Most of these men had come from the central regions of the country or from the bigger cities. At about the same time Potter, who had noticed the relatively large number of goitre patients among the inhabitants of the city of Utrecht, conducted experiments with rats, which showed that animals given water from the Utrecht waterworks, taken from deep moorland wells, developed enlarged thyroids after a while. Those rats which had had to quench their thirst with Amsterdam tap water showed no signs of enlarged thyroids. It seemed likely, then, that the development of hypertrophied thyroids depended on the quality of the tap water, but since the differences in composition of the water had not been sufficiently examined, Potter could not draw any definitive conclusions as to the exact cause. It was noticed that after the construction of water mains in the town of Culemborg more cases of goitre were found than before, especially amoung young girls.[40] At this stage, however, no one had thought of iodine deficits.

9.4.6. *Urology*

As in so many other fields of surgery, important changes also occurred in urology. The incidence of vesical calculus, which had since the era of Hippocrates been one of the most common afflictions of Western man, had shown a very considerable decrease in the course of the nineteenth or even the eighteenth century. Now, however, more and more cases were reported of ureteric calculi, rarely mentioned in the early literature. In the pathology of the urogenital system, tuberculosis played an important role. The treatment of the tuberculous kidney sometimes included nephrectomy, an operation first performed in 1869 by Gustav Simon (1824—76) at Heidelberg, for a case of ureteric fistula of the abdominal wall, resulting from a gynaecological operation during which the ureter had been severed. The electrically lighted cytoscope, devised in 1879 by Max Nitze (1848—1906) at Vienna, meant a considerable extension of the urological diagnostic possibilities. Soon afterwards it also became possible to inspect the inside of other hollow organs using specially adapted endoscopes. The operation cystoscope introduced by Nitze twenty years later enabled surgeons to excise small bladder tumours without cystotomy.

During the early years of the twentieth century, Dutch surgeons made important contributions in the field of urology.[41] Hiddo Jan Brongersma (1869—1945), who in 1906 was to become the first Dutch lecturer in urology at Amsterdam, diagnosed a tumour of the renal pelvis on the basis of abnormal cells in urine obtained by ureteric catheterization; the second case of cell diagnostics in the literature. In 1906, Willem Jacob van Stockum (1860—1913), surgeon at the Coolsingel Ziekenhuis at Rotterdam, made an artificial bladder out of a segment of the small intestine. In the following year he proposed the method of retropubic, extravesical prostatectomy, which was described again in 1945 by Terence John Millin of Dublin as a 'new extravesical method'. Nephrectomy and nephrotomy were performed in Holland from the turn of the century. In 1915, L. D. van Hengel performed an extirpation of the urinary bladder in a case of papillomatosis at Arnhem.

In the first decade of the century, Zaayer of Leyden performed a uretero-ileo-cutaneostomy, which is now associated with the name of Bricker. Zaayer made another spectacular achievement when in 1908 he managed to transplant a dog's kidney into its own fossa iliaca. After he had removed the other kidney eight months later, the dog, named Jan, lived on in good health for another eight years. The animal was shown in demonstrations in many places, until it finally became ill and died in 1918. The cause of death was found to be chronic nephritis; the anastomoses had functioned perfectly.[42]

9.4.7. *Vascular Surgery*

Among the many great innovations realized by nineteenth-century antiseptic surgery, the suture of blood vessels may be regarded as one of the most brilliant.[43] At the 11th German Congress of Surgery in 1882, Max Schede (1844—1902) of Hamburg reported that he had sutured a defect in a femoral vein without subsequent haemorrhage. The practicability of vascular repair was thus demonstrated. Between 1882 and 1900, some 35 case reports on clinical venous sutures appeared in the literature. After 1882, a great deal of experimental work was done in this field as well. An outstanding example was the thesis entitled *Die Arteriennaht*, submitted in 1889 at the university of Dorpat in Estonia by A. Jassinowski. This thesis presented experimental proof of the feasibility of closing partial artery wounds by interrupted end-on coaptation stitches.

Mathieu Jaboulay (1860—1913) and E. Briau of Lyons described a circular anastomosis by means of interrupted everting mattress sutures passing through the entire wall, as a result of which an intima-to-intima approximation was achieved. The latter principle also underlay the method devised by Alexis Carrel (1873—1944), who was still working at Lyons when he developed it in 1902. In this technique the essential feature is a number of traction sutures to facilitate adaptation. Carrel's suture became the procedure of choice.

Whereas surgical reports regarding the blood vessels in the nineteenth century were almost exclusively concerned with surgical and traumatic wounds, aneurysmorrhaphy was frequently carried out after 1903. After the development of a reliable method of vascular suture, the transplantation of vessels and organs became the subject of a large series of experimental studies — 'surgery of the blood vessels and consequently transplantations of organs are the order of the day', wrote Tuffier in 1907. The name of Carrel, in particular, will remain attached to this research. After the first clinical applications by José Goyanes Capdevila (1876—1964) at Madrid in 1906, and by Erich Lexer (1867—1937) at Königsberg in 1907, using a venous autograft, vascular transplantation for a time occupied a secure if modest place in surgical treatment. The technique of renal transplantation was brought to perfection many years before the outbreak of the First World War:[42] Jaboulay even performed two clinical transplantations in 1906. But as the problem of immunological rejection was still unsolved, organ transplantation fell into disuse.

Blood vessel anastomosis was used by George Washington Crile (1864—1943) at Western Reserve University in the direct type of blood transfusion, but attempts at embolectomy or disobliterative endarteriectomy failed because of recurrent thrombosis. Further developments in vascular surgery appeared impossible as long as anticoagulant therapy was not available. In the early years of the present century it became clear that the further surgery evolves, the more it becomes dependent on conditions outside the discipline proper. Vascular transplantation was practically abandoned after World War I. In the early history of vascular surgery, no major Dutch achievements can be reported.

9.4.8. *Treatment of Fractures*

Among the changes in the surgery of the extremities made possible by the introduction of antisepsis, the most important was that in the treatment of fractures. It was now possible to refrain from immediate amputation in compound fractures. In fact, the first clinical case in which Lister demonstrated the efficiency of his method was a compound fracture in a lower leg. Thus on the one hand fracture treatment became more conservative, but on the other hand attempts were made at operative reduction — even of closed fractures — and osteosynthesis. A pioneer in this field was Sir William Arbuthnot Lane (1856—1943), who worked at Guy's Hospital at London. Initially he preferred wire and screws, but in 1907 he introduced plates and screws. The Belgian surgeon Albin Lambotte (1866—1955) of Brussels was probably the most versatile protagonist of the operative treatment of fractures. He introduced all kinds of screws, plates and metal bands, which he initially made with his own hands. He also suggested a method for external fixation.[44]

As in most other areas of medicine, the introduction of roentgenology had important consequences for the treatment of fractures (Fig. 113). Whereas before, surgeons had settled for a well functioning limb, now anatomical considerations began to outweigh the functional ones. For a while this resulted in an increase in the number of operations, or the use of Lambotte's 'fixateur externe'. But after the risks of these methods, antiseptic precautions notwithstanding, had become clear, Dutch surgeons generally returned to conservative treatment with plaster or

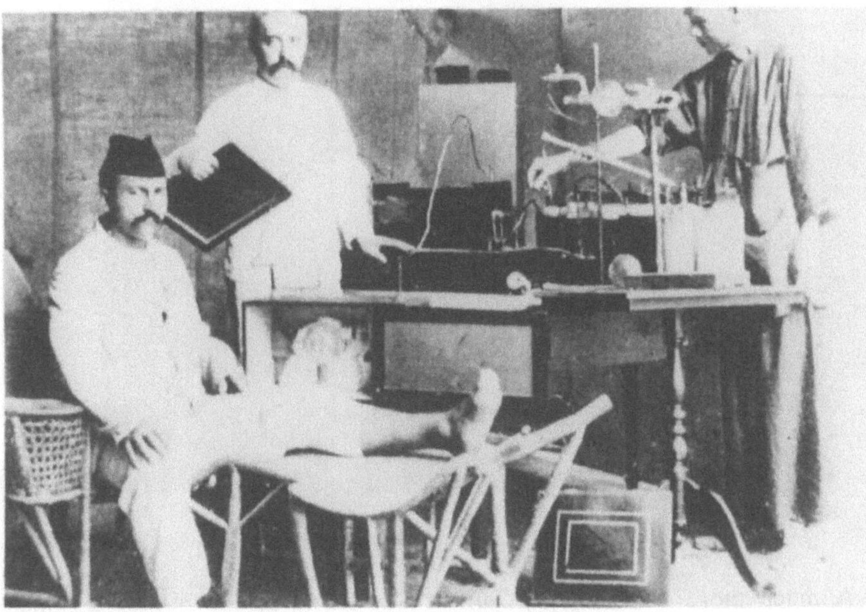

Fig. 113. First X-ray machine in the former Dutch East Indies. It was placed in the military hospital at Koeta-Radja in Achin in 1898. It is being operated by the Military Pharmacist First Class Douwes with the assistance of a Chinese technician.

continuous traction. Cerclage treatment was used occasionally, especially for the tibia, the patella and the olecranon.

At the Coolsingel Ziekenhuis in Rotterdam, which for years was known as one of the best accident hospitals in Europe, Van Stockum introduced an interesting new treatment for compound fractures in 1904. He left the wound open, filled it up with balsam of Peru, tamponed loosely and applied an immobilizing plaster cast. His results were amazing, and the treatment with peruvian balsam found many supporters in Holland. When, during the First World War, this material became scarce it was discovered that ordinary treacle gave similar results.[45]

An almost uninterrupted debate was held over fractures of the neck of the femur.[46] Their treatment by means of continuous extension, which dated from the previous century, gave poor results. The same was true of the continuous suspension traction recommended in 1903 by Leendert Marie Metz (1871—1945) for the treatment of femoral shaft fractures (Fig. 114).[47] And the well-known leg-splint introduced in 1875 by Hugh Owen Thomas (1834—91) of Liverpool, which made it possible to mobilize the patient without the leg bearing weight, or even with continuous traction, was also found to be ineffective in the treatment of such fractures.

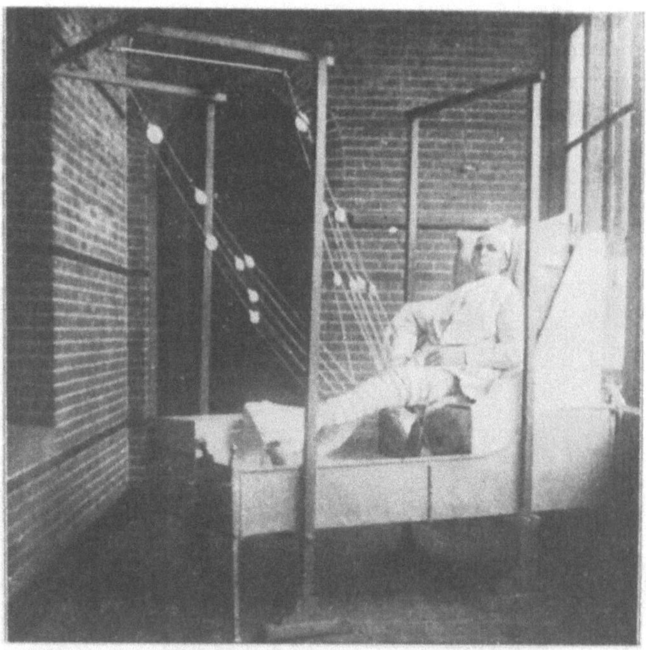

Fig. 114. The 'Balkan frame' devised by Dr. L. M. Metz.

A much more satisfactory treatment was found in the plaster treatment in abduction and slight internal rotation, which was made popular especially by Royal Whitman (1857—1946) in New York. As early as the second half of the nineteenth century, attempts were occasionally made to fixate intracapsular fractures surgically by means of screws or metal nails. The results, however, were not very encouraging. One of the problems of this technique was that the bone did not accept the foreign material introduced into it. Hence in 1908 Erich Lexer, then professor at Königsberg, attempted the internal fixation by means of a bone peg taken from the patient's tibia. This led to a revival of the interest in surgical treatment of femoral neck fractures. A point of debate in this connection was whether or not the hip joint should be laid bare. Before the First World War, the first guiding apparatuses were introduced, which were designed to enable the surgeon to introduce a nail into the neck of the femur without exposing it. The use of autogenous bone transplants was stimulated particulary by Fred Albee (1876—1945) of New York.

9.5. ANAESTHESIA AND SHOCK MANAGEMENT

Beneficial as anaesthesia had proved to be since its introduction, it was not entirely without its dangers, as had soon become clear. Moreover, it was often followed by an 'postanaesthetic hangover'. Before World War II, only a few doctors in the world had specialized in administering narcosis. The Netherlands had exactly one physician-anaesthetist. His name was Theodoor Hammes (1874—1951), who, after having been an assistant at Korteweg's surgical clinic for some years, had received his training in anaesthetics in London. Around 1904, he settled in Amsterdam, where he was admitted into the teaching staff of the university as an unsalaried lecturer. Soon he was nicknamed 'the town stupefyer' (de stadsbedwelmer). His textbook on the subject, *De narcose*, written in 1906, was reprinted several times.

In the great majority of operating theatres, anaesthesia was induced by one of the assistants or by a nurse, who could choose between chloroform, ether, or the so-called Billroth mixture, using the open method (Fig. 115).[48] Morphine and scopolamine were the usual premedication. In view of the abovementioned risks, local anaesthesia was increasingly used, even in major operations. The history of modern local and regional anaesthesia begins in 1884, when Carl Koller (1857—1944) of Vienna reported on the anaesthetizing action of a cocaine solution, when applied in the eye.[49] It was not long before subcutaneous injection of such solutions could be used to interrupt temporarily the conduction of impulses in sensory nerves, and even anaesthetize large areas of the skin and underlying tissues. It was soon discovered, however, that cocaine is a dangerous agent, so that it was an important improvement when in 1899 the chemist Alfred Einhorn (1856—1917) of Munich managed to provide a replacement in the form of the far less dangerous and non-addictive synthetic novocaine.

Around the turn of the century surgeons, especially in Britain and the United States, began to pay attention to the phenomenon of surgical shock. Although surgeons have been acquainted with this phenomenon since time immemorial, the first coherent description of its complex of symptoms was given by Henri Le Dran — who used the word 'secousse' — in his *Traité ou reflexions tirées de la pratique sur les playes d'armes à feu* of 1737. This treatise was also published in German

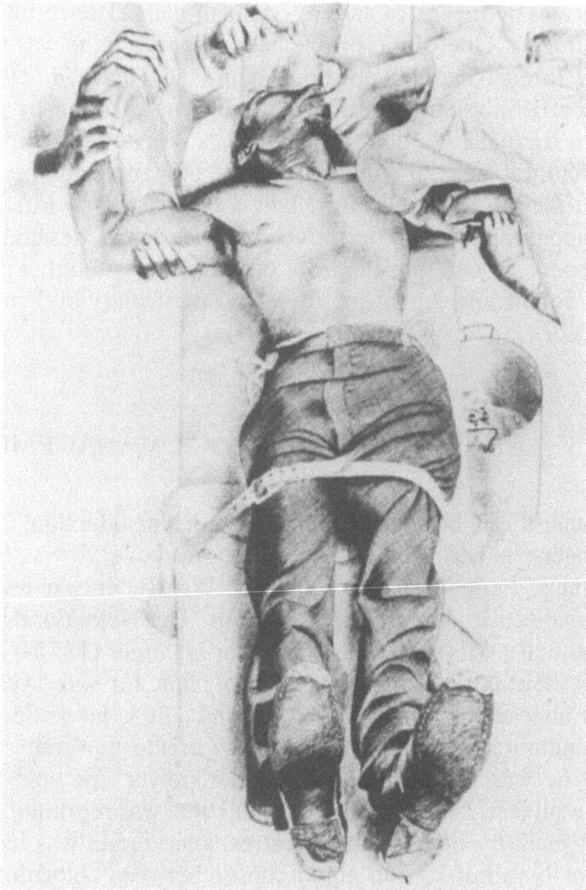

Fig. 115. Open drip anaesthesia in the Utrecht university surgical clinic in the early 1940s.

and in Dutch.[50] The word 'shock' was widely used in connection with wounds by the beginning of the nineteenth century.

In the years before the Great War, the most important development in the field of shock management was the experimental work of George W. Crile, already mentioned on page 320. This work led to an improved understanding of the phenomenon and a more causal treatment by administering parenteral fluid. The *Nederlandsch Tijdschrift voor Geneeskunde* (Dutch Journal of Medicine) gave little attention to Crile's important studies, nor to publications in the English journal *The Lancet* by William Arbuthnot Lane in 1891 and by Peter Horrocks (1852–1909) in 1893, in which they reported good results after administering intravenous saline. It is something of a surprise, therefore, to find in a Dutch textbook of nursing, dating from 1907, a description of the administering of subcutaneous physiological saline (0.7 per cent NaC1): 'usually, ½—1 litre is given at a time, sometimes several times a day. It is astonishing how quickly the introduction of so much water under the skin can improve the action of the heart' (Fig. 116).

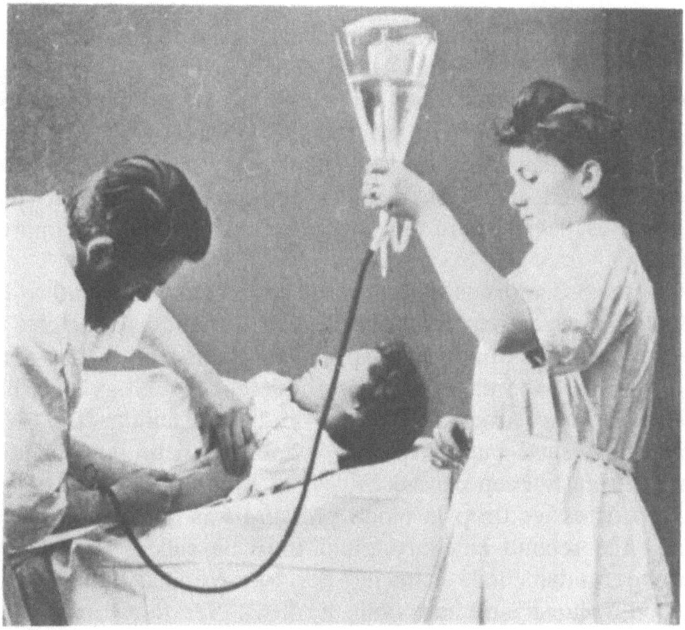

Fig. 116. Hypodermoclysis, 1907.

Intravenous administration is also mentioned in the textbook.[51] These events took place at a time when the majority of surgeons — and certainly not only in the Netherlands — had no interest whatsoever in pathophysiological problems.

All in all, in the history of surgery, and especially operative surgery, the years before the First World War may be regarded as a period extremely rich in original ideas. However, many of these could as yet not be realized, as the required material resources and tools were lacking. But the rise of antiseptic surgery taught the surgeon, through all the centuries eminently an individualist, to work in a surgical team.

9.6. THE FIRST WORLD WAR

The First World War confronted the surgeons of the belligerent nations with enormous problems, because it resulted in 19 million wounded soldiers who had to be taken care of. Surgical exigencies are different in every war; experiences gained in the Balkan Wars or in South Africa were of little use on the battlefields of Europe. On the western front in particular, fragments of shells, land mines and hand grenades caused lacerated, deep and soiled wounds such as had never been seen before.

Aseptic wound treatment as this had developed since the days of Lister, was of little avail. Life-threatening tetanus and gas gangrene were frequent complications. There was a sharp drop in the incidence of tetanus after the introduction of routine prophylactic treatment with administration of tetanus antitoxin, but apart from early amputation, no preventive was known against gas gangrene, which was seen for the first time at a large scale in this war. After much experimental work the Carrel-Dakin treatment was introduced in 1915. It consisted of a wide excision of the wound, with removal of all lacerated tissue and any foreign bodies, to be followed by repeated irrigations with a sodium hypochloride solution. New antiseptics such as flavine were developed for the treatment of more superficial lesions.

One of the major causes of death on the battlefield was found to be shock. In order to study this phenomenon more closely, the Medical Research Committee of the British Privy Council appointed a special committee, consisting of a number of well-known surgeons, as well as eminent physiologists such as Sir William Bayliss (1860—1924) and the American Walter Bradford Cannon (1871—1945). This committee distinguished between cases where the depressed condition of the circulation had clearly been caused by loss of blood, and those cases where the cause of the progressive drop in blood pressure was unclear. In the committee's opinion, only the second category could truly be called 'shock'. Their studies revealed some fundamental characteristics, viz. capillary haemoconcentration, reduced blood volume, and metabolic acidosis. Yet the committee refused to identify shock as acidosis, since it had been found in animal experiments that an intravenous injection of an extract of the animal's own crushed muscle tissue led to a decrease in blood pressure as well as to haemoconcentration. The committee ascribed these findings to loss of fluid from the bloodstream as a result of increasing capillary permeability. Since it was already known that histamine could induce both phenomena, the conclusion was that shock resulted from histamine intoxication. If, then, shock basically arises from increased permeability of the capillaries, therapy should not consist of giving saline, but of administering solutions of high viscosity, with molecules too large to pass through the interstices in the damaged capillary wall.[52]

By the time the committee had come to this conclusion, however, the war was over, and their advice has probably not been put into practice very often. Blood transfusion did not play a significant role in World War I. This was to change in the Spanish Civil War.

Fractures of course were far more often compound or comminuted than in civil practice. The Thomas' splint reduced the mortality in compound fractures of the femur from 80 per cent to somewhere in the neighbourhood of 20 per cent.[53] Operative treatment assumed large proportions. X-ray diagnosis came into more general use.

Orthopaedics and prosthetics, too, made rapid strides, and continued to do so for quite a while after the cessation of hostilities. The same is true of plastic surgery. On the side of the Allies in the 1914—18 War, Sir Harold Gillies (1882—1960) was the acknowledged leader in this field; in the opposite camp this was Erich Lexer, together with the Dutchman Jan Esser (1877—1946). Holland did not participate in the war; its only medical commitment was the sending of Red Cross ambulances. Ever since the Red Cross was founded in 1864, the Netherlands, while observing the strictest neutrality, sent ambulances to many

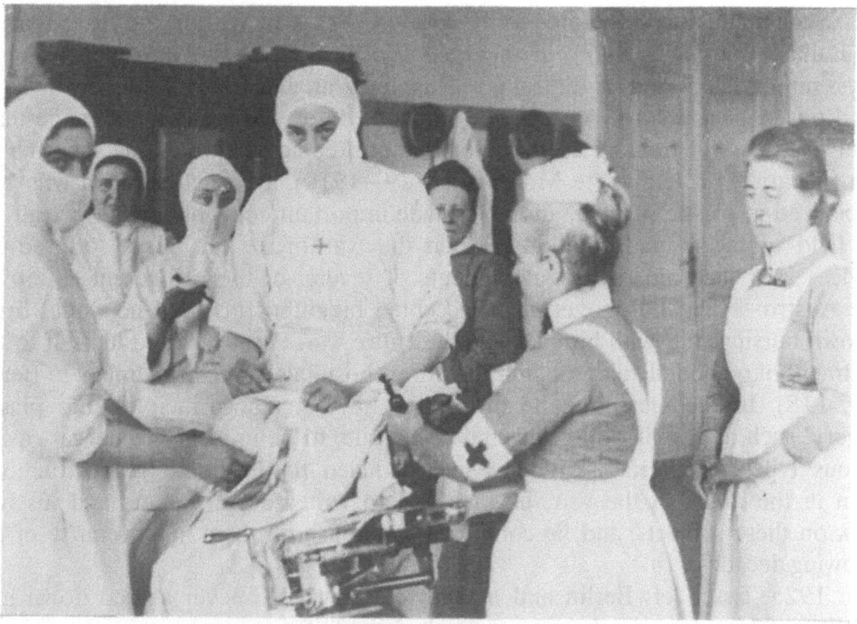

Fig. 117. Dutch Red Cross surgical team in Salonika, Greece, during the First Balkan War (1912–13), directed by Dr. Offerhaus and Dr. Ittmann.

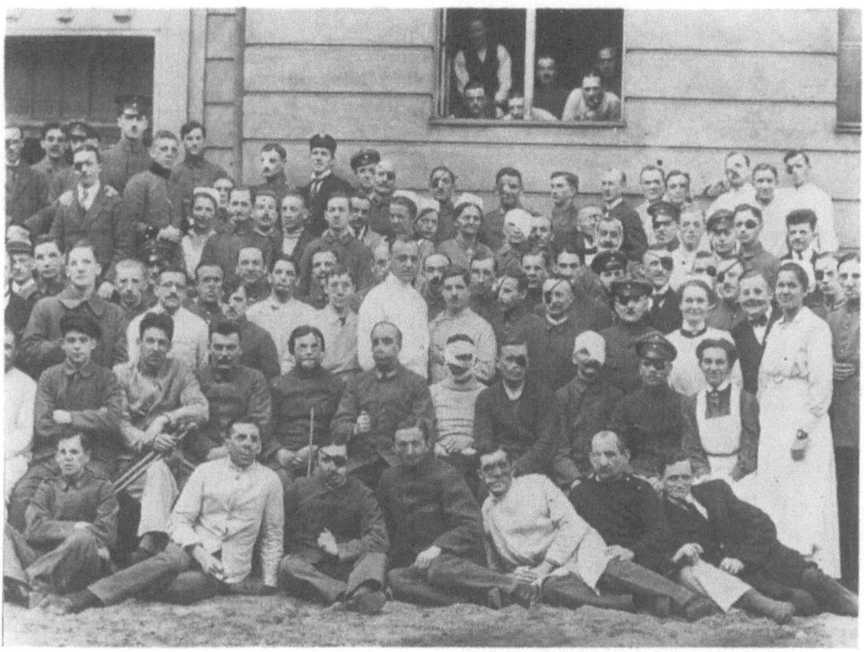

Fig. 118. Dr. Jan F. S. Esser in the midst of soldiers requiring plastic surgery in Berlin in the early twenties.

wars. Such ambulances operated in the Franco—Prussian War, in the Boer War, in the Balkan Wars (Fig. 117), in the First World War, in the Italian invasion of Abyssinia of 1935, and in the Finno—Russian War. Jan Esser, however, in 1914 acted on his own accord. As a plastic surgeon, Esser was really a self-made man. After two years of training at professor Laméris' clinic in Utrecht, he spent half a year in Paris with Hippolyte Morestin (1869—1919), a French surgeon who had specialized in plastic surgery, and who made important contributions, especially in the field of facial malformations. When the war broke out, Esser offered his services as a surgeon to the governments of several of the belligerent countries. The Austro—Hungarian government accepted his offer, provided he would bring his own nursing staff with him. During the entire war, Esser devoted himself to the treatment of wounded soldiers, first in various hospitals in Austria, finally in Berlin (Fig. 118). In the meantime he introduced several new principles into plastic surgery, such as a split skin graft inlay technique, to be used in the buccal cavity, various types of arterial skin flaps and pedicled toe-to-thumb reconstructions. Even in the midst of the war, he managed to write several papers and his first book on these subjects, and he continued to publish on them in the course of the following decades.

In 1925, Esser left Berlin and moved to France. He never settled down in a practice of his own, but he was a much sought-after consultant in the field of reconstructive surgery all over Europe.[54]

CHAPTER 10

Surgery in the Past 75 Years

10.1. BETWEEN THE TWO WORLD WARS

10.1.1. *Social Background*

The armistice of November 11, 1918, was unfortunately not followed by a lasting peace in Europe. Individual countries were faced with major political and economic problems, which often led to social unrest. Although the United States, after having contributed so much to the Allied Forces' victory, showed a tendency towards a degree of political isolationism, the American life-style nevertheless began to penetrate Europe. On both sides of the Atlantic Ocean, jazz music, the charleston and foxtrot, cocktails, the cinema and short skirts were a part of the cheerful life-style of the 'roaring 'twenties', which did its best to forget the preceding years in superficial entertainment. More profound social changes resulted from the fading of traditions, the rise of the trade union movement, and, last but not least, the changed position of women, who during the war had acquired a degree of independence they were unwilling to relinquish. Technological developments such as the telephone, wireless broadcasting, the automobile, and even to a certain extent aviation — KLM opened its first regular air service in 1920 — contributed to the development of a way of life sharply different from before the war.

New art forms came to the fore, such as surrealism and 'Art Déco', the typical artistic mode of the twenties and thirties. Few people realized that through the war Europe had lost its hegemony over the world, and the dramatic events of October 1929 in Wall Street showed to what extent the Old World had come to depend on the American economy. The Great Depression put an end to the careless optimism of the 1920s. German democracy collapsed during the economic recession with the takeover by the National Socialists in 1933. Unemployment and poverty are the key words characterizing the thirties in many people's memories, and there was a general feeling that war was looming ahead. This crisis notwithstanding, mortality rates for infants and elderly persons fell in the Western countries, and a decrease in the incidence of tuberculosis could be observed. Rickets was still common. Cancer was found to have shown an alarming increase since the 1914—1918 war, and this increase could not be attributed solely to the ageing of the population. On the other hand, myocardial infarction was rare, causing barely 200 deaths per million people each year, a number which was to rise to nearly 3500 million over the next twenty years.

10.1.2. *Medical Science in the 1920s and 1930s*

In medical science, technological progress continued. Thus, direct writing, portable electrocardiographs were constructed which, thanks to technical devices derived from radio technology, had far greater sensitivity than their predecessors. Through the application of other leads in addition to those already in use, the utility of electrocardiography was greatly enhanced in the second half of the 1930s. Another contribution to cardiological diagnosis was made by the German surgeon Werner Forsmann (1904—79) at Eberswald, who in 1929, experimenting on himself, showed that heart catheterization was a practicable technique. However, this method of examination was not clinically applied until after the Second World War.

The years between the two World Wars also saw the rapid development of endocrinology, which had immediately found a therapeutic application in 1921 with the discovery of insulin, thus revolutionising the treatment of diabetes. Within two years of this discovery, a pharmaceutical company, bearing the appropriate name of *Organon*, was founded in Oss in the Netherlands, having at that time the novel aim of scientifically producing drugs from animal glands.

Vitamin research was also making rapid progress during this period. Vitamins were soon accepted by the general public, and daily diets were gradually changed to include them. From 1926 onwards, the treatment of pernicious anaemia, which until then had consisted of a great variety of techniques, including extraction of all the teeth, could be undertaken successfully by means of liver extracts.[1]

10.1.3. *Surgery: General Characteristics*[2]

Unlike the developments seen in our own days, social changes between the two World Wars did not affect the surgical scene. Notwithstanding a steady increase in the number of female doctors, surgery remained exclusively a man's profession. Its hierarchical structures were strictly upheld, and in general, surgery has not been the worse for this. However, European clinics were being less frequently visited by Americans, while more Europeans than ever before went on study tours across the Atlantic. And after the war, American professional journals, for which *Surgery, Gynecology and Obstetrics*, with its fine illustrations by Max Brödel is a good example, were read in Europe with greater attention than hitherto. German surgery slowly began to lose its position of supremacy. International contacts were encouraged by world congresses, organized by the 'Societé International de Chirurgie', founded in 1902, and the 'International College of Surgeons', dating from 1935.

The results of surgical treatment were influenced favourably by improvements in the diagnostic tools offered by the rapidly developing science of radiology, which by means of contrast media succeeded in making more and more hollow organs accessible to X-ray examination. Refinements in instrument design especially benefitted endoscopy. And after the 1920s, laboratory tests came to play an ever-increasing diagnostic rôle: in addition to the introduction of the erythrocyte sedimentation test, the new liver function tests proved especially valuable for surgery in the ensuing years.

10.1.3.1. Surgery as a Recognized Speciality

At its 81st general meeting in 1930, the Dutch 'Maatschappij tot Bevordering der Geneeskunst' (Dutch Medical Association) decided to initiate the registration of specialists.[3] A committee was created which had to register recognized specialists, as well as specify the training requirements for the various specialities. This committee proposed to set the duration of the surgeon's training at two years — probably as a confirmation of current usage — but at the request of the faculties this period was extended to three years. This remained the required period of training until 1948.

10.1.3.2. Operative Surgery

As far as practical surgery is concerned, the 1930s were in many respects more interesting than the preceding decade, despite austerity measures which affected the clinics as well.[4]

Abdominal Surgery

In the twenties and thirties, developments in abdominal surgery concentrated particularly on refinements of indications for treatment and in operative techniques, as well as the improved treatment of postoperative complications.

After its introduction by Billroth, partial gastric resection was at first only sporadically practised. Until the 1920s, pyloric stenosis, together with carcinoma, were the most common indications. The non-obstructive peptic ulcer was — insofar as operative treatment was considered at all — preferably treated by means of pyloroplasty or gastroenterostomy. Since the results of these techniques did not always live up to expectations, the alternative of partial gastric resection more and more met with support, especially in Germany, even during the First World War. In the 1920s, this principle became generally accepted in Holland, but opinions were seriously divided over the question of which type of resection, Billroth I gastrectomy or Pólya gastrectomy with gastrojejunal anastomosis (Billroth II), ought to be used. There were heated, at times even emotional debates on this subject at the meetings of the 'Nederlandsche Vereeniging voor Heelkunde' (Dutch Surgical Society). In Germany the situation was no different.[5]

Eventually, the peculiar situation arose in which the university clinics at Amsterdam, Groningen and Utrecht fully supported the Pólya variant while the school of The Hague followed the Billroth I technique.

A most important part in the history of Dutch gastric surgery was played by Jan Schoemaker (1871—1940), from 1902 onwards surgeon at the Gemeente Ziekenhuis (Municipal Hospital) at The Hague. With its 300 beds, this hospital was at the time one of the largest in the country. Schoemaker seems to have been an impressive personality. Hans Haberland of Cologne, by no means the least among the German surgeons of his day, described him as follows:

Seine grosse, schlanke, elastische, vornehme und elegante Erscheinung, seine angeborene weltmännische Art und Weise, ein offener, geradliniger Charakter, temperamentvolles, ungezwungenes, niemals gekünsteltes Benehmen, taktvoll, schnellstes Einfühlen und Respektieren des Sentiments der einzelnen Nationalitäten, Beherrschen vieler Sprachen in Wort und Schrift kennzeichnen etwa seine überragende Persönlichkeit.[6]

Schoemaker is said to have been a brilliant surgeon: systematic, self-assured and elegant: 'I pencil with the knife', as he liked to express it. Surgeons came to The Hague from other European countries and even from the United States to see Schoemaker at work, especially when he performed the Billroth I gastric resection which had contributed so much to his world-wide fame since the early 1920s (Fig. 119). At a time when in some clinics mortality rates for resection of benign ulcers

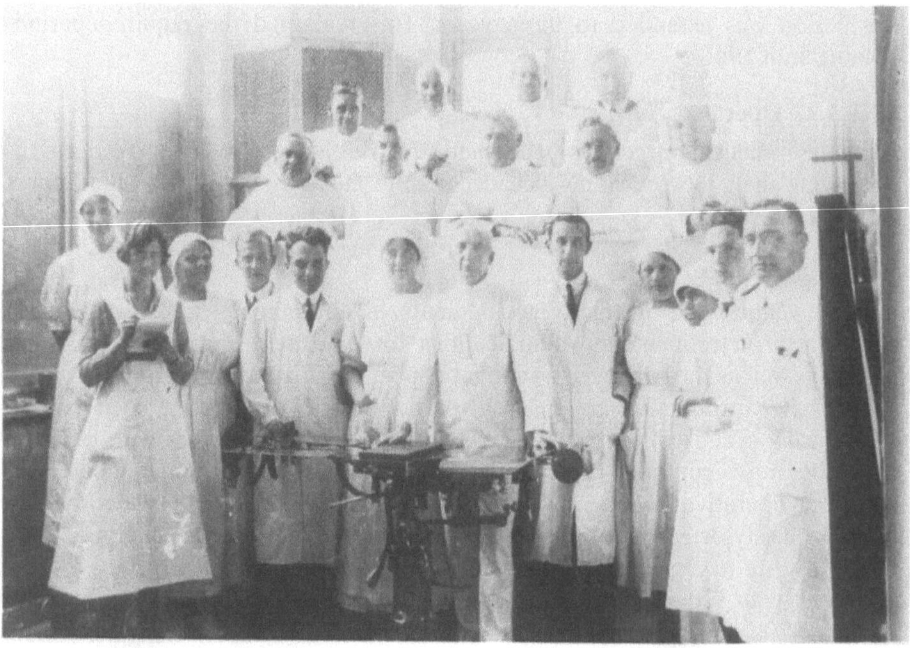

Fig. 119. Dr. Jan Schoemaker with assistants, nurses and American visitors.

was still almost 25 per cent, Schoemaker could pride himself on a mortality rate of no more than 5.5 per cent. He published a great deal, and on many different subjects. He was one of the few Dutch surgeons in the years before the Second World War who managed to get articles accepted by leading German and American journals. Characteristically for those days, all his publications dealt with practical surgery. His pragmatic nature is also evident from the numerous instruments and devices of all kinds that he designed. Some of these remained part of the standard equipment of Dutch operating theatres until well after World War II. Like so many other pre-war clinical specialists, Schoemaker for years did his own radiology work. As a result, he developed a skin cancer on his hands, and died from its metastases.

At Rotterdam in 1929, Boevé treated four cases of chronic inflammation of the terminal part of the ileum, a disease which Burill Bernard Crohn (1884—1983) in New York was to term 'ileitis regionalis' in 1932. Inflammation of the large intestine posed a serious problem for the surgeon, far more so than was the case with tumours, for which Schoemaker established an aseptic resection method. For rectal carcinoma, extirpation was preferred to resection.

Meanwhile, appendectomy had turned out to be an operation involving relatively small risks. It may have been partly for this reason that removal of the appendix, like tonsillectomy, became more or less a fashionable operation for a while, an operation apparently not always performed on the strictest indications; surgery is by no means free of modish trends. Malicious tongues have suggested that 'chronic remunerative appendicitis' may have been the indication in some instances.

Another early subject of debate at the meetings of the 'Nederlandsche Vereeniging voor Heelkunde' was surgery of the gall-bladder and bile ducts. In the 1920s an important discussion centred round the question whether or not a cholecystectomy should routinely be combined with choledochotomy. The latter course was especially advocated by Hiddo Jan Laméris (1872—1948), professor of surgery at Utrecht from 1906 onwards. Laméris was one of the most prominent characters in Dutch surgery between the wars. With his impressive moustache, he made a striking figure of a man. He was a born teacher (Fig. 120). His lectures

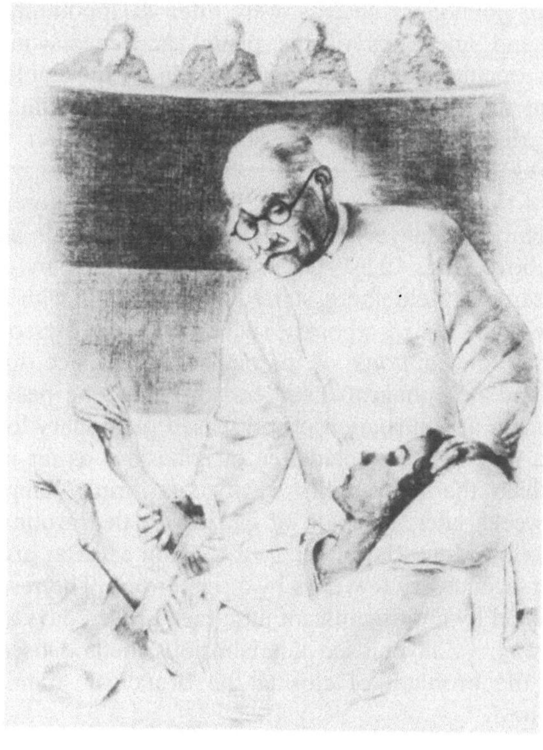

Fig. 120. Professor H. J. Laméris lecturing.

were often sheer theatrical performances, sprinkled with pithy maxims, which became winged words in Dutch surgery. 'He who opens a cold abscess, opens the gates of death,' was one of them. He furthermore liked to recite Celsus' famous stipulations for a good surgeon (see p. 12). In addition, Laméris was a surgeon of God-given talent: 'An operation should be a symphony of the hands,' he emphasized. He bequeathed his particular interest in gallbladder surgery to his pupil and successor Nuboer, which ensured that the Utrecht university clinic remained an important centre for this field of surgery until after the Second World War.

Thoracic Surgery

Sauerbruch's low pressure chamber, which was briefly mentioned on page 314, and which made it possible to open the thoracic cavity without the risk of an immediate pulmonary collapse, had in practice encountered a number of problems. To my knowledge, the low pressure chamber was never used in the Netherlands. Even before World War I it was being replaced by anaesthetic techniques of intralaryngeal insufflation in which Zaayer was one of the pioneers.[7]

The major concern of thoracic surgery between the wars was still with tuberculous cavities, which were treated by pneumolysis, artificial pneumothorax or thoracoplasty. Sauerbruch, in particular, also ventured into lobectomy as early as the twenties. The results of this operation, usually undertaken for treatment of bronchiectasis or pulmonary abscess, were often disappointing because of tension pneumothorax and infections of the pleura and mediastinum, resulting from leakage of the bronchial stump, apparently an almost inevitable complication.[8] The pleural cavity at that time was not drained after the operation, but all kinds of methods were tried to obliterate the dead space left after resection. The hilar structures were ligated en masse.

In the field of thoracic surgery of the 1920s, special reference should be made to Johannes Henricus Zaayer (1876—1932), who has already been mentioned several times above (Fig. 121). Zaayer, who received part of his training from Vincenz von Czerny at Heidelberg, started as an assistant with Lanz in Amsterdam, and with Korteweg in Leyden, whom he succeeded as a professor in 1914.

Zaayer made contributions of particular importance to the treatment of bronchiectasis and oesophageal disorders.[9] In 1927, he became the first Dutch surgeon to perform an extirpation of a diseased pulmonary lobe with a left lower lobectomy. The lobe was dissected free of adhesions as far as possible up to its hilum, after which the surrounding cavity was firmly tamponed. In a second session, three weeks later, a length of gauze was tied around the hileum of the affected lobe, followed ten days later by a Nelaton catheter around the gauze. The catheter was replaced every few days by a tighter one. The result was that the lobe gradually atrophied to 'an insignificant little rag'. Fifteen days after being tied off, it could be cut away.[10] Zaayer used this laborious method because, as Sauerbruch also admitted, the problem of closing the bronchial stump had not yet been satisfactorily solved.

Zaayer's interest in oesophageal surgery focussed on cardiospasm — which he regarded as resulting from a weakening of the cardiac sphincter — and benign and

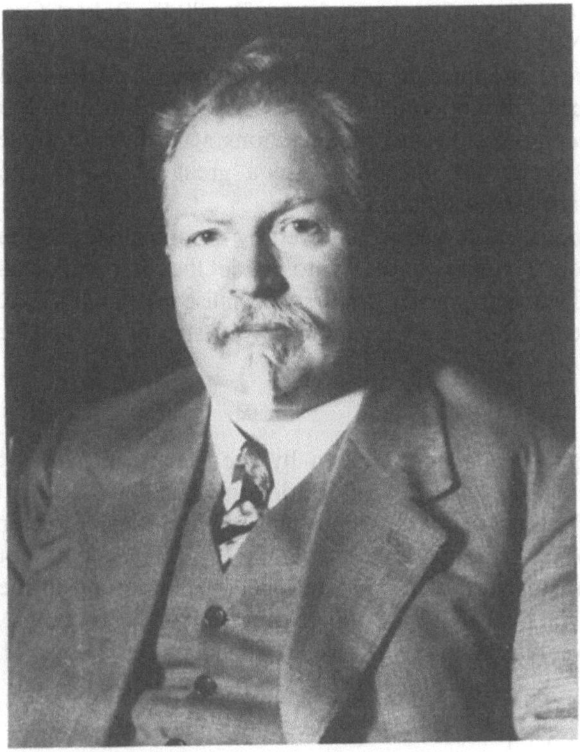

Fig. 121. Professor J. H. Zaayer.

malignant stenoses. As for benign stenoses, he was able to report a successful case of an antethoracic oesophagoplasty by the Heller technique, which he had performed in 1917 for relief of a sulphuric acid burn. He was never very successful in his attempts at oesophageal resection for carcinoma, even though he had shown the feasibility of this operation in animal experiments (see p. 315). He also engaged in the then customary surgical treatment of pulmonary tuberculosis. Zaayer performed his thoracic operations under positive pressure nitrous oxide narcosis in combination with local anaesthesia of the skin.[11]

During the 1930s, the technique of total and partial pulmonary resection was refined by anatomical dissection of the hilar structures, and the prognosis was improved by drainage of the pleural cavity. In Holland, the first pneumonectomy for bronchiectasis was performed in 1940 by Hendrik Wamsteker (1900—59) of Haarlem, a pupil and son in law of Zaayer. Rudolf Nissen, at Sauerbruch's clinic in Berlin, had pioneered this technique in 1931.[12]

Operations on the heart and intrathoracic blood vessels were very rarely performed between the wars: there was a complete pericardiectomy by Victor Schmieden in 1924; an embolectomy from the pulmonary artery — an operation already suggested by Trendelenburg in 1907 — by Martin Kirschner in the same year; a digital commissurotomy to relieve mitral stenosis by Sir Henry Souttar in London in 1925; a resection of an aneurysm of the right ventricle by Sauerbruch in 1931; and the closure of an open ductus Botalli by Robert Gross at Boston in 1938.[13] In the Netherlands, professor C. F. A. Koch (1859—1950) of Groningen managed to cure a suppurating pericarditis by means of drainage, while he and some others successfully operated on cases of pericarditis calculosa in the 1920s, by means of decompression and rib resections according to Brauer's method. At the time, such operations did not cause a great deal of excitement, as their practical importance seemed limited.

With his oesophageal resection followed by oesophagogastrostomy in 1933, the Japanese surgeon T. Ohsawa of Kyoto made the first important non-Western contribution.[14] Two years earlier the first specialist journal in this subject had been published as the *Journal of Thoracic Surgery*, a sign of the heightened interest in this field.

Urology

Studies using Uroselectan, undertaken by the American Moses Swick during a fellowship at Hamburg-Altona and Berlin in 1928 and 1929, resulted in the development of intravenous urography. This important examination technique was introduced in the Netherlands as early as 1930, by M. Roeper at Groningen.

Transurethral resection of the prostate became important in the 1920s, mainly as a result of the activities of the young Hippolyte E. M. Houtappel of Amsterdam, who had learnt this technique from Hugh Hampton Young (1870—1945) at Baltimore.

The Endocrine System

We have already encountered thyroidectomy for cases of hyperthyroidism in the era of Kocher as an example of an operation not primarily meant to remove the diseased organs or parts of them as such, but rather aiming at the consequences of such removals, viz. restoring a disordered physiology. In the nineteen-twenties, other operations with this purpose were added: the removal of adrenal tumours to cure virilism, extirpation of parathyroid adenomata in osteitis fibrosa and of adenomata of the islets of Langerhans in hypoglycemia. In 1924, the above-mentioned Boevé was the first Dutch surgeon to remove a parathyroid tumour in a patient suffering from osteitis fibrosa generalisata.

Vascular Surgery; Interruption of Nervous Pathways

The interest in direct operations on the peripheral arteries which existed before the First World War had largely subsided in the period between the wars.

With his lumbar and periarterial sympathectomy, the spirited French surgeon René Leriche (1879—1955) gave a new, physiological impulse to the treatment of peripheral vascular diseases. Such periarterial sympathetic resections were also the most important blood vessel operations performed in this country until the period following World War II.

In 1924, Willem Frederik Suermondt (1890—1976), a pupil of Zaayer, made a thorough empirical study of the effect of vagotomy on peristalsis. In 1911, Exner had suggested that bilateral vagotomy might be a possible treatment for 'gastric crises', but there were contradictory reports in the literature on its outcome. On the basis of his study using dogs, Suermondt concluded that after complete disruption of the vagus the animal is at first very ill, but gradually makes a complete clinical recovery. On radiological examination, however, atony of the stomach and delayed evacuation persisted. On the basis of his results, he expressed the opinion that atony of the stomach might have a favourable effect, insofar as the mucosa would not be so easily damaged mechanically, but he also held the belief that vagotomy alone would certainly not suffice to cure this condition since so many other factors were involved in the aetiology of peptic ulcer. Suermondt did not establish the level of acidity in the stomach.

J. G. Kopp and Suermondt, in 1926 and 1933 respectively, performed a cervical sympathectomy as a treatment for angina pectoris. Chordotomy was carried out for the first time in this country in 1939, but Egaz Moniz' prefrontal leucotomy of 1936, which sought to influence the psyche favourably by neurosurgical intervention, was rarely copied here, except in cases of unmanageable behaviour due to mental subnormality. During the late sixties, this operation became obsolete, largely because modern psychopharmacological drugs became available.

10.1.3.3. Treatment of Fractures

Between the wars, the therapeutic approach to fractures was, especially on the European continent, dominated by Lorenz Böhler (1885—1973) of Vienna. He strongly advocated a conservative form of treatment, consisting of careful reduction and strict immobilization, combined with simultaneous active exercise of all non-immobilized joints. Immobilization was achieved by means of continuous traction as well as by encasing in plaster (Fig. 122). A significant improvement of the extension treatment was made by Martin Kirschner (1879—1942) of Tübingen, a technically highly skilled surgeon, when in 1927 he modified the wire extension method invented in 1907 by Fritz Steinmann (1872—1932).[15]

The Vienna Accident Hospital, led since 1925 by Böhler, had a worldwide reputation, and set an example to numerous emergency surgery clinics and departments elsewhere. For several decades, Böhler's masterly book *Technik der Knochenbruchbehandlung* was a generally respected standard work. It was translated into many languages and was reprinted time and again until the 1950s. For many Dutch surgeons, this was the bible of fracture treatment. It was not until after the Second World War that Sir Reginald Watson-Jones' *Fractures and joint injuries*, which was also conservative in its approach, became a close second.

As far as the treatment of intracapsular fractures of the femoral neck is concerned, the third decade of the century was dominated by the question which of two methods was to be preferred: the plaster cast or operative fixation using autogenous bone. In Holland, too, opinions were sharply divided on this issue. Plaster treatment was tenaciously defended by Schoemaker, while the operation using the patient's own bone was ardently advocated by Willem Noordenbos (1875—1954), professor of surgery with Otto Lanz since 1920. The introduction, in 1925, of the triflanged stainless steel nail by Marius Smith Petersen (1886—1953) of Boston, settled the dispute in favour of the operation. Up to the 1970s, this operative technique was to remain the standard treatment.

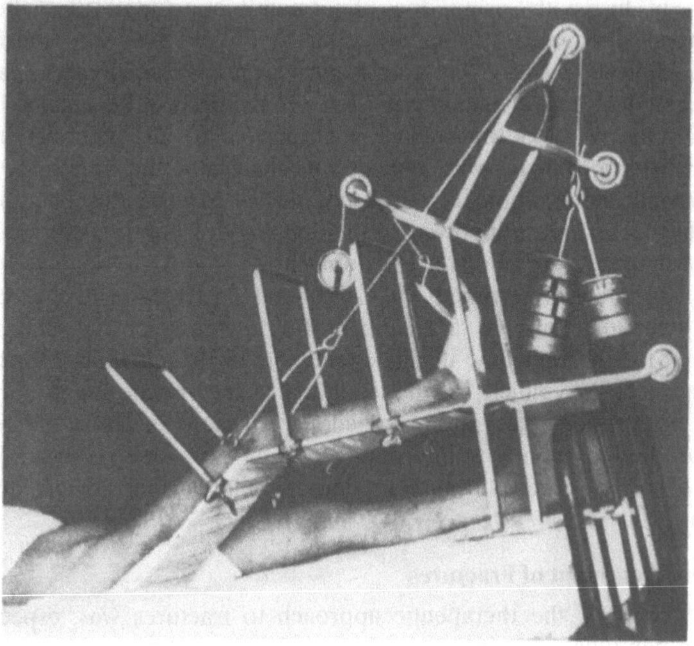

Fig. 122. Continuous traction by the wire extension method in general use for the treatment of femoral shaft fractures in the first half of the present century.

10.1.3.4. Anaesthesiology

The art of administering local and regional anaesthesia reached unprecedented heights between the wars. Many surgeons used this form of anaesthesia by preference, even though new narcotics such as ethylene, Avertin and Evipan had been introduced in the late twenties and early thirties. In operations for inguinal hernia or goitre, this method of anaesthesia was more or less standard procedure. It is not unlikely that the surgeons, who were still fully responsible for the anaesthesia, were glad to be relieved of the obligation to keep a watchful eye on the narcosis, administered by a nurse or assistant, during the operation. Specialized anaesthetists were still rare, although their numbers slowly grew during the 1930s. One of the factors stimulating the development of anaesthesiology as a distinct specialty was the fact that opening the thoracic cavity became more and more common practice. In English speaking countries, conduction anaesthesia was apparently less common. In England, endotracheal narcosis was occasionally applied from 1921 onwards, and in 1928 the principle of the closed circuit was developed in America. The world's first academic chair of anaesthesiology was created in 1941, at Harvard University in the United States, with Henry K. Beecher as its first professor.

10.1.3.5. Postoperative Care, Shock Management and Blood Transfusion

Until far into the 1930s, the papers submitted to the 'Nederlandsche Vereeniging voor Heelkunde' dealt almost exclusively with surgical techniques and case reports.

It was only after operative methods had become more or less standardized that it dawned on surgeons that further improvements had to be sought in the hitherto neglected field of postoperative care. The word 'shock' was probably first uttered at the society's meetings in 1941, when Wamsteker stated that he gave blood transfusions routinely in all thoracotomies as a prevention of this complication. It was only shortly before this time that a reliable method of indirect transfusion of conserved blood became available.

Although the risks had decreased considerably as a result of the discovery of blood groups by Karl Landsteiner in 1900, blood transfusion was not yet a routine procedure in the 'twenties and 'thirties. It was only used in cases of serious loss of blood or chronic anaemia, but its technical implementation, directly from donor to recipient, was laborious and time-consuming (Fig. 123). Surgeons, at least those in

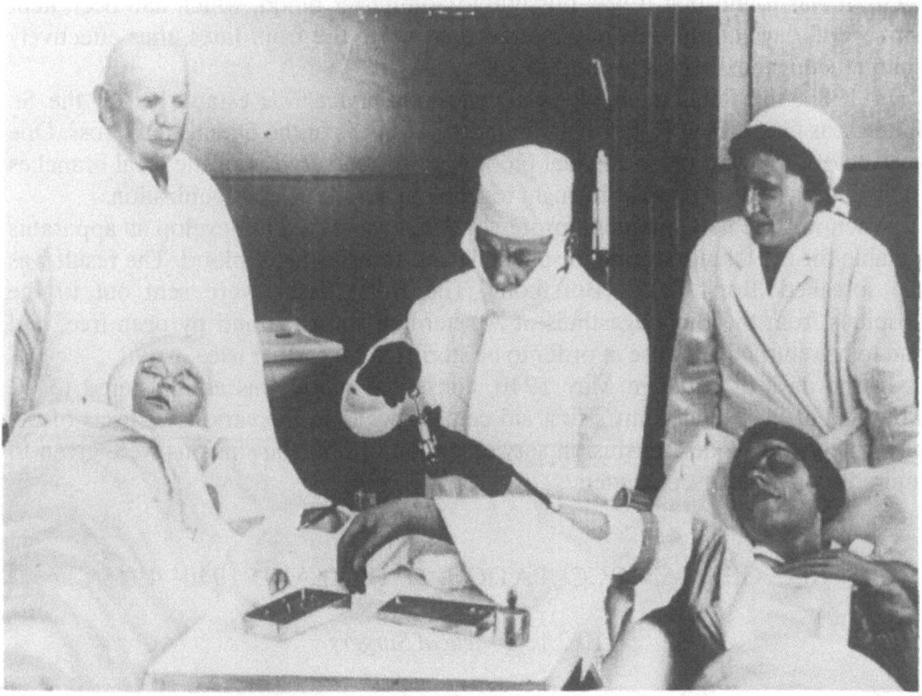

Fig. 123. Direct blood transfusion in 1933, probably in the Westeinde Hospital at The Hague. The transfusion is performed by means of Jubé's apparatus. A nurse acts as donor. Since the donor is a ruddy-complexioned woman whereas the recipient is pale as death, the indication cannot be in doubt.

this country, felt they rarely needed it. The number of publications on this subject which appeared in the *Nederlandsch Tijdschrift voor Geneeskunde* between 1900 and 1930 can be counted on the fingers of two hands.[16]

As late as the 1930s, the management of shock consisted of administering cardiotonics and salt or glucose solutions subcutaneously or intravenously. The well-known Amsterdam professor of internal medicine Jacobus Gerardus Gerbrand Borst (1902—75) took the view that solutions which were to be administered intravenously had to contain large molecules (proteins). He must be credited with having pointed out to Dutch surgeons the life-saving effect of blood transfusions in cases of serious shock.

In 1914 and 1915, the Belgian Albert Hustin, the Argentinian Louis Agote and the American Richard Lewisohn independently discovered that sodium citrate can prevent the coagulation of blood. In principle, this opened the way to improved methods of indirect blood transfusion, but it was only after the introduction of the slow-drip method by Hugh Marriot and Alan Keckwick in 1935 that the indirect method started to oust the direct method. This also made it possible to keep the blood, taken from a donor, in stock for a prolonged period of time, provided it was collected under sterile conditions and stored at 4°C. In 1937 the first 'blood bank' with blood conserved in this manner was established at Cook County Hospital in the United States. At the 'testing ground' of the Spanish Civil War in 1938, it was found that it was possible to administer blood, which had been kept for several days, to the severely injured right up to the front lines, thus effectively counteracting the dreaded 'wound shock'.

In 1930, the first Dutch blood transfusion service was established at the St. Franciscus Gasthuis at Rotterdam, under the auspices of the Dutch Red Cross. One year before the war, the individual blood transfusion services of the local branches of the Dutch Red Cross were brought together in a centralized organization.

When war seemed imminent, professor Borst was asked to develop an apparatus suitable for the taking, storing, dispatching and transfusing of blood. The result was the so-called 'Borst flask' (Borstkolf). The Borst flasks were sent out to the hospitals from the Binnengasthuis at Amsterdam sterilized and pyrogen-free, and had to be returned after use in order to be sterilized for further use.

In the days of battle in May 1940, conserved blood was administered to 22 wounded at the Dutch army's first aid centres, while in the various districts of the now integrated blood transfusion service a total of 650 transfusions were given to injured civilians and servicemen.[17]

10.2. GERMAN OCCUPATION OF HOLLAND 1940—1945

10.2.1. *Practical Surgery*

During the years of the German occupation remarkable changes occurred in the prevalence of surgical diseases. Soon after the beginning of the occupation, the incidence of duodenal ulcer and volvulus of the large intestine started to rise. The number of patients with tuberculous cervical glands also increased sharply, as did that of patients with pulmonary tuberculosis. Anal fissure and strangulated hernia occurred more frequently as well. On the other hand, the number of cases of acute appendicitis and gallstones fell considerably. Thrombosis and pulmonary embolism were hardly encountered any more. These changes were on the one hand presumably related to the increased stress people lived under, on the other to the severely restricted diet.

The circumstances under which surgeons had to work were often far from easy. Many hospital beds had been confiscated by the occupying forces, which meant that more operations had to be performed on an outpatient basis, including even cases of peritonitis and fractures of the femoral neck. Sometimes people who were hiding from the Germans had to be operated on in cellars or attics, without heating or adequate lighting.[18] At the Canisius Hospital in Nijmegen, a city which was in the front line from February 1944 until March 1945, hundreds of war wounded were operated on during that period. After bombing raids, the surgical staff sometimes worked at seven tables simultaneously, under the direction of Carel Hendrik ten Horn (1884—1964), a former associate of Sauerbruch.[19] Blood was administered on a large scale in these operations, while Küntscher's intramedullary nail was used for the first time in the Netherlands during this same period.[20]

10.2.2. *Underground Research*

During the German occupation of Holland, medical research sometimes went underground, especially if the results could be expected to be of practical use in warfare. Thus the 'Delftse Gist- en Spiritusfabrieken' managed, secretly, to produce penicillin and prepare it for practical use.[21]

When it was rumoured that during the Battle of El Alamein, in October 1942, the British had successfully applied dried plasma, equipment for the production of freeze-dried plasma was built at the Central Laboratory of the Red Cross blood transfusion service which was started in all secrecy at the Binnengasthuis in Amsterdam in January, 1943.[22] A large stock of dried plasma was available when on September 17, 1944, British and Polish parachutists carried out their ill-fated airborne landing near Arnhem. During the fierce fighting which ensued, the Allied Forces were supplied with blood plasma by staff of the Amsterdam laboratory, who had crossed the enemy lines.

Of great long-term consequence was the development of the so-called 'artificial kidney', the extracorporeal haemodialysis machine, which was designed and put into clinical use in 1942/3 by Willem Johan Kolff, at that time internist at the relatively small hospital at Kampen.[23]

10.3. SURGERY AFTER THE SECOND WORLD WAR

10.3.1. *General Aspects*

The years after the Second World War were initially characterized by Europe's being scientifically considerably behind the United States. It took a great deal of effort and a number of years for Europe to catch up with that country, but the scientific centre of medicine remained in America.[24] German surgery has now largely lost its leading position in the world.[25]

Since the Second World War, the scope of surgery has enlarged considerably. Like the intestinal suture in the last century, the suture of blood vessels has opened up a whole new territory. During the 1950s the latter technique first went through an experimental phase comparable to that in the early years of the century, but thanks to the introduction of anti-coagulants it could now gain a firm position in operative surgery. This nicely illustrates how surgery came to depend more and more on factors which lie outside the field of surgery proper. On the other hand, the new possibilities of vascular surgery have greatly stimulated the development of the diagnosis of congenital and acquired heart diseases. The history of cardiovascular surgery, with vascular anastomosis as its basis, reveals the most spectacular surgical development of our time, and can be traced in a straight line all the way to the heart transplant carried out by Christiaan Barnard at Cape Town on December 2, 1967. It also made possible the transplantation of other organs, and here again the results are dependent on the non-surgical contributions of anaesthesia, and immunosuppresive and antibiotic drugs. The surgeon, who towards the end of last century had learnt to work in a surgical team, now had to adapt himself to forms of close cooperation with non-surgical disciplines as well.

For the moment, transplantation surgery constitutes the climax of the development of surgery in our century, a development from extirpation to restitution. But before this culminating stage could be reached, the surgeon had to allow physiological and biophysical elements to enter his initially almost purely morphological way of thinking. An illustration of successful assimilation was the development of the pump oxygenator in the 1950s, a development involving many names, in particular those of John H. Gibbon and C. Walton Lillehei.

Another significant contribution was that made by, among others, Henry T. Randall, toward a better understanding of the fluid and electrolyte balance of the 'milieu intérieur' — a result of shock studies during the war. For a while, the state of metabolism following accidents or operations was a cherished theme in experimental surgery. An improved understanding of metabolic processes has led to an effective pre- and postoperative surveillance of the patient (Fig. 124). This form of patient control and especially the further developments in anaesthesia, have made it possible to push age limits upward as well as downward, so that nowadays even very old and very young patients can be submitted to surgery. The cooperation between surgeon and anaesthetist is no longer limited to the work inside the operation theatre, but has expanded beyond it to include resuscitation, which is playing an increasingly important part in modern traumatology. Owing to the growth in motorized traffic, the surgeon has still not been able to bid farewell to his original task, that of wound-healing; in many respects, the polytraumatized patient forms a major problem for modern practical surgery.

10.3.2. *Surgery in the Netherlands After World War II: The American Era*

After this general survey when we take a rapid glance at developments in the Netherlands, it must be said that during the early post-war years, the interest of the Dutch surgeons was mainly technical, just as it had been before the war. In 1946, postoperative treatment, shock management and pathophysiology were still in their initial stages. It was not until the 'fifties that the first Dutch contributions were made in this area, while intensive care units did not become generalised until the late 'sixties.

Thoracic Surgery

In the post-war years, interest in the relatively new area of pulmonary surgery was

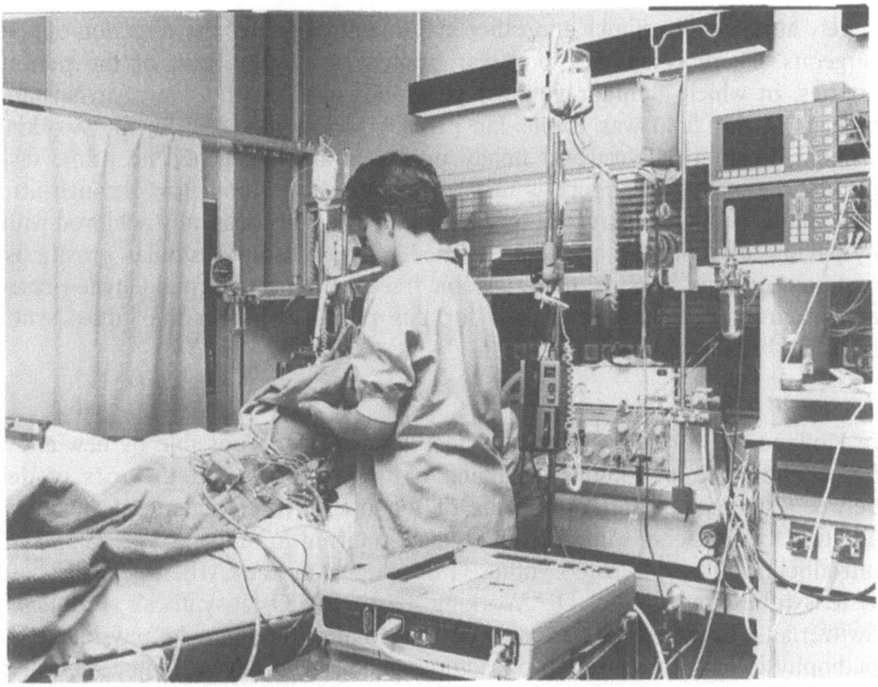

Fig. 124. A department for intensive care, 1986.

taken up especially by the professors Leendert Daniël Eerland (1897—1977) at Groningen and Johannes Franciscus Nuboer (1900—79) at Utrecht. In 1958, Eerland reported on 1447 patients operated on during the period 1943—1957, and the following year Nuboer gave a survey of 1481 resections. In all cases, tuberculosis was the indication. Another important centre of lung surgery was the St. Antonius Ziekenhuis at Utrecht, where Dr. Marie Chrétien Albert Klinkenbergh (1891—1985) headed the department of surgery. At this hospital, and at Eerland's clinic, the foundation was laid for the development of the surgery of the heart and intrathoracic blood vessels in the Netherlands. In 1950 Dr. A. G. Brom, a pupil of Klinkenbergh, became the first Dutch professor with a special chair at Leyden in thoracic surgery. The pump oxygenator came into use at the end of the 1950s. At present most Dutch universities and several other large hospitals have clinics for heart surgery; the demand especially for coronary artery surgery at first greatly exceeded the capacity for treatment. As a result, 'air lifts' were organized, partly at the instigation of the 'Vereniging van Hartpatiënten' (Dutch Association of Heart Patients), which took patients from Holland to heart centres in the United States, Britain and Switzerland. Particularly in the early 'eighties, large numbers of patients have been transported abroad. These air lifts have since been largely discontinued: as a result of the creation of more and more cardio-surgical units, there is at the moment even a tendency towards cardio-surgical overcapacity in this country.

Vascular Surgery

The development of pulmonary, cardiac, and oesophageal surgery has taken place largely at university clinics and other major centres, under the direction of leading surgeons. There is another post-war branch of surgery, that of the peripheral arteries, in which a rather younger generation has led the way. An outstanding pioneer in this field was Emile Jan ('Dick') Moeys (1918—65), first working at Utrecht, later at Tilburg and finally professor at Nijmegen. The prime task of present-day vascular surgery is that of restoring the blood flow through arteries which have become obstructed by atherosclerosis. This is usually achieved with the by-passing or replacing of the obstructed segment using a tubular prosthesis. At first, autogenous venous materials or freeze-dried or formaldehyde-preserved arteries from cadavers were used for this purpose, but in the 'fifties synthetic materials became available.

Treatment of Fractures

In Holland, as in other countries, osteosynthesis, made possible by new alloys — for example the well-known vitallium of the 1930s — led to years of debate between supporters and opponents of the operative treatment of fractures. In addition to Küntscher's intramedullary nail, referred to on page 341, 1958 saw the introduction of 'stable osteosynthesis', developed by the 'Arbeitsgemeinschaft für Osteosynthesefragen' (A. O., Working Party for Osteosynthesis Problems) in Switzerland. Its principles had been developed after fundamental physiological and pathophysiological research into fracture healing, by applying biomechanical laws. In the course of the next ten years or so, clear indications and contraindications for an operative approach have taken shape. New plastic materials have enabled surgeons by the late seventies to supplement nailing methods of treatment of hip fractures, with replacement by prosthetic devices of several types.

Gastrointestinal Surgery

In 1947, Lester Reynold Dragstedt (1893—1975) and associates published their excellent results of section of the vagus nerves to the stomach in the treatment of peptic ulcer in 212 patients; ulcer symptoms had persisted in only five cases, probably due to incomplete division. Dutch surgeons, however, were reluctant to abandon the time-honoured resection, and it was only in the 1970s that selective vagotomy became the preferred method in this country as well.

Modern treatment of ulcerative colitis by colectomy and construction of a permanent ileostomy or ileorectostomy had made its entry twenty years before.

Oncological Surgery

In addition to 'radical' methods in the treatment of carcinoma of the breast, based on Halsted's technique, whether followed by radiotherapy or not, other less drastic operations, combined with radiation treatment, have been introduced in Holland, just as they were elsewhere.[26] It is still a matter of debate on which is the best treatment, and this will inevitably remain so until more is known of the aetiology of cancer. Radiographic mass screening for breast cancer, first undertaken in this country, has been shown to be most worthwhile.

Experimental Surgery

Apart from Zaayer's and Suermondt's animal experiments in the early decades of the present century and a few other examples, experimental surgery was rarely practised in Holland before the Second World War. This was to change rapidly afterwards.

Experimental surgery started at Boerema's clinic in Amsterdam. It was here that it was shown to be possible to interrupt for 10—15 minutes the circulation of a dog in a state of hypothermia, in order to carry out intracardiac operations. With Bigelow in Canada, Boerema (1902—80) was the first to apply this principle in practice; among post-war surgeons he was the one to exhibit the greatest degree of originality, both in the field of experimental and that of operative surgery (Fig. 125).[27]

Organ Transplantation

In 1950, R. Küss and his associates in Paris, and J. E. Murray with colleagues in

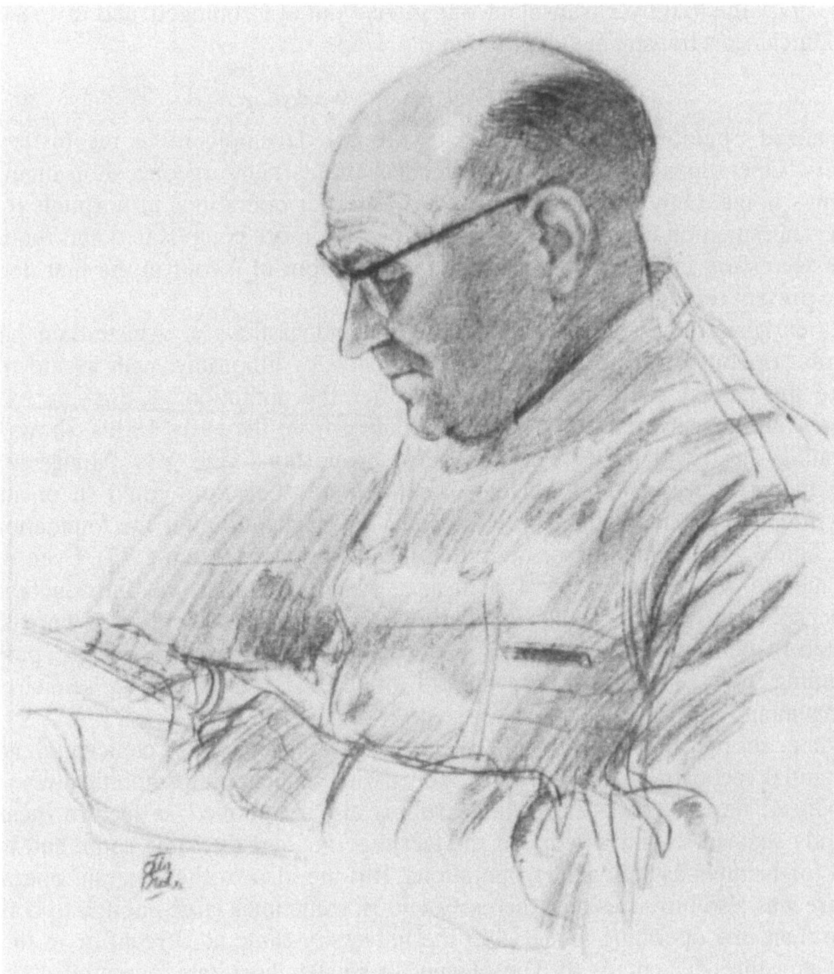

Fig. 125. Professor Ite Boerema.

Boston, transplanted the first kidneys from deceased persons into patients. These operations were technically successful, but the patients then died as a result of the rejection of the foreign organs by their bodies. In Leyden, the first kidney from a living donor was successfully transplanted eleven years later. This meant the start of clinical organ transplants in Holland.[28] In the intervening years, thanks to the work of the English biologist Sir Peter Medawar, and the Australian immunologist Sir Frank M. Burnet, and others, a better insight had been gained into the nature of the immune barrier, and chemical and other immunosuppressants had been developed. Largely at the instigation of Johannes Joseph van Rood, professor of immunohaematology, a wonderful organization was founded at Leyden, under the name of Eurotransplant, which takes charge of the optimal distribution of available cadaver kidneys on a European level. The management of immunological problems of transplantation is continually improving.

In 1979, the first liver transplant was carried out at Groningen, and in 1984 the first Dutch heart transplant at Rotterdam.[29]

10.3.3. *The Surgeon's Workshop*

Specialized operating rooms are a fairly recent development in the history of surgery. Operations used to be performed in the barber-surgeon's shop or in the patient's home. Only the very poor underwent their operations in hospitals (cf. p. 121). This situation changed as operations became more complicated and required more secondary facilities: operations at home fell out of favour in the first decade of the present century.[30]

As early as the eighteenth century, the Binnengasthuis at Amsterdam had a separate operating theatre, intended specifically for lithotomy, with a side room where the patient could stay before and after the operation. A drawing by the Amsterdam artist Christiaan Andriessen, dating from the early 1800s, shows this operating theatre to have been of modest proportions (Fig. 93). Alongside the walls there were ascending benches, on which the spectators could sit or stand. This principle was maintained when in 1834 C. B. Tilanus, after the foundation of the Clinical School, had a new operating theatre installed (see p. 272). Even when this theatre was replaced by a new one, which was after the introduction of antisepsis, the principle of allowing space for spectators was kept up. Whereas the spectator's benches in Dutch hospitals of the last century were in straight, parallel ascending rows, large hospitals abroad often had benches in a semicircular arrangement.

When, shortly after the turn of the century, Dutch university clinics underwent substantial reconstruction, operating rooms with semicircular amphitheatres were introduced here as well. These large rooms also functioned as lecture theatres. Nobody seemed to take offence at the fact that one and the same room had to be used for lectures as well as for operations. But the idea of the separate operating theatre was also introduced in the early 1900s; sometimes large enough to contain more than one operating table, as in the university clinic at Utrecht or in that of the Gemeente Ziekenhuis at The Hague. In smaller hospitals, operating theatres were for a long time to remain very simple in their equipment. Thus the theatre at Tilburg was until the 1920s heated by means of a coal-fired stove, even though the anaesthetic was administered by open drop. Sterilization facilities there were so limited, that the surgeon had to complete his operating programme without changing his one and only sterilized gown and one pair of gloves.[31]

New insights on antisepsis in the early 1900s led to the use of easy-to-clean iron furniture, painted a brilliant white (Fig. 126).[32] Between 1900 and 1910, electric light was introduced.

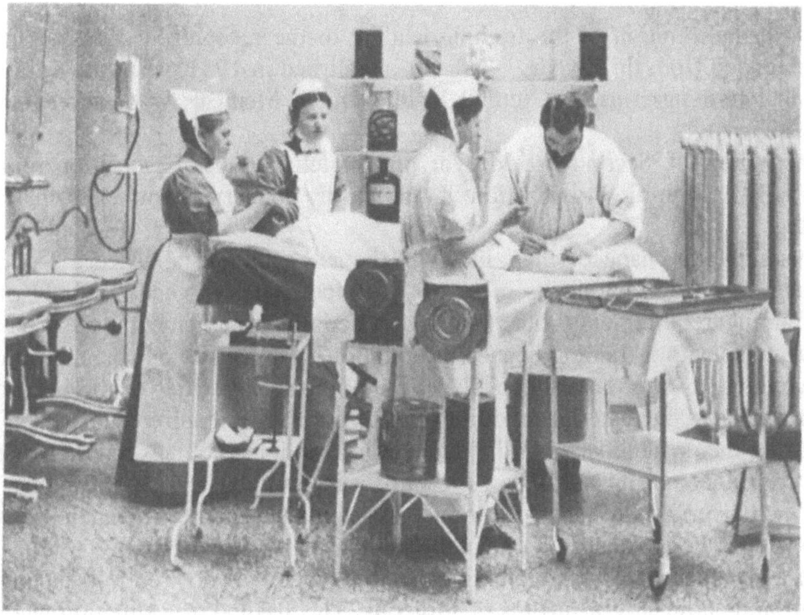

Fig. 126. An operation in the Deaconess Hospital, Utrecht, c. 1907. White furniture, but no masks or gloves.

Further developments in the design of the operating theatre were highly dependent on the antiseptic views of the time, and on the development in anaesthesia.[33] During the second and third decades of this century, the steady rise in the number of operations led to new innovations: the 'twin-set' operating theatre became popular. Wash basins, instrument cases and scalding pans were removed to adjoining rooms, while nitrous oxide apparatus was brought in. Lighting, heating and ventilation steadily underwent technical improvements.

During the post-war years anaesthesia developed very rapidly.[34] One of the results of this advance was the appearance of more and more technical equipment in the operating theatre. Subspecialities demanded, and got, specially designed operating theatres adapted to their particular requirements. Recovery rooms and intensive care units came into being, all liberally provided with a variety of equipment.

A wave of hospital infections which swept the world in the 1950s and 1960s made it clear that technical equipment and antibiotics could not replace the rules of asepsis.

Increasingly, disposable materials have come into use. One no longer sees the once familiar sight of theatre nurses occupying themselves when no operation was in progress, in a room set aside for that purpose, with the cleaning of gloves, the checking of them by means of inflation, the repairing and powdering of them, and in the folding of a seemingly endless supply of pieces of gauze.

10.3.4. *Training*[35]

In 1948, the duration of the training leading to the recognized status of surgeon was extended from three years — a term established in 1931, when the duration of specialist trainings was first settled by the Dutch Medical Association — to six years.

Until after the Second World War, the Dutch Surgical Association remained essentially a scientific organization: it was hardly concerned with such matters as training.

This situation changed when, in 1948, the association established a 'Concilium Chirurgicum' from among its members. This council has since not only drafted the training requirements, but also supervised their implementation in surgical departments with a training licence. In addition to university clinics, these include departments in other large hospitals where both the capacities of the head of the department and the material conditions meet a number of requirements.

During the ensuing years, individual surgical training courses have increasingly been coordinated. Thus 1974 saw the start of institutionalized basic training, to be given by university clinics, for all trainee assistants in a particular region, including those who wished to qualify in one of the surgical sub-disciplines.

As a result of too much training capacity, which was not reduced in time, the Netherlands now have a surplus of surgeons. This has led to a situation where the individual heads of departments qualified to train prospective surgeons are no longer free to decide how many and which young doctors they will accept for training. A national committee now selects a number of doctors from among the applicants each year, maintaining a strict numerus clausus, and assigns them to the various training clinics.

10.3.5. *Nederlandse Vereniging tot Bevordering der Chirurgische Wetenschappen* (Dutch Society for the Advancement of Surgical Sciences)[36]

In order to raise the scientific level of surgical disciplines, the societies for general surgery, orthopaedics, urology, neurosurgery, and later also those for thoracic surgery and others, joined forces in 1947 to form the 'Nederlandse Vereniging tot Bevordering der Chirurgische Wetenschappen', later renamed 'Collegium Chirurgicum Neerlandicum'. Within this coordinating institution, each of the affiliated associations was to retain its independance, but had to contribute to the common purpose for which it had been set up. This aim was pursued by means of regular conferences on themes of general interest to all surgeons, whatever their specialties, and by the publication of a common journal in the English language, the *Archivum Chirurgicum Neerlandicum*.[37] In 1980, the name of this journal, published since 1949, was changed to *Netherlands Journal of Surgery*. However, since 1957 this is no longer a publication of the 'Nederlandse Vereniging tot Bevordering der Chirurgische Wetenschappen', but is subsidized exclusively by the 'Nederlandse Vereniging voor Heelkunde' (Dutch Surgical Society).

10.3.6. *Surgical Subspecialties*[38]

The steady increase in the practical possibilities for operative treatment stimulates the development of 'subspecialties', whether officially recognized or not. Although on the one hand this fragmentation is a regrettable development, it should be recognized on the other hand that it is precisely this specialised interest which has made the recent progress in surgery possible. But the sense of fellowship between the various surgical disciplines is gradually weakening, as each of them engages in close cooperation with the corresponding subdiscipline of internal medicine, just as neurosurgery and neurology did before the war. Major specialties dissolve into multi-disciplinary organ specialities, and the traditional dinstinction between medicine and surgery is progressively blurred.

During the last few decades of the previous century, some of the now familiar surgical specialties were beginning to take shape. Thus the 'Nederlandsche Gynaecologische Vereeniging' (Dutch Gynaecological Society) was founded as early as 1887, while the 'Nederlandsche Orthopaedische Vereeniging, vereeniging van artsen ter beoefening van orthopaedie, mechanotherapie, geneeskundige gymnastiek en massage' (Dutch Orthopaedic Society, a society of physicians for the practice of orthopaedics, mechanotherapy, remedial gymnastics and massage) dates from 1898. The latter society, however, only began to flourish after 1909, and the first professor of this subject — Dr. G. M. San Giorgi (1910—69) — was not appointed until 1962, at Nijmegen. Defining the spheres of activity of orthopaedics and surgery has led to a good deal of friction, especially after the Second World War. The main problem was which of these specialties should be entrusted with the treatment of fractures. Unlike the situation in many other countries, where the treatment of fractures has been laid entirely in the hands of the orthopaedist, this area is in the Netherlands covered by both orthopaedic and general surgeons. It was not until after World War II that the orthopaedist as an independent specialist managed to earn himself a place on the medical staff of Dutch hospitals.

The same is true for urology, although a 'Vereeniging voor Urologie' (Urological Society) was founded as early as 1908. Just as in the case of the orthopaedic society, it counted several general surgeons among its membership. In 1906 and 1910, unsalaried lectureships for urology were created in Amsterdam and Leyden, but nearly half a century was to pass before academic teaching in this discipline was resumed. Chairs of urology were not created until 1965. The first chair in Holland, that at Nijmegen was held by Dr. W. A. Moonen, that at Leyden shortly afterwards by Dr. P. J. Donker. The introduction, after the Second World War, of the resectoscope, a device which can only be used after special training, contributed a great deal to the growth of urology toward its independence.

Neurosurgery in the Netherlands originated in the 1920s and 1930s. The first neurosurgeons were initially general surgeons, who specialized not only in its typical technical aspects, but also in neuropathology and diagnosis. On the other hand there were also neurologists who started to operate themselves. It may therefore be said that this specialist interest stems both from neurology and from surgery. The oldest departments of neurosurgery in the Netherlands were founded in cooperation with neurological clinics, the first one in 1929 at the Wilhelmina Gasthuis in Amsterdam. The 'Nederlandse Vereniging voor Neurochirurgen' (Dutch Neurosurgical Society) was founded in 1952, although a study group for neurosurgery had existed since 1937, and is still active today. In 1955 the first chair in neurosurgery was established at Groningen; it was held by Dr. C. H. Lenshoek (1902—69).

Plastic surgery was not recognized as an independent subspecialty in Holland until 1950. Yet one of the pioneers of modern plastic and reconstructive surgery was a Dutchman, Jan Esser, whose biography has been briefly sketched on page 328. Esser, however, worked outside his native country all his life.

The first specialists in this field to work inside the Netherlands had received their training in England, where during World War II a great deal of experience had been gained in the treatment of burns and frostbite, injuries especially common in members of the Royal Air Force. For years afterwards, a one to two years in-service training in a foreign clinic was required for the completion of one's specialist training. In 1962, Dr. C. A. Honig became the first university lecturer in the new discipline, at Utrecht.

As was discussed above, thoracic surgery was started in this country in the 1930s. The 'Nederlandse Vereniging voor Thoraxchirurgie' (Dutch Society for Thorax Surgery) was founded in 1947. Initially, its members were general surgeons. But as increasingly specialized knowledge and experience came to be required, especially for heart surgery, this became less and less compatible with the practice of general surgery. Hence, it was deemed useful to raise the status of heart surgery to that of an independent subspecialty. Since it was feared that revenues from heart surgery alone might not provide a reasonable income, its practitioners also made a claim to pulmonary surgery, so that the new subspecialty was established in 1973 as cardiopulmonary surgery.

Presumably, future historiographers will consider the period 1950—1970 to have been just as revolutionary as the years following the introduction of antisepsis in the last century.

10.4. EPILOGUE

We have now come to the end of our long journey through Time, a journey in which we have covered some 2500 years of surgical tradition. The last six centuries were travelled mainly through a Dutch timescape but with glimpses from Italy, France, Germany, Britain and America. That 'scape was basically similar, though its colours were often fainter, rarely brighter, than abroad. We came to see the common history of Western surgery in its foundations and practical elaboration, where even the social position of its practitioners through the centuries has been comparable; perchance now one country or even one city took

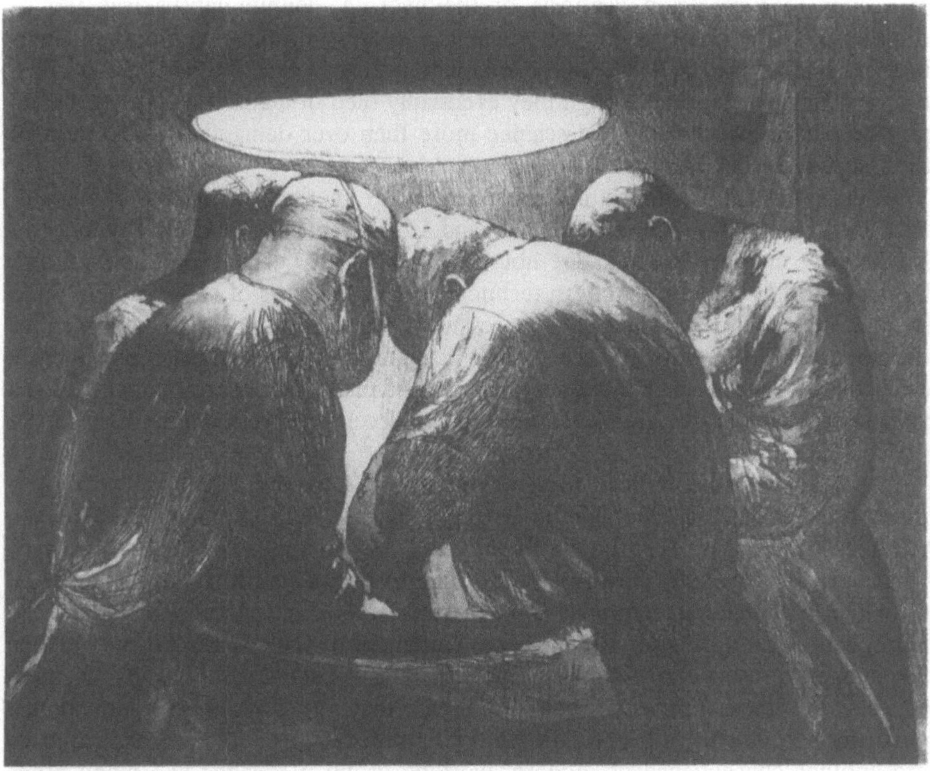

Fig. 127. Operative surgery, 1959.

the lead and then again another. As Goethe put it: 'Die Geschichte der Wissenschaften ist eine grosse Fuge, in der die Stimmen der Völker nach und nach zum Vorschein kommen'.[39]

The general character of surgery remained by and large the same all through the ages, until Joseph Lister by his introduction of the antiseptic wound treatment brought about its First Great Revolution. Surgery, until then primarily occupied with the treatment of wounds and fractures, was then to enter on the epoch of extirpation, which ended with no organ being able to resist the surgeon's determination to excise. Great was the reaping, with which the social position of the surgeon rose concomitantly. Jürgen Thorwald spoke of 'Das Jahrhundert der Chirurgen'.

And yet, twentieth century surgery has by no means been an uninterrupted triumph. Numerous operations have been attempted, used for a period, and then abandoned. Examples are Von Eiselsberg's unilateral exclusion of the pylorus, gastrorraphy as a treatment of gastroptosis, nephropexy to fix a floating kidney, or decapsulation of this organ in cases of chronic nephritis and eclampsia, implantation of fatty tissue in the brain to treat epilepsy resulting from scar formation, sympathectomy against essential hypertension, ligation of the mammary artery or cardio-omentopexy in angina pectoris, or Talma's operation in cases of ascites resulting from cirrhosis of the liver. A definite lapsus was the — translumbar — hemicorporectomy, which was 'successfully' carried out a few times in the United States in 1962 and 1964: successfully in that the patients survived the gruesome operation although they eventually died of metastases. The technical possibilities of modern medical science more than ever demand consideration of the associated ethical problems.[40]

In the early 1960s surgery has entered into yet another epoch, that of Restitution. Defective parts or even whole organs are now being replaced. This Second Revolution, unlike the First, did not have its primary origins in surgery itself, but was brought about by modern technology using all sorts of new synthetics and by the introduction of immunosuppressive drugs. This illustrates that further developments in operative surgery have become largely dependent upon factors other than the surgeons, although such further refinements of surgical technique as microsurgery have also greatly contributed to recent progress, particularly in the surgical subspecialties.

Recent developments have forced the surgeon into now becoming more and more a participant in therapeutic working parties. This is exemplified in the treatment of cancer. For the past ten years, the treatment of malignancies of whatever type is usually performed according to protocols which have often been drawn up in regional, national or even international consultations, e.g. in the European Organization for Research on Treatment of Cancer. Besides its obvious advantages, protocol medicine, so typical of the 1980s, also has its negative aspects, the most important being the fact that the physician in attendance delegates a large part of his responsibility to a schedule. Randomized clinical trials are another consequence of modern 'working group medicine': like many other recent developments in medicine it may raise ethical questions which are not always easy to answer.

One of the distinguishing features of the Second Surgical Revolution which started between the 1950s and the 1970s, is the ever-mounting cost. At first this did not seem to matter, but now we are gathering the bitter fruits of these two decades of prosperity. There are at present too many medical faculties in this country, too many hospital beds and too many surgeons. Unlike the eighteenth century, modern unemployed surgeons cannot fall back on their barber shops as they once had been able to do in Amsterdam. It would perhaps have been better if we had never given up barbering!

Notes and References

CHAPTER I: THE ROOTS OF WESTERN SURGERY

[1] Since the Middle Ages and the Renaissance, when Latin translations of classical medical texts became available, these are usually referred to by their Latin title. For an annotated English version of 'On ulcers' see *The genuine works of Hippocrates* transl. by Adams, vol. 2, pp. 789—809.
[2] 'But every person acquainted with practice is aware that a healthy suppuration is one of the best means of preventing inflammation', was Adams' personal comment. *Hippocrates*. Ed. Adams, p. 795, n. 1.
[3] Hippocrates was slightly more explicit in the treatise *On wounds in the head*, where he understood by inflammation a sort of fever occurring in the flesh which becomes full of burning heat. Ed. Jones, vol. 3, p. 37.
[4] See e.g. 'Prognostic' in *Hippocrates*. Ed. Jones, vol. 2, p. 19. Hippocrates' description, of course, reminds us of the current expression 'pus bonum et laudabile'. Its precise source is unknown, but it may be connected with the Italian surgeon Nicolaus Florentinus (d approx. 1411) who stated: 'Dividitur autem sanies — pus — in saniem laudabilem et bonam et illaudabilem et malam'. Gurlt, *Gesch. Chir.*, vol. 1, p. 825.
[5] A cataplasma or emplastrum — plaster in English — is an external, solid glutinous medicament which softens with the heat of the skin and which sticks to the part of the body to which it is applied. Up till the 19th century, such medicated poultices were in common use, as appears from the numerous prescriptions which occur in surgical literature.
[6] Gurlt: *Gesch. Chir.*, vol. 1, p. 245.
[7] *Hippocrates*. Ed. Jones, vol. 4, p. 25.
[8] Rubin Pinault: 'How Hippocrates cured the plague'.
[9] *Hippocrates*. Ed. Adams, vol. 1, pp. 423—66; Ed. Jones, vol. 3, 1—51.
[10] The existence of the fracture by contrecoup was a moot point far into the 19th century.
[11] *Hippocrates*. Ed. Jones, vol. 3, p. 43. Since no trepans from Graeco—Roman times seem to have survived and Hippocrates does not describe them, we have only a vague idea of what they looked like. They were probably instruments of two types. One, like the modern trephine having a crosswise handle for turning, the other modelled after the carpenter's augur, turned around by a bow the cord of which encompasses the stem. The head could be pointed as in the perforating trepan, or — even in Hippocrates' days — carry a sharp-toothed crown.
[12] *De affectionibus*, Hippocrates, Ed. Littré vol. 6, p. 215; *De morbis II*. Ed. Littré vol. 7, p. 47.
[13] *De affectionibus internis*. Ed. Littré, vol. 7, p. 227.
[14] *De Morbis I*. Ed. Littré, vol. 6, p. 151; *De Morbis II*. Ed. Littré, vol. 7, pp. 93—5, 153.
[15] Prognostic. Ed. Jones, vol. 2, p. 35.
[16] *De affectionibus*. Ed. Littré, vol. 6, p. 233.
[17] *Prognostic*. Ed. Jones, vol. 2, p. 9.
[18] *Airs, waters, places*. Ed. Jones, vol. 1, pp. 95—7.
[19] *The oath*. Ed. Jones, vol. 1, p. 299.
[20] *Epidemics II*. Ed. Littré, vol. 5, p. 83.
[21] *On fractures, On joints*. Ed. Jones, vol. 3, pp. 95—397. Around 1870 Petrequin, who provided a French translation of the surgical writings of Hippocrates, stated that he considered 'Hippocrates, as far as fractures and dislocations of the lower arm are concerned, to be more complete than Boyer, and as far as congenital dislocations are concerned, richer than Dupuytren'. Littré called *On Fractures* and *On Joints* 'the greatest surgical monument from Antiquity'.

22 *Mochlikon*. Ed. Jones, vol. 3, pp. 399—449.
23 *On Joints*. Ed. Jones, vol. 3, p. 349.
24 *In the surgery*. Ed. Jones, vol. 3, pp. 63—73.
25 *Aphorisms*, VI, 38. Ed. Jones, vol. 4, p. 189.
26 *De Morbis*. Ed. Littré, vol. 6, p. 151.
27 Choulant: *Handbuch der Bücherkunde*, lists on pp. 33—34 six different 17th-century editions.
28 Van Gesscher: *De heelkunde van Hippocrates*. Amsterdam: J. B. Elwe, 1790—92. *Die Wundarzneikunst des Hippocrates*. Leipzig: E. Fleischer, 1795.
29 An inventory of references and the fragments is provided by M Michler: *Die alexandrinischen Chirurgen*.
30 Daremberg: 'De Paul d'Egine et des médecins compilateurs dans le Bas-Empire'. In his: *La médecine*, pp. 99—122.
31 *Celsus*. Ed. Spencer, vol. 2, pp. 2—175; vol. 3, pp. 294—471.
32 *Op. cit*., vol. 2, pp. 67—129.
33 *Op. cit*., vol. 2, p. 79. His well-known description of the inflammation with the symptoms 'rubor et tumor cum calore et dolore', however, is to be found in Book III, which is not discussed here.
34 *Op. cit*., vol. 3, p. 405.
35 By 'dietetics' the Ancients understood more than merely a regulation of diet: rather it comprised an entire health regimen.
36 Adapted from Spencer's translation: *Op. cit*., vol. 3, p. 295.
37 Spencer's translation. The surgeon who, although filled with pity, elegantly cuts and burns his patient, whilst deaf to his cries and curses during the performance of the task, was taken as an example by the Church Fathers. Saint John Chrysostom, patriarch of Constantinople in the 4th century, explains that treatment of the soul although this too is beneficial, can also be a painful event. Frings: *Medizin u Arzt bei den griechischen Kirchenvätern*, p. 75.
38 By means of the table of contents of Spencer's edition the interested reader will have no difficulty in finding on pp. 294—471 in Celsus the subjects shortly referred to here.
39 Vesalius was the first to describe the thyroid gland in 1543: *De humani corporis fabrica*. Lib. II, c. 22; Lib. VI, c. 4.
40 The significance of the Latin word 'hernia' is unknown. Celsus only states that it is an improper but commonly used designation.
41 '. . . but since a doubtful hope is preferable to certain despair . . .'.
42 Plutarch relates as a curious example of self-control how the consul Marius let himself be operated on for varicose veins while standing up, without having been bound. He refused, however, to have the other leg undergo similar treatment since whatever the improvement, it was not worth the pain. *Plutarch's Lives*. Ed. Perrin, vol. 9, p. 476.
43 See Temkin: *Galenism* for an excellent survey of this subject.
44 Setaceum or seton (Du: fontanel or etterdracht): a strip of woven material or a thick thread introduced subcutaneously or if needs be right through a pathologic process by way of two small stab incisions. The ends are left hanging out of the puncture track to allow the escape of issue.

Vesicatory or issue (Du: etterblaar): artificial blister brought about by the application of a vesicant after removal of the epidermis.

45 Paulus Aeginata: *The seven books*, transl. Adams, vol. 2, pp. 52—3, 64, 68—69, 81, 84, 85.
46 Here we come across a viewpoint which remained current far into the 19th century. An eruption ('uitslag') is an accumulation of morbid matter in and underneath the skin. With the treatment of complaints which are characterized by lesions of the skin one should beware that the morbid matter is not driven inward because it is then that the situation becomes really dangerous.
47 Neuburger: *Gesch. Med*., vol. 1, p. 395. We really come across revulsion and derivation as apparently current notions in Hippocrates, e.g. in *Epidemics VI*, Ed. Littré, vol. 5, p. 277.
48 For Galen's place in Hellenistic surgery, see Michler: *Das Spezialisierungsproblem*, pp. 50—62.
49 *Galen*. Ed. Kühn, vol. 10, pp. 1—1021.
50 Aretaeus: *The extant works*. transl. Adams, p. 306.
51 Walsh: 'Galen's writings', gives a picture of Galen's own surgical activities.
52 Galen appears only to know of the traumatic aneurysm. His therapy of this dangerous affliction is a conservative one.
53 In the Middle Ages the word 'apostema' was often used for a pathological swelling of any kind.
54 Oribasius, an alumnus of the medical school of Alexandria, was court physician to the Byzantine emperor Julian the Apostate. His extensive medical compilation, in which he accorded a very prominent place to Galen, contributed to the latter's later stature as the authority in the field of medicine. Neuburger: *Gesch. Med*., vol. 2, p. 48.
55 *Paulus Aegineta*, transl. Adams, vol. 2, pp. 247—511. By means of Adams' table of contents the interested reader may easily find the subjects referred to in our text.

[56] The first medical author who clearly distinguished the true from the false variety of aneurysms was probably Antyllus, an outstanding surgeon in Roman imperial times (fl. 140 AD). Only fragments of his published works have been preserved. De Moulin: 'Aneurysms in Antiquity'.
[57] Adams gives in his commentary a fine summary of the technique of the lithotomy of the classical writers and of the Arabians. *Paulus Aegineta*, vol. 2, pp. 356–63.
[58] Homer: *Iliad*, XI, 514–15.
[59] Temkin: 'Byzantine medicine'. In: *The double face of Janus*, pp. 202–24.
[60] *Isagoge Johanitii ad tegni Galeni*. Neuburger: *Gesch. Med.*, vol. 2, pp. 149, 204, 459.
[61] Ten Doeschate: 'Rolduc als Middeleeuwse voorpost', p. 133. Pp. 133–9 contain a brief summary.
[62] Hippocrates, Galen, Oribasius, Aëtius, Paul. Neuburger: *Gesch. Med.*, vol. 2, p. 170.
[63] Charles of Anjou was a cultured monarch who employed a staff of translators, scribes, illuminators and bookbinders. Fischer: 'Moses of Palermo'.
[64] The 'Ad regem Mansorem libri' is in Latin transl. by Gerard of Cremona included in the volume *Abubetri Rhazae Maomethi opera exquisitiora* . . . Basiliae: in officina H. Petri, 1544 [Repr. Bruxelles: Culture et Civilisation, 1973].
[65] Gurlt: *Gesch. Chir.*, vol. 1, pp. 670–2. Modern editions of the surgical part: J. Pagel: Eine bisher unveröffentlichte lateinische Version der Chirurgie der Pantegni . . . Latin text only. *Langenb. Arch. klin. Chir.* **81**: 733–86, 1906. M. T. Malato, L. Loria: Chirurgia. Costantino l'Africano. Lat. text with Italian transl., *Pagine di Storia della Scienza e della Tecnica* **13**: 61–211, 1960.
[66] The famous story of the clever slave girl named Tawaddud in *The Arabian Nights*, who astonishes an assembly of scholars by her extensive knowledge of medicine and other scientific disciplines, could not have been written if the author had lacked an accurate knowledge of Avicenna. Kirchmair: 'Die kluge Sklavin Tawaddud'. The discussion centred on anatomy, physiology and health sciences, surgery was not referred to.
[67] Choulant: *Handbuch der Bücherkunde*, pp. 362–6.
[68] There exists no complete edition of the *Canon* in any of the modern languages. A reprint of the Venice edition of 1507 was published in 1972. (Bruxelles: Culture et Civilisation).
[69] *Albucasis*. Ed. Spink and Lewis, pp. 346–61.
[70] Brief summaries in Gurlt: *Gesch. Chir.*, vol. 1, pp. 659–60 and in Neuburger: *Gesch. Med.*, vol. 2, pp. 186 and 220–1.
[71] *Albucasis*. Ed. Spink and Lewis, p. 528. He does not explain how to distinguish between wounds that have been altered by the air and those that have not.
[72] Probably only the diaphysis.
[73] Urology is the subject of a separate work by Rhazes, of which an Arabic manuscript is in the collection of the library of Leyden University. A French translation, which is accompanied by the Arabic text was published by P. de Koning: *Traité sur le calcul* . . . par Abū Bakr Muhammad Ibn Zakarīya ar-Rāzī. Leyden, 1896.

CHAPTER 2: THE WESTERN MIDDLE AGES

[1] Pirenne: *De Middeleeuwen*, Introduction, Ch. 1–3.
[2] Neuburger: *Gesch. Med.*, vol. 2, pp. 241–78: Die Medizin im frühen Mittelalter.
[3] See Beccaria A: *I codici di medicina del periodo presalernitano*. Roma: Ed. di Storia e Letteratura, 1956, for a survey of the 9th through the 11th centuries. Beccaria's study did not involve the codices held by libraries in Spain.
[4] Most of the translations which appeared from the 5th through the 7th centuries probably originated in Sicily.
[5] For a more detailed analysis I refer to my *Heelkunde in de vroege Middeleeuwen*, pp. 23–109.
[6] De Moulin: *Op. cit.*, 120–5.
[7] Dioscorides (1st cent. AD) is the author of the oldest textbook of pharmacology that has been preserved; Caius Plinius Secundus, who lived in the same century, wrote a large encyclopaedia.
[8] One of the tales in Bocaccio's *Decameron*, which was written between 1348 and 1358, is about a surgeon who prepared a narcotic potion the day before he was to perform an operation. This medicine was swallowed by mistake by his wife's lover, who thereupon lost consciousness. Readers who are interested in how the story ends are referred to the ninth novel of the fourth day in the book mentioned above.
[9] Cockayne: *Leechdoms*, vol. 2, pp. 83–7. For surgery in Anglo-Saxon times see also: Bonner: *Medical background of Anglo-Saxon England*, pp. 98–108.

[10] Sudhoff: 'Salerno'. Baader: 'Die Schule von Salerno'.
[11] Constantine's translations did not appear in print until the 16th century.
[12] Corner: 'Bamberg surgery'.
[13] The Hague Royal Libr. Ms 78 C 27, ff. 91r—140r.
[14] The extremely valuable *Ars chirurgica*, which first appeared in Venice in 1498, and which was afterwards reprinted by various publishers at least five times, contains in one volume writings of Guy de Chauliac, Roland, Bruno, Theoderic, Lanfranc, William of Saliceto. The contents of the various editions may differ slightly: William of Saliceto did not appear in this collection until the fifth and last edition in 1546. Roger and the Four Masters have been reprinted by ES de Renzi: *Collectio salernitana . . .*, 5 vols. Napoli: Filiatre-Sebezio, 1852—59 [Reprint Bologna: Forni, 1967], vol. 2, pp. 426—96 (*Rogerii . . . chirurgia*, in Roland's adaptation derived from *Ars chirurgica*. Venetiis: apud Iuntas, 1546), pp. 497—724 (*Glossulae Quatuor Magistrorum super chirurgiam Rogerii et Rolandi*, edited by Ch. Daremberg). Vol. 4 contains an adaptation of Roger and the Four Masters in Latin verse, edited by Daremberg (pp. 39—176).
[15] Gurlt: *Gesch. Chir.*, vol. 1, pp. 704—20.
[16] The surgeons of the school of Salerno were the first since Antiquity to illuminate their texts with illustrative case-histories.
[17] The popular superstition that sexual abstinence is a prerequisite for the successful performance of certain activities derives from pre-Christian times, but was still alive in the Middle Ages, not only in Italy, but in Germany and possibly elsewhere in Europe as well. It is expressed in *Jonghe Lanfranc*, cf. p. 63. The use of garlic etc. allegedly poisoned the breath so that the wound might start to putrify. While both these ideas have a magical origin, the prescription to be sober — which is often mentioned expressis verbis — and to wash one's hands are of a more practical nature, even though they conform to the idea of cleanliness, with which one liked to associate the surgeon. Eis: 'Kultische Keuschheit'.
[18] See e.g. Neuburger: *Gesch. Med.*, vol. 2, p. 306. This view may have taken root as a result of the division which Guy de Chauliac made in the surgeons of his day, based on their methods of wound treatment. See summary on p. 54.
[19] Red powder is part of the Galenic—Arabic tradition, see pp. 19 and 31; it was used by many mediaeval — and later — surgeons, albeit not always with exactly the same composition. Bolus armenicus, mastic, incense, were its usual components. Other dessicating and astringent simples which were traditionally used for the treatment of wounds are Graecian pitch, mummia, the fur of hare very finely cut, roasted nut shells and others. Dragon's blood — the resin of fruit of the palm Daemonorops which gave the powder its red colour — seems to be an Arabic addition: Albucasis: *On surgery* (Ed. Spink and Lewis, p. 528).
[20] Vienna, Österreich Nat. Bibl. 2818, ff. 156r—200v.
[21] Gurlt: *Gesch. Chir.*, vol. 1, pp. 726—40.
[22] I have not been able to trace the origin of this current tripartition which also occurs in Theodoric, Lanfranc, Mondeville, Chauliac. The pseuso-Galenic *Introductio s medicus* only mentions 'synthesis' and 'diaeresis' as the basic proceedings. As late as 1748 we meet a surgical tripartion, albeit a dissimilar one, in the frontispiece of Scultetus *Armamentarium*, see Fig. 84.
[23] The treatment of lacerated wounds with suppurative medicaments, already recommended by Hippocrates, was the rule until the introduction of antisepsis.
[24] Real surnames were still unknown at that time. Thus, often the city or even the country of origin functions as such, sometimes the person's profession.
[25] Gurlt: *Gesch. Chir.*, vol. 1, p. 742.
[26] Cf. note 14. The modern English transl. provided by Campbell and Colton has an unsatisfactory introduction.
[27] Campbell, Colton: *Surgery of Theoderic*, vol. 1, pp. 16, 49, 54, 138.
[28] Galen *Methodus medendi*, bk. 4, ch. 5 (Ed. Kuhn vol. 10, p. 278). This principle can actually be traced back to Hippocrates, see page 3.
[29] In anatomical representations of that time the brains are shown with three cavities located behind one another: the cellula fantastica, the cellula rationalis and the cellula memorialis. In these were located respectively imagination, logical reasoning and memory.
[30] Galen reported a similar occurrence. See Gurlt: *Gesch. Chir.*, vol. 1, p. 436.
[31] Campbell, Colton: *Surgery of Theoderic*, vol. 2, p. 11.
[32] *Fasciculus medicine houdende in hem dese navolghende tractaten*. . . Een alder-excellenste ende expertse anothomie van meester Mondinus (Fascicle of medicine containing the following tracts . . . a most excellent and expert anatomy by Master Mondinus). Antwerp: C. die Grave, 1512, ff. lxllv—cir. This compilation is a translation by a certain Petrus Antonianus of *Fasciculus medicinae Joannis de Ketham*. Venetiis: Di Gregori, 1491. Johannes de Ketham was a German physician living in Italy. Van Dongen: 'Incunabelen' VIII, *Med. Contact* **20**: 448—50, 1965.

[33] It is said that the Church opposed the development of anatomy by prohibiting the dissection of human cadavers. The papal bull *De sepulturis* of 1300 which is usually quoted in this connection, only opposed the habit, which had originated during the Crusades, of cutting up and boiling persons who had died a long way from home, to facilitate transportation of the bones to their native country. Neuburger: *Gesch. Med.*, vol. 2, p. 432.
[34] Neuburger: *Op. cit.*, vol. 2, p. 384.
[35] Talbot: *Medicine in medieval England*, p. 55.
[36] Elaut: 'Ecclesia abhorret a sanguine'.
[37] Fabbri: 'Della litotomia antica'.
[38] Nicaise: *Guy de Chauliac*, pp. LIV—LVII.
[39] Many surgeons' guilds in the Netherlands have also been named after Cosmas and Damian. The fact that the holy twins successfully conducted a leg transplant, is likely to have been the basis for that. Together the two brothers, one of whom was allegedly the physician and the other the surgeon, symbolize the indivisibility of medicine. Lanfranc, who was himself both a physician and a surgeon, strongly advocated this indivisibility.
[40] Nicaise: *Guy de Chauliac*, p. LXIV. While in the 14th century there existed, at least in Paris, qualified female surgeons, they had all but vanished by the 16th century.
[41] Gurlt: *Gesch. Chir.*, vol. 1, 765—6.
[42] Keil, Müller: 'Deutsche Lanfrank-Übersetzungen'.
[43] Their reference numbers are: Univ. Libr. Amsterdam MG 11 F39; Univ. Libr. Ghent 1272; Univ. Libr. Uppsala Kod Waller 132; Darmstadt Hess Landes- u. Hochschulbibl. ZU 2201; Cologne Stadtarchiv GB Kasten A 57; Cologne Univ. u. Stadbibl. S 9; London Brit. Libr. Harley 1648, fol. 140r (I owe these references to professor R. Jansen-Sieben in Brussels).
[44] London Brit. Libr. Harley 1648, fol. 105r—126v; Paris Bibl Arsenal 8216, fol. 59v—73v. *Chyrurgie meester Lanfrancks van Meylanen*. Leuven: Conrad Braem, 1481; *Idem*, Antwerpen: Willem Vorsterman, 1529.
[45] Gurlt: *Gesch. Chir.*, vol. 1, pp. 766—90.
[46] The last three subjects together form the trivium, the threefold way which leads to wisdom, part of the seven Liberal Arts, which since Antiquity formed the curriculum of secondary education and the preliminary course of higher education. The *Artes liberales* consisted of the 'trivium' — grammar, logic, rhetoric — and the 'quadrivium' — arithmetic, geometry, astronomy, music.
[47] This type of deontological advice which, starting with Bruno, we come across in most mediaeval surgical treatises, is most probably derived from *The guide for doctors* by the Egyptian oculist Isaac Judaeus (d. 932) which was instrumental in the shaping of mediaeval medicine. Neuburger: *Gesch. Med.*, vol. 2, pp. 176—7.
[48] Lanfranc apparently aims at recovery by first intention. It is by no means always clear from the writings of the mediaeval surgeons whether by means of their wound suture they aimed at primary wound healing, or at reduction of the wound.
[49] Dulieu: *La chirurgie à Montpellier*, pp. 17—32.
[50] Apart from doctors, there also existed since the Middle Ages baccalaureates and licentiates of medicine. A baccalaureate could be obtained after two to three years of university training by taking an examination. The licentiate's examination preceded that for the doctorate, and entitled the holder to practise medicine. Graduates in a medical faculty initially received the title of 'magister', so one occasionally comes across 'masters of medicine', who should however not be confused with the qualified surgeons. Neuburger: *Gesch. Med.*, vol. 2, pp. 346—7. In the 19th century, graduates from the Clinical Schools in Holland were sometimes also called 'geneesmeesters': masters of medicine.
[51] Brit. Libr. Cotton Galba E XIII, 151 parchment leaves.
[52] It is not clear why that obviously popular work never appeared in a Renaissance edition.
[53] As late as 1676 the 'anatomico-chirurgicus' C. van de Voorde used an analogous expression, when he wrote in his *Lichtende Fakkel der Chirurgie* that the surgeon should know the human body as the sculptor knows his wood or stone.
[54] Probst: 'Der Weg des ärtzlichen Erkennens'.
[55] Mondeville quotes 59 authors in all, including about 40 medical writers, of which predominantly Galen (431x), Avicenna (307x), Hippocrates (68x), Rhazes (38x), Albucasis (18x). His immediate Italian predecessors are mainly represented by Theodoric (113x) and Lanfranc (17x). The latter would have been his main guide in the last three tracts which were only partly completed. Gurlt: *Gesch. Chir.*, vol. 2, p. 36. It is striking that in most cases he supplies relatively careful references to his sources, a practice which was not common in the Middle Ages.
[56] Nicaise: *Henri de Mondeville*, pp. 97—8.
[57] A Latin translation of the *Ars medica* appeared fairly early although it is not known exactly when. Mondeville attached much significance to the 'res naturales', 'res non-naturales' and 'res contra naturam' which are described in this treatise. The 'things natural', seven in all, concern the elements,

the temperament, the humours, the organs, the faculties or properties, the functions, the vital spirits: they are more or less summarized by the modern concepts of anatomy and physiology. The 'non-naturales', of which there are six, relate to the ways of life and hygiene: air, food and drink, sleeping and waking, excretion and retention, passions and emotions. The 'counter-naturals' concern pathology and consist of diseases, their causes and their symptoms. Nicaise: *Henri de Mondeville*, p. 121. Although the notions as such are Galenic, the Latin terminology is coming from the *Isagoge* by Johanitius, see p. 355, n 60. 'Res non-naturales' is an unfortunate transl. of 'conserving causes'. Rather: 'The six things non-natural'. The 'six non-naturals' occupied an important position in the therapeutical considerations of the better surgeons, including Cornelis van de Voorde in the 17th century. Until the mid 19th century they formed the pattern for popular works on hygiene.

58 Nicaise: *Henri de Mondeville*, pp. 117—20.

59 *Op. cit.*, p. 184.

60 *Op. cit.*, p. 100.

61 *Op. cit.*, p. 170.

62 *Op. cit.*, e.g. pp. 112—3, 197—202.

63 *Op. cit.*, pp. XVI—XIX.

64 As late as the 17th century we repeatedly find the dialectic line of argument in the medical-scholarly literature whereby the notions of the author, who of course includes himself amongst the moderns, are opposed to not always clearly defined 'ancients'.

65 *Henri de Mondeville*, pp. 308—9. Cf. n. 71 for 'digestives'.

66 *Op. cit.*, p. 242.

67 *Op. cit.*, p. 252.

68 *Op. cit.*, pp. 257—8.

69 *Op. cit.*, p. 273.

70 *Op. cit.*, pp. 566—9.

71 This antidotary, like the one in the work of Guy de Chauliac mentioned on p. 58, gives an exellent survey of the surgical medicines in use in the Middle Ages, divided into:

Repercursiva: remedies which repel humours that cause a part to swell toward the interior of the body.

Resolutiva: resolving agents.

Maturativa or *digestiva*: stimulating agents which promote purulence in phlegmonous inflammations. They may be applied as cataplasma, emplastrum or unguentum.

Abstersiva or *mondificativa*: cleansing medicaments used to remove viscid or putrid matter from organic surfaces.

Incarnativa or *regenerativa* promote the regeneration of soft parts.

Consolidativa or *cicatrisativa* assist the cicactrization.

72 Nicaise: *Guy de Chauliac*, p. XLVIII. According to Michler the real Galenism in mediaeval medicine started with Guy. Michler: 'Guy de Chauliac als Anatom'. In his days Guy had access not only to Latin translations, which Gerard of Cremona had made of Arab editions of Greek authors in Toledo in the 12th century, but also to direct translations by Nicolas de Reggio in the 14th century, made on the basis of Greek manuscripts which had been sent to Robert of Sicily by the Byzantine emperor Andronicus. Neuburger: *Gesch. Med.*, vol. 2, p. 440. Guy must have had access to the papal library. He was not, however, familiar with Celsus.

73 Nicaise: *Guy de Chauliac*, p. CLX.

74 Of the two Middle Dutch copies (Ms 1356 University Library Utrecht and Ms 10 c 17 of the Museum Meermanno-Westreenianum in The Hague) the first one is likely to have originated in the Southern Netherlands. The origin of the second one is completely unknown.

75 Apart from this there are numerous manuscript and printed editions of abridged versions and separate chapters.

76 This will be done on the basis on Nicaise's critical edition but, in order to limit the number of notes, we will summarize the separate books without providing any further pagination.

77 The image of the *nanus in humero gigantis*, which apart from Guy de Chauliac we have come across in a few other medical writers from 13th and 14th centuries, for example Henri de Mondeville (Nicaise, pp. 215, 745), apparently originates from Bernard of Chartres, who in the 12th century was chancellor of the famous abbey school in that place. John of Salisbury (ca. 1115—50), *Metalogicon*. If Bernard wished to signify with this, that we are all dependent on the classical authors for our own knowledge, the mediaeval physicians on the other hand emphasized with this metaphor the 'little bit more' which each successive generation adds to total knowledge. Steudel: 'Zwerg auf der Schulter des Riesen'.

78 The founder of the dry method is, as has already been mentioned, Theodoric's father Hugo, and not Bruno. Actually it was already proposed by Hippocrates in cases of fresh wounds as we have seen.

[79] Michler: 'Guy de Chauliac als Anatom'.
[80] *Pentateuchos chirurgicum* was e.g. the title of one of Fabricius' books, published in Frankfurt am Main in 1592. Cf. p. 365, n. 102.
[81] And fortunately so, because soon after he was rid of this stone by natural means at the intercession of Saint Gerard. De Moulin: 'Cutting for the stone'.
[82] *Mirakelen van Onse Lieve Vrouwe tot sHertogenbosch*, p. 291.
[83] Municipal Archives Utrecht, city archives 1, no. 22.
[84] Van Ginneken: 'Geert Groote's levensbeeld', p. 359.
[85] Van Herwaarden: 'Medici in de Nederlandse samenleving', p. 365.
[86] Ten Doesschate: *Rolduc als middeleeuwse voorpost*, p. 139.
[87] Professor R. Jansen-Sieben, personal communication.
[88] This hospital is one example of the secularization of these institutions in the 13th century. Formerly founded in direct or indirect connection with the Church, they were now endowed by lay persons. The city government was often responsible for the care of the patients, which it would usually entrust to nuns or related groups, preferably women. Van Herwaarden: *Medici in de Nederlandse samenleving*, p. 360. Cf. p. 125.
[89] Van Leersum: *Jan Yperman*, pp. 223—33.
[90] Brussels Royal Libr. Ms 15624—41 (1351); Ghent Univ. Libr. Ms 1273 (between 1450 and 1460); London Brit. Libr. Ms Harley 1684 (second half 15th cent.); Cambridge, St. John's College Libr. Ms A19 (15th cent.), incomplete. These four codices also contain other Middle Dutch medical treatises.
[91] A sworn master or 'chirurgus iuratus' acted as expert witness in cases of bodily harm. Van Herwaarden: *Medici in de Nederlandse samenleving*, p. 351.
[92] The Hague Royal Libr. Ms 78 C 27; London Brit. Libr. Ms Harley 1648.
[93] Van Leersum: 'Book of surgeries', pp. 49—50.
[94] Jansen-Sieben: 'Jonghe Lanfranc'. See Müller: *Jonghe Lanfranc*, pp. 75—103 for a transcription of Cod A 19, St. John's Coll, Cambridge.
[95] Jansen-Sieben, Keil: 'Eine chirurgische Glossensammlung'.

CHAPTER 3: THE RENAISSANCE

[1] The word 'guild' is probably derived from 'gildan' from ancient German which means deposit or offering. Van Eeghen: *Gilden*, p. 8.
[2] Baumann: *Dokter en geneeskunde*, pp. 95—6.
[3] Apparently the use of similar instruments was the motive behind bringing several crafts together under one guild. Van Herwaarden: 'Medici in de Nederlandse samenleving', p. 371.
[4] Van Lieburg: 'Genees- en heelk. in de Noordelijke Nederlanden'.
[5] It should not be concluded that barbers only conducted barber's work and blood-letting. In a medico-legal attestation of 1550 two 'beard-shavers' appear as surgical attendants of someone who died as a result of penetrating spear wounds to the head. 'Visum repertum of Master Arent and Master Albert, barbers. June 1550': *Opuscula*, vol. XIII, 1935, pp. 4—7. A strict line of demarcation could not as yet be drawn.
[6] The phlebotomy examination also appears to have formed part of the surgical examination in other places in Europe. It was e.g. mentioned as such in the statutes of the Confraternité des Chirurgiens de Saint-Côme et de Saint-Damian in Montpellier. Dulieu: *La chirurgie à Montpellier*, p. 26.
[7] The Dutch translator of Vesalius' *Epitome* for instance, Jan Wouters of Veere, calls himself in 1569 'Medicyn ende Chirurgyn' ('Physician and Surgeon') on the title page (Fig. 20).
[8] Municipal Archives Amsterdam. Surgeons' Guild record no. 227. Consent of Philip II to annual dissection (1555). According to the 'anatomy book' of the surgeons' guild, a dissection had already taken place in Amsterdam before this privilege was granted. The subject was a notorious thief. 'een fameuse dief'. This statement has not been confirmed by other contemporaneous sources, but the stripped and prepared 'skin of a felon' was one of the curiosities preserved and exhibited in the anatomical theatre in Amsterdam (cf. Fig. 41 in the foreground to the right).
[9] Putscher: 'Ein Totentanz von Titian', refutes the tradition that the woodcut illustrations of the *Fabrica* were made by the Flemish artist J. S. van Calcar.
[10] O'Malley: *Andreas Vesalius*, p. 184.
[11] Luyendijk-Elshout: 'Introduction of Juan Valverde's and Bartholomy Cabrol's anatomy'.
[12] Nuyens: 'Ontleedk onderwijs Amsterdam', p. 54. Such lists seem also to have existed in other places in Holland and Germany.

13 Van Rompaey: 'Bourgondische periode', p. 325.
14 *Vijfhonderdste verjaring van de boekdrukkunst*, pp. 90—5.
15 Klebs: *Incunabula scientifica*, p. 166. The only copy known to have existed was burnt in Louvain in 1914.
16 'Medizijn ende Prelecteur der Chirurgijen, binnen de vermaerde coopstadt van Antwerpen'.
17 Van Dongen: 'Incunabelen', XIII, 1965, pp. 853—5.
18 Franco: *Chirurgie*, p. xxxiv.
19 Da Vigo: *Chyrurgylick werck*, fol. LV^{r}: '. . . vander locht niet ghealtereert'.
20 *Op. cit.*, fol. LVII^{r}.
21 *Op. cit.*, fol. CXII^{v}.
22 *Op. cit.*, fol. LXXVIII^{v}.
23 *Op. cit.*, fol. XLIX^{v}: 'den wiltfancken ende loopende cyrurginen die dese cure hantieren'.
24 Du: Scheel-Hans, i.e. squinting Hans.
25 Hippocrates had already advised young surgeons to attach themselves to mercenary troops in order to gain experience in surgery. *De medico* Ch. XIV, Ed. Jones vol. 2, p. 305.
26 We will present a paragraph on surgical instruments from the 16th up till the 18th century on pp. 256—9.
27 Grabert KW: cited by Keil & Müller: 'Deutsche Lanfrank-Übersetzungen', p. 92.
28 Brunschwig: *Cyrurgia*, p. 262.
29 Brunschwig: *Op. cit.*, p. 37. Gersdorff: *Feldtbuch*, p. XXIII^{v}.
30 Brunschwig: *Op. cit.*, p. 46. Gersdorff: *Op. cit.*, p. XXIX^{v}.
31 Although authoritative surgeons like Paré and Fabricius denied the poisonousness of gunshot wounds, the subject continued to be a theme of discussion until well into the 17th century.
32 Brunschwig: *Op. cit.*, pp. 56—58.
33 Gersdorff: *Op. cit.*, p. XLII^{r}.
34 Brunschwig: *Op. cit.*, p. 91.
35 *Op. cit.*, pp. 192—3.
36 *Op. cit.*, pp. 180—2.
37 *Op. cit.*, p. 138.
38 Ergotism, poisoning caused by eating bread made from ergotized flour, occurred frequently in the Middle Ages especially in rural areas. It can lead to a kind of dry gangrene of the limbs. In iconography, St. Anthony the Abbot, the patron saint of sufferers from this disease, is often surrounded by worshippers from whose arms flames are leaping. The unfortunate people who so often appear in mediaeval paintings or sculpture moving on knee crutches, will in many cases have been left cripples by 'Saint Anthony's fire' (Fig. 30).
39 Brunschwig: *Op. cit.*, p. 50. Gersdorff: *Op. cit.*, 3rd unnumbered page after p. LXX.
40 Scheel-Hans: *Veldt Boeck*, transl. by J. P. Phrisius. This was the best book to be had in Dutch, in the opinion of Pieter Volck Horst, the surgeon who translated the first three books of Paracelsus' *Grosse Wundarzney*, where it was superseded by the latter text. Horst did not think much of French and Italian standard-works like the books by Lanfranc, Guy or Giovanni da Vigo 'which even today surgeons drag around like the cat her kittens'. He was apparently not aware of the influence of Lanfranc and Guy on the two Strasbourg authors (cf. p. 78).
41 *Dits dat hantwerck der cirurgien.* In the preface to the German edition B states to belong to the family of the Sauler. He is certainly not a scion of a Salernitan lineage, as the Dutch version might suggest.
42 The noble experyence of the vertuous handywarke of surgeri practysyd & compyled by . . . Mayster Jherome of Bruynswyke . . . Billings: *Hist. and lit. of surg*, p. 41.
43 It seems that Paracelsus enjoyed some popularity in Holland. Apart from his *Chirurgia magna* — of which, however, only the first three treatises of the first book were translated — his *Chirurgia parva* (*Cleyne chirurgie*), his hospital book (*Tgasthuys boeck*), as well as a compilation entitled *Die peerle der chirurgijen* have been turned into Dutch. Only very few copies, however, have survived.
44 Paracelsus, *Die groote chirurgie*, fol. 1^{v}.
45 *Op. cit.*, fol. xv^{r}—xxviii^{r}.
46 *Op. cit.*, fol. xxx^{r}—xxx^{v}.
47 *Op. cit.*, fol. xxxvi^{r}.
48 *Op. cit.*, fol. xiii^{v}.
49 Arceus: *Kortbondige middel en kunst*, p. 5.
50 *Op. cit.*, p. 26.
51 *Op. cit.*, pp. 19—20.
52 *Op. cit.*, pp. 94—7.
53 *Op. cit.*, pp. 130—48.

[54] *Op. cit.*, pp. 154—5.
[55] Unguentum diachylon, today consisting of equal parts of lead plaster and sesame oil, is a very old remedy. As its Greek name indicates, it also formerly contained plant juices (chylos = juice or slime).
[56] Arceus: *Op. cit.*, pp. 165—7.
[57] Arceus' balsam, composed of mutton and pork fat with terpentine and resina elemis, was used until the second half of last century as an excitant.
[58] Emplastrum de Vigo consisted of emplastrum de ranis (a decoction of frogs, earth worms and several herbs), boiled with fat, oil and litharge. Schelenz: *Gesch Pharm*, p. 409. For Unguentum basilicum cf. p. 363, n. 53.
[59] Arceus: *Kortbondige middel en kunst*, p. 215.
[60] *Op. cit.*, p. 223—33.
[61] About 25 years previously, scholars had started to translate the classic writers into French. Montpellier took the lead in this. Gurlt: *Gesch. Chir.*, vol. 2, p. 689.
[62] Paré met Vesalius in person at the sick-bed of the French king Henry II, in 1559. Gurlt: *Op. cit.*, vol. 2, p. 684. Paré's great interest in anatomy was imparted to him in the four years that he worked as a surgeon's apprentice in the large Hôtel-Dieu in Paris. There he had been able to study anatomy on an inexhaustible supply of subjects. Yet he contributed nothing to that discipline.
[63] Through his annotated text edition of Paré's complete works in 1840—41, the French surgeon Joseph-François Malgaigne has contributed, more than anyone else, to the general recognition of the great significance of that Renaissance author as founder of a more modern surgery. Rogge: *Ambroise Paré*, p. 9.
[64] *De chirurgie ende alle de opera*, pp. 236—75, 'tracterende van de onnaturelicke gheswellen int generale'.
[65] *Op. cit.*, pp. 291—300, 'Van de ghenesinghe der breucke ofte gescheurtheyt'.
[66] *Op. cit.*, pp. 307—87.
[67] 'Syncope of de groote beswijmenisse', *Op. cit.*, p. 319.
[68] *Op. cit.*, p. 337.
[69] *Op. cit.*, pp. 387—427.
[70] *Op. cit.*, p. 399.
[71] *Op. cit.*, pp. 449—54.
[72] *Op. cit.*, pp. 503—4.
[73] 'tracterende van diversche accidenten ende particuliere operatien'.
[74] Paré: *Op. cit.*, p. 1102.
[75] *Geka Sôden*, 1706. Huard *et al.*: *La médecine japonaise*, pp. 55—56.
[76] In Dordrecht two more translations appeared from Dutch into English:

1 Guillemeau, *The Frenche chirurgerye* . . . With dedication to 'Ladye Elisabeth . . . Queene of Englande, Fraunce, and Irelande', signed by her 'wellwillinge subjecte . . . Maximiliane Bouman chirurgian at Dort' who 'causede . . . [the work] to be translatede both into Englishe and Lowdutch', by A. M. Dort: Isaac Canin, 1597 (the colophon states 1598).

2 Oswald Gabelkover (1539—1616) *The boock of physicke* . . . [*Arzneybuch* . . . Tübingen, 1594], transl. out of High-duche (German) by . . . Charles Battus . . . and now nuelyc translatede out of Low-duche into Englishe by A. M. Dorte: Isaack Caen, 1599.

(*Catalogue of sixteenth cent. printed books in the Nat. Libr. of Med.*, Bethesda (Md), 1967).
[77] Baten: *Handboeck d. chirurgyen*, p. 242.
[78] 'One should endure to endure'. This small treatise is reprinted in Rohlfs *Dtsch. Arch. Gesch. Med.*, vol. 4 (1881) and 5 (1882).
[79] Franco: *Chirurgie*. As the interested reader will have no difficulty in finding the subjects summarized in the following with the help of the indexes in Nicaise's edition, we will usually refrain from supplying page references.
[80] Nicaise (Franco: *Chirurgie*, p. 60, n. 2) is inclined to believe that Franco was referring here to what latter would become known as femoral hernia. Franco's additional statement that this type of hernia is the easiest to reduce makes his supposition improbable.
[81] Franco was familiar with the sign of translucency, using a candle, in cases of hydrocele. Pneumatocele: a gaseous swelling of the scrotum. According to Fock: *Natuur- en geneesk woordenboek*, this condition is an accumulation of air in an intestinal loop that in a pre-existing hernia has descended into the scrotum. By humoral hernia Franco probably understood orchitis.
[82] Some modern authors — Fischer (p. 522), Shelley and others — believe that Franco improved on the Marian operation by cutting through the prostate. Franco did indeed devise scissors with external cutting edges which should cut bilaterally through the prostate when they were opened and redrawn from the bladder in which they had been introduced when closed via an incision of the urethra. He conceded, however, never to have used this instrument in practice.

[83] *Chyrurgylick werck*, preface. The post-Hippocratic tripartion of therapy in pharmacotherapy, dietetics and surgery, was mentioned in so many words by Celsus (Ed. Spencer, vol. 1, p. 7) and since repeated by many authors.
[84] Wound potions were supposed to influence favourably the composition of the humours.
[85] Van Lieburg: 'De 'Materia Chirurgica'', pp. 1395—7.

CHAPTER 4: THE GOLDEN AGE

[1] Huizinga: *Nederland's beschaving*, p. 4.
[2] Barge: *Geneesk onderwijs*, pp. 8—9.
[3] Bauman: *Dokter en geneesk.*, vol. 2, pp. 37—8.
[4] King: *Med. enlightenment*, pp. 93—136.
[5] Rothschuh: *Konzepte*, pp. 230-2.
[6] Lindeboom: *Med. wetensch. Nederl.*, pp. 52, 55.
[7] Schrader: *Decades quattuor*, pp. 207—8. We will enter more fully into Swammerdam's discovery on p. 231.
[8] Haeser: *Gesch. Med.*, vol. 2, pp. 416—22. For the earliest history of blood transfusion see De Moulin: 'Some remarks'.
[9] Lower's *Tractatus* was reprinted in Latin in Amsterdam in 1671. Glazemaker's anthology (see n. 11) includes on pp. 1—6 a transl. of the report of Lower's work which appeared in the Paris *Journal des Scavans* **1**: 57, 1667. Samuel Pepys in his well-known *Diary* records to have seen 'the person who had his blood taken out': the man said he felt just fine. When asked why he had precisely the blood of a lamb transfused to him, he answered: 'Sanguis ovis symbolicam quandam facultatem habet cum sanguine Christi, quia Christus est agnus Dei'. Pepys: *The diary*. Ed. Wheatley: vol. VI, pp. 60—1, 63; vol. VII, pp. 195—6, 203.
[10] Denis: 'Receuil de quelques nouvelles observations', pp. 87—94, 182—85.
[11] Glazemaker: *Verz nieuwe waarn*, pp. 6—10.
[12] Lindeboom: *Reinier de Graaf*, p. 82.
[13] Van Helmont: *Ortus medicinae*, pp. 604—5. '*Splen primorum conceptuum sedes* . . . in splene, jam alias demonstravi, imaginativam primorum conceptuum, eamque inde ad stomachum, duumviratus socium, etiam & hinc facile ac primordialiter (in altero sexu) ad uterum distendi. Splen ergo, tam fons est idearum conceptarum in imaginativa hominis, quam ipsius Archei.'
[14] Jarcho: '17th cent. medical journalism', p. 68.
[15] In England, the revival of this ancient experiment — it was recorded by Pliny in his *Historia naturalis*, Lib. XI, cap. 80 — was undertaken by the Helmontian physician George Thomson in 1655 or 1656 according to Webster: 'The Helmontian Thomson'.
[16] De Moulin: 'Barbette', p. 511.
[17] Van Lamzweerde: *Chirurgiae veteris*, p. 49.
[18] Solingen: *Manuale operatien*, part 4, p. 369.
[19] De Heide: *Anatome mytuli*, obs. 55, pp. 123—6.
[20] The English philosopher Francis Bacon, a contemporary of William Harvey, postulated that science should be separated from theology, that knowledge should be based on empiricism, that one should arrive at generally valid laws by way of induction, that negative data too should be included when judging the results and that the scientist should guard himself against the drawing of hasty conclusions and being prejudiced.
[21] Bauman: *Dokter en geneesk*, vol. 1, p. 77.
[22] Van Beverwyck: *Heel-konste*, p. 140.
[23] King: *Med. enlightenment*, pp. 140—5. Rothschuh: *Konzepte*, pp. 151—2.
[24] Van Beverwyck relates that he was once visited by Sir Kenelm Digby, who told him about his magnetic cure ('seyl-steenige genesinge') at a distance, just like a magnet can attract from afar. Van Beverwyck: *Heel-konste*, p. 140. Since Van Beverwyck died in 1647, Digby must have already used his powder before that year.
[25] Haeser: *Gesch. Med.*, vol. 2, p. 430.
[26] Gelfand: *Training of surgeons*, pp. 2, 23, 28—9. Gelfand's book is an excellent social history of surgery in Paris during the 17th and 18th centuries.
[27] Osteology encompassed the anatomy of bones as well as fractures. It was a separate subject in the surgeons' examinations in most countries.
[28] Billings: *Hist. and lit. of surg.*, p. 54.

[29] Hoffmann: *Medicus politicus*, pars I, cap. 1, regula 8.
[30] Towns in which a surgeons' guild existed were:

Alkmaar	's-Gravenhage	Rotterdam
Amsterdam	Groningen	Schiedam
Arnhem	Haarlem	Schoonhoven
Bergen op Zoom	Harderwijk	Sneek
Bolsward	Harlingen	Steenwijk
Breda	's-Hertogenbosch	Tholen en Schakerloo
Brielle	Hoorn	Utrecht
Delft	Hulst	Veere
Deventer	Kampen	Vlissingen
Dordrecht	Leeuwarden	Weesp
Enkhuizen	Leyden	Workum (Fr)
Goes	Maastricht	Zaltbommel
Gorkum	Middelburg	Zierikzee
Gouda	Nijmegen	Zwolle

Slenders: *Theatrum anat.*, p. 141.
[31] Hilte: 'Chir. gilde in Nijmegen', p. 23.
[32] Slenders: *Theatrum anat.*, p. 69.
[33] Nuyens: 'Ontleedk onderwijs Amsterdam', p. 57. Van Eeghen: *Gilden*, pp. 90—1.
[34] Van Nierop: 'Dagboek', p. 150.
[35] Van Lieburg: *Med. onderwijs Rotterdam*, p. 19.
[36] Van Eeghen: *Gilden* p. 73; Van Nierop: 'Dagboek', p. 135; Cohen: 'Amsterd. Joodsche chirurgijns', p. 114.
[37] Hilte: 'Chir. gilde in Nijmegen', p. 23.
[38] Daniëls: 'Een dominé-operateur'.
[39] Cohen: 'Amsterd. Joodsche chir', pp. 115, 117—20.
[40] The guild's board at Middelburg, e.g., consisted of a 'deken' (dean) and two 'beleeders' (assessors), at Nijmegen of two 'meesters-in-de-tijd' (masters serving their term of office), at Gouda of an 'overman' and four deans. Schoute: *Middelburgsche chir. gilde*, p. 7; Hilte: 'Chir. gilde in Nijmegen', p. 21; Schouten: *Chir. kamer Gouda*, p. 16.
[41] Hilte: 'Chir. gilde in Nijmegen', p. 27.
[42] *Op. cit.*, p. 27.
[43] Van Lieburg, personal communication. A polder is a tract of low land reclaimed from the sea.
[44] See e.g. Brouwer Ancher: 'Oude ordonnantiën', pp. 1188—9; Schoute: *Middelburgsche chir. gilde*, pp. 32—3; Van Lieburg: 'Instrument coll. of P. Vink', p. 212.
[45] Schoute: *Middelburgsche chir. gilde*, p. 34; van Loon: 'Rotterd chir. gilde', p. 3912; Van Andel: *Chirurgijns*, p. 142.
[46] van Andel: *Chirurgijns*, pp. 44—5.
[47] Baumann: *Dokter en geneesk.*, vol. 1, pp. 100, 102.
[48] Van Eeghen: *Gilden*, p. 75.
[49] *Op. cit.*, p. 77. Amongst the contracting parties one finds quite a few names that belong to former Hugenots.
[50] The 'leerknecht' was left entirely to the tender mercies of his master. According to a notary's act dated April, 1672, the Hague surgeon Solingen once tied his 13-year old 'leerknecht' to a chair and beat him with a length of rope so badly that the boy later had to be bandaged and bled. Van Andel: 'De chirurgijn Solingen', p. 50.
[51] Bontekoe: *Nieuw gebouw*, vol. 1 unpaged preface.
[52] Van Eeghen: *Gilden*, p. 79. Cf. note 50!
[53] For reasons given on page 76 the well-advised candidate had recourse to Tagault's surgery book in preparing for this part of the interrogation. At the beginning of his work, Tagault gave a general summary of the different classifications which can be made in surgery. One of these bears on the five basic ointments the surgeon should always have ready to hand. They represent an age-old tradition as their names betray and were in common use way into the 18th or even the 19th century: the digestive *Unguentum basilicum*, the resolving *Ung. apostolicum*, the incarnative *Ung. aureum*, the consolidative *Ung. album* and the emollient *Ung. dialtheum*. Cf. note 71 of Ch. 2.
[54] Boesman: *Examens*, pp. 25, 57—8. By this oath the surgeon undertook to care for the patient in the best way he could without doing him any harm by design and moreover to observe professional secrecy, except in cases of injury caused by criminal violence which he was obliged to report to the bailiff. But in the wording of the Middelburg oath of 1589, there is no question of any professional secrecy. Fokker: 'Losse bladen', p. 362.

[55] Leuftink: *Geneesk bij 's lands oorlogsvloot*, p. 35.
[56] Suringar: 'Ontleedk onderwijs te Leiden', p. 385.
[57] For obvious reasons public dissections — which lasted up to a whole week — only took place in the winter season.
[58] Slenders: *Theatrum anat.*, pp. 15—27. In 1673 even in far-off Batavia an anatomical theatre was established and a 'doctor anatomicus' appointed. Römer: *Hist. schetsen*, pp. 190—1.
[59] Geijl: 'Titsingh', p. 34.
[60] Slenders: *Theatrum anat*, pp. 67—9. The smaller theatres may not have consisted of circular galleries but of straight parallel rows.
[61] *Op. cit.*, p. 94.
[62] At times an anatomical object could be obtained in a more direct way. A sad example is provided by a short entry in the cash book of the anatomy department at Harderwijk: 'November 8, 1617. The treasurers pay to Jan Ketelbuyter eight guilders for having his daughter anatomized'.
[63] Hellinga: 'Beteekenis Amsterd St. Pietersgasth'.
[64] In 1681, the governors of the Amsterdam gasthuis prohibited any corpses being taken away from the hospital for public dissection or private anatomising in doctors' residences without their written consent. Hellinga: 'Uit de qeschied. der Amstrraamsche qasthuiun'.
[65] De Moulin: 'Natuurhist. verzameling Rotterd.' pp. 131—7. There also existed at the time many private collections of curiosities. The celebrated collection of Frederik Ruysch will be described below (p. 142).
[66] See Endtz: *Hage-professoren* for a survey of the tuition of anatomy at The Hague.
[67] Slenders: *Theatrum anat.*, pp. 54—62, 89—94.
[68] Thiels: 'De Leidse chirurgijns', p. 215.
[69] Orlers: *Beschrijving der stad Leyden*, p. 148.
[70] Thiels: 'De Leidse chirurgijns', pp. 216—9.
[71] Nuyens: 'Ontleedk onderwijs Amsterd', pp. 57—85.
[72] See Houtzager: *Medicyns, vroedwyfs*, pp. 84—97 for a description of the paintings by Van Mierevelt and De Man.
[73] Slenders: 'Anat les Dr de Jager'.
[74] Taking over a surgeon's shop was a costly affair. At Amsterdam in the 18th century the price was 1000 guilders on average. Van Eeghen: *Gilden*, p. 86.
[75] Antvelink: 'Goodwill', pp. 1507—8.
[76] Van Andel: *Chirurgijns*, p. 77.
[77] Breen: 'Een barbierswinkel in 1669'.
[79] **Solingen: *Manuale operatien*, p. 368. Not rarely patients had, even as late as the 19th century,** their operation in a room at an inn.
[80] Coopmans: *Rechtstoestand*, p. 13.
[81] Probably the first major operation to be performed here, was an arm amputation in 1429. *Sint Janshospitaal Brugge*, p. 74, n. 129. In 1976, after more than eight centuries, this hospital moved to new buildings outside the town. The former hospital is now a magnificent museum of mediaeval art but also keeps relics of its medical past.
[82] For details the reader is referred to the memorial volumes published by the various hospitals.
[83] Brondgeest: *Balye van St. Catharina*, p. 83.
[84] There does not seem to be a proper English equivalent for it. Yet 'Gasthuis', literally 'guesthouse' or 'house for strangers' has some relation to hospital in sofar that the latter word is derived from 'hospes', meaning stranger as well as host. As late as the 19th century, 'gasthuis' was in common use.
[85] The non-aristocratic Order of the Holy Ghost was founded in the 13th century in Montpellier. It established Houses of the Holy Ghost for the sick, for travellers, orphans and foundlings, in France and Italy in particular, but also in North-West Europe.
[86] Kunz: *Oude en Nieuwe Gasthuis*, p. 35. Only in 1854 the Delft hospital surgeons were formally relieved from the obligation to barber the male patients.
[87] Schoute: 'Gasthuis te Middelburg', p. 16.
[88] *Op. cit.*, pp. 15, 28. The regulations for the hospital surgeons, as laid down in this hospital's rule book of 1604 are reproduced on pp. 68—9.
[89] Van Eeghen: 'Van gasthuis tot acad ziekenhuis', p. 50.
[90] *Op. cit.*, pp. 51—2. All through the 'ancien régime', major operations required official permission, the concurrence of a town physician and the presence of wardens of the guild.
[91] Hellinga: 'Gasthuis-chirurgijns', p. 31.
[92] *Op. cit.*, p. 32.
[93] Kerkhoff: *Geneesk verzorging Staatse leger*, pp. 51—8.
[94] Leeflang: 'Chirurgijnen te Enkhuizen', p. 1235.

[95] Van Lieburg: 'Med. stadsgesch. Rotterdam', p. 118.
[96] Banga: *Gesch. geneesk. in Nederl.*, pp. 240, 273, quoting Tulp and Van Meekeren.
[97] Bitter: 'De beul', afl. 3. In Germany too, some public executioners enjoyed a reputation as healers. Haeser: *Gesch. Med.*, vol. 2, p. 433. Frederick the Great granted skilful executioners in Prussia permission to treat fractures, wounds and ulcers. Billings: *Hist. and lit. of surg.*, p. 64.
[98] The number of appointed executioners was limited to one per province, only very few towns like Dordrecht enjoyed the ancient privilege of having such a functionary of their own. The public executioner of the province of Holland resided at Haarlem. Van Eeghen: 'Beul in Amsterdam', p. 120.
[99] Haneveld: 'Ledezetters'.
[100] At Enkhuizen, the physicians were even entitled to practise surgery, according to the byelaws of the surgeons' guild enacted in 1636. From 1636 to 1644 the doctors of that place went so far as to join the guild. Leeflang: 'Chirurgijnen', pp. 1234—5. In Middelburg a society of physicians and surgeons was established in 1658, called 'Collegium anatomico-chirurgicum', for the advancement of medical science and anatomy in particular. Schoute: *Middelburgsche chir. gilde*, pp. 43—4.
[101] Johannes van Horne is one of those who, after having studied medicine at home, went to Italy to receive his M.D. from Padua. In Naples he stayed for a while with the celebrated surgeon Marco Antonio Severino. After eight years he returned to his native country via Switzerland, France and England.
[102] Girolamo Fabrizio d'Acquapendente's *Opera chirurgica*, first published in 1617, consists of two parts. The first one deals with operative surgery, the second with surgical pathology and treatment classified according to the traditional five sections. This part had previously been edited by one of Fabricius' German pupils under the title *Pentateuchos chirurgicum*. The *Opera chirurgica* went through several editions, one in Leyden as late as 1723. Fabricius' surgery is strongly influenced by the Ancients, by Celsus and Paulus in particular, as he acknowledges himself. The Arabs too, are frequently cited: his strong aversion to bloody interventions he probably acquired from them.
[103] Wilhelm Fabry, born in Hilden in Germany, published six volumes of case histories, entitled *Observationum et curationum chirurgicarum centuriae* in Basel, Frankfurt and Lyons between 1606 and 1641. The different places in which they appeared bear testimony of the interest they created all over Europe. A Dutch translation never appeared but the one of Fabry's book on military surgery was successful. He is also the author of books on burns, gangrene and lithotomy. He is sometimes regarded as the founder of scientific surgery in Germany and Switzerland, because he furnished the craft with a firm anatomical basis.
[104] Fabricius Hildanus and Thomas Bartholin were in fact no strangers to Holland. The first mentioned visited Leyden with the anatomist Pieter Pauw, with whom he afterwards carried on correspondence, whereas Bartholinus (Thomas Bertelsen), the discoverer of the thoracic duct, was a student at Leyden for three years.
[105] Beverwyck: 'Treatise on the stone', *Opuscula*, pp. 39, 41, 57—67.
[106] Beverwyck quotes on p. 67 a poem on a stone which had made its appearance, composed by Carel van Malepert, in the manner of the poem made by Catullus on a ship:

> This little stone, which hurts your hand, asserts
> That once upon a time it was Dutch cheese
> And could provoke a thirst in any glutton
> No matter whether he was wont to slake it
> With French or with Iberian wine. And both
> These kinds of wine are furnished by the market
> Of Amsterdam, . . . etc.
>
> English transl. by Van Andel.

[107] It was so, indeed, in Beverwyck's own family. He and his brother inherited it as a child from their grandfather: his brother died from it. 'Treatise on the stone', *Opuscula*, p. 69.
[108] Beverwyck: *Heel-konste*, p. 129.
[109] *Op. cit.*, p. 156.
[110] De Moulin: 'Barbette'.
[111] Barbette: *Praxis*, pp. 125, 176, 180, 125.
[112] *Op. cit.*, p. 206.
[113] Krul: 'Argumentatio fustis'.
[114] Van Andel: 'De chirurgijn Solingen', p. 52.
[115] Solingen: *Alle de werken*, pp. 1—34.
[116] *Op. cit.*, pp. 25—31.
[117] *Op. cit.*, pp. 138—63.

[118] *Op. cit.*, pp. 172–92.
[119] *Op. cit.*, pp. 195–208.
[120] *Op. cit.*, p. 197. A price list of J. van Musschenbroek's is printed in Erndl: *De itinere suo*, p. 79. Nicolas de Blegny M.D. (1652–1722), originally a truss maker, was the author of *l'Art de guérir les hernies*. Paris: 1676. His appreciation of Solingen's trusses is not expressed in this work.
[121] Solingen: *Alle de werken*, pp. 240–66.
[122] Bartholomaeus Maggius (1516–52), professor of anatomy and surgery at Bologna, was the author of *De vulnerum a bombardarum et sclopetorum globulis illatorum*, Bologna, 1552, of which there were many later editions. Maggi indeed mentioned the possibility of amputation at a joint as an alternative method, but was not quite such a champion of it as appears from his relevant chapter, cited in large part by Gurlt: *Gesch. Chir.*, vol. 2, pp. 320–1.
[123] Solingen: *Alle de werken*, pp. 324–40.
[124] Rustingh: *Nieuw gebouw*, preface, p. 270. Steven Blankaart, M.D. (1650–1704) was a medical practitioner in Amsterdam and a prolific writer on anatomy, paediatrics, sundry diseases, materies medica, surgery etc. His works are not particularly valuable since their author was a compiler rather than an original thinker. He is best remembered for his Greek–Latin medical lexicon which went into many editions. Blankaarts *Nieuwe hervormde anatomie*, which first appeared in Dutch in 1678 and afterwards in Latin, was strongly condemned by the Louvain professor of anatomy and surgery Philippe Verheyen who charged Blankaart of having reproduced many of his own anatomical drawings without making any mention of their provenance. Since Blankaart published another book on anatomy in 1688, it is not sure which work Rustingh was referring to. In his cryptic allusion to the Rotterdam publication, Rustingh possibly referred to Dionis *Verhandelingen van alle de chirurgicale operatien*, although this was not in quarto. W. K. Gnirrep, personal communication.
[125] The age of the apprentices for whom Van de Voorde had been writing was 15 or 16, according to a passing reference.
[126] Van de Voorde: *Lichtende fakkel*, p. 8. Simple or homogenous parts remain the same matter upon being cut into ever so small particles, dissimilar parts are what we nowadays call tissues. The distinction between homogenous and heterogenous parts was first made by Aristotle: *De partibus animalium* part I, ch. 1. Galen upheld it in *On the usefulness of the parts*, vol. 2, p. 67.
[127] It should be pointed out, that Van de Voorde mentions 'membranes' among the examples of less simple parts, *Op. cit.*, p. 13. Their existence, therefore, was appreciated long before Bichat. Nerves apparently still were believed to be hollow structures with vital spirits or a particular nerve juice passing through them.
[128] Van de Voorde: *Lichtende fakkel*, p. 10. Adriaan van den Spieghel (1578–1625), born at Brussels, was professor of anatomy and surgery at Padua. He was the author of *De humani corporis fabrica libri decem*, a highly valued textbook on anatomy (Venice, 1627).
[129] *Op. cit.*, pp. 77–8.
[130] Galen: *Usefulness of the parts*, vol. 1, p. 215. Galen's fencing master was actually a gladiator. The Ancients regarded digestion as a process of boiling. His being an iatrochemist may explain why Van de Voorde stuck to this pre-Galenic conception.
[131] Van de Voorde: *Op. cit.*, p. 56. Albertus Kyper (c. 1614–55), born in Königsbergen in Prussia was personal physician to prince Frederik Hendrik and since 1648 professor of medicine in Leyden. He was a confirmed upholder of the Aristotelian–Galenic tradition in medicine. Van de Voorde was one of his students.
[132] Van de Voorde: *Lichtende fakkel*, p. 70.
[133] *Op. cit.*, p. 74. 'Innate heat' is yet another surviving ancient physiological conception. It was supposed to be the driving force behind the functions of life and to have its seat in the heart. Cf. p. 99 for Sylvius' explanation of innate heat! For a thorough review of the conceptions of lymph physiology at the time, the reader is referred to Van Lieburg: 'Nicolaas Zas'.
[134] They are Nathaniel Highmore (1613–85) — 'een deftigh Engels anatomicus' — and Thomas Wharton (1614–73) — misspelled as Wortonius — without specification of their works. From the text it may be inferred that the books concerned are *Corporis humani disquisitio anatomica*, published at The Hague in 1651, and the well-known *Adenographia* from 1656, respectively.
[135] Van de Voorde: *Lichtende fakkel*, pp. 222–34.
[136] *Op. cit.*, p. 225.
[137] *Op. cit.*, pp. 178–93.
[138] *Op. cit.*, pp. 334–6.
[139] *Op. cit.*, pp. 364–78.
[140] *Op. cit.*, pp. 415–33.
[141] *Op. cit.*, pp. 468–508.
[142] *Op. cit.*, pp. 508–22.

[143] *Op. cit.*, pp. 578—92.
[144] Tulp: *Observ. med.*, preface.
[145] Lindeboom: 'Ruysch's anat. preparaten'.
[146] Ruysch: *Alle de werken*, vol. 1, pp. 82—3.
[147] *Op. cit.*, vol. 2, pp. 654, 770, 793, 806—7.
[148] Titsingh: *Verdonkerde heelkonst*, pp. 700—1.
[149] Schreiber: 'Verhaal van het leven', pp. 102—3.
[150] De Moulin: preface to reprint van Meekeren.
[151] Van Roonhuyze: *Aanmerkingen*, pp. 3—12.
[152] *Op. cit.*, pp. 194—226.
[153] Sprengel: *Gesch. Chir.*, vol. 1, p. 159.
[154] Van Roonhuyze: *Aanmerkingen*, pp. 145—6.
[155] *Op. cit.*, 2nd part, p. 1—85.

CHAPTER 5: THE AGE OF ENLIGHTENMENT

[1] At that time haemorrhoids were very common and the current inadequate methods of treatment must indeed have made bleedings a usual occurrence.
[2] Gelfand: *Training of surgeons*, p. 52.
[3] *Op. cit.*, pp. 21—3.
[4] *Op. cit.*, pp. 101—3.
[5] *Op. cit.*, p. 114.
[6] *Op. cit.*, p. 153.
[7] *Op. cit.*, p. 208.
[8] In the Paris Hôtel-Dieu in the second half of the eighteenth century the nursing conditions were deplorable. This is also apparent from stories which Du Pui told his successor Jacob Cornelis Broers. Although the hospital was dedicated to God it seemed instead to serve the devil. Each bed held two or more patients. The corpses of the deceased were removed only once a day. Du Pui remembered two patients playing at cards while a dead body was lying in between them. The care of the sick was in the hands of people of low repute or beginners. The physicians were in a great hurry when visiting the sick. Nervous fevers and hospital gangrene caused great carnage. Broers: *Oratio de Puteano*, p. 8.
[9] Gelfand: *Op. cit.*, p. 214.
[10] *Op. cit.*, pp. 33, 179—80.
[11] Crosse: *A surgeon in the early 19th cent.*, pp. 39—41.
[12] Bishop: *Early hist. of surgery*, pp. 118—23.
[13] Bromfeild: *Chir. obs.*, pp. 214—28, 347—50.
[14] See Risse: *Hospital life in Enlightenment Scotland* for an excellent survey of patient care and clinical teaching at the Royal Infirmary in the 18th cent. Edinburgh never became a training centre for Dutch surgeons and physicians. From the works of Van Gesscher and others it appears, however, that Edinburgh medical publications were read in Holland.
[15] Among these, his grandson Philipp Franz Balthasar von Siebold (1796—1866), who as a medical officer in the Dutch colonial army worked in Japan for many years where he laid the foundations of education in Western medicine. The anthropological collection, which he brought back from Japan, forms the nucleus of the Ethnographical Museum in Leyden.
[16] Their number cannot be accurately determined. In 1759 to 1760 Matthias van Geuns lived in a Dutch student hostel in the Rue Mazarin. He occupied the house together with some ten other Dutch students and two Danes, who had studied at Leyden. Sypkens Smit: *Matthias van Geuns*, p. 28.
[17] Haver Droeze: *Coll. med. Amstelaedamense*, p. 133.
[18] Van der Zwaag: *Wouter van doeveren*, p. 14. 4000 livres tournois would have amounted to 1900 Dutch guilders, 3 louis d'or to about 12 guilders.
[19] Dionis: *Verhandelingen*; (De la Faye): *Aanmerkingen op de chirurgicale operatien van den Heere Dionis.*
[20] Van der Haar: *Verhandelingen over kankergezwellen*, p. 21.
[21] Titsingh: *Verdonkerde heelkunst*, preface. In this work, Titsingh repeatedly marks his dislike of French surgery: 'it is better to walk on Dutch legs, than on French stilts', p. 96. 'French surgeons are knife-happy', pp. 332, 617 etc. Yet Johannes de Vries (c. 1720—post 1794) was enabled by the province of Friesland to study anatomy and lithotomy in Paris for three years, prior to his appointment in 1753 as 'lecturer in anatomy, surgery and obstetrics'. Kulsdom: 'Landschapsmedici', p. 1583.
[22] *Aanmerkingen op de chirurgicale operatien van den Heere Dionis.*

[23] Van Wijck: *Waarneming rakende eenen fungus*, first unnumbered page. Far into the first half of the nineteenth century many Dutch surgeons expressed their criticism of careless after-treatment by the French in letters and diary entries.
[24] Delprat: *Genootsch ter Bevord. Natuur- Genees- en Heelkunde*, p. 22.
[25] Smellie: *Vroedkunde*, autobiogr. introduction.
[26] De Gorter: *Gezuiverde heelknost*, preface.
[27] Van Lieburg: *Med. onderwijs*, p. 21. Far from all apprentices eventually took their master's degree.
[28] Thiels: *De Leidse chirurgijns*, p. 228.
[29] The well-known Haarlem surgeon Johannes Daams translated Richter's *Abhandlung von den Brüchen* as well as De la Faye's *Principles de la clinique* into Dutch. The Dutch edition of the latter work was translated into Japanese (not by Daams, however).
[30] Van Nierop: 'Dagboek', p. 176.
[31] Frijhoff: 'Non satis dignitatis', p. 402.
[32] Van Nierop: 'Dagboek', p. 175.
[33] *Op. cit.*, p. 138.
[34] Rogier: 'Uit de geschiedenis', p. 11.
[35] Van Nierop: 'Dagboek', p. 149.
[36] Geyl: 'Titsingh', p. 43.
[37] Bruneel: 'Livre de comptes', p. 256.
[38] Ringoir: *Plattelandschirurgijns*, pp. 268, 284—7.
[39] The father of the Middelburg lecturer De Wind as a physician also had a dairy shop. Verkroost: 'Paulus de Wind en zijn proefschrift', p. 1034. In the village of Ransdorp in the Province of North Holland the local surgeon was at one and the same time burgomaster and butcher. Ringoir: *Plattelandschirurgijns*, p. 297. In 1742 there were in Rotterdam six physicians and surgeons who derived another income from a shop or had a sideline as a bargeman. Oldewelt, quoted by Frijhoff: 'Non satis dignitatis', p. 391, n. 42. In Amsterdam and elsewhere surgeons are known to have kept inns, while some physicians held public posts, etc.
[40] Van Nierop: 'Dagboek', p. 169.
[41] Van Andel: 'Spectatoriale vertoogen', p. 485. Schlichting confirms this by stating that in some German countries and in Italy, Dutch medical doctoral degrees were no longer recognized because it had become known that such diplomas could be had for money. Schlichting: *Traumatologia*, footnote in preface. Harderwijk might have been largely responsible for that awkward reputation.
[42] Geyl: 'Titsingh', p. 32. Schlichting was an 'associé étranger' of the Académie royale de Chirurgie in Paris and a member of the Academia Caesareo-Leopoldina. This he probably owed to his diligence in reporting interesting Amsterdam case histories to these august societies. The same two memberships were held by his contemporary Joannes Grashuis (1699—1772), who was also from Amsterdam. Other Dutch associates of the Paris Académie were Van Swieten and Camper; in 1774 the total number of associés étrangers amounted to 17.
[43] Schlichting: *Traumatologia*, p. 8, n. 12. Words of like import occur at several other places.
[44] The surgeon and obstetrician Jacob van der Haar (1717—99), who lived in 's-Hertogenbosch and who previously had been surgeon-general of the army of the Dutch Republic, held the very opposite view: 'A proficient surgeon can easily become a competent physician, but a physician with an ordinary degree can become a good surgeon only with difficulty'. Mulder: *Redevoering*, p. 26.
[45] Lindeboom: *Herman Boerhaave*, pp. 302 ff.
[46] Boerhaave: *Kortbondige spreuken*. His pupil Gerard van Swieten (1700—72), personal physician to the empress Maria Theresa of Austria and reformer of university education in medicine in that country, published an extensive, five-part commentary on those *Aphorisms*. This work too has been frequently reprinted in several European countries. Van Swieten was a staunch advocate of the promotion of Austrian surgery which, when he came to Vienna in 1745, appeared to be very backward. His ideal in this was the eventual union of surgery with medicine. Lesky: 'Van Swieten und die Chirurgie'.
[47] Barge: *Geneesk onderwijs*, pp. 11, 12, 16.
[48] Apart from his already mentioned *Natuur- en Geneesk Bibliotheek* Eduard Sandifort published a three part Latin bibliography of academic dissertations and other selected works relating to medicine.
[49] Thiels, Luyendijk-Elshout: 'De Leidse chirurgijns', pp. 228, 235 n 39, 227, 230.
[50] Corn. Henr. Velse: *De mutuo intestinorum ingressu*. Thesis Leyden, 1742. Quoted by Cope: *Hist of the acute abdomen*, p. 85.
[51] Leporin: 'Ausführlicher Bericht', pp. 9—24.
[52] Johannes Jacobus Rau (1668—1719) was a German who spent a three year apprenticeship with a surgeon in Strassbourg and ended up in Amsterdam after many wanderings. He went to sea as a

ship's surgeon and after having served in that capacity for some years he saved up enough money to study medicine in Leyden. Before his graduation in 1694, he spent some time in Paris in order to acquire further proficiency in anatomy and surgery. He attended the lectures and dissections of Joseph Duverney and Jacques Petit. After having received his M.D. he established himself in Amsterdam where he soon taught a private course in anatomy and surgery. Rau was widely recognized as a good anatomist and an excellent operator. Christianus Henricus Erndl later to become court physician in Poland (d. 1734), who in 1707 spent five months with Rau together with Heister (see p. 166), called him an incomparable anatomist and surgeon, with an insight and experience in dissecting which almost surpassed the experience and dexterity of Vesalius. E(rndl): *De itinere suo*, pp. 95—6. In 1713 Rau succeeded Govert Bidloo as professor of medicine, anatomy and surgery in Leyden. He died insane six years later. He left his large collection of instruments and anatomical specimens to the university where it formed the nucleus of the large educational collection which was started in the eighteenth century. Some items are still preserved. In 1725 B.S. Albinus published a catalogue of the anatomical instruments Rau had bequeathed to the University (*Index supellectilis anatomicae*). Albinus prefaced this list with a biography of the donator, in which he paid attention to Rau's method of cutting for the stone.

53 Like Heister, Ulhoorn was present at the siege of Tournai in the spring of 1709 and the battle of Malplaquet in September of the same year and was charged with the care of great numbers of injured soldiers on both occasions. Ulhoorn settled in Amsterdam in 1715 on passing the master-surgeon's examination in Leyden, after a study tour in Paris. Here he acquired a good reputation on account of his didactic talents, which he showed so clearly during his collegia anatomico-chirurgica that the burgomasters permitted him to dissect cadavers in the dissecting room of the hospital for the instruction of surgeons. The city even awarded him an annual salary for this in 1731.

54 Heister: *Heelkundige onderwijzingen.*

55 Van Gesscher: *Hedend oeffenende heelk*, vol. 3, p. 73.

56 Van Nierop: 'Dagboek', pp. 133—9. Geyl: 'Titsingh', pp. 22, 25—31. Krul: 'Titsingh', pp. 436—9.

57 Serving in a ship provided the opportunity to save money for buying a shop.

58 Krul: 'Titsingh', pp. 440—2. The Roonhuysian secret was disclosed in 1753 by its then owners. Depictions of several versions of that lever drawn by Petrus Camper were added to his article on difficult deliveries in *Mém. Acad. roy. Chir.* **5**: 729—46, 1774.

59 Antonius Nuck M.D. was an unusually able anatomist who earned general recognition by his description of the lymphatic system in particular. In 1687 he became professor of medicine and anatomy at Leyden. Nuck also left a fine work on surgery entitled *Operationes & experimenta chirurgica*, which was published posthumously in Leyden in 1692 and was reprinted several times in the Netherlands as well as in Germany. It was moreover translated into German and Dutch.

60 Govert Bidloo was a qualified surgeon before he graduated in medicine. He is particularly remembered by his *Anatomia humani corporis*, a magnificent anatomical atlas, illustrated by the well-known Amsterdam artist Gerard de Lairesse, published in 1685. He was successor to Nuck, first in The Hague, later in Leyden. Bidloo became physician in ordinary to king William III of Orange, whom he accompanied to England. He was a member of the Royal Society. Endtz: *Hage-professoren*, pp. 45—71.

61 Schwencke was probably the first to describe a case of post-traumatic hygroma as a late sequal of a head injury. Endtz: *Op. cit.*, pp. 81—95.

62 Leporin: *Ausführlicher Bericht*, p. 14.

63 Here, and in a few other places in the preface, De Gorter proves to have adopted the ethical notions which developed under the influence of the Enlightenment.

64 A similar representation we also find in Robert Boyle and Anton Nuck.

65 Schoute: *Middelburgsche Chir. Gilde*, p. 43.

66 The Provincial Library in Middelburg holds a manuscript (P12 B48) in which Paulus de Wind kept note of 98 lithotomies, performed between 1739 and 1770. He used the lateral method according to Rau, described on p. 248. Verkroost: 'Paulus de Wind als steensnijder'.

67 Slenders: *Theatrum anat.*, pp. 29—33.

68 Van der Zwaag: *Wouter van Doeveren*, pp. 14—5, 28.

69 The origin of this well-known Goethe quotation is unknown to the present writer.

70 William Smellie (1697—1763) was one of the leading obstetricians of the eighteenth century: in 1752 he was to publish a textbook which acquired great fame, with superb illustrations by the Dutch draughtsman Jan van Riemsdijk and several equally fine illustrations by Petrus Camper. A Dutch translation of this work was edited by the Amsterdam surgeon and obstetrician Matthijs van der Haage. In 1748 William Hunter (1718—83), anatomist, surgeon and obstetrician, had opened his own school of anatomy in Litchfield Street.

Pringle was physician-general of the British army between 1744 and 1752. His book on diseases prevalent in the army, which was published in 1752, was translated into many languages, including Dutch. Cf. p. 378, n. 9.

Sloane was an enthusiastic collector; after his death in 1753 his collections formed the nucleus of the British Museum.

71 Louis A.: 'Eloge de Camper', *Eloges de l'Académie royale de Chirurgie*. Ed. E. F. Dubois d'Amiens, 1859, p. 382. Quoted and transl. by Gelfand: *Training of surgeons*, p. 213.

72 Latin ms Univ. Libr. Leyden BPL 247.19.

73 Doets: *Heelk van Petrus Camper*, p. 173.

74 Such courses differed from the collegia anatomico-chirurgica already discussed, in that they were not given at the home of the individual lecturer but in the Theatrum anatomicum. Desault introduced the anatomy practice by students in Paris only in 1785. Gelfand: *Training of surgeons*, p. 299.

75 *Academia groningana*, p. 291, n. 3.

76 For his English journeys, see 'Petri Camperi Itinera in Angliam 1748—1785', *Opuscula selecta*, vol. XV, 1939. Dutch and Latin, with English transl.

77 It is not possible to date this drawing, but since Hunter in 1770 moved his dissecting school to Great Windmill Street it must have been made during Camper's last visit.

78 Ringoir: 'Plattelandschirurgijns', pp. 320—59.

79 Doets: *Heelk van Petrus Camper*, p. 25.

80 Gelfand: *Training of surgeons*, pp. 40—2.

81 *Verhandelingen van het Genootschap ter Bevordering der Heelkunde* te Amsterdam **2**: VI—XV, 1793.

82 Bonn: 'Tegenwoordige staat', p. 7 footnote. Cf. p. 377, n. 37.

83 Rau's significance for lithotomy, Verduin's for the amputation of the lower leg and the importance of Jan Palfijn (1650—1730) of Ghent for the development of the obstetric forceps, had probably escaped the young professor.

84 Van Lieburg: *Med. onderwijs Rotterdam*, p. 31.

85 Slenders: *Theatrum anat.*, p. 33—4.

86 Delprat: 'Wording van het Genootschap', p. 20.

87 The society still exists today, although it is now called 'Genootschap ter Bevordering van Natuur-, Genees-, en Heelkunde te Amsterdam (Society for the advancement of physics, medicine and surgery at A'dam). The society soon had a salutary influence. Niewenhuys in his medical topography of Amsterdam, noted in 1816 that in that city, due to scientific societies, surgery 'albeit learnt without proper training and abased by its association with a meaner craft', had now 'surpassed medicine by far'. Nieuwenhuys: *Geneesk. plaatsbeschrijving Amsterdam*, vol. 1, p. 372.

88 Amsterdam was very energetic in this, because on 25 May 1798 the Representative Body (Parliament) decreed that the existing ordinances concerning the guilds were still in force pending further regulations. In several other cities the guilds would continue their activities for a few more years.

89 Van der Weyde: 'Eed voor een heelmeester'.

90 Van Gesscher: *Heelk. ziektekunde*, p. 27.

91 De Moulin: 'Natuurhist verzameling te Rotterdam', p. 136.

92 Nieuwenhuys: *Geneesk plaatsbeschrijving Amsterdam*, vol. 1, p. 357.

93 Haneveld: *Path. anat. in Utrecht*, pp. 113—36.

CHAPTER 6: PRACTICAL SURGERY IN THE 17TH AND 18TH CENTURIES

1 De Gorter: *Gezuiverde heelkonst*, p. 306.

2 Hunter: Cited by Fischer: *Chir. vor hundert Jahren*, p. 389. Hunter's famous book was not translated into Dutch.

3 Petit: *Traité des maladies chirurgicales*, vol. 3, p. 164.

4 Van Roonhuyze: *Genees- en heelk aanmerkingen*, obs. 26.

5 Solingen: *Manuale operatiën*, p. 255.

6 De Gorter: *Gezuiverde heelkonst*, p. 312.

7 Van de Voorde: *Lichtende fakkel*, p. 434.

8 See e.g.: Guy de Chauliac, p. 56.

9 Van de Voorde: *Op. cit.*, p. 451.

10 De Gorter: *Gezuiverde heelkonst*, p. 313.

[11] Heister: *Heelkundige onderwijzingen*, vol. 1, p. 62.
[12] Schlichting: *Traumatologia*, pp. 140–511.
[13] Van der Haar: Cited by Mulder: *Redevoering*, p. 14.
[14] Purmann, M. G.: *Chirurgia curiosa*. Francoforti, 1694, book 2, ch. 1. Cited by Churchill: 'Healing by first intention'.
[15] Van de Voorde: *Lichtende fakkel*, pp. 455–6.
[16] Fischer: *Chir. vor hundert Jahren*, p. 394.
[17] Doets: *Heelk. van Camper*, pp. 147–9.
[18] Barbette: *Chirurgie*, p. 168.
[19] See p. 357, n. 57.
[20] Solingen: *Manuale operatien*, p. 270.
[21] Quesnay thought nothing of bleeding a patient three or four times in the course of a day. In one case, 160 ounces were taken in nine days but, he gravely added, 'two years elapsed before she was quite well again'. In the figure of Dr. Sangrado, the French novelist Alain-René le Sage sharply denounced extreme bloodletting in his *The adventures of Gil Blas of Santillane* (1715–35). Sir Astley Cooper mentioned an instance in which 208 ounces were abstracted from a patient. Adams: *Hippocrates*, vol. 1, p. 444.
[22] Kerkhoff: *Staatse leger*, pp. 25–6, p. 190, n. 160.
[23] Haneveld: 'Medische aspecten van de slag bij de Doggersbank'.
[24] Full quotation in Zimmerman, Veith: *Great ideas*, pp. 351–4.
[25] De Moulin: 'Dominique Anel'.
[26] Eau d'arquebuscade: a wound water introduced by the Prussian army surgeon Theden, consisting of a decoction of sorrel, spirit of wine, sugar, spirit of vitriol. Theden: *Genees- heelk. onderw.*, pp. 395–6.
[27] Fischer: *Chir. vor hundert Jahren*, p. 453.
[28] Full quotation in English in: Zimmerman, Veith: *Great ideas*, pp. 380–3.
[29] Bonn: *Descriptio thesauri ossium morbosorum Hoviani.*
[30] For a historical survey of the treatment of fractures of the long cylindrical bones, Dutch readers are referred to Van Loon's *Historisch overzicht van de fractuurbehandeling der lange pijpbeenderen.*
[31] Reichel G. Ch.: *Dissertatio de epiphysium ab ossium diaphysios diductione*. Thesis Leipzig, 1759. Quoted by Fischer: *Chir. vor hundert Jahren*, p. 414.
[32] Earle: 'Short account of the life of the author (P. Pott)'.
[33] Heister: *Heelk. onderwijzingen*, vol. 1, p. 200.
[34] 'From the muscles then, and from them only, proceeds all the difficulty which we meet with in making our extension; and by the resistance of these, and of these only, are we prevented from being always able to put the ends of a fractured bone immediately into the most apt contact.' Pott, P.: 'Some few general remarks on fractures and dislocations', *Chir. Works*, vol. 1, pp. 362–3.
[35] Ravaton: *Chirurgie d'armée*, pp. 363–8.
[36] Posch: *Beschreibung einer sehr bequemen Maschine das Fussbette genannt*. Haller: *Bibl. Chir.*, vol. 2, p. 588. Van Loon: *Fractuurbehandeling*, p. 179.
[37] Veraart: 'Bidloo's verhaal'.
[38] Brasdor: 'Fracture de la clavicule'.
[39] Bichat: *Oeuvres chirurgicales . . . de Desault*, vol. 1, pp. 63–90.
[40] Icart: 'En réponse au Mémoire de M. Pujol', pp. 172–3.
[41] Camper, P.: *Dissertatio de fractura patellae et olecrani*. Hagae Comitum: I van Cleef, 1789.
[42] Van Gesscher: *Hedendaagsche heelk.*, vol. 1, p. 270.
[43] Ruysch: *Alle de werken*, vol. 2, pp. 654, 770.
[44] Geyl: 'De ontdekking van de breuk van den hals van het dijbeen'.
[45] Petit: *Ziekten der beenderen*, part 2, pp. 118–24.
[46] Van Gesscher: *Hedendaagsche heelk*, vol. 1, p. 275.
[47] *Op. cit.*, vol. 1, p. 273.
[48] Van Loon: *Fractuurbehandeling*, p. 175.
[49] Camper: Cited by Doets: *Heelk. v. Petrus Camper*, pp. 32–41.
[50] Van Montfort: *Omstandig verhaal*, pp. 9–15.
[51] Munniks: *Alle de wercken*, p. 433. These observations probably date from the late 17th century.
[52] Pott: *Some few general remarks*, vol. 1, pp. 409–11. Quoted in Zimmerman, Veith: *Great ideas*, pp. 330–1.
[53] Van Loon: *Fractuurbehandeling*, p. 165. Fischer: *Chir. vor hundert Jahren*, p. 413.
[54] Ten Haaff: 'Eene kwalyk geneezene breuk'.
[55] Du Hamel du Monceau, H. L.: *Mén. Acad. roy. Sci. de Paris*, 1741. Cited by Sprengel: *Pragm. Gesch. Med.*, vol. 5, p. 76.

56 Detlef, P.: *Ossium calli generatio et natura per fracta in animalibus rubiae radice pastis ossa demonstrata.* Thesis Göttingen, 1753. Cited by Haller: *Bibl. Chir.*, vol. 2, p. 380.
57 Cited by Doets: *Heelk. v. Petrus Camper*, pp. 98—100.
58 'The way in which this all happens is unknown'. Bonn: *Descriptio thesauri*, pp. 149—200.
59 Fischer: *Chir. vor hundert Jahren*, pp. 429—34.
60 In the seventeenth century the clinical picture of rickets was first and most often described by English physicians. Hence the original Dutch designation 'lendenvang' was superseded by 'the English disease'. De Knecht-van Eekelen: *Naar een rationele zuigelingenvoeding*, p. 152.
61 Brockband: 'The crookedness clinic of Nicholas and Peter Schot'.
62 Haneveld: *Mr Arnoldus Fey*, pp. 67—73. Fey also was reputed to be able to cure cancer. He was amongst those who were summoned to the French court to advise on the treatment of the breast cancer of Anne of Austria, the mother of king Louis XIV.
63 Van Deventer, H.: *Beschrijving van de ziektens der beenderen, insonderheit van de rhachitis . . .* (Description of the diseases of the bones, in particular of rickets). Leyden: J. A. Langerak, 1739; 1765^2.
64 Van Gesscher: *Over de wangestalten der ruggegraat*, tab. II.
65 Camper: 'Verhandeling over den schoen'.
66 Valentin, B.: *Geschichte der Orthopädie.* Stuttgart: G. Thieme, 1961.
67 Van Beverwyck: *Heelkonste*, p. 156. These amputations were done a handbreadth below the knee.
68 Van Roonhuyze: *Genees- en heelk. aanmerkingen*, p. 99.
69 Van de Voorde: *Lichtende fakkel*, p. 373.
70 Verduin: *Nouvelle méthode.*
71 Vergniol: Preface to Verduin: *Nouvelle méthode.*
72 Ruysch: *Alle de werken*, vol. 1, pp. 406—16.
73 Koenerding: *Nutte beschrijving*, preface.
74 Heister: *Heelk. onderwijzingen*, vol. 1, pp. 586—7; Sharp: *Oordeelk aanm*, pp. 488—9 De la Faye: *Aanm op de operatien van Dionis*, p. 259;.
75 See also Bishop: *Early hist.*, p. 96.
76 Verduin: *Nouvelle méthode*, p. 13. Leaving the matter of priority for what it is worth, this bit of information discloses that at the end of the century the foreign relations of Dutch surgeons also began to span the North Sea. This is corroborated by the fact that some of them — amongst whom was Van Roonhuyze — started to make study trips to England.
77 De Gorter: *Gezuiverde heelkonst*, pp. 158—161. Constituents of the plaster are the traditional mastic, la(b)danum (Cistus creticus), terra segillata, ship's tar, turpentine, white wax. Burnt lead, incense and attar of roses may form part of it too, according to different recipes given by De Gorter.
78 Petit: *Ziekten der beenderen*, vol. 3, pp. 111—209.
79 Doets: *Heelk. v. Petrus Camper*, p. 227.
80 Fischer: *Chir. vor hundert Jahren*, p. 405.
81 Dionis: *Alle de operatien*, pp. 564—6.
82 Bromfeild: *Chirurgical cases*, vol. 1, p. 161. Bromfeild also introduced the method of drawing the skin upwards before making an incision to remove a joint mouse from the knee. After letting the skin go, there was no longer any direct connection between the joint and the atmospheric air. *Op. cit.*, vol. 1, p. 334.
83 Solingen: *Manuele operatien*, p. 253.
84 Richter: *Beginselen*, pp. 126—43.
85 Van de Voorde: *Lichtende fakkel*, p. 157.
86 Dionis: *Alle de operatien*, p. 562.
87 Heister: *Kort begrip*, p. 234.
88 Van Wyck: *Waarneminge rakende eenen fungus*, article XXXIII.
89 Morand: *Opuscules*, part 1, pp. 76—84. The essays by Wohlert — Volher, according to Morand — and Puthod were reprinted in Morand: *Op. cit.*, pp. 189—98 and 199—238. Morand, however, cites no instance of clinical application.
90 Barbet: 'Mémoire sur l'amputation de la cuisse'.
91 Anon: 'Gewichtig heelkundig voorval', *Nieuwe algemene Konst- en Letter-bode* voor meer- en min-geöeffenden, vol. X, no. 248, pp. 97, 1798.
92 Mulder, C.: Letter to the Editor, *Op. cit.*, N.S. vol. 1, pp. 161—2, 1824.
93 White: 'An account of a case'.
94 Park: *An account of a new method.*
95 De Moulin: 'Treatment of compound fract.'.
96 Dionis: *Alle de operatien*, p. 555.
97 Boucher: 'Observations'.

[98] Faure: 'Mémoire sur la question'.
[99] Bilguer: *Verhand over het seldsaam gebruik van het afsetten*, pp. 60—4, 83—6.
[100] Morand: *Opuscules*, part 1, pp. 232—53. De La Martinière: 'Mémoire sur le traitement des playes d'armes à feu'.
[101] Pott: 'Remarks on the necessity of amputation. In: *Chir. works*, vol. 3, pp. 371—407.
[102] Van Gesscher: *Verhandeling over de afzetting*. It is worthy of note that, some hundred years earlier, Van de Voorde in his discussion of the treatment of a compound leg fracture, made no mention of amputation as a possible approach (p. 140).
[103] Larrey: *Mémoires de chirurgie militaire*, vol. 4, p. 49.
[104] Van Nierop: 'Dagboek', p. 178.
[105] Doets: *Heelk. v. Petrus Camper*, p. 94.
[106] Schouten: *Het gewonde hoofd.*
[107] Van de Voorde: *Lichtende fakkel*, p. 475.
[108] Dionis: *Alle de operatien*, pp. 370—2.
[109] Stalpart vander Wiel: *Observ.*, vol. 1, pp. 1—2.
[110] De Gorter: *Gezuiverde heelkonst*, p. 76.
[111] Van Meekeren: *Heel- en geneesk. aenmerkingen*, pp. 29—39.
[112] De Gorter: *Gezuiverde heelkonst*, p. 76.
[113] In contrast to Dutch idiom, English has two different nouns to designate the act of making burr holes in the skull, viz *trepanation* and *trephination*. One might assume that in the first case the *trepan* is being used, an instrument resembling the carpenter's bit and brace, in the latter instance a *trephine*, a small circular saw with a pivot. It seems, however, that English authors use the two words somewhat indiscriminately.
[114] Van de Voorde: *Lichtende fakkel*, p. 490.
[115] Pott: *Twee heelk. verhand.*, p. 80.
[116] Dionis: *Alle de operatien*, p. 386.
[117] Schouten: *Het gewonde hoofd*, p. 178.
[118] One of Schouten's patients was a four-year old girl in whom he made a burr hole next to the depression through which he introduced an elevator by which he raised the impacted fragment to level. Fourteen years later she appeared to be in good health. *Op. cit.*, p. 156.
[119] Cf. p. 69.
[120] Tulp: *Observat medicae*, pp. 8—9.
[121] Suspected haematoma was the indication. Van den Spiegel made 3 burr holes on the first day, 2 on the third day and 3 more a few days later. The patient, a coachman, was reported to have been cured. Glandorp: *Speculum chirurgorum*, pp. 21—2.
[122] Dionis: *Alle de operatien*, p. 396.
[123] This impressive instance of surgical perseverance is related by Solingen *Manuele operatien*, p. 29, as well as by Stalpart vander Wiel *Observ. centuriae*, vol. 1, pp. 36—38. The latter disposed of an attestation drawn up by Philip of Nassau himself. Unfortunately the count did not go into details.
[124] Dionis: *Alle de operatien*, p. 387.
[125] Schmucker: *Heelk waarnemingen*, vol. 1, p. 2. All 12 cases are described in extenso, as well as a number of trepanations which were attended with success.
[126] Desault: *Oeuvres chir.*, vol. 2, pp. 40—56.
[127] See Adams: *Hippocrates*, vol. 1, pp. 432—39, for a short survey of trepanation in Britain in the late 17th and early 18th cent.
[128] De Moulin: 'Aneurysms in Antiquity'.
[129] Lancisi: *Aneurysms*, p. 147.
[130] De Moulin: 'More historical notes on aneurysms'.
[131] Hunter: Cited by Home: 'An account of Mr. Hunter's method'. Two specimens of such cases obtained 1½ and 40 years after operation by Hunter, are still on display in the Hunterian Collection of the Royal College of Surgeons in London. They show obliteration of the artery distal to the ligation, the sac has almost completely disappeared. In England in the 18th century, relatively many publications on the ligation of big arteries appeared.
[132] Heister: *Kort begrip*, p. 205.
[133] Van Gesscher: *Verhand over de afzetting*, p. 70.
[134] Valsalva: Quoted by Morgagni: *De sedibus et causis morborum*, vol. 1, p. 138.
[135] Sandifort: *Heel- en ontleedk verhand. over eenen slagaderbreuk.*
[136] Ruysch: *Alle de werken*, vol. 2, pp. 49—50.
[137] De Moulin: 'Hist. notes on vascular surgery I'.
[138] Asman: *De aneurysmate*, §§ XXV—XXXI.
[139] Verduin: 'Twee-en-twintig waarnemingen', obs. III, VIII, XVII.

[140] Van Roonhuyze: *Genees- en heelk aanmerkingen*, first observation.
[141] Baumann: 'Hendrick van Roonhuyse', p. 858.
[142] De Moulin: *Short history of breast cancer*, chapt. 4.
[143] De Gorter: *Gezuiverde heelkonst*, pp. 401—2.
[144] Camper: 'Over den waren aart der kankervorming'.
[145] Tulp: *Observat medicae*, pp. 307—9.
[146] De Moulin: 'Hist. notes on breast cancer I'.
[147] De Moulin: de Groot: 'The cancer operation by Romeyn de Hooghe'.
[148] De Moulin: 'Hist. notes on breast cancer II'.
[149] Fabricius Hildanus: *Observationum centuriae*, cent. II, obs. 79, pp. 150—1.
[150] De Moulin: 'Hist. notes on breast cancer I, II'.
[151] Ulhoorn in: Heister: *Heelk. onderwijzingen*, vol. 2, p. 846.
[152] Doets: *Heelk. v. Petrus Camper*, p. 25.
[153] Van der Haar: *Verhand. over kankergezwellen.*
[154] Bidloo: *Opera omnia*, p. 160.
[155] Van de Voorde: *Lichtende fakkel*, p. 429.
[156] Van Wij: 'kunnen wij ons overtuigd houden', p. 119.
[157] Camper: 'Oorzaaken der breuken'.
[158] Rombach: 'Vergelijking'. Rombach's excellent article gives a detailed overview of herniology between c. 1750 and c. 1850.
[159] Monnikhoff: *Over de scheursels.* The influence of a humid climate owing to which membranes and fibres tend to be more flaccid, was stressed by several authors. This belief may have been inspired by Hippocrates, who in § VII of his *Airs, waters, places* wrote that children are very subject to hernia in regions where waters were bad.
[160] Schrader: *Observationum anatomico-medicarum decades IV*, obs. V, pp. 207—8.
[161] Boerhaave, H.: Cited by Schierbeek: *Jan Swammerdam*, p. 35.
[162] Méry, J.: *Mém. Acad. roy. Sci.*, 1701. Quoted by Haller: *Bibl. chir.*, vol. 1, p. 474.
[163] Reneaulme de la Garanne: *Vertoog ter opening van het School der heelk*, pp. 125—40.
[164] Croissant de Garengeot: *Traité des opérations*, vol. 1, pp. 300—355.
[165] Benevoli, Tacconi: *Heelk. waarnemingen*, p. 127.
[166] Pott: *Twee heelk. verhand.*, pp. 113—245.
[167] [Arnaud de Ronsil G]: *Traité des hernies*, pp. 108—18.
[168] Richter: *Verhand. over de breuken*, vol. 1, pp. 13—22.
[169] Scarpa, A.: *A treatise on hernia.* Transl. by J. U. Wishart. Edinburgh: Longman, Hurst et al., 1814. His description of sliding hernia is reprinted in Zimmerman, Veith: *Great Ideas*, pp. 390—3.
[170] Camper: *Oorzaaken der breuken*, p. 260.
[171] Richter: *Verhand. over de breuken*, vol. 1, pp. 78—87.
[172] Heister: *Acta medico-physica Naturae Curiosorum*, vol. 10, obs. 2, p. 4. Quoted by Camper: 'Oorzaaken der breuken', p. 259—60.
[173] Rombach: 'Vergelijking der breuken', p. 49.
[174] Barbette: *Chirurgie*, pp. 27, 34.
[175] Ulhoorn: Cited by Rombach: 'Vergelijking', p. 33.
[176] Van Foreest, P.: Cited by Banga: *Gesch. Geneesk. in Nederland*, p. 123.
[177] Dionis: *Alle de operatien*, pp. 255—6.
[178] Solingen: *Manuele operatiën*, p. 200.
[179] Vink: Preface to (de la Faye) *Aanmerkingen op de chir. operatien van Dionis.*
[180] Doets: *Heelk. v. Petrus Camper*, pp. 46—51.
[181] Ulhoorn: Cited by Rombach: 'Vergelijking', p. 39.
[182] [Van Musschenbroek]: *Catalogus instrumentorum*, pp. 79—80.
[183] 'De operateurs die overal door het land lopen, zijn zeer behending deze deelen (testes) uit te halen zonder dat het de omstanders gewaar worden . . . verbergen het in haare hand, om in haare tas te steeken, zonder dat het iemand gezien heeft. Men heeft een van die operateurs gekent, die zijn hond nergens anders mee voede, als met de klootjes . . .' Dionis: *Alle de operatien*, p. 252.
[184] Gorus, G.: *Medicina contempta propter ignorantium medicorum.* Lugd.-Bat. 1700. Cited by Van Andel: 'J. H. Francken', p. 354. Gerard Gorus (1657—post 1711) was a physician at Leyden.
[185] Van Andel: *Op. cit.*, p. 376.
[186] Van Andel: *Op. cit.*, p. 380.
[187] Helfreich: *Gesch. Chir.*, p. 263.
[188] Van Gesscher: *Hedendaagsche heelk.*, vol. 3, p. 258.
[189] Van Meekeren: *Heel- en geneesk. aanm.*, pp. 460—2.
[190] Van Dyck: Cited by Van Zuiden: 'Op welke voorwaarden'.
[191] Doets: *Heelk. v. Petrus Camper*, p. 64.

192 Cyprianus: Cited by Napjus: 'De hoogleraren in de geneeskunde . . . te Franeker. XIII Abraham Cyprianus'. Cf. n. 202.
193 Helfreich: 'Gesch. Chir.', pp. 268—70.
194 Tulp: *Observ. medicae*, pp. 209—10.
195 Doets: *Heelk. v. Petrus Camper*, p. 25: 'het snyden van verstropte breuken'.
196 Van Meekeren: *Heel- en geneesk. aanm.*, pp. 261—69.
197 Dekkers, F.: *Exercitationes practicae circa methodum medendi* . . . . Amsterdam: 1673. Cited by Banga: *Gesch. geneesk. in Nederland*, p. 702.
198 Van Roonhuyze: Cited by Baumann: 'Hendrick van Roonhuyse', pp. 865—6.
199 Heister: *Chirurgie*, pp. 733—4.
200 Wintgens: *Johannes Monnikhoff en zijn legaat.*
201 Van Beverwyck: *Steen-stuck*, Ch. 2, ed. Van Andel: *Opuscula selecta* XVII, pp. 36—7.
Amongst those who were suffering from gravel, was Erasmus of Rotterdam. In two letters dating from 1526 he vividly described the torture he had to endure. These Latin letters were edited and translated into English by Van Andel: *Op. cit.*, pp. 2—9.
202 Muffett, Th.: Cited by Drummond and Wilbraham: *The Englishman's food*, p. 154. A few Dutch lithotomists were active in London. Amongst them was Joannes Groeneveld M.D. (1647—1710), who after his emigration for unknown reasons to England in 1675, anglicized his name into Greenfield. He was trained in the operation for the stone at Amsterdam by the renowned lithotomist Hendrik Velthuis. Greenfield, who was in favour of the suprapubic approach, published several works on his specialty. Another Dutch M.D.—surgeon who practised in London as a lithotomist was the celebrated Abraham Cyprianus. He settled in London in 1695 and although he only stayed for some five years, he amassed riches and reputation in the British capital. One of his patients there was Thomas Millington, physician to king-stadtholder William III. Cyprianus became a member of the Royal Society.
203 Van Foreest: Quoted by Banga: *Gesch. Geneesk. in Nederland*, pp. 123, 140.
204 Barbette: Quoted by Banga: *Op. cit.*, p. 264.
205 Gelfand: *Training of surgeons*, p. 12.
206 From a letter of Claude Pouteau (1725—75), surgeon at Lyons, quoted by Desnos: 'Hist. d'urologie', p. 175. The operation for the stone inspired the court musician Marin Marais (1656—1728) to compose a piece of music for viola da gamba and harpsicord entitled 'L'opération de la taille' (1725).
207 Nieuwenhuys: *Geneesk. plaatsbeschrijving Amsterdam*, vol. 2, p. 95.
208 Titsingh: *Heelk. verhand. over den steen*, pp. 65, 76, 91.
Titsingh in this book continuously attacks the Leyden lithotomist Jacob Denijs — to whom fuller reference will be made below — whose proficiency he evidently did not value highly. The work contains many items of human interest, like the sad case of a widow who lost three sons after being cut for the stone (p. 97). It appears that Dutch children were sent all the way from Batavia to Amsterdam to be operated upon: Ulhoorn treated two such boys within one year (p. 24).
209 Camper: 'Steensnyden in twee reizen', pp. 346—59.
210 Van der Berge: *Privilegiën*, p. 24.
211 Camper: *Steensnijden in twee reizen*, pp. 358—9.
212 An example of this, regarding Haarlem in 1694, is given by Bitter: 'Stadsoperateurs en steensnijders'.
213 Titsingh: *Heelk. verhand. over den steen*, p. 58.
214 *Aenteekeningen omtrent operatiën van den steen*, gehouden door stads-doctoren en overluyden van het chirurgijnsgilde (Notes on operations for the stone, kept by town physicians and aldermen of the surgeons' guild). Municip Archives Amsterdam. The Amsterdam list has been published by Van Staveren: *Aenteekeningen omtrent operatiën van den steen*. It cannot be anything like complete.
215 Van de Ven: 'Een steensnijding in 1653'. Van Dyck and the attending physicians received a truly princely fee in this case. It is known that Noach Smaltius (1629?—?), town surgeon at Haarlem and a prominent lithotomist, charged 30 guilders for patients under 20 years of age and 42 guilders for older ones, cf. Bitter: 'Stadsoperateurs en steensnijders'. In 1678 a surgeon attached to the hospital in Amsterdam, drew 400 guilders a year for which he had twice a day to go there to see the patients, cf. Hellinga: 'De positie der 17de en 18de eeuwsche gasthuis-chirurgijns'.
216 Van der Weyde: 'Iets over steensnijden'.
217 Numerous articles and textbook-chapters have been written on this colourful person. Dutch readers are referred to Moonen: 'Frère Jacques de Beaulieu'.
218 This case made a stir at the time. A portrait painted shortly afterwards representing Jan de Doot, proudly holding the corpus delicti in his hand, is kept in the Pathological Department of the University of Leyden, together with the knife he used and the stone he took out. Tulp devoted a chapter to this memorable event in his *Observationes medicae*.

[219] Banga: *Gesch. Geneesk. in Nederland*, p. 782.
[220] Heister: *Chirurgie*, p. 853.
[221] Leporin: *Ausführlicher Bericht*, p. 11.
[222] Erndl: *De itinere suo*, pp. 119—21.
[223] Titsingh: *Heelk. verhand. van den steen*, p. 11.
[224] Rau, J. J.: *De methodo anatomen docendi et discendi*. Lugd.-Batav. 1713. Quoted by Albinus: *Index suppellectilis*, Ed. Van Andel: *Opuscula selecta* XVII, pp. 198—9. Rau's claim lacks underpinning. The Amsterdam list referred to in note 214 discloses that in the period between March 1700 and May 1705, he did only 33 lithotomies (with four deaths). It is true, however, that since in this inventory for unknown reasons the years 1704—1725 are missing, we have no official record of the number of operations he did between May 1705 and September 1713 when he assumed his post in Leyden. Furthermore it is known that he also operated outside his place of residence. Charles Bell characterized Rau as 'the greatest lithotomist that ever lived'. 'On lithotomy', p. 773.
[225] Cheselden, W.: *The anatomy of the humane body*. London: C. Hitch & R. Dodsley, 1756, pp. 325—34. Cheselden's historical account is quoted in full by Zimmerman & Veith: *Great ideas*, pp. 307—12.
[226] Denos: 'Hist. d'urologie', p. 162.
[227] Hossard: 'Le Cat, lithotomiste', p. 156.
[228] Sermes: *Aanmerkingen over de twee manieren*.
[229] Francken: 'Over het steensnijden'.
[230] Denijs: *Heelk. aanmerkingen*.
[231] Billings: *Hist. and lit. of surg*., p. 96.
[232] Nieuwenhuys: *Geneesk. plaatsbeschrijving Amsterdam*, vol: 3, p. 178.
[233] Francken: 'Over het steensnijden, pp. 308—9.
[234] Denos: 'Hist. d'urologie', p. 230.
[235] Schechter: 'Role of the humane societies'.
[236] Gorter: *De tabaksrook-klisteer*. The Amsterdam society exhibits a small collection of fine 18th and 19th centuries tobacco smoke clysters.
[237] De Moulin: 'Tobacco smoke in the treatment of intussusception'.
[238] Meyer-Steineg: *Chir. Instrumente des Altertums*.
[239] Gurlt: *Gesch. Chir*., vol. 2, p. 262.
[240] Fellows: 'Hist. of some surgical instruments'.
[241] Fabricius Hildanus: quoted by Gurlt: *Gesch. Chir*., vol. 3, p. 145.
[242] Solingen: *Manuale operatiën*, Introduction. Solingen held that a surgeon should have sufficient draughtmanship to make clear to a blacksmith or any other mechanic the exact instrument he wishes him to make. A surgeon should moreover have some cognizance of iron and steel and be familiar with how these materials should be worked. Ulhoorn, too, added 15 large plates of surgical instruments after his own drawings to his translation of Heister.
[243] Schoute: *Schets. Middelb. Chir. Gilde*, p. 33.
[244] Van Gesscher: *Hedend. oeffenende heelk*., preface to vol. 1.
[245] Erndl: *De itinere suo*, pp. 79—80.
[246] Van Nierop: 'Dagboek', p. 169.

CHAPTER 7: THE BEGINNING OF MODERN SURGERY

[1] Ackerknecht: 'Pariser Chirurgie'.
[2] The word 'morphology' was coined by Goethe.
[3] Bichat, M. F. X.: *Anatomie générale, appliquée à la physiologie et à la médecine*. 2 vols. Paris: Brosson, Gabon & Cie (1801).
[4] Corvisart des Marets, J. N.: *Essai sur les maladies . . . du coeur . . .*. Paris: Méquignon-Marvis, 1806.
[5] Laennec, R. Th. H.: *De l'auscultation médiate*. 2 vols. Paris: J. A. Brosson & J. S. Chaudé, 1819.
[6] Crosse: *A surgeon in the early nineteenth century*, p. 33.
[7] Rothschuh: *Konzepte*, pp. 385—96.
[8] Rochard: *Hist. de la chir. française*, p. 55.
[9] Malgaigne, J. F., quoted by Rochard: *Op. cit*., p. 58.
[10] Logger: 'Aanteekeningen op eene wetenschappelijke reize'.
[11] De Moulin: 'Guillaume Dupuytren'.

[12] The Pathological Anatomy Museum which he founded in Paris still bears his name.
[13] The diary Tilanus kept on that journey was in part and not very satisfactorily published in English in 1925.
[14] Casper: *Charakteristik der französischen Medicin*, pp. 148–9.
[15] Roux, Ph. J.: *Relation d'un voyage à Londres en 1814*. Paris: Méquignon-Marvis, 1815.
[16] Rochard: *Hist. de la chir. française*, p. 93.
[17] *Op. cit.*, p. 439.
[18] Bishop: *Early hist. of surg.*, p. 143.
[19] The operating theatre of the old St. Thomas's Hospital which had been built in 1821 in the loft of the adjacent Church of St. Thomas, opposite Guy's Hospital in London, was bricked up in 1872 when the hospital moved to its present site. The old hospital buildings were subsequently torn down, but the church still stands. Restored to its original condition, this operating theatre is the only surviving example of its kind dating from the third decade of the 19th century.
[20] Keith, Keys: 'The anatomy Acts of 1831 and 1832'. On the European mainland there were far less general objections against anatomical dissection. However, occasional cases of body snatching occurred there too. The well-known Utrecht professor of chemistry Gerrit Jan Mulder (1802–80), son of a surgeon, remembered how at the tender age of about ten years his passion for anatomy had led him to exhume the dead body from a freshly-dug grave. He subsequently managed to wheel his acquisition home in a barrow, without being detected. Mulder: *Levensschets*, p. 20. It is not recorded what his mother had to say.
[21] De Moulin: 'Fracture of the lower end of the radius'.
[22] Billings: *Hist. and lit. of surg.*, pp. 118–31.
[23] Machiel Polano at Rotterdam was the first to perform an ovariotomy in the Netherlands in 1865. 'Ovariotomie. Waarneming van een genezen geval' (Ovarectomy. Observations in a case of complete recovery), *Nederl. Tijdschr. Geneeskd.* **1** (II), 1865: 109–33.
[24] Haeser: *Gesch. Med.*, vol. 2, pp. 683, 957–65.
[25] Küster: *Gesch. n. dtsch. Chir.*, p. 60.
[26] Schönbauer: *Das medizinische Wien*, p. 178.
[27] Nieuwenhuys: *Geneesk plaatsbeschrijving der stad Amsterdam*, vol. 4, pp. 350–65.
[28] Van Eeghen: 'Anthonie van den Hout en Pieter Klases Pel'.
[29] Nieuwenhuys: *Geneesk plaatsbeschrijving der stad Amsterdam*, vol. 1, p. 372.
[30] *Op. cit.*, vol. 1, pp. 357–8.
[31] There appears to have been a huge number of surgeons in Amsterdam. In Rotterdam there were only 45 master-surgeons and a similar number of medical doctors at the end of the 18th century, for something more than 50000 inhabitants.
[32] Vosmaer: *Het leven van meester Maarten Vroeg*, p. 127. These delightful sketches of the life of a village barber-surgeon first appeared separately in the journal *Vaderlandsche Letteroefeningen* in 1821–2.
[33] *Camera obscura*, written by Hildebrand (ps. of N. Beets) in 1839, is a Dutch literary classic. It consists of a number of short stories and sketches, 'The barber' being one of them. The letter is a parody, supposedly written by a barber-surgeon whose name (literally: 'scrape him') is indicative of the author's profession.
[34] [Greidanus]: *Een dorpsdokter uit de Friese Wouden vertelt*, pp. 13, 11.
[35] Nieuwenhuys: *Geneesk plaatsbeschrijving der stad Amsterdam*, vol. 1, p. 362. A Cayenne catheter was a flexible instrument made of resin of Cayenne.
[36] Van der Klaauw: 'Het eertijds verplichte instrumentarium'.
[37] Like the 'Ecoles centrales de Médecine', which had already been founded during the French annexation of Belgium in Brussels, Ghent, Antwerp and Bruges in 1804 and 1805, their origins can probably be found in the training establishments of 'officiers de santé' in France. These second-rate doctors received their tuition at specially founded schools outside the university. They were only permitted to practise in the 'département' for which they had passed the examination, taken before a jury which had been specifically set up for the purpose. The husband of Madame Bovary was such an 'officier de santé' and the reader might remember how much the couple were burdened by his inferior status. The idea of special schools for country doctors had already existed for some time. The journal *Göttinger Anzeigen von gelehrten Sachen* of July 14, 1792, 112. Stück, p. 1122, contained a short summary of a prize-winning entry to a competition for finding the best method of providing adequate obstetric care in the country. The author recommended either to give village doctors an annual income, or to establish practical schools at the hospitals for country doctors and surgeons. Cited by Bonn: 'Tegenwoordige staat' p. XII, footnote. Such schools were indeed opened in Germany in the early 19th century — in Breslau, Magdeburg, Königsberg, Greifswald and Münster — but were closed again in 1849. Haeser: *Gesch. Med.*, vol. 2, p. 1062.

[38] Lindeboom: 'De Clinische School te Rotterdam'.
Van Lieburg: 'Gasthuis en Clinische School'.
[39] Hulsman, Zwaveling: 'Frederik Willem Krieger'.
[40] Zwaveling, Hulsman: 'Machiel Polano'.
[41] De Moulin: *Vier eeuwen Amsterdams Binnengasthuis*, p. 20.
[42] Anonymous, obit. *Nederl. Tijdschr. Geneeskd.* **19** (II): 626—8, 1983.
[43] Anonymous: 'Levensschets van G. D. Schröder'.
[44] Van Leuven, S.: *Bundel van heelkundige operatien*, gedicteerd door de WelEd. Heer Schröder, stads chirurgijn te Amsterdam. (Collection of surgical operations, dictated by S, town surgeon at A). Handwritten notes, Institute for the History of Medicine, Catholic University Nijmegen. S.a. (1833—4).
[45] Hellinga: 'Van 'Verbanthuys' tot dubbele chirurgische cliniek'.
[46] Kerkhoff: *Geneeskundige verzorging in het Staatse leger.*
[47] Romeyn: *Onze militair-geneesk dienst*, pp. 70—1.
[48] Blondeau: 'De negentiende en twintigste eeuw', p. 315.
[49] Romeyn: *Onze militair-geneesk dienst*, pp. 61—9.
[50] Spoelstra: *Antonius Mathijsen*, pp. 290—308.
[51] A number of alumni, amongst whom were Jonkheer Johannes Lydius Catharinus Pompe van Meerdervoort (1829—1908) and Antonius Franciscus Bauduin (1822—85), worked in Japan for some years where they played a leading part in introducing Western medicine to that country. When in 1862 the first Japanese young men came to Holland to study medicine, they chose the Military Medical School in Utrecht for this purpose.
[52] Van Lieburg: 'De Nederlandse medische tijdschriften', p. 8.
[53] De Moulin: 'Die Medizin zur Zeit der Regierung des Königs Wilhelm I', pp. 33—5.
[54] Chelius, M. J.: *Leerboek der heelkunde.* 4 vols., Ed. by G. J. Pool, Amsterdam: C. G. Sulpke, 1830—2.
[55] De Knecht-van Eekelen: *Naar een rationele zuigelingenvoeding*, p. 31.
[56] Trent: 'Surgical anaesthesia 1846—1946' and many more publications on this subject.
[57] *Algemeen Handelsblad*, 10th March, 1847, p. 2.
[58] Korteweg: 'De ontwikkeling der heelk gedurende de laatste halve eeuw'.
[59] Mathijsen: *The plaster of Paris bandage.*
[60] De Moulin: 'Heelk. onderwerpen in het Nederl. Weekblad'.
[61] New growths and inflammation depended on particular 'blastemas' which, in their turn, reflected a particular 'crasis' — state — of the blood. King: *The growth of medical thought*, pp. 196—207.
[62] Virchow: 'Rokitansky, Handbuch'.
[63] 'One will rarely find the two men necessary for the operation', Korteweg: 'De ontwikkeling der heelk gedurende de laatste halve eeuw'.
[64] Charles-Gabriel Pravaz (1791—1853) at Lyons was also the inventor of the hypodermic syringe.
[65] Schrant: *Prijsverhandeling over de goed- en kwaadaardige gezwellen.*
[66] Schroeder van der Kolk: 'Over de vorming en verspreiding van kankercellen'.
[67] Virchow: *Die krankhaften Geschwülste*, vol. 1: a, p. 47; b, p. 92.
[68] Tilanus: *Overzigt van de chirurgicale gebreken.*
[69] Van Goudoever: 'Verslag der chirurgische kliniek'.

CHAPTER 8: ANTISEPSIS, A TURNING POINT IN SURGERY

[1] [Greidanus]: *Een dorpsdokter*, pp. 23—34.
[2] Küster: 'Gesch. n. dtsch. Chirurgie', pp. 15—6.
[3] Greidanus: *Op. cit.*, p. 11.
[4] Küster: *Op. cit.*, pp. 10—5.
[5] Pouteau: *Oeuvres posthumes.* Lyon, 1783, vol. 3. Quoted by Helfreich: 'Gesch. Chir.', p. 27.
[6] Brugmans: 'Verhand over de gesteldheid van den dampkring'.
[7] Delpech: *Précis des maladies chirurgicales*, vol. I, 123—32.
[8] Küster: 'Gesch. n. dtsch. Chirurgie', p. 13.
[9] Sir John Pringle (1707—82) therefore advised that the wards should be adequately ventilated. His well-known book *Observations on the diseases of the army*, London: Royal Society, 1752, enlarged with a description of the hospitals by Donald Monro, was also brought out in Dutch. Pringle, who had graduated at Leyden, served as physician-general to the British army during the War of the

Austrian Succession. He was a pioneer of the idea that military hospitals should be regarded as neutral and immune from attack. In his paper *Experiments upon septic and antiseptic substances*, read before The Royal Society in 1750, the word 'antiseptic' was used for the first time in history. Mercer: 'Some Edinburgh pioneers', pp. 345—6.

10 Temkin: 'A historical analysis of the concept of infection'. In: *The double face of Janus*, p. 461.

11 Heister: *Heelk. Onderwijzingen*, vol. 1, pp. 75—6.

12 Rotgans: 'Eenige bladzijden', p. 582.

13 Fischer: *Chir. vor 100 Jahren*, pp. 394, 393.

14 Camper, P.: *Essai fur les influences que l'air par ses diverses qualités peut avoir dans les maladies chirurgicales*. 1775, Univ. Libr. Leyden Ms BPL 247/51 & 52).

15 Rotgans: 'Eenige bladzijden', p. 582.

16 Fischer: *Chir. vor 100 Jahren*, pp. 556—7.

17 In 1872, Rudolf Ulrich Krönlein, at the time assistant of Rose at Zürich, later of Billroth, published statistical evidence showing that the postoperative death rate had been reduced by 60% through the method of open wound treatment. Rotgans: 'Eenige bladzijden', pp. 583—4.

18 Rotgans: *Op. cit.*, p. 583.

19 Brugmans: 'Verhand. over den dampkring', p. 18.

20 *Op. cit.*, p. 45.

21 *Op. cit.*, pp. 56—7, 61. Fumigating hospital wards with hydrochloric acid vapours to combat hospital fever was first used in 1773 by the Frenchman Guyton Morveau. Seven years later James Carmichael Smyth used nitric acid fumes for the same purpose. Zambon: 'Brugmans'.

22 Clendening: *Source book*, p. 603.

23 Holmes: 'Contagiousness of puerperal fever'.

24 Semmelweis: *Die Aetiologie des Kindbettfiebers*, pp. 103—8.

25 *Op. cit.*, pp. 310—3.

26 Van Tussenbroek: *Ontwikkeling der aseptische verlosk.*, pp. 61—87.

27 Pasteur: 'Mémoire sur les corpuscles organisés', pp. 60—4.

28 Lister: 'On the antiseptic principle'.

29 Temkin: 'A historical analysis of the concept of infection'. In: *The double face of Janus*, pp. 456—71; p. 462.

30 Van Iterson: 'Geneeskundig Congres te Londen'.

31 Ravitch: *Century of surgery*, vol. 1, pp. 24—33.

32 Dermatitis on the hands of one of his nurses, produced by solutions of mercuric chloride, was the reason why, in 1889, professor William Stewart Halsted introduced the use of rubber gloves in his operating room at The Johns Hopkins Hospital in Baltimore. Randers-Pehrson: *The surgeon's glove*, p. 54. Although disinfection of the hands soon became a recognized problem, it took some time before gloves were universally worn. Twenty years later in Groningen only the professor was entitled to wear them at the operating table, the residents were not. Boerema: 'De aard van het werk in de Vereeniging voor Heelkunde', p. 132.

33 Von Bruns: 'Fort mit dem Spray!'.

34 Tilanus, J. W. R.: *Herinneringswoord*, p. 7.

35 Tilanus, J. W. R.: 'Vernieuwing der stedelijke ziekenhuizen', p. 96.

36 De Leng: *Verslag . . . 1873—1874*, first thesis. Among the cases described, there is a patient who had four sebaceous cysts removed from his scalp. After the operation ice bags were placed on his head to prevent irritation of the brain. The patient died of erysipelas. De Leng's dissertation gives interesting additional information. It appears, for instance, that subcutaneous injections of morphine were given to alleviate pain, but that 'issues' (see p. 354, n. 44) and hirudines were still in use. A case of bladder stone was treated with lateral lithotomy.

37 Ten Doeschate: *De Utrechtse Universiteit*, p. 155.

38 Klasen: 'Hans Rudolph Ranke'.

39 Brieger: *Medical America*, p. 235.

40 Kouwer, Laméris: *Gesch. Klinieken te Utrecht*, p. 73.

CHAPTER 9: THE GERMAN PERIOD IN DUTCH SURGERY

1 Küster: 'Gesch. n. dtsch. Chir.', pp. 103—5.

2 Klasen: 'Hans Rudolph Ranke'.

3 Ten Doeschate: *De Utrechtse Universiteit*, pp. 156—7.

[4] Kuijjer: 'Oprichting van de Vereniging', pp. 68–75.
[5] In the two first decades of the present century, Jakob Rotgans (1859–1948) was one of the most prominent Dutch surgeons. He studied at clinics in Berlin and Jena. In 1893, Rotgans was appointed professor of surgery at Amsterdam. His special interest was gastroenterostomy. In 1913, he initiated the founding of the 'Nederlandsch Kankerinstituut' (Dutch Cancer Institute) at Amsterdam, later renamed, for obscure reasons, the 'Antoni van Leeuwenhoekhuis'.
[6] For the history of surgery in the Netherlands during the first 75 years of this century, Dutch readers are referred to Kuijjer et al.: *Nederlandse Vereniging voor Heelkunde 1902–1977.*
[7] Grond: 'De positie van de geneeskundigen in Nederland', p. 33.
[8] Among the members of the 'Nederlandsche Maatschappij tot bevordering der Geneeskunst', 'specialists' are first mentioned in 1883. However, these were physicians who dealt exclusively with one particular aspect of one of the three major subjects. They would nowadays be called 'sub-specialists'.
[9] Veltheer: 'Dawn of gastric resection'. Billroth was also highly musical, and a good friend of the Viennese composer Brahms, many of the latter's piano compositions and lieder were performed for the first time at the Billroth family home.
[10] Boerema: 'Aard van het werk', p. 107.
[11] Westerman: 'Behandeling van de peritonitis'. This principle was named after O. H. Wangensteen who, in 1932, reported three successful applications in cases of bowel obstructions. Cornelis Willem Johan Westerman (1868–1925) was surgeon at the Elisabeth of Groote Gasthuis at Haarlem.
[12] Leriche: *Souvenirs*, p. 35.
[13] An English transl. of Schenk's clinical description can be found in Glenn, Grafe: 'Hist. events in biliary tract surgery'.
[14] Petit: 'Remarques sur les tumeurs formées par la bile retenue'.
[15] As early as 1867, John Stough Bobbs (1809–70) of Indianapolis, Indiana, operated on a woman thought to have an ovarian cyst. He found, however, a huge hydropic gall-bladder, from which he removed a number of stones and much fluid. The incision in the gall-bladder was closed by a stitch. His patient survived for many years. Sparkman: 'Dr. John S. Bobbs'.
[16] Taubert: '75 Jahre Cholezystektomie'.
[17] De Moulin: 'Hist. notes on appendicitis'.
[18] Van Capellen: 'In memoriam Prof. Dr. Otto Lanz'. The diagnosis of acute appendicitis is characterized by the large number of 'points' which have been defined for it over the years. In addition to McBurney's well-known point and Lanz's, Dorland's *Illustrated medical dictionary* mentions points indicated by Cope, Kümmell, Lanzmann, Lotheisen and Morris.
[19] 'The art of medicine lies wholly in observations'. De Moulin: 'Hernias in history'. We have met the Halle professor of medicine above on p. 149.
[20] Trendelenburg: *Die ersten 25 Jahre*, pp. 291–2. It is difficult nowadays to imagine the dimension which neglected hernias can assume: we met with a few impressive specimens on p. 145 and 239. Friedrich Trendelenburg (1844–1924), professor of surgery at Leipzig, recalled that 'scrotal herniae hanging almost to the knees were in the days of my apprenticeship still occasionally seen, a great burden for the sufferer and a difficult problem for the tailor'. Much earlier, Gaius Lucilius (149–103 B.C.), the Roman satirist, joked about the scrotal hernia of one Dionysius, which was so big that by floating on it he managed to be the sole survivor of a shipwreck. Quoted by A. G. J. Hermans: Grote hernia als reddingsboei (Big hernia as a lifebuoy), *Med. Contact* **14**: 207, 1959.
[21] This operation, whereby the inguinal canal is obliterated and the spermatic cord rendered subcutaneous, differs little in essentials from that of Josef Fabricius, who closed the inguinal canal in two layers (1894).
[22] The relatively high infection rate reported by this author is somewhat surprising in view of the thorough preparation of the patients. On admission, they were bathed and shaved. On the eve of the operation, a wet compress soaked in Burow's solution was applied to the abdomen. Immediately before the operation, they were thoroughly washed once again with hot water and soap, shaved once more, and dried with a sterile towel. Thereupon the operative field was rubbed with ether, then with 60 or 70% alcohol, and finally with mercury bichloride 1 : 1000. Boerema: 'De aard van het werk', pp. 107–9.
[23] To give a comparison: William B. Coley at New York had in 1901 4% wound infections after hernioplasty: after the introduction of the surgical glove the percentage fell to 0.5%. Ravitch: *A Century*, vol. 1, p. 258.
[24] Scarff: 'Fifty years of neurosurgery'. Sir Victor Horsley (1857–1916) was the father of British neurosurgery. Alexander H. Bennett and Sir Rickman Godlee, however, must be credited with the first successful removal of a tumour of the brain, in 1885.
[25] Nissen, Wilson: *Pages in the history of chest surgery*, pp. 10–77.

[26] Zimmerman, Veith: 'Ferdinand Sauerbruch and the explosive expansion of thoracic surgery'. In: *Great ideas*, pp. 536–47.
[27] Tuffier: *Chirurgie du poumon*, p. 31.
[28] Nissen, Wilson: *Pages in the history of chest surgery*, pp. 51–66.
[29] Mann: *Zauberberg*, vol. 1, p. 184.
[30] Westerman: 'Intrathorakale oesophagusresectie'. Murphy's button, introduced by the Chicago surgeon John Benjamin Murphy (1857–1916), was a metal device for intestinal anastomosis, more or less based on the principle of the snap fastener.
[31] Zaayer: 'Overdruknarcose'; 'Eenige gevallen van thoraxoperatie'.
[32] Moore: 'On the influence of inadequate operations'.
[33] Westerman: 'Thorax-excisie bij recidief van carcinoma mammae'.
[34] Von Winniwarter: *Beiträge zur Statistik der Carcinome*, p. 44. Numerically, breast cancer yielded only to carcinoma of the face, with 278 cases. Characteristic of that time, 34 breast cancer patients died after the operation because of pyaemia or erysipelas.
[35] De Moulin: 'Hist. notes on breast cancer III', p. 197.
[36] De Moulin: *Op. cit.*, p. 198.
[37] Van der Goot: 'Bijdrage tot de radiotherapie'.
[38] 'Quis tumidum guttur miratur in Alpibus?' (Who is astonished at a swollen neck in the Alps?), the Roman satirist Juvenal wondered in *Sat.* XIII, 162. For the history of endemic goitre the reader is referred to the magnificent book by Merke: *Geschichte des Kropfes.*
[39] Zimmerman, Veith: 'Theodor Kocher and the surgery of the endocrine system'. In: *Great ideas*, pp. 499–518.
[40] Brand: 'Het voorkomen van struma in Nederland'. Potter: 'Proefondervindelijk onderzoek der veranderingen der ratten'.
[41] Boerema: 'De aard van het werk', pp. 127, 138–9. Boer et al.: *Nederlandse Vereniging voor Urologie.*
[42] Roegholt: 'Niertransplantatie in 1908'.
[43] De Moulin: 'Hist. notes on vascular surgery' I, II, III.
[44] Matti: *Die Knochenbrüche*, vol. 1, pp. 311–4.
[45] Boerema: 'De aard van het werk', p. 122. Treacle is sterile and is strongly hygroscopic, which means that it draws out the tissue fluid, and along with it the bacteria that have invaded the wound.
[46] De Moulin: 'De dijbeenhalsbreuk'.
[47] Metz: 'Behandeling der schuine dijbeenbreuken'. Metz was with Dutch Red Cross ambulances in the Boer War, in the 1913 Balkan War, and in Germany during World War I. Other foreign surgeons, who saw Metz apply his frame, copied it and took it back with them to their own countries. This suspension traction apparatus became known the world over as 'Balkan frame'.
[48] Billroth's mixture: alcohol 1, chloroform 3, ether 1.
[49] Bochalli: 'Geschichte der örtlichen Betäubung'.
[50] Le Dran: *Verhand van de geschote wonden*, pp. 1–5. The French term 'commotion' for the condition of shock, was rendered into Dutch as 'dreuning'.
[51] Laan: *Chirurgische zieken*, p. 235.
[52] Hunter: 'Old unhappy far off things', pp. 291–4.
[53] Mercer: 'Some Edinburgh pioneers'.
[54] Haeseker: *Dr. J. F. S. Esser*, pp. 77–110.

CHAPTER 10: SURGERY IN THE PAST 75 YEARS

[1] In his book *Organon*, Tausk gives a fascinating description of the developments summarized in this paragraph.
[2] De Moulin: 'Heelkunde sinds de eeuwwisseling', pp. 19–25.
[3] Grond: 'Opleiding', p. 239.
[4] For a short but masterly survey of surgery in the first half of this century, the reader is referred to Nissen: 'Chirurgie einst und jetzt'. Until the publication, in 1949, of the surgical journal *Archivum Chirurgicum Neerlandicum*, nearly all publications by Dutch surgeons except those published in foreign journals — which were few — are to be found in the *Nederlandsch Tijdschrift voor Geneeskunde.* It is only in the past few years that there has been a growing tendency, partly as a result of the pressure exercised by the abominable *Citation Index*, to publish in major foreign journals. I. Boerema has presented a general survey of the Dutch contributions of the period 1902–1947 in Kuijjer *et al.*:

Nederlandse Vereniging voor Heelkunde. H. Muller did the same for the years from 1947 to 1972. Since the publications they mention can easily be traced in the two above-mentioned journals, the present author has decided not to provide an extensive bibliography for the next two paragraphs. The author gratefully acknowledges his debt to Boerema's and Muller's articles in the writing of the final chapter of this book. The same is true in the case of other aspects of Dutch surgery which have been extensively and carefully described by other authors in the commemorative book; their work, too, has been a source of inspiration to me.

[5] Guleke: 'Fünfzig Jahre Chirurgie', p. 34.

[6] Haberland: 'Jan Schoemaker'.

[7] Zaayer: 'Overdruknarcose'.

[8] In 1923, Graham in the United States was able to find records in the literature of only 48 cases of patients treated for bronchiectasis by lobectomy, with 25 deaths. Graham himself was one of the pioneers of pulmonary surgery, being the first to remove successfully an entire lung in a case of bronchial cancer in 1933. He died of pulmonary cancer.

[9] The diagnostic problems of lungs and oesophagus have been greatly facilitated by the discovery and use of contrast media such as bismuth (1898) and lipiodol (1921) in radiology.

[10] Zaayer: 'Heelkundige behandeling van bronchiectasen'.

[11] Zaayer was a surgeon of wide interests. Apart from thoracic surgery, his publications include numerous other subjects, including a fair number of neurosurgical ones.

[12] Nissen: *Helle Blätter*, pp. 131–4.

[13] See the chapter 'Surgery of the heart' in Nissen, Wilson: *Pages in the history of chest surgery.*

[14] *Op. cit.*, pp. 116–8.

[15] Peltier: 'A brief history of traction'.

[16] Spaander: *Het bloedtransfusiewezen in Nederland*, pp. 7–27.

[17] Spaander: 'Dutch blood-transfusion service'.

[18] Boerema: 'Het werk in de Vereeniging voor heelkunde', p. 145.

[19] Hommerson: 'De afdeling Nijmegen tijdens de Tweede Wereldoorlog', p. 55.

[20] Moeys, E. J.: *Osteosynthesis with a long intramedullary metal pin* (*Küntscher's method*). Thesis Utrecht, 1948. Gerhard Küntscher (1900–1972) of Kiel had already published his method in 1940, but due to the war situation it had not become widely known outside Germany. In fact, military doctors with the Allied Forces were quite surprised when during the later stages of the war they saw prisoners of war treated with this method.

[21] Elema: *Honderd jaren gistfabriek*, pp. 34–9.

[22] Spaander: *Het bloedtransfusiewezen in Nederland*, pp. 21–23.

[23] Kolff: *De kunstmatige nier* (The artificial kidney). Engl summary. Thesis Groningen, 1946.

[24] Den Otter: 'Internationale contacten', pp. 273–8.

[25] A gradual displacement of the world's great centres of medical science can be discerned over the centuries. In the late Middle Ages and the Renaissance, Italy set the trends, especially at Padua. This was succeeded by Paris, Leyden and Edinburgh in the 17th and 18th centuries, by London and once more by Paris during the first half of the 19th, then by German and Austrian centres, and finally by the United States.

[26] De Moulin: *Short hist. breast cancer*, pp. 94–104.

[27] In addition to hypothermia, Boerema's experimental work included preoperative haemodilution and autotransfusion during the operation, using blood taken from the patient a week before the operation. After 1956, further experiments were carried out using atmospheric hyperpressure, which considerably improves the oxygen saturation level of the tissues. This also increases the solubility of oxygen in circulating fluids, which reduces the haemoglobin demand. In December, 1958, an astonished meeting of the 'Vereniging voor Heelkunde' saw a pig, which some weeks before had lived for fifteen minutes with a haemoglobin level of 0.5%, run merrily around the lecture theatre. In 1960, the hyperpressure tank at the Wilhelmina Gasthuis at Amsterdam was put into use. In it, many experimental and clinical studies and treatments were undertaken by Boerema and his co-workers. Especially in the treatment of gas gangrene, this hyperpressure tank has proved invaluable. Muller: 'Wetenschap en Vereniging v. Heelk.', p. 237.

[28] Persijn: 'Verleden, heden en toekomst van de orgaantranspl. in Nederland'.

[29] The Rotterdam heart transplants are the result of a cooperation of the university hospitals at Rotterdam and Leyden, and the St. Antonius Ziekenhuis at Nieuwegein.

[30] The well-known Dutch man of letters and columnist Henri Knap reports that his mother once told him the moving history of his great-aunt Ida, who was operated on for a strangulated hernia, in the green room of her parental home in Amsterdam, around 1880, at the age of twenty. 'First the doctor burnt a hundred candles in the room for an hour, in order to purify the air. Certainly, aunt Ida was given anaesthesia, chloroform, and she was operated on by a very clever doctor. But during the operation she was suddenly dead'. *P*(arool) *S*(upplement), January 5, 1974, p. 3.

[31] Beukers, A. C. M. (1885—1969), personal communication to the author.
[32] From the days of the Psalmist (Ps. 51 : 9) and the Vestal Virgins, to our days of 'Detergent Commercials', white has ever been considered the colour of purity. It is no coincidence, therefore, that asepsis too was clad in white for many decades. It was not until after the Second World War that the white linen in the operating theatre was replaced by blue, green or grey fabrics, which were easier on the eyes of the operating team, although the well-known British surgeon Berkeley Moynihan had already advocated this change as early as 1915.
[33] Dutch readers are referred to the excellent article by Bauer: 'Veranderingen in de operatiekamer'.
[34] The first Dutch anaesthetic training was established after the war, in Boerema's clinic in Amsterdam.
[35] Grond: 'Opleiding'.
[36] Bax: 'Nederl. Ver. Bevord. Chir. Wetensch.'. Meijne: 'Van Stichting tot Collegium Chirurgicum'.
[37] Meijne: 'Het *Archivum Chirurgicum Neerlandicum*'.
[38] Eeftinck Schattenkerk: 'Heelk. specialismen'.
[39] *Goethes Gespräche I.* Quoted by G. Baumans: *Goethe Lektüre für Augenblicke.* Frankfurt/Main: Insel, 1982, p. 65.
[40] Van den Berg: *Medische macht*, pp. 29—31.

Bibliography

Academia groningana MDCXIV–MCMXIV (Commemorative volume Univ. of Groningen). Groningen: P. Noordhoff, 1914.

Ackerknecht, E. H.: Pariser Chirurgie von 1794 bis 1850. *Gesnerus* **17**: 137–44, 1960.

Adams, F.: *See* Hippocrates; Paulus of Aegina; Aretaeus.

Albinus, B. S.: *Index supellectilis anatomicae* quam ... legavit ... Rau ... Lugd-Batav: H. Mulhovius, 1725 [Re-edited with Engl. transl. by M. A. van Andel. In: *Opuscula selecta*, vol. XVII, 1943, pp. 184–217].

Albucasis: *Albucasis on surgery and instruments.* Arab text with Engl. transl. and commentary by M. S. Spink and G. L. Lewis. London: Wellcome Inst. Hist. Med., 1973.

Van Andel, M. A.: Spectatoriale vertoogen over de geneeskundige praktijk in het laatst der 18de eeuw (Spectatorial representations on medical practice at the end of the 18th cent.). *Med. Weekbl.* **25**: 481–90, 497–505, 513–20, 1918–19.

Van Andel, M. A.: J. H. Francken, een reizend meester in de 18de eeuw (J.H.F., a travelling surgeon in the 18th cent.). *Med. Weekbl.* **26**: 349–56, 361, 373–81, 1919.

Van Andel, M. A.: De chirurgijn Cornelis Solingen en zijn instrumentarium. *Ned. Tijdschr. Geneeskd.* **80**(I): 47–55, 1936.

Van Andel, M. A. (Ed.): De lithotomia, *Opuscula selecta*, vol. XVII, 1943.

Van Andel, M. A.: *Chirurgijns, vrije meesters, beunhazen en kwakzalvers* (Surgeons, interlopers and quacks). 's-Gravenhage: M. Nijhoff, 1981[3].

Anonymous: Levensschets van G. D. Schröder (Biographical notes on G.D.S.). *Ned. Lancet* **1**: 514–6, 1838–9.

Antvelink, J. G.: Goodwill in het verleden (Goodwill in the past). *Med. Contact* **40**: 1507–8, 1985.

Arcaeus, F.: *Kortbondige ende rechte middel en kunst, om allerhande zoorten van wonden ... te genezen* (Concise and proper means and art to cure all sorts of wounds). Uit Lat ... d Jac Geusius. Leeuwarden: Yvo Takes Wielsma, 1667, 68[2].

Aretaeus: *The extant works of Aretaeus the Cappadocian* (81–138? AD). Ed. and transl. by F. Adams. London: Sydenham Soc., 1856 [Repr. Boston (Mass): Mitford House, 1972].

[Arnaud de Ronsil, G.]: *Traité des hernies ou descentes*, 2 vols. Paris: P. G. le Mercier, 1749.

Asman, C.: *De aneurysmate.* Thesis Groningen, 1773.

Baader, G.: Die Schule von Salerno. *Med.-hist. J.* **13**: 124–45, 1978.

Banga, J.: *Geschiedenis van de geneeskunde en van hare beoefenaren in Nederland ... tot aan den dood van Boerhaave* (History of medicine and its practitioners in the Netherlands ... up to the death of B.). Leeuwarden: W. Eekhoff, 1868 [Repr. Schiedam: Interbook, 1975].

Barbet: Mémoire sur la question suivante: Dans le cas où l'amputation de la cuisse dans l'article paroîtroit l'unique ressource pour sauver la vie à un malade, déterminer si l'on doit pratiquer cette opération. ... *Recueil des pièces, qui ont concouru pour le prix de l'Academie Royale de Chirurgie* **4**: 1–18, 1759.

Barbette, P.: *Praxis Barbettiana* of genees-oeffening. Met aentekeningen ... door Frederik Dekkers. Rotterdam: F. van Hoogstraeten, 1669.

Barbette, P.: *Chirurgie.* Nae de hedendaegsche practijk beschreven (Surgery, according to contemporary practice). Amsterdam: J. Lescailje, 1672.

Barge, J. A. J.: *Het geneeskundig onderwijs aan de Leidsche universiteit in de 18de eeuw* (Medical education at Leyden University in the 18th century). Leiden: van Doesburgh, 1934.

Baten, C.: *Handtboeck der Chirurgyen.* Amsterdam: H. Laurentsz, 1620[3].

Bauer, M. G. M.: Veranderingen in de operatiekamer (Changes in the operating room). In: Kuijjer *et al.*: *Ned. Ver. Heelk.*, pp. 285—312.
Baumann, E. D.: *De dokter in de geneeskunde* (Doctor and medicine), 2 vols in 1. Amsterdam: H. Meulenhoff, 1915.
Baumann, E. D.: Hendrick van Roonhuyse. *Ned. Tijdschr. Geneeskd.* **66**(1): 856—74, 1922.
Bax, H. R.: De Nederlandse Vereniging tot Bevordering der chirurgische Wetenschappen (The Dutch Society for the Advancement of surgical Sciences). In: Kuijjer *et al.*: *Ned. Ver. Heelk.*, pp. 149—64.
Bell, C.: On lithotomy. *The Lancet* **12**: 699—776, 1826—27.
Benevoli, A., Tacconi, G.: *Heelkundige waarnemingen* (Annotated transl. by J. B. Sandifort of 'Tre dissertazioni: ernia intestinale . . .'. Firenze, 1747). 's-Gravenhage: O. van Thol, 1770.
Van den Berg, J. H.: *Medische macht en medische ethiek* (Medical power and medical ethics). Nijkerk: C. F. Callenbach, 1969.
[Van der Berge P.]: *Privilegiën, willekeuren en ordonnantiën betreffende het Collegium Chirurgicum Amstelodamense* (Privileges, acts and ordinances regarding the Amsterdam surgeon's guild). Amsterdam: P. van den Berge, 1736.
Van Beverwyck, J.: *Heel-konste, ofte derde deel van de Genees-konste, om de uytwendige gebreecken te heelen* (Surgery, or third part of the art of healing, to cure the external disorders). Amsterdam: J. J. Schipper, 1671^2. Also in the collected works — *Alle de wercken* — Amsterdam: J. J. Schipper, 1680.
Van Beverwyck, J.: Steen-stuck (Treatise on the stone). *Alle de wercken.* Amsterdam: J. J. Schipper, 1680, pp. 228—87. Re-edited with Engl. transl. by M. A. van Andel: *Opuscula selecta*, vol. XVII, 1943, pp. 10—129.
Bichat, X.: *Oeuvres chirurgicales . . . de P. J. Desault*, 3 vols. Paris: Mequignon, 1801—3.
Bidloo, G.: *Opera omnia anatomico-chirurgica.* Lugd. Batav: S. Luchtmans, 1715.
Bilguer, J. U.: *Verhandeling over het seldsaam en bijna onnodig gebruik van het afsetten der ledemaaten van het menschelijk lichaam.* Na den 2e verb. Hoogd. dr., vert. + verm. met voorre. + aanmerk. uit de Franse vert. van [S.A.] Tissot (door P. N. Lotichius) (Treatise on the rare and almost unnecessary use of the amputation of the limbs of the human body. Dutch transl. from the 2nd High-German ed. enlarged by . . . remarks . . . Tissot). Nijmegen: I. van Campen, 1770.
Billings, J. S.: 'The history and literature of surgery'. In: F. S. Dennis: *System of Surgery.* New York/ Philadelphia: Lea Brothers, 1895—96, 1, 17—144.
Bishop, W. J.: *The early history of surgery.* London: R. Hale, 1960.
Bitter, H.: De beul te Haarlem als chirurgijn in de 17de en 18de eeuw (The public executioner at Haarlem as a surgeon in the 17th and 18th cent.). *Maandbl. Ver. Bestrijd. Kwakz.* **34**, issues 3, 5, 9, 1914.
Bitter, H.: Stadsoperateurs en steensnijders in de 17de en 18de eeuw in Haarlem (Specialized town surgeons and lithotomists in the 17th and 18th cent. at H.). *Ned. Tijdschr. Geneeskd.* **58**(II): 568—76, 1914.
Blondeau, R. A.: De negentiende en twintigste eeuw (The 19th and 20th century). In: A. Nauwelaerts (ed.), 'Kunst en Wetenschap' (Art and Science), vol. 12 of *Twintig eeuwen Vlaanderen.* Hasselt: Heideland-Orbis, 1974.
Bochalli, R.: Zur Geschichte der örtlichen Betäubung. *Med. Monatschr.* **14**: 121—5, 1960.
Boer, P. W., Felderhof, J., Moonen, W. A., Schreinemachers, L. H. M.: *Nederlands Vereniging voor Urologie* (Dutch Society for Urology). Private print: 1983.
Boerema, I.: De aard en het wetenschappelijk peil van het werk in de Vereeniging voor Heelkunde, 1902—1947 (The nature and the scientific level of the work in the Association of Surgeons, 1902—47). In: Kuijjer *et al.*: *Ned. Ver. Heelk.*, pp. 106—48.
Boerhaave, H.: *Kortbondige spreuken wegens de ziektens* (Aphorisms). Dutch transl. by K. Love. Amsterdam: J. Gysies, 1741 [Repr. Alphen aan den Rijn: Stafleu, 1979, with introd. by G. A. Lindeboom].
Boesman, Th.: *De examens in de chirurgijnsgilden.* Thesis Utrecht, 1942.
Boevé, J.: Verenigingsleven van 1947 tot 1977 (Social life from 1947 till 1977). In: Kuijjer *et al.*: *Ned. Ver. Heelk.*, pp. 173—200.
Bonn, A.: Descriptio thesauri ossium morbosorum Hoviani, adnexa est dissertatio de callo. 3 fascicles. Amsterdam: J. C. Sepp, 1783.
Bonn, A.: De tegenwoordige staat der heel- en verloskunst in ons vaderland (The present state of the surgical and obstetrical arts in our country). *Verhand. Genootsch. Bevordering Heelk. Amsterdam* **2**: VI—XV, 1793.
Bonn, A.: *Tabulae anatomico-chirurgicae doctrinam herniarum illustrantes.* Ed. by G. Sandifort. Lugd-Bat: S. et J. Luchtmans, 1828.

Bonner, W.: *The medical background of Anglo-Saxon England.* London: Wellcome Hist. Med. Library, 1963.
Bontekoe, C.: *Niew gebouw van de chirurgie . . . stuksgewijse opgetimmert . . .* Alwaar de gemene praktijk der chirurgijns van een menigte van abuisen en verkeertheden, mitsgaders van wreedheid en moordadigheid overtuigd word (New building of surgery piece by piece erected . . . in which the common practice of surgeons is shown to contain a multitude of oversights and errors, as well as cruelty and murderousness), 2 vols. in 1. 's-Gravenhage: P. Hagen, 1680—81.
Bornewasser, J. A., Van Caenegem, R. C., Jansen, H. P. H., Schöffer, I., Van der Wee, H. (Eds.): *Winkler Prins Geschiedenis der Nederlanden* (Winkler Prins History of the Netherlands), 3 vols. Amsterdam, Brussel: Elsevier, 1977.
Boucher, [P. J.]: Observations sur des playes d'armes à feu, compliquées de fracture. . . . *Mém. Acad. roy. Chir.* **2**: 287—307, 1753.
Brand, B.: Het voorkomen van struma in Nederland (Incidence of goitre in Holland). *Ned. Tijdschr. Geneeskd.* **63**(I): 1053—4, 1919.
Brasdor, P.: Mémoire sur la fracture de la clavicule, et description d'un nouveau bandage pour cette fracture. *Mém. Acad. roy. Chir.* **5**: 575—91, 1774.
Breen, J. G.: Een barbierswinkel in 1669 (A barber-surgeon's shop in 1669). *Amstelodamum* **13**: 1—6, 1920.
Bremer, G. J.: *See* Mathijsen.
Brieger, G. H.: *Medical America in the nineteenth century.* Baltimore, London: Johns Hopkins Press, 1972.
Brockband, W.: The crookedness clinic of Nicholas and Peter Schot. *J. Bone Jt. Surg.* **41B**: 413—7, 1959.
Broers, J. C.: *Oratio de Puteano* [M. du Puy], *chirurgiae et obstetriciae doctore et professore . . .* Lugd-Bat: private print, 1835.
Bromfeild, W.: *Chirurgical observations and cases*, 2 vols. London: T. Cadell, 1773.
Brondgeest, P. Q.: *Bijdragen tot de geschiedenis van het Gasthuis, het Klooster en de Balije van St Catherina der Johanniter-ridders . . . te Utrecht* (Contributions to the history of the hospital, the monastery and the priory of St Catherine of the knights of St John . . . at Utrecht). Hilversum: Nonhebel, 1901.
Brouwer Ancher, A. J. M.: 'Oude ordonnantiën betreffende genees-, heel- en verloskundigen, apothekers, kwakzalvers enz' (Old ordinances on physicians, surgeons, pharmacists, quacks etc.). *Ned. Tijdschr. Geneeskd.* **35**: 1173—97, 1899.
Brugmans, S. J.: Verhandeling over de gesteldheid en samenstelling van den dampkring, in welke de zoogenaamde hospitaalversterving bij gewonden plaats heeft (Treatise on the state and composition of the atmosphere in which the so-called hospital gangrene takes place). *Natuurk. Verhand. Hollandsche Maatsch. Wetensch.* (Haarlem) **7**(II): 3—68, 1814. German transl. in S. J. Brugmans & J. Delpech: *Ueber den Hospitalbrand.* Jena: Manke, 1816.
Bruneel, C.: Le livre de comptes d'un chirurgien rural en Brabant (1758—1788). *Bijdr. tot de Geschied.* **62**: 254—66, 1979.
Von Bruns, V.: Fort mit dem Spray! *Berl. klin. Wschr.* **17**: 609—11, 1880.
Brunschwig, H.: *The book of cirurgia of Hieronymus Brunschwig.* Facsimile of 'Dis ist das buch der Cirurgia. Hantwirckung der Wundartzny von Hyeronimo brunschwig'. Strassburg: Grüninger, 1497. With a study on H. B. and his work by H. E. Sigerist. Milano: R. Lier, 1925.
ps-Brunschwig, H.: *Dits dat hantwerck der cirurgien ende leert alle wonden, gehouden gesteken . . . cuereren* . . . . Utrecht: Jan Bernts, 1535.

Cabrol, B.: *Het anatomiicke ABC.* Du transl. by C. Nollens. 's-Gravenhage: H. I. van Wouw, 1630.
Campbell, E.: *See* Theodoric.
Camper, P.: *Praelectiones chirurgiae inchoatae A° 1751.* Ms in C's handwriting containing the text of his Amsterdam lectures of 1751. Univ. Libr. Amsterdam.
Camper, P.: Verhandeling over de oorzaken der meenigvuldige breuken in de eerstgeboorene kinderen (Treatise on the causes of the frequent ruptures in the newly-born). *Verhand Holl Maatsch Wetensch* **6**: 235—65, 1761.
Camper, P.: Het steensnyden in twee reizen (Cutting for the stone in two stages). *Hedendaagsche vaderlandsche Letteroefeningen*, vol. 6, 1777. Re-edited with Engl. transl. by M. A. van Andel, *Opuscula selecta*, vol. XVII, 1943, p. 346—59.
Camper, P.: Over den waren aart der kankervorming en over een zeer zakelijk en onfeilbaar teken van onherstelbaren borstkanker (On the true character of cancer formation and on a most material and infallible sign of incurable breast cancer). *Genees- Natuur- Huishoudk Kabinet* **1**: 193—208, 1779.

Camper, P.: Verhandeling over den besten vorm van den schoen (Treatise on the best shape of the shoe). *Genees- Natuur- Huishoudk Kabinet* **3**: 275—308, 1781.
Camper, P.: *Dissertatio de fractura patellae et olecrani.* Hagae Com.: I. van Cleef, 1789.
Camper, P.: *Icones herniarum.* Ed. by S. T. Sömmerring. Francof.a.M.: Varrentrapp et Wenner, 1801.
Van Capellen, D.: In memoriam Prof. Dr. Otto Lanz. *Ned. Tijdschr. Geneeskd.* **79**(I): 1366—8, 1935.
Celsus, A. C.: *De Medicina.* Latin text with an Engl. transl. by W. G. Spencer, 3 vols. Loeb Classical Library. Cambridge (Mass): Harvard Univ. Press & London: W. Heinemann, 1948—53.
De Chauliac: *See* Guy.
Choulant, L.: *Handbuch der Bücherkunde für die ältere Medizin.* Leipzig: L. Voss, 1841 [Repr. Graz: Akad. Druck- u. Verlagsanstalt, 1956].
Churchill, E. D.: Healing by first intention and with suppuration. Studies in the history of wound healing. *J. Hist. Med. all Sci.* **19**: 193—214, 1964.
Clendening, L.: *Source book of medical history.* New York: Dover, 1960.
Cockayne, T. O.: *Leechdoms, wortcunning and starcraft of early England,* 3 vols. London: Longman, Green & Co., 1864—66.
Cohen, D. E.: De Amsterdamsche Joodsche chirurgijns (The Jewish surgeons of Amsterdam). *Ned. Tijdschr. Geneeskd.* **74**(I): 2234—56, 1930.
Colton, J.: *See* Theodoric.
Cooper, A.: *The anatomy and surgical treatment of abdominal hernia,* 2 pts. London: Longman, 1804—7.
Coopmans, J. P. A.: De rechtstoestand van de Godshuizen te 's-Hertogenbosch vóór 1629 (The legal status of the Hospices at 's-H.). Thesis Nijmegen, 1964. 's-Hertogenbosch: Zuid Ned. Drukkerij, 1964.
Cope, Z.: *A history of the acute abdomen.* London: Oxford Univ. Press, 1965.
Corner, G. W.: On early Salernitan surgery and especially the 'Bamberg Surgery'. *Bull. Inst. Hist. Med.* **5**: 1—32, 1937.
Croissant de Garengeot, R. J.: *Traité des opérations de chirurgie,* 3 vols. Paris: Huart, 1731^2.
Crosse, V. M.: *A surgeon in the early nineteenth century.* Edinburgh, London: Livingstone, 1968.

Daniëls, C. E.: *Een dominé-operateur in de zeventiende eeuw en nog iets* (A minister-surgeon in the 17th cent. and something more). Populair Wetenschappelijk Nederland No. 7. Amsterdam: Iepenbuur & van Seldam, 1913.
Daremberg, Ch.: *La médecine,* histoire et doctrines. Paris: Didier et J. B. Baillière, 1865.
Dekkers, F.: *Geneeskonstige of werk-stellige oeffeningen* omtrent de manier van geneesinge .... Uit het Latin vertaald (Medical or executable practices in the way of healing .... Transl. from the Latin). Leiden: J. du Vivie, 1717.
Delpech, J. M.: *Précis élémentaire des maladies réputées chirurgicales,* 3 vols. Paris: Méquignon-Marvis, 1816.
Delprat, C. C.: *De wording en de geschiedenis van het Genootschap ter Bevordering van Natuur-, Genees- en Heelkunde te Amsterdam, 1790—1915* (Origin and history of the Society for the Advancement of Physics, Medicine and Surgery at Amsterdam). Amsterdam: Kruyt, 1916.
Denis, J.: Receuil de quelques nouvelles observations des effects très considérables de la transfusion du sang .... *Journ. d. Scavans*: 87—94, 182—5, 1667.
Denos, E.: Histoire de l'urologie. In: *Encyclopédie française d'urologie,* publiée sous la direction de A. Pousson et E. Denos. Paris: Oct Doin et fils, 1914, vol. 1, 1—294.
Denys, J.: *Heelkundige aanmerkingen* (Surgical observations). Leyden: J. à Kerckhem, 1730, Ch. 8. Re-edited with Engl. transl. by M. A. van Andel, *Opuscula selecta,* vol. XVII, 1943, pp. 256—89.
Dionis, [P.]: *Verhandelingen van alle de chirurgicale operatien* (Treatises of all surgical operations). Rotterdam: J. Hofhout, 1710.
Ten Doesschate, G.: *Rolduc als middeleeuwse voorpost der wis-, natuur- en geneeskunde in de Nederlanden* (R. as mediaeval outpost of mathematics, physics and medicine in the Netherlands). Lochem: Tijdstroom, 1948.
Ten Doesschate, G.: *De Utrechtse Universiteit en de geneeskunde 1636—1900* (The University of Utrecht and medicine). Nieuwkoop: B. de Graaf, 1963.
Doets, C. J.: *De heelkunde van Petrus Camper* (The surgery of P.C.). Thesis Leyden, 1948.
Van Dongen, J. A.: De incunabelen en postincunabelen in de bibliotheek van de Maatschappij (Incunables and postincunables in the library of the Royal Dutch Society for Medicine). Series of 52 descriptive articles in *Medisch Contact,* 1964—1970.
Le Dran, H. F.: *Verhandeling van de geschote wonden* ... Uit het Fr. vert. d. Hendrik Korp, chirurgijn in Amsterdam (Treatise of shot wounds. Transl. from the French by H. Korp, surgeon). Amsterdam: Van Gerrevink e.a., 1748.

Drummond, J. C., Wilbraham, A.: *The Englishman's food.* London: J. Cape, 1939.
Dulieu, L.: *La chirurgie à Montpellier.* Avignon: Presses Universelles, 1957.

Earle, J.: *See* Pott, P.
Eeftinck Schattenkerk, J. C. P.: Ontwikkeling van de heelkundige specialismen (Development of the surgical specialties). In: Kuijjer *et al.*: *Ned. Ver. Heelk.*, pp. 45—67.
Van Eeghen, I. H.: Beul in Amsterdam (Public executioner in A.). *Amstelodamum* **41**: 120—7, 1954.
Van Eeghen, I. H.: *De Gilden.* Theorie en praktijk. Bussum: de Haan, 1974[2].
Van Eeghen, I. H.: Anthonie van den Hout en Pieter Klases Pel, of de opleiding in de genees-, heel- en verloskunde (A.v.d.H. and P.K.P., or the training for medicine, surgery and obstetrics). *Amstelodamum* **61**: 1—5, 1974.
Van Eeghen, I. H.: Van gasthuis tot academisch ziekenhuis (From 'gasthuis' to university hospital). In: D. de Moulin, I. H. van Eeghen, R. Meischke: *Vier eeuwen Amsterdams Binnengasthuis* (Four centuries of Amsterdam Inner Hospital). Wormer: Inmerc, 1981, pp. 47—104.
Eis, G.: Kultische Keuschheit in der mittelalterlichen Wundarznei. *Med. Mschr.* **10**: 617—9, 1956.
Elaut, L.: Ecclesia abhorret a sanguine. Terugslag op de medische praktijk sinds de Middeleeuwen (E.a.a.s. In reference to medical practice since the Middle Ages). In: *Recht in beweging* (Law in motion). Festschr. for R. Victor Kt. Deurne, Antwerp: Kluwer, 1973, pp. 473—83.
Elema, B.: *Opkomst, evolutie en betekenis van research gedurende honderd jaren Gistfabriek* (Rise, evolution and significance of research during a hundred years Yeast-factory). Delft: Kon. Ned. Gist- Spiritusfabriek, 1970.
Endtz, L. J.: *De Hage-professoren.* Geschiedenis van een chirurgische school (The professors at The Hague. History of a surgical school). Amstelveen: Specia, 1972.
Erndl, Chr. H.: *De itinere suo anglicano et batavo annis 1706 et 1707 facto, relatio.* Amstelodami: apud Janssonio-Waesbergios, 1711.
Eulner, H. H., Mann, G., Preiser, G., Winau, R., Winkelmann, O.: *Medizingeschichte in unserer Zeit.* Festgabe für Edith Heischkel-Artelt und Walter Artelt zum 65 Geburtstag. Stuttgart: F. Enke, 1971.

Fabbri, G. B.: Della litotomia antica e dei litotomi ed oculisti Norcini e Preciani. *Mem. Accad. Sci. Istor. Bologna*, ser. 2, **60**: 239—66, 1869.
Fabricius Hildanus, G.: *Opera quae extant omnia.* Francofurti ad Moenum: Sumptibus J. Beyeri, 1646. Observationum centuriae I—VI, pp. 1—634; Lithotomia vesicae, pp. 700—67.
Fabrity ab Aquapendente, H.: *Heelkonstige werkingen* (Surgical operations); B. Cabroly: *ABC der ontledinge* (ABC of dissection); I. Fernely: *Beschrijvinge des menschelijken lichaams* (Description of the human body), 1 vol. Rotterdam: Joannes Naeranus, 1661.
Faure, [J. L.]: Mémoire sur la question proposée par l'Académie Royale de Chirurgie . . .: L'amputation étant absolument nécessaire . . . déterminer les cas où il convient de différer . . . . *Recueil des pièces, qui ont concouru pour le prix de l'Académie royale de Chirurgie* **3**: 489—520, 1759.
[De La Faye, G.]: *Aanmerkingen op de chirurgicaale operatien van den Heere Dionis*, uit 't Fransch vertaalt . . . en vermeerdert door P. Vink (Comments on the surgical operations of Mr. Dionis, transl. from the French and enlarged by P. Vink). Rotterdam: J. D. Beman, 1740.
Fellows, E. W.: The history of some surgical instruments. Part 1. *The General Practitioner* **22**: 277—9, 1954.
Fischer, G.: *Chirurgie vor hundert Jahren.* Leipzig: Vogel, 1876 [Repr. with introduction by R. Winau. Berlin, Heidelberg, New York: Springer, 1978].
Fischer, K. D.: Moses of Palermo, translator from the Arabic at the court of Charles of Anjou. *Hist. Sci. méd.* **27**: 278—81, 1982.
Fock, L. C. E. E.: *Natuur- en geneeskundig etymologisch woordenboek* (Physical and medical etymological dictionary). Gorkum: J. Noorduyn, 1855.
Fokker, A. A.: Losse bladen uit de geschiedenis van het chirurgijnsgilde te Middelburg (Loose leaves from the history of the surgeons' guild at M.). *Ned. Tijdschr. Geneeskd.* **13**(II): 333—72, 1877.
Francken, J. H.: Over het steensnyden, zo boven als onder het schaambeen (On the excision of stones, both above and below the pubic bone). Second exercise from *Nieuwe oeffenings verhandelingen der vier hoofdhandgrepen* (New instructive treatise on the four principal manipulations). Amsterdam: J. Helm, 1733. Re-edited with Engl. transl. by M. A. van Andel, *Opuscula selecta*, vol. XVII, 1943, pp. 290—345.
Franco, P.: *Chirurgie de Pierre Franco* composée en 1561. Nouv. éd. avec une introduction historique, une biographie et l'histoire du Collège de Chirurgie, par E. Nicaise. Paris: F. Antan, 1895.

Frings, H. J.: *Medizin u Arzt bei den griechischen Kirchenvätern bis Chrysostomos*. Thesis Bonn, 1959.
Frijhoff, W.: Non satis dignitatis . . . Over de maatschappelijke status van geneeskundigen tijdens de Republiek (On the social status of medical practitioners during the Republic). *Tijdschr. Geschied.* **96**: 379—406, 1983.

Galen: *Opera omnia*. Editionem curavit C. G. Kühn. Gr. text with Lat. transl. by R. Chartier, 20 vols. Lipsiae: C. Cnobloch, 1821—33 [Repr. Hildesheim: Olms, 1964—65].
Galen: *On the usefulness of the parts of the body* (De usu partium). Transl. introd. comment. by M. T. May, 2 vols. Ithaca, N.Y.: Cornell Univ. Press, 1968.
Gelfand, T.: *The training of surgeons in eighteenth-century Paris and its influence on medical education*. Thesis The Johns Hopkins University, 1973. Xerox University Microfilms. Ann Arbor, Michigan, USA/London, England, 1979.
Von Gersdorff, H.: *Feldtbuch der Wundtartzney*. Strassburg: J. Schott, 1517. Facsimile-reprint with introd. by J. Steudel. Darmstadt: Wissenschaftl Buchgesellschaft, 1967.
(Von Gersdorff, H.), Scheel-Hans: Veldt Boeck van den chirurgia. Overgheset uyt den Hoochduytsche in onse Nederlantsche tale, door Jan Pauwelszoon Phrisius. Amstelredam: Cornelis Claesz, 1593.
Van Gesscher, D.: *Verhandeling over de bestaanbaarheid en noodzaaklykheid der afzetting in verscheidene heelkundige gebreken* (Treatise on the practability and necessity of the amputation in several surgical ailments). Amsterdam: F. de Kruyff, 1771.
Van Gesscher, D.: *Hedendaagsche oeffenende heelkunde* (Contemporary practical surgery). 3 vols. Amsterdam: Jan Doll, 1781—86.
Van Gesscher, D.: *Aanmerkingen over de wangestalten der ruggegraat en de behandeling der ontwrichtingen en breuken van het dyebeen* (Remarks on the deformities of the spine and the treatment of dislocations and fractures of the thigh bone). Amsterdam: J. B. Elwe, 1792.
Van Gesscher, D.: *Schets der heelkundige ziektekunde*, ten gebruike zijner toehoorders (Sketch of surgical pathology). Amsterdam: Elwe en Werlingshoff, 1803.
Geyl, A.: De ontdekking van de breuk van den hals van het dijbeen door den Amsterdamschen chirurgijn Borst in 1680 (The discovery of the fracture of the neck of the thigh bone by the Amsterdam surgeon B. in 1680). *Ned. Tijdschr. Geneeskd.* **55**(II): 1613—9, 1911.
Geyl, A.: Abraham Titsingh, de deken der Amsterdamsche chirurgijns (A.T., dean of the Amsterdam surgeons). *Geneesk. Bladen.* **16**: 1—44, 1912.
Van Ginneken, J.: Geert Groote's levensbeeld naar de oudste gegevens bewerkt (G.G.'s biography adapted to the oldest data). *Verh. Ned. Akad. Wetensch.*, afd. Letterk, N.R., vol. 47, nr. 2.
Glandorp, M. L.: Speculum chirurgicorum. In: *Opera omnia*. Londini: C. Davis and A. Vandenhoeck, 1729, pp. 1—114.
Glazemaker, J. H.: *Verzameling van verscheide nieuwe waarneemingen van zeer gewichtige uitwerkselen der overstorting van 't bloet uit het een in 't ander lighaam* . . . (Compilation of various recent observations of very important effects of pouring blood from one body into another). Amsterdam: P. Arentsz, 1668.
Glenn, F., Grafe, W. R.: Historical events in biliary tract surgery. *Arch. Surg.* **93**: 848—52, 1966.
Van der Goot, D. H.: Bijdrage tot de radiotherapie (A contribution to radiotherapy). *Ned. Tijdschr. Geneeskd.* **53**(I): 882—6, 1909.
Gorter, D. A.: *De tabaksrook-klisteer voornamelijk als reanimator* (Fumigation chiefly for resuscitation, with Engl. summaries). Amsterdam: Maatschappij tot Redding van Drenkelingen, 1953.
De Gorter, J.: *De gezuiverde heelkonst*, ter onderwijzinge van den leerenden en konstoeffenenden heelmeester (Purified surgery for the instructions of students and practitioners of surgery). Leiden: De Janssoons van der Aa, 1735.
Van Goudoever, L. C.: Verslag der chirurgische kliniek aan de Utrechtsche Hoogeschool, gedurende de academiejaren 1849—1858 (Report on the surgical clinic at the University of Utrecht for the academic years 1849—58). *Nederl. Tijdschr. Heel- Verloskd.* **6**: 85—166, 244—389, 1854.
[Greidanus, S.]: *Een dorpsdokter uit de Friese Wouden vertelt* (Memoirs of a country-doctor from F.W.). Leeuwarden: A. M. van Seyen, 1974^2.
Grond, J. Th.: Opleiding (Training). In: Kuijjer *et al.*: *Ned. Ver. Heelk.*, pp. 239—68.
Grond, J. Th.: De positie van de geneeskundigen in Nederland in de tweede helft van de negentiende eeuw (The position of the doctors in Holland in the second half of the 19th cent.). In: Kuijjer *et al.*: *Ned. Ver. Heelk.*, pp. 29—44.
Guleke, N.: *Fünfzig Jahre Chirurgie*. Berlin, Göttingen, Heidelberg: Springer, 1955.
Gurlt, E. J.: *Geschichte der Chirurgie und ihrer Ausübung*, 3 vols. Berlin: Hirschwald, 1898 [Repr. Hildesheim: Olms, 1964].

Guy de Chauliac: *La grande chirurgie* de Guy de Chauliac. Annotated transl. by E. Nicaise. Paris: F. Alcan, 1890.

Ten Haaff, G.: Eene kwalijk geneezene breuk van het dyebeen, door kunst herbroken (A badly healed fracture of the thighbone, refractured by the art). *Verhand. Holl. Mij. Wetensch.* (Haarlem) **3**: 158—82, 1775.

Van der Haar, J.: *Verhandeling over de natuur en aart van de klier-, knoest-, en kankergezwellen* (Treatise on the nature of glandular, scirrhus and cancerous tumours). Amsterdam: J. Heun, 1761.

Haberland, H.F.O.: Jan Schoemaker. *Zentralbl. Chir.* **45**: 2098—9, 1940.

Haeseker, B.: *Dr. J. F. S. Esser and his contributions to plastic and reconstructive surgery.* Thesis Rotterdam, 1983.

Haeser, H.: *Lehrbuch der Geschichte der Medizin*, 3 vols. Jena: G. Fischer, 1875, 1881, 1882 [Repr. Hildesheim: Olms, 1971].

Von Haller, A.: *Bibliotheca chirurgica*, 2 vols. Bernae: E. Haller, Basileae: J. Schweighauser, 1774—75 [Repr. Hildesheim: Olms, 1971].

Von Haller, A.: *Haller in Holland.* Het dagboek van Albrecht von Haller van zijn verblijf in Holland (1725—27) (A.v.H.'s diary of his stay in Holland). Introduced and annotated by G. A. Lindeboom. Delft: Kon. Ned. Gist- en Spiritusfabriek, 1958.

Hanbury, E. M., Jr., Boyd, D. P.: History of thyroid surgery. *Surgery* **54**: 550—6, 1963.

Haneveld, G. T.: De ledezetters van Jisp (The bonesetters from Jisp). *Spiegel historiael* **12**: 514—7, 1977.

Haneveld, G. T.: *Mr. Arnoldus Fey, chirurgijn tot Oirschot.* Amsterdam: Meyster, 1977.

Haneveld, G. T.: *Pathologische anatomie in Utrecht*, circa 1800—1850. Thesis Utrecht, 1978.

Haneveld, G. T.: Medische aspecten van de slag bij de Doggersbank (Medical aspects of the Battle near the Dogger Bank). *Tijdschr. Geschied. Geneesk. Natuurw. Wisk. Techn.* **5**: 78—88, 1982.

Haver Droeze, J. J.: *Het collegium medicum Amstelaedamense.* Haarlem: Bohn, 1921.

De Heide, A.: *Anatome mytuli, belgicè mossel . . . Subjecta est centuria observationum medicarum.* Amstelod: Apud Jansonio Waesbergios, 1683.

Heister, L.: *Heelkundige onderwijzingen* (Dutch transl. from the German 'Chirurgie', Nuremberg, 1718, with notes and comments by H. Ulhoorn), 2 vols. Amsterdam: Janssoons van Waesbergen, 1741.

Heister, L.: *Kort begrip der heelkonst.* Naar den tweeden druk uit het Hoogduitsch vertaald (Epitome of surgery. Transl. from the 2nd High German ed.). Amsterdam: J. Morterre, 1764.

Heister, L.: *Chirurgie.* Nürnberg: G. N. Raspe, 1763 [Repr. Osnabrück: R. Kuballe, 1981].

Helfreich, F.: Geschichte der Chirurgie. In: Puschmanns *Handbuch der Geschichte der Medizin.* Jena: G. Fischer, 1905, vol. 3, pp. 1—306.

Hellinga, G.: Een en ander uit de geschiedenis der Amsterdamsche gasthuizen (het Sint Pieters-Gasthuis en Pesthuis) (Something of the history of the Amsterdam hospitals: St. Pieter's Gasthuis and Plague-Hospital). *Ned. Tijdschr. Geneeskd.* **67**(I): 43—7, 1923.

Hellinga, G.: Een en ander over de positie der 17e en 18e eeuwsche gasthuis-chirurgijns in Amsterdam (Something of the position of the 17th and 18th century hospital-surgeons at Amsterdam). *Ned. Tijdschr. Geneeskd.* **70**(II): 30—41, 1926.

Hellinga, G.: De beteekenis van het Amsterdamsche St. Pietersgasthuis voor het ontleedkundig onderwijs in ons land in vroeger tijden (The significance of the Amsterdam St. Pietersgasthuis for the teaching of anatomy in our country in former times). *Ned. Tijdschr. Geneeskd.* **77**(III): 3042—52, 1933.

Hellinga, G.: Van 'Verbanthuys' tot dubbele chirurgische cliniek (From 'dressing house' to double surgical clinic). *Ned. Tijdschr. Geneesk.* **83**(IV): 4857—64, 1939.

Van Helmont, J. B.: *Ortus medicinae* . . . . Amsterod: L. Elzevier, 1648.

Henri de Mondeville: *Chirurgie* de maître Henri de Mondeville. Annotated transl. by E. Nicaise. Paris: F. Alcan, 1893.

Herls, C.: *Examen der chirurgie*, seer nut . . . alle jonge chirurgijns ende insonderheyt die haer begeven na Oost-ofte West-Indien (Examination of surgery, very profitable for all young surgeons, in particular for those who will make for the East or West Indies). Amsterdam: B. Jansz, 1645[3].

Van Herwaarden, J.: Medici in de Nederlandse samenleving in de late Middeleeuwen (veertiende—zestiende eeuw) (Medical practitioners in Dutch society in the late Middle Ages, 14th—16th cent.). *Tijdschr. Geschied.* **96**: 348—78, 1983.

Hilte, A. J. M.: Over het chirurgijnsgilde in Nijmegen (The surgeon's guild at Nijmegen). *Numaga* **20**: 17—36, 1973.

Hippocrates: *Oeuvres complètes d'Hippocrate*. Greek text with French transl. by E. Littré, 10 vols. Paris: J. B. Ballière, 1834—61 [Repr. A. M. Hakkert, Amsterdam, 1961—62].
Hippocrates: *The genuine works of Hippocrates*. Transl. from the Greek with . . . annotations by F. Adams, 2 vols. London: Sydenham Society, 1849.
Hippocrates: *Hippocrates*. Greek text with an English transl. by W. H. S. Jones (vols. 1, 2, 4) and E. T. Withington (vol. 3), 4 vols. Loeb Classical Library. Cambridge (Mass): Harvard Univ. Press and London: W. Heinemann, 1957[4], 1952[3], 1959[4], 1953[3].
Hoffmann, F.: *Medicus politicus* s Regulae . . . secundum quas medicus iuvenis studia sua . . . dirigere debet. Lugd-Batav: Ph. Bonk, 1738.
Holmes, O. W.: On the contagiousness of puerperal fever. *New Engl. quart. J. Med. Surg.* **1**: 503—30, 1842—3. Partly reprinted in Clendening: *Source book*, pp. 605—6.
Home, E.: An account of Mr. Hunter's method of performing the operation for the popliteal aneurysm. *London med. J.* **7**: 391—406, 1786.
Homer: *The Iliad*. Greek text with Engl. transl. by A. T. Murray, 2 vols. Loeb Classical Library. London: W. Heinemann and Cambridge (Mass): Harvard Univ. Press, 1924—25.
Hommerson, M.: De Afdeling Nijmegen en Omstreken tijdens de Tweede Wereldoorlog (The Department Nijmegen and Surroundings of the Dutch Medical Association during the Second World War). In: De Moulin (ed.): *De geschiedenis van de Afdeling Nijmegen*, pp. 40—61.
Hoogvliet, J.: *See* Petit, J. L.
Hossard, J.: Le Cat, lithotomiste et les remèdes de Mlle Stephens *Rev. Hist. Pharm.* **22**: 155—62, 1970.
Houtzager, H. L.: *Medicyns, vroedwyfs en chirurgyns*, schets van de gezondheidszorg in Delft en beschrijving van het Theatrum Anatomicum aldaar in de 16de en 17de eeuw (Physicians, midwives and surgeons. An outline of health care at Delft and description of the anatomical theatre at that place in the 16th and 17th centuries). Amsterdam: Rodopi, 1979.
Huard, P., Ohya, Z., Wong, M.: *La médecine japonaise*. Paris: R. Dacosta, 1974.
Huizinga, J.: Duitschland's invloed op de Nederlandsche beschaving (Germany's influence on Dutch culture). *Verzamelde Werken*. Haarlem: Tjeenk Willink, 1953, vol. 2, pp. 304—13.
Huizinga, J.: *Nederland's beschaving in de 17de eeuw* (Civilization of the Netherlands in the 17th cent.). Groningen: H. D. Tjeenk Willink, 1972[4].
Hulsman, G., Zwaveling, A.: Frederik Willem Krieger, heelmeester (F.W.K., surgeon). *Ned. Tijdschr. Geneeskd.* **110**: 18—20, 1966.
Hunter, A. R.: Old unhappy far off things. Some reflections on the early work on shock. *Ann. roy. Coll. Surg. Engl.* **40**: 289—305, 1967.

Icart: En réponse au Mémoire de M. Pujol . . . sur une amputation naturelle de la jambe . . . *J. Méd. Chir. Pharm.* **44**: 164—81, 1775.
Van Iterson, J. E.: Mededeelingen omtrent het Geneeskundig congres te Londen (An account of the Medical Congress in London). *Ned. Tijdschr. Geneeskd.* **17**: 769—76, 1881.

Jansen-Sieben, R.: 'Jonghe Lanfranc'. In: *Die deutsche Literatur des Mittelalters-Verfasserslexicon*. Berlin, New York: W. de Gruyter, 1978[2]—, vol. 4, column 836—38.
Jansen-Sieben, R., Keil, G.: Eine chirurgische Glossensammlung des frühen 14. Jahrhunderts. *Zschr. dtsche. Sprache* **27**: 129—46, 1971.
Jarcho, S.: Seventeenth-century medical journalism. *J.A.M.A.* **220**: 64—8, 1972.
Jones, W. H. S.: *See* Hippocrates.

Keil, G., Müller, R.: Deutsche Lanfrank-Übersetzungen des 14. und 15. Jahrhunderts. Zur Wertung der Lanfrank-Zitate in Brunschwigs 'Chirurgie'. In: Eulner *et al.*: *Medizingeschichte in unserer Zeit*, pp. 90—110.
Keith, N. M., Keys, Th. E.: The Anatomy Acts of 1831 and 1832. *Arch. int. Med.* **99**: 679—94, 1957.
Kerkhoff, A. H. M.: *Over de geneeskundige verzorging in het Staatse leger* (Medical provisions in the army of the Dutch Republic). With summary in English. Thesis Nijmegen, 1976.
Kings, L. S.: *The growth of medical thought*. Chicago, London: Univ. of Chicago Press, 1963.
King, L. S.: *The road to medical enlightenment*. London: MacDonald; New York: American Elsevier, 1970.
Kirchamir, H.: Die Kluge Sklavin Tawaddud. *Med. Klinik* **52**: 470—72, 1957.
Van der Klaauw, C. J.: Het eertijds verplichte instrumentarium van den heelmeester (Instruments formerly made compulsory for the surgeon). *Ned. Tijdschr. Geneeskd.* **83**(III): 3343—53, 1939.

Klasen, H. J.: Hans Rudolph Ranke, professor of surgery at Groningen, and the conditions in which he worked 100 years ago. *Arch. chir. neerland* **30**: 191—7, 1978.
Klebs, A. C.: Incunabula scientifica et medica. *Osiris* **4**: 1—359, 1938 [Reprint Hildesheim: G. Olms, 1963].
De Knecht-van Eekelen, A.: *Naar een rationele zuigelingenvoeding.* Voedingsleer en kindergeneeskunde in Nederland 1840—1914 (Towards a rational infant diet. Dietetics and paediatrics in the Netherlands 1840—1914). Engl. and Germ. summary. Thesis Nijmegen, 1984.
Koenerding, A.: *Nutte beschryving van het heet en koud vuur, neffens het afsetten van scheen- en kuyt beenderen . . .* (Useful description of inflammation and gangrene, together with the amputation of shin and splint-bones). Rotterdam: H. Kentlink, 1739^2.
Korteweg, J. A.: De ontwikkeling der heelkunde gedurende de laatste halve eeuw (The development of surgery during the last half-century). *Ned. Tijdschr. Geneeskd.* **51** (I): 28—35, 1907.
Kouwer, B. J., Laméris, H. J.: *Iets uit de geschiedenis der klinieken voor heel- en verloskunde der Rijks-Universiteit te Utrecht met een beschrijving der nieuwe inrichting* (Something of the history of the clinics for surgery and obstetrics of the State University at Utrecht, with a description of the new establishment). Kampen: Stads Boek- en Courantdrukkerij, 1908.
Krul, R.: Argumentatio fustis. Bijdrage tot het leven van de broeders Stalpert van der Wiel en Cornelis Solingen (Argumentatio fustis. Contribution to the biography of the brothers St.v.d.W. and C.S.). *Ned. Tijdschr. Geneeskd.* **19**: 871—4, 1883.
Krul, R.: Abraham Titsingh. Harrewarrerijen en schermutselingen tusschen Amstels doctoren en chirurgen, in verband met het gildewezen (A.T. Squabbles and skirmishes between doctors and surgeons of Amsterdam connected with the guild system). *Ned. Tijdschr. Geneeskd.* **27** (II): 429—48, 1891.
Van Kulsdom, M. E.: De landschapsmedici en operateurs van Friesland in de achttiende eeuw (The district physicians and surgeons in F. in the 18th cent.). *Ned. Tijdschr. Geneeskd.* **99**(II): 1582—91, 1955.
Kunz, G. G.: *Oude- en Nieuwe Gasthuis 1252—1977.* Delft: Elmar, 1977.
Küster, E.: *Geschichte der neueren deutschen Chirurgie.* Vol. 15 in the monograph series 'Neue deutsche Chirurgie'. Ed. by P. v. Bruns. Stuttgart: F. Enke, 1915.
Kuijjer, P. J.: Oprichting van de Vereeniging in 1902 en het verenigingsleven tot 1947 (Foundation of the Association in 1902 and club life until 1947). In: Kuijjer *et al.*: *Ned. Ver. Heelk.*, pp. 68—105.
Kuijjer, P. J., Boevé, J., Eeftinck Schattenkerk, J. C. P., Grond, J. T. H., De Moulin, D. (Eds.): *Nederlandse Vereniging voor Heelkunde 1902—1977* (Association of surgeons of the Netherlands 1902—1977). Utrecht: Bohn, Scheltema & Holkema, 1977.

Laan, H. A.: *Chirurgische zieken en hunne verpleging* (Surgical patients and their nursing). Utrecht: A. W. Bruna & Zn., 1907.
Van Lamzweerde, J. B.: *Chirurgiae veteris ac modernae promptuarium . . .* Amstelodami: J. à Someren, 1672.
Lancisi, G. M.: *Aneurysms.* The Latin text of Rome, 1745, revised, with transl. and notes by W. C. Wright. New York: Macmillan, 1952.
Larrey, D. J.: *Mémoires de chirurgie militaire, et campagnes*, 4 vols. Paris: J. Smith, 1812—7.
Leeflang, M.: De Chirurgijnen en de 'Gemeene Faculteit der Medicijnen' te Enkhuizen (The surgeons and the 'Common Faculty of Medicine' at E.). *Med. Contact* **22**: 1233—7, 1967.
Van Leersum, E. G.: *See* Yperman, Jan and Scellinck, Thomas.
De Leng, T. A. T.: *Verslag der chirurgische polikliniek en kliniek aan de Leidsche Hoogeschool gedurende de academische cursus 1873—1874* (Report on the surgical clinic and outpatients clinic of the Leyden University, 1873—74). Thesis Leiden, 1875.
Leporin, C. P.: *Ausführlicher Bericht vom Leben und Schriften des . . . Herrn D. Laurentii Heisteri.* Quedlinburg: J. G. Sievert, 1725 [Repr. Dr. F. J. Schmidt, private print, 1981].
Leriche, R,: *Souvenirs de ma vie morte.* Paris: Ed. du Seuil, 1956.
Lesky, E.: Van Swieten und die Chirurgie. In: *Circa Tiliam.* Studia historiae medicinae Gerrit Arie Lindeboom septuagenario oblata. Leiden: E. J. Brill, 1974, pp. 140—9.
Leuftink, A. E.: *De geneeskunde bij 's lands oorlogsvloot in de 17e eeuw* (Medicine in the Dutch navy in the 17th cent.). Thesis Groningen, 1952.
Lewis, G. L.: *See* Albucasis.
Van Lieburg, M. J.: Gasthuis en Clinische School (1828—1832) (Hospital and Clinical School). *Maandbl. Acad. Ziekenhuis Rotterdam* **4**: 45—8, 1975.
Van Lieburg, M. J.: Uit de medische stadsgeschiedenis van Rotterdam. XV De chirurgijns en hun gilde (From the medical town history of Rotterdam. XV The surgeons and their guild). *Monitor* **5**: 117—9, 1976.

Van Lieburg, M. J.: *Het medisch onderwijs te Rotterdam* (1407—1967) (Medical teaching at Rotterdam). Amsterdam: Rodopi, 1978.
Van Lieburg, M. J.: The instrument-collection of Peter Vink. A chapter in the development of the surgical profession in the Netherlands during the 18th century. *Janus* **67**: 207—19, 1980.
Van Lieburg, M. J.: De 'Materia Chirurgica' in de ordonnanties en examens der Noord-Nederlandse chirurgijnsgilden vóór 1600 ('Materies chirurgica' in the ordinances and examinations of the surgeons' guilds in the North Netherlands before 1600), *Pharm. Weekbl.* **116**: 1393—8, 1981.
Van Lieburg, M. J.: Dé genees- en heelkunde in de Noordelijke Nederlanden, gezien vanuit de stedelijke en chirurgijnsgilde-ordonnanties van de 16de eeuw (Medicine and surgery in the Northern Netherlands, as seen from 16th century municipal and surgeons' guild regulations). *Tijdschr. Geschied. Geneesk. Natuurw. Wisk. Techniek* **6**: 179—84, 1983.
Van Lieburg, M. J.: Nicolaas Zas (1610—68). Een biografische bijdrage tot de geschiedenis van de chylus- en lymfefysiologie (N. Zas. A biographic contribution to the history of the chyle and lymph physiology. With English summary). In: A. H. M. Kerkhoff, A. M. Luyendijk-Elshout, M. J. D. Poulissen (Eds.): *De novis inventis*, essays in the history of medicine in honour of Daniel de Moulin. Amsterdam & Maarssen: A.P.A.-Holland Univ. Press, 1984, pp. 231—57.
Van Lieburg, M. J.: De Nederlandse medische tijdschriften en de wetenschappelijke geneeskunde 1840—70 (The Dutch medical journals and scientific medicine). In: D. de Moulin (Ed.): *Kracht en stof.* Amsterdam: Rodopi, 1985, pp. 1—19.
Lindeboom, G. A.: Ruysch's anatomische preparaten in Leningrad. *Ned. Tijdschr. Geneeskd.* **106**: 32—3, 1962.
Lindeboom, G. A.: De Clinische School te Rotterdam. *Ned. Tijdschr. Geneeskd.* **109**: 2095—8, 1965.
Lindeboom, G. A.: *Herman Boerhaave.* The man and his work. London: Methuen, 1968.
Lindeboom, G. A.: *De geschiedenis van de medische wetenschap in Nederland* (The history of medical science in the Netherlands). Bussum: Fibula-Van Dishoeck, 1972.
Lindeboom, G. A.: *Reinier de Graaf.* Delft: Elmar, 1973.
Lister, J.: On the antiseptic principle of the practice of surgery. *Brit. Med. J.* **ii**: 246—8, 1867. Reprinted in Clendening: *Source Book*, pp. 615—21.
Littré, E.: *See* Hippocrates.
Logger, H. J.: Aanteekingen op eene wetenschappelijke reize naar Parijs in den jare 1818 (Notes on a scientific journey to P. in 1818). *Geneesk. Bladen* **1**: 96—146, 1826.
Van Loon, L.: *Historisch overzicht van de fractuurbehandeling der lange pijpbeenderen* (Historical survey of the treatment of fractures of the long cylindrical bones). Thesis Leyden, 1935.
Van Loon, L.: Het Rotterdamsche chirurgijnsgilde 'St Cosmos et Damianus' van 1467—1798. *Ned. Tijdschr. Geneeskd.* **83**(III): 1485—92; 3911—8, 1939.
Luyendijk-Elshout, A. M.: De duisternis rondom Vesalius (The darkness around V.). *Tijdschr. Gesch.* **85**: 390—409, 1972.
Luyendijk-Elshout, A. M.: The introduction of Juan Valverde's and Bartholomy Cabrol's anatomy into the Low Countries between 1568—1633. *Actas XXVII Congreso Internacional de Historia de la Medicina*, 2 vols. Barcelona: Acadèmia de Ciències Mèdiques de Catalunya i Balears, 1981, pp. 298—303.

Mann, Th.: *Der Zauberberg.* 2 vols. Frankfurt a.M.: Fischer Taschenbuch, 1975.
De la Martinière [G. P.]: Mémoire sur le traitement des playes d'armes à feu. *Mém. Acad, roy. Chir.* **4**: 1—39, 1768.
Mathijsen, A.: *The plaster of Paris bandage.* Its invention by Antonius Mathijsen. Two facsimiles (1852 and 1854) with an introduction by G. J. Bremer. Nieuwkoop: B. de Graaf, 1962.
Matti, H.: *Die Kochenbrüche und ihre Behandlung*, 2 vols. Berlin: J. Springer, 1918.
Van Meekeren, J.: *Heel- en geneeskonstige aenmerkingen* (Surgical and medical remarks). Rotterdam: J. Hofhout, 1728^2 [Repr. with introduction by D. de Moulin. Stafleu: Alphen aan den Rijn, 1979].
Mercer, W.: Some Edinburgh pioneers in orthopaedic surgery. *Ann. roy. Coll. Surg. Engl.* **26**: 339—61, 1960.
Merke, F.: *Geschichte und Ikonographie des endemischen Kropfes und Kretinismus.* Bern, Stuttgart, Wien: H. Huber, 1971.
Metz, L. M.: De behandeling der schuine dijbeenbreuken (Treatment of oblique fractures of the femur). *Geneesk. Bladen* **10**, no. 8, pp. 217—44, 1904.
Meyer-Steineg, Th.: *Chirurgische Instrumente des Altertums.* Jenaer medizin-hist. Beiträge Heft 1. Jena: G. Fischer, 1912.
Meijne, N. G.: Het *Archivum chirurgicum neerlandicum*, spiegel van de Nederlandse chirurgie (The journal A.C.N., reflection of Dutch Surgery(. In: Kuijjer *et al.*: *Ned. Ver. Heelk.*, pp. 279—84.

Meijne, N. G.: Van Stichting via Vereniging der chirurgische Wetenschappen tot Collegium chirurgicum neerlandicum (From Foundation via Society for surgical Sciences to Coll. chir. neerl.). In: Kuijjer *et al.*: *Ned. Ver. Heelk.*, pp. 165—72.
Michler, M.: Guy de Chauliac als anatom. *Med. Mschr.* **18**: 306—11, 1964.
Michler, M.: *Die alexandrinischen Chirurgen.* Eine Sammlung u. Auswertung ihrer Fragmente. Die hellenistische Chirurgie Teil I. Wiesbaden: F. Steiner, 1968.
Michler, M.: *Das Spezialisierungsproblem u. die antike Chirurgie.* Stuttgart, Wien: H. Huber, 1969.
Van der Minne, A.: *Bijdrage tot de kennis der herniologie* (Contribution to the science of herniology). Thesis Utrecht, 1900.
Mirakelen van Onze Lieve Vrouwe te 's-Hertogenbosch 1381—1603 (Register containing the miracles ascribed to the Holy Virgin of 's-Hertogenbosch). Ed. by Hens, H., Van Bakel, H., Van Dyck, G. C. M., Frantzen, J. H. M. Series Bijdr. Gesch. Zuiden van Nederland, XLII. Tilburg: Stichting zuid hist. Contact, 1978.
De Mondeville: *See* Henri.
Monnikhoff, J.: *Ontleed-, heel- en werktuigkundige zamenstelling . . . over de scheursels of breuken* (Anatomical, surgical and mechanical composition . . . on ruptures or herniae). Amsteldam: J. Hazeu Cornelisz, 1792[2].
Van Montfort, F.: *Omstandig verhaal ofte korte dog nauwkeurige beschrijving eener schuynsche onherstelbaare en beswaarlijke beenbreuk* gered met de binding van eenen gouden draad (Elaborate account or short but accurate description of an oblique irreparable and difficult fracture saved by ligature with a golden thread). Antwerpen: C. H. de Vos, n.d. [c. 1796]. 19 pp.
Moonen, W. A.: Frère Jacques de Beaulieu, een veel omstreden periodeut (1651—1714), (F. J. de B., a controversial itinerant). *Ned. Tijdschr. Geneeskd.* **112**: 24—32, 1968.
Moore, C. H.: On the influence of inadequate operations on the theory of cancer. *Med.-chir. Transact.* **50**: 245—80, 1867.
Morand [S. F.]: *Opuscules de chirurgie*, 2 parts. Paris: G. Desprez, 1768.
Morgagni, G. B.: *De sedibus et causis morborum per anatomen indagatis libri quinque*, 2 vols. Pativii, sumpt Remondinianis, 1765[2].
De Moulin, D.: Historical Notes on vascular surgery I, II, III. *Arch. chir. neerl.* **7**: 218—26; 321—30, 1955 and **8**: 31—42, 1956.
De Moulin, D.: Some remarks on the early history of blood transfusion. *Arch. chir. neerl.* **10**: 176—83, 1958.
De Moulin, D.: Dominique Anel and his operation for aneurysm. *Bull. Hist. Med.* **34**: 498—507, 1960.
De Moulin, D.: Aneurysms in Antiquity. *Arch. chir. neerl.* **13**: 49—63, 1961.
De Moulin, D.: Some more historical notes on aneurysms. *Arch. chir. neerl.* **15**: 277—84, 1961.
De Moulin, D.: *De heelkunde in de vroege Middeleeuwen* (Early medieval surgery, with summary and conclusions in English). Leiden: E. J. Brill, 1964.
De Moulin, D.: De natuurhistorische verzameling in het voormalige theatrum anatomicum te Rotterdam (The natural-history collection in the former anatomical theatre at Rotterdam). *Rotterdams Jaarboekje* 1972, pp. 129—39.
De Moulin, D.: Historical notes on appendicitis. *Arch. chir. neerl.* **27**: 97—103, 1975.
De Moulin, D.: Fracture of the lower end of the radius: an obscure injury for many centuries. *Arch. chir. neerl.* **29**: 213—6, 1977.
De Moulin, D.: De heelkunde sinds de eeuwwisseling (Surgery since the turn of the century). In: Kuijjer *et al.*: *Ned. Ver. Heelk.*, pp. 9—28.
De Moulin, D.: Hernias in history. *Arch. chir. neerl.* **30**: 129—40, 1978.
De Moulin, D.: Die Medizin zur Zeit der Regierung des Königs Wilhelm I in den Niederlanden. *Janus* **65**: 21—44, 1978.
De Moulin, D.: Historical notes on breast cancer, with emphasis on the Netherlands. I Pathological and therapeutic concepts in the 17th century. *Neth. J. Surg.* **32**: 129—34, 1980.
De Moulin, D.: Heelkundige onderwerpen in het Nederlandsch Weekblad voor Geneeskundigen (Surgical subjects in the N.W.v.G.). *Ned. Tijdschr. Geneeskd.* **125**: 1427—30, 1981.
De Moulin, D. (Ed.): *Vier eeuwen Amsterdams Binnengasthuis* (Four centuries Binnengasthuis hospital at Amsterdam). Wormer: Inmerc, 1981.
De Moulin, D.: Historical notes on breast cancer . . . . II. Pathophysiological concepts, diagnosis and therapy in the 18th century. *Neth. J. Surg.* **33**: 206—16, 1981.
De Moulin, D.: Historical notes on breast cancer . . . . III. The growth of scientific surgery in the 19th century. *Neth. J. Surg.* **34**: 193—200, 1982.
De Moulin, D.: *A short history of breast cancer.* Boston, The Hague, Dordrecht, Lancaster: M. Nijhoff, 1983.
De Moulin, D.: Guilleaume Dupuytren in Paris Hôtel-Dieu. Eye witness reports by foreign visitors.

In: O. Baur, O. Glandien: *Zusammenhang*, Festschrift für Marielene Putscher. Köln: Wienand, 1984, pp. 633—52.
De Moulin, D.: The value of tobacco smoke in the treatment of intussusception. *Neth. J. Surg.* **36**: 57—8, 1984.
De Moulin, D.: Paulus Barbette M. D.: a seventeenth century Amsterdam author of best-selling textbooks. *Bull. Hist. Med.* **59**: 506—14, 1985.
De Moulin, D.: The treatment of compound fractures in the eighteenth century. *Neth. J. Surg.* **37**: 54—9, 1985.
De Moulin, D.: De dijbeenhalsbreuk: historisch overzicht (Fracture of the neck of the femur: a historical survey). In: J. B. van Mourik (Ed.): *Heupfracturen bij bejaarden* (Hipfractures in the elderly). Utrecht: Bunge, 1986, pp. 55—61.
De Moulin, D. (Ed.): *De Afdeling Nijmegen en Omstreken van de K.N.M.G.* (History of the dept. Nijmegen and surroundings of the Royal Dutch Medical Association). Nijmegen: Not for sale, 1986.
De Moulin, D., De Groot, I. M.: The cancer operation by Romeyn de Hooghe. *Organorama* **5**(II): 22—3, 1974.
Mulder, G. J.: *Levensschets van G. J. Mulder, door hem zelven geschreven* (Sketch of G. J. M.'s life, written by himself). Utrecht: vd. Post, 1883.
Mulder, J.: Redevoering over de redenen, waarom de Nederlanders in het algemeen zeer weinig tot verbetering en uitbreiding van de heel- en verloskunde hebben toegebragt . . . (Oration on the causes why the Dutch in general contributed very little to the improvement and expansion of surgery and obstetrics). Leeuwarden: D. van der Sluis, 1797.
Muller, H.: De Wetenschap en de Vereniging voor Heelkunde, 1947—72 (Science and the Association of Surgeons, 1947—72). In: Kuijjer *et al.*: *Ned. Ver. Heelk.*, pp. 201—39.
Müller, R.: *Der 'Jonghe Lanfranc'*. Thesis Bonn, 1968.
Munniks, J.: *Alle de wercken van den heer J. Munniks M.D.* (The collected works of Mr. J. M. M.D.). Amsterdam: J. Hartog, 1740.
[van Musschenbroek, J.]: *Catalogus instrumentorum, quae apud Joann van Musschenbroek veneunt Lugd Bat 1707.* Amstelodami: apud Janssonio-Waesbergios, 1711.

Napjus, J. W.: De hoogleeraren in de geneeskunde aan de hoogeschool en het Athenaeum te Franeker (1585—1843), XIII Abraham Cyprianus (The professors of medicine at the University and the Athenaeum at Franeker (1585—1843) XIII: A.C.), *Ned. Tijdschr. Geneeskd.* **83**(II): 2625—31, 1939.
Neuburger, M.: *Geschichte der Medizin*, 2 vols. Stuttgart: F. Enke, 1906—11.
Nicaise, E.: ***See*** **Guy de Chauliac, Henri de Mondeville; Franco, P.**
Van Nierop, L.: Het dagboek van Jacob Bicker Raye' 1732—1772. Van geneesheren (The diary of J. B. R. 1732—72. On medical men). *Jaarboek Amstelodamum* **35**: 131—78, (1938).
Nieuwenhuys, C. J.: *Proeve eener geneeskundige plaatsbeschrijving der stad Amsterdam* (Attempt at a medical topography of the city of Amsterdam), 4 vols. Amsterdam: J. van der Hey, 1816—20.
Nissen, R.: Chirurgie einst und jetzt. *Deutsch. med. J.* **9**: 91—6, 1958.
Nissen, R.: *Helle Blätter — dunkle Blätter.* Erinnerungen eines Chirurgen. Stuttgart: DVA, 1969.
Nissen, R.: Wilson, R. H. L.: *Pages in the history of chest surgery.* Springfield Illinois: Ch. C. Thomas, 1960.
Nuyens, B. W. Th.: Het ontleedkundig onderwijs en de geschilderde Anatomische lessen van het Chirurgijns Gilde te Amsterdam, in de jaren 1550 tot 1798 (Anatomical tuition and the painted anatomical lessons of the Surgeons' Guild at Amsterdam, 1550—1798. *Jaarverslag . . . Kon. Oudheidk. Genootsch.* **71**: 45—90, 1928.

O'Malley, C. D.: *Andreas Vesalius of Brussels.* Berkeley, Los Angeles: Univ. Calif. Press, 1964.
Opuscula selecta neerlandicorum in arte medica. Series of Dutch medical classics, published by *Ned. Tijdschr. Geneeskd.*, 19 vols. Haarlem: F. Bohn, 1907—58.
Orlers, J. J.: *Beschrijving der stad Leyden* (Description of the town of L.). Leyden: H. Haestens, J. Orlers, J. Maire, 1614.
Den Otter, G.: Internationale contacten. In: Kuijjer *et al.*: *Ned. ver. Heelk.*, pp. 273—8.

Paracelsus [Ph. A. Th.]: *Die groote chirurgie* . . . ghetransl. wt den hoochd. . . . duer Pieter Volck Horst, 1556 (The great surgery transl. from the High-German by P. V. H.). Antwerpen: G. van Diestle, 1555.
Paracelsus [Ph. A. Th.]: *De cleyne chirurgie ende 'tgasthuysboeck*, nu eerst wten Hoochd in ons Nederl Duytsche overgheset duer M. Everaert (The small surgery and hospitalbook, now for the first time transl. from the High-German by M. E.). Thantwerpen: Wed. H. de Laet, 1568, 1567.

Paracelsus [Ph. A. Th.]: *Die peerle der chirurgijen*, inhoudende den rechte(n) gront ... om alle versche wonden, oude seeren, verbrantheyt ... te ghenesen .... Ghetrocken ... uit den boecken Domini Doctoris Paracelsi ... van Meester Philippus Hermanni enz. (The pearl of surgery, containing the two grounds to cure all fresh wounds, old ulcers, burns, excerpted from the books of D. D. P. by master P. H.). Thantwerpe: J. A. Roela(n)ts, 1553.
Paré, A.: *De Chirurgie ende alle de opera*. Transl. by Carolus Battus. Dordrecht, Jan Canin, 1592.
Park, H.: *An account of a new method of treating diseases of the joints of the knee and elbow*. London: J. Johnson, 1733 (misprint for 1783).
Pasteur, L.: Mémoire sur les corpuscules organisés qui existent dans l'atmosphère. *Ann. Sci. nat.* (Zool.) 4e Série, **16**: 5—98, 1861.
Paulus of Aegina: *The seven books of Paulus Aegineta*. Transl. from the Greek with a commentary ... by F. Adams, 3 vols. London: Sydenham Society, 1844—47.
Peltier, L. F.: Percivall Pott and Pott's fracture. *Surgery* **51**: 280—6, 1962.
Peltier, L. F.: A brief history of traction. *J. Bone Jt. Surg.* **50**—A: 1603—17, 1968.
Pepys, S.: *The diary of Samuel Pepys*. Ed. by H. B. Wheatly, 8 vols. London: G. Bell & Sons, 1926.
Petit, J. L.: Remarques sur les tumeurs formées par la bile retenue dans la vésicule du fiel, qu'on a souvent prises pour des abcès au foye. *Mém. Acad. roy. Chir.* **1**: 155—87, 1743.
Petit, J. L.: *Verhandeling van de ziekten der beenderen*. Waarin men vertoont de verbanden en konsttuigen tot derselver genezing behoorende (Treatise on the diseases of the bones, in which are shown the bandages and appliances proper to their cure). Transl. from the French by J. Hoogvliet. Rotterdam: Ph. & J. Losel, 1736; 1751[2].
Petit, J. L.: *Traité des maladies chirurgicales et des opérations qui leur conviennent*. Nouv. éd., 3 vols. Paris: Mequignon, 1790.
Persyn, G. G.: Verleden, heden en toekomst van de orgaantransplantatie in Nederland (Past, present and future of organ-transplantation in Holland). *Med. Contact.* **41**: 1343—5, 1986.
Pirenne, H.: *De middeleeuwen* (The Middle-Ages). Transl. from the French by J. A. Meijers. Amsterdam: L. J. Veen, n.d., 2nd ed.
Plutarch: *Plutarch's parallel lives*. Greek text with Engl. transl. by B. Perrin, 11 vols. Loeb Classical Library. London: W. Heinemann, Cambridge (Mass): Harvard Univ. Press, 1959, vol. 9.
Pott, P.: *Twee heelkundige verhandelingen* van den heere Percival Pot. De eerste over de natuur en de gevolgen der wonden en kneuzingen van het hoofd ..., de andere over de breuken ('Obs. on the ... wounds and contusions of the head ...', and 'On ruptures'). Rotterdam: R. Arrenberg, 1768.
Pott, P.: *The chirurgical works of Percivall Pott* ... to which are added, a short account of the life of the author ... by Sir James Earle, 3 vols. London: J. Johnson, G. G. J. and J. Robinson and others, 1790.
Potter, A.: Proefondervindelijk onderzoek der veranderingen der ratten, die het diepe heidewater te Utrecht en enkele andere wateren dronken (An experimental investigation into changes in rats which drank the deep moor-water in Utrecht and some other waters). *Ned. Tijdschr. Geneeskd.* **63**(I): 2238—40, 1919.
Probst, C.: Der Weg des ärztlichen Erkennens bei Heinrich von Mondeville. In: G. Keil *et al.* (Eds.): *Fachliteratur des Mittelalters*. Festschr. for G. Eis. Stuttgart: J. B. Metzler, 1968, pp. 333—57.
Pujol, A.: Amputation naturelle de la jambe. *J. Méd. Chir. Pharm.* **43**: 160—72, 1775.
Putscher, M.: Ein Totentanz von Tizian. Die 17 grossen Holzschnitte zur Fabrica Vesals (1538—42). In: W. Göpfert, H. H. Otten (Eds.): *Metavoeite — wandelt euch durch neues Denken*. Festschr. H. Schadewaldt. Düsseldorf: Triltsch, 1983.

Randers-Pehrson, J.: *The surgeon's glove*. Springfield, Illinois: C. C. Thomas, 1960.
Rather, J. L.: The 'Six things non-natural': a note on the origins and fate of a doctrine and a phrase. *Clio medica* **3**: 337—47, 1968.
Ravaton, H.: *Chirurgie d'armée* ou traité des plaies d'armes à feu et d'armes blanches. Paris: P. Fr. Didot le jeune, 1758.
Ravitch, M.: *A century of surgery*, 2 vols. Philadelphia, Toronto: J. B. Lippincott, 1982[2].
Reneaulme de la Garanne, M. L.: *Vertoog ter opening van het School der heelkunde, benevens een verhandeling der scheursels* (Address at the inauguration of the School of Surgery, together with a treatise on ruptures). In 't Nederd. gebragt door J. van der Hulst. Haarlem: Geertruyd van Kessel, 1724.
Richter, A. G.: *Verhandeling over de breuken*. Uit 't Hgd. door J. Daams (Treatise on ruptures. Transl. from the High-German by J. D.), 2 vols. Haarlem: C. van der Aa, 1780—84.
Richter, A. G.: *Beginselen der heelkunde*. Uit't Hoogd. vert. (Fundamentals of Surgery. Transl. from the High-German). Amsterdam: A. J. van Toll, 1784.

Ringoir, D. B. J.: *Plattelandschirurgijns in de 17de en 18de eeuw*. De rekeningboeken van de 18e eeuwse Durgerdamse chirurgijn Anthony Egberts (Rural surgery in the 17th and 18th cent. The account book of the 18th cent. Durgerdam surgeon A.E.). Thesis Free University Amsterdam, 1977.
Risse, G. B.: *Hospital life in Enlightenment Scotland*. Cambridge etc.: Cambridge Univ. Press, 1986.
Rochard, J.: *Histoire de la chirurgie française au XIXe siècle*. Paris: J. B. Baillière, 1875.
Roegholt, M. N.: Niertransplantatie in 1908 (Renal transplantation in 1908). *Ned. Tijdschr. Geneeskd.* **110**: 1877, 1966.
Rogge, C. W. L.: *De betekenis van Ambroise Paré* (The significance of A.P.). With Engl. abstract. Thesis Groningen, 1973.
Rogier, L. J.: Uit de geschiedenis van de beoefening der geneeskunde, inzonderheid te Nijmegen (On the history of medical practice, in Nijmegen in particular). *Numaga* **7**: 3—69, 1961.
Rombach, K. A.: Proeve eener vergelijking van onze kennis der breuken (herniologie) met die van de vorige eeuw (Essay on a comparison of our knowledge of ruptures — herniology — with that of the last century). *Ned. Tijdschr. Geneeskd.* **4**(II): 25—101, 1868.
Von Römer L. S. A. M.: *Historische schetsen*. Batavia: Javasche Boekhandel en Drukkerij, 1921.
Romeyn, D.: *Onze militair-geneeskundige dienst voor honderd jaren en daaromtrent* (Our army medical service some 100 years ago). Haarlem: F. Bohn, 1913.
Van Rompaey, J.: De Bourgondische periode. In: *Winkler Prins Geschiedenis der Nederlanden*, 3 vols. Amsterdam, Brussel: Elsevier, 1977, vol. 1, pp. 263—327.
Van Roonhuyse, H.: *Genees- en heelkonstige aanmerkingen*. Amsterdam: Th. J. Lootsman, 1672.
Rotgans, J.: Eenige bladzijden uit de geschiedenis der chirurgie dezer eeuw (A few pages from the history of surgery in this century). *Ned. Tijdschr. Geneeskd.* **35**(I): 573—93, 1899.
Rothschuh, K. E.: *Konzepte der Medizin* in Vergangenheit und Gegenwart. Stuttgart: Hippokrates, 1978.
Rubin Pinault, J.: How Hippocrates cured the plague. *J. Hist. Med. all. Sci.* **41**: 52—75, 1986.
Van Rustingh, S.: Nieuw gebouw der heelkonst, gegrondvest op reeden en ervarentheyt (New structure of surgery based on reason and experience). Amsterdam: Jan ten Hoorn, 1709.
Ruysch, F.: *Alle de ontleed-, genees- en heelkundige werken*. Vertaald in Nederduyts door Y. Arlebout (Collected anatomical, medical and surgical works, transl. into Low German [i.e. Dutch] by Y.A.), 3 vols. Amsterdam: J. van Waesberge, 1744.

Sandifort, E.: *Heel- en ontleedkundige verhandeling over eenen slagader-breuk in de groote slag-ader, uitwendig opengebarsten* (Surgical and anatomical treatise on an arterial rupture in the great trunk artery, burst outwardly). 's-Gravenhage: P. van Cleef, 1765.
Sandifort, J. B.: *See* Benevoli, A., Tacconi, G.
Scarff, J. E.: Fifty years of neurosurgery, 1905—55. *Int. Abstr. Surg.* **101**: 417—513, 1955.
Scellinck, Thomas: The 'Book of Surgeries' of master Thomas Scellinck from Thienen. Ed. with Engl. introd. by E. C. van Leersum after Mss in the Hague and London, *Opuscula selecta*, vol. VII, 1928.
Schechter, D. C.: Role of the humane societies in the history of resuscitation. *Surg. Gyn. Obst.* **129**: 811—5, 1969.
Schelenz, H.: *Geschichte der Pharmazie*. Berlin: Springer, 1904 [Repr. Hildesheim: Olms, 1962].
Schierbeek, A.: *Jan Swammerdam*. Zijn leven en werken (J. S. His life and works). Lochem: De Tijdstroom [1946].
Schlichting, J. D.: *Traumatologia nov' antiqua* ofte vernieuwde wondheelkunde. Amsterdam: J. van Heun, 1748.
Schmucker, J. L.: *Heelkundige waarnemingen* (Surgical observations). Transl. from the German by J. B. Sandifort, 2 vols. Leiden: P. van der Eyk, D. Vijgh, 1775—76.
Schoute, D.: *Schets van het Middelburgsche chirurgijnsgilde* (A short history of the Middelburg surgeon's guild). For private circulation [1913].
Schoute, D.: De levensloop van een ziekenhuis. Geschiedenis van het Gasthuis te Middelburg (The life story of a hospital. History of the Gasthuis at Middelburg). *Ned. Tijdschr. Geneeskd.* **61**(II): 3—64, 1917.
Schouten, J.: *De chirurgijnskamer in het Catharinagasthuis te Gouda* (The surgeons' hall at the Catherine Hospital at Gouda). Gouda: Stedelijke Musea, n.d.
Schouten, W.: *Het gewonde hooft*, of korte verhandeling van de opper-hooftswonden . . . (The wounded head, or short treatise on the wounds of the scalp and fractures of the skull). Amsterdam: A. van Someren, 1694.
Schrader, J.: *Observationes et historiae . . . ut et observationum anatomico-medicarum decades IV*. Amstelodami: A. Wolfgang, 1674.

Schrant, M. J.: *Prijsverhandeling over de goed- en kwaadaardige gezwellen.* Nieuwe verhandelingen bekroond met de gouden eereprijs van het Legaat van Joh. Monnikhof VII (Prize-winning essay on benign and malignant tumours. New essays awarded a gold medal to by the Legacy of J. M., no. VII). Amsterdam, n.d. [1851].
Schreiber, J. F.: Verhaal van het leven en de verdiensten van Frederik Ruysch (Account of the life and the merits of F. R.). In: Ruysch: *Alle de werken*, vol. 1, pp. 5—104.
Schroeder van der Kolk, J. C.: Over de vorming en verspreiding van kankercellen in den omtrek van kanker en het gewigt ervan bij het doen eener operatie (On the formation and spread of cancer cells in the adjacent tissues of cancer and its weight in performing an operation. *Ned. Lancet* 3rd Ser **3**: 129—58, 1853—4.
Seilberger, J. R.: Mededeeling omtrent een zeer eenvoudigen en doelmatigen toestel ter inademing van den zwavel-aether (Communication on a most simple and effective apparatus for the inhalation of sulphur-ether). *Boerhaave*, tijdschr. v. genees-, heel-, verlos- en artsenijkunde NS **6**: 456—9, 1847.
Semmelweis, I. Ph.: *Die Aetiologie, der Begriff und die Prophylaxis des Kindbettfiebers.* Pest, Wien & Leipzig: C. A. Hartleben, 1861.
Sermes, J.: *Aanmerkingen over de twee manieren van steensnyden van de heren J. J. Rau en J. Douglas* (Comments on the two methods of lithotomy of Mr. J. J. R. and Mr. J. D.). Utrecht: J. Visch, 1726. Re-edited with Engl. transl. by M. A. van Andel, *Opuscula selecta*, vol. XVII, 1943, pp. 218—25.
Sharp, S.: *Oordeelkundige aanmerkingen over de heelkunde in 't algemeen*, en de behandeling der operatien in 't byzonder, benevens de instrumenten daartoe dienende (Critical inquiry into the present state of surgery, Dutch transl. of the 3rd ed. and Treatise on the operations of surgery). Amsterdam: F. Houttuyn, 1751.
Shelley, H. S.: Cutting for the stone. *J- Hist. Med. all. Sci.* **13**: 50—67, 1958.
Sigerist, H. E.: *See* Brunschwig.
Sint Janshospitaal Brugge 1188—1976. Tentoonstelling georganiseerd door de Commissie van Openbare Onderstand te Brugge. Brugge: COO, 1976.
Slenders, J.: *Het Theatrum Anatomicum in de Noordelijke Nederlanden* (1555—1800). Extended student's essay, Nijmegen, 1978. Regrettably, this important paper never appeared in print.
Slenders, J.: De anatomische les van Dr. Zacheus de Jager (1640). With English summary. *Tijdschr. Geschied. Geneeskd. Natuurw. Wisk. Techniek* **4**: 159—67, 1981.
Smellie, W.: *Verhandeling over het bespiegelend en bewerkend deel der vroedkunde* . . . na den derden druk in 't Hollandsch gebracht . . . door Matthijs van der Haage, heel- en vroedmeester te Amsterdam (Treatise on the theory and practice of midwifery, transl. after the third ed. by M. van den Haage, surgeon and male-midwife at Amsterdam). Amsterdam: J. Morterre, 1765.
Solingen, C.: *Manuale operatiën der chirurgie* beneffens het ampt . . . der vroedvrouwen (Manual operations of surgery together with the office of the midwives). Amsterdam: J. Bouman, 1684.
Solingen, C.: Manuale operatiën der chirurgie. In: *Alle de medicinale en chirurgische werken* . . . . Amsterdam: J. ten Hoorn, 1698, pp. 1—396.
Spaander, J.: Dutch blood-transfusion service during the German occupation. *The Lancet* **1**: 494—5, 1947.
Spaander, J.: *Het ontstaan en de ontwikkeling van het bloedtransfusiewezen in Nederland* (The origin and development of organized blood-transfusion in the Netherlands). Nijmegen: Stichting Rode Kruis Bloedbank Nijmegen en Omstreken, 1983.
Sparkman, R. S.: Dr. John S. Bobbs of Indiana. *J. Indiana State med. Assn.* **60**: 541—8, 1967.
Spink, M. S.: *See* Albucasis.
Spoelstra, D.: *Antonius Mathijsen*, uitvinder van het gipsverband (A. M. inventor of the plaster-of-Paris bandage). Thesis Amsterdam, 1970.
Sprengel, K.: *Geschichte der Chirurgie.* Geschichte der wichtigsten Operationen, 2 vols. Halle: K. A. Kümmel, 1805—19.
Sprengel, K.: *Versuch einer pragmatischen Geschichte der Arzneykunde*, 6 vols. in 7. Halle: Gebauer, 1821—28 (vol. 1—5), Wien: C. Gerold, 1840 (vol. 6, I, II).
Stalpart vander Wiel, C.: *Observationum rariorum medic. anatomic. chirurgicarum centuriae I, II*, 2 vols. Leidae: J. à Kerkem, 1727.
Van Staveren, C.: *Aenteekeningen omtrent operatiën van den steen* (Records of operations for the stone). Thesis Amsterdam, 1934.
Steudel, J.: *See* Gersdorff.
Steudel, J.: Zwerg auf der Schulter des Riesen. *Sudhoffs Arch. Gesch. Med. Naturw.* **27**: 394—9, 1953.

Sudhoff, K.: Salerno, eine mittelalterliche Heil- und Lehstelle am Tyrrhenischen Meere. *Sudhoffs Arch. Gesch. Med.* **3**: 43—62, 1921.
Suringar, G. C. B.: De vroegste geschiedenis van het ontleedkundig onderwijs te Leiden (The earliest history of anatomical tuition in L.). *Ned. Tijdschr. Geneeskd.* **5**: 385—94, 1861.
Sylvius, P.: *Tfundament der medicinen ende chyrurgien.* Antwerpen: Willem Vorsterman, 1540.
Sypkens Smit, J. H.: *Leven en werken van Matthias van Geuns M.D.* (Life and works of M. v. G.). Thesis Groningen, 1953.

Talbot, H.: *Medicine in medieval England.* London: Oldbourne Book, 1967.
Taubert, E.: 75 Jahre Cholezystektomie. *Zentralbl. Chir.* **82**: 2058—63, 1957.
Tausk, M.: *Organon.* The story of an unusual pharmaceutical enterprise. Oss: Akzopharma, 1984.
Temkin, O.: *Galenism,* rise and decline of a medical philosophy. Ithaca, London: Cornell Univ. Press, 1973.
Temkin, O.: *The double face of Janus.* Baltimore, London: Johns Hopkins Univ. Press, 1977.
Theden, J. C. A.: *Genees- en heelkundig onderwijs voor land- en zee-chirurgijns* (Medical and surgical textbook for land and sea surgeons). Uit het Hoogduitsch vert. en met de gewoone ziekten ter ZEE . . . verrijkt door A. Schrage. Amsteldam: J. B. Elwe, 1782.
Theodoric: *The Surgery of Theoderic.* Transl. from the Latin by E. Campbell and J. Colton, 2 vols. New York: Appleton-Century-Crofts, 1955—60.
Thiels, Ch., Luyendijk-Elshout, A. M.: De Leidse chirurgijns en hun kamer boven de Waag (The Leyden surgeons and their hall over the Weighhouse). *Ned. Kunsthist. Jb.* **31**: 215—38, 1980.
Tilanus, C. B.: *Overzigt van de chirurgicale gebreken behandeld in het Binnen Gasthuis . . . gedurende den cursus 1852—1853* (Handwritten tables of the surgical cases treated in the Binnen Gasthuis in the academic year 1852—53). Amsterdam: Municipal Archives, 'Archief Klinische School'.
Tilanus, C. B.: *Surgery a hundred years ago.* Extracts from the diary of Dr. C. B. Tilanus. Ed. by prof. H. T. Deelman. London: G. Bles, 1925.
Tilanus, J. W. R.: *Herinneringswoord over wijlen Prof. C. L. Wurfbain* (In commemoration of the late Prof. C. L. W.). Amsterdam, 1905 (private print).
Tilanus, J. W. R.: De vernieuwing der stedelijke ziekenhuizen te Amsterdam in de 19de eeuw (The renovation of the municipal hospitals at Amsterdam in the 19th century). *Ned. Tijdschr. Geneeskd.* **51**(I): 85—112, 1907.
Titsingh, A.: *De verdonkerde heelkunst der Amsterdammers . . .* (The obscured surgery at Amsterdam). Alkmaar: G. Hazemaker, 1730; 1735^2.
Titsingh, A.: *Heelkundige verhandeling over den steen en het steensnijden . . .* (Surgical treatise on the stone and lithotomy). Amsterdam: G. Bouman, 1731.
Trendelenburg, F.: *Die ersten 25 Jahre der Deutschen Gesellschaft für Chirurgie.* Berlin: J. Springer, 1923.
Trent, J. C.: Surgical anaesthesia 1846—1946. *J. Hist. Med. all. Sci.* **1**: 505—26, 1946.
Trioen, K.: Genees- en heelkundige waarneemingen, Leide: P. van der Eyk & J. van der Kluis Pz., 1743.
Tuffier, Th.: *Chirurgie du poumon* en particulier dans les cavernes tuberculoses et la gangrène pulmonaire. Paris: Masson, 1897.
Tulp, N.: *Observationes medicae.* Editio nova, libro quarto auctior. Amstelredami: L. Elzevir, 1652.
Van Tussenbroek, A. P. C.: *De ontwikkeling der aseptische verloskunde in Nederland* (The development of aseptic obstetrics in Holland). Haarlem: F. Bohn, 1911.

Ulhoorn, H.: *See* Heister, L.

Veltheer, W.: The dawn of gastric resection. *Neth. J. Surg.* **38**: 107—14, 1981.
Van de Ven, A. J.: Een steensnijding in 1653 (A lithotomy in 1653). *Ned. Tijdschr. Geneeskd.* **79**(III): 3300—7, 3750—60, 1935.
Veraart, B. A. G.: G. Bidloo's verhaal van de laatste ziekte en het overlijden van Willem III, koning van Engeland (G. B.'s account of the last illness and the death of W. III, king of E.) *Ned. Tijdschr. Geneeskd.* **78**(IV): 5057—64, 1934.
Verduin, P. A.: *Nouvelle méthode pour amputer les membres.* Trad. en Fr. par Joseph Vergniol. Amsterdam: J. Wolters, 1697.
Verduin, P. A.: Twee en twintig heelkonstige waarnemingen. In: J. Scultetus: *Vermeerderde wapenhuis der heelmeesters* (Twenty-two surgical observations. In: J. Scultetus: Augmented arsenal of the surgeons), 2 vols. Amsterdam: Janssoons van Waesberge, 1748, vol. 2, pp. 987—1021.

Vergniol, J.: *See* Verduin: *Nouvelle méthode.*
Verkroost, C. M.: Paulus de Wind als steensnijder (P. de W. as lithotomist). *Med. Contact* **30**: 967—8, 1975.
Verkroost, C. M.: Paulus de Wind en zijn proefschrift (P. de W. and his thesis). *Med. Contact* **33**: 1034—6, 1978.
Vesalius, A.: *De humani corporis fabrica* libri septem. Basileae: ex. off. Ioannis Oporini, 1543 [Repr. Bruxelles: Culture et Civilization, 1964].
Da Vigo, G.: *Dat chyrurgylick werck* D. Johanis de Vigo Genuensis. Antwerpen: Claes de Grave, 1533.
De vijfhonderdste verjaring van de boekdrukkunst in de Nederlanden (The 500th anniversary of printing in the Netherlands). Catalogue of an exhibition. Brussel: Kon. Bibl. Albert I, 1973.
Vink, P.: *See* [De la Faye, G.].
Virchow, R.: Rokitansky. Handbuch der allg. path. Anatomie. *Preuss. med. Ztg.* **15**: 237—8, 1846.
Virchow, R.: *Die krankhaften Geschwülste*, 3 vols. Berlin: A. Hirschwald, 1863—7.
Van de Voorde, C.: *Lichtende fakkel der cheirurgia* (Illuminating torch of surgery). Amsterdam: J. Vinckel, 1668.
Vosmaer, J.: *Het leven en de wandelingen van meester Maarten Vroeg* (Life and strolls of Master M.V.). New annotated ed. by J. Wagelaar. Culemborg: Tjeenk Willink/Noorduyn, 1978.

Walsh, J.: Galen's writings and influences inspiring them. *Ann. med. Hist.* NS **9**: 34—61, 1937.
Webster, Ch.: The Helmontian George Thomson and William Harvey: the revival and application of splenectomy to physiological research. *Med. Hist.* **15**: 154—67, 1971.
Westerman, C. W. J.: Over intrathorakale oesophagusresectie (On intrathoracical oesophagus resection). *Ned. Tijdschr. Geneeskd.* **41**: 1621—5, 1905.
Westerman, C. W. J.: Thoraxexcisie by recidief van carcinoma mammae (Excision of the thorax in a case of recurrent mammary cancer). *Ned. Tijdschr. Geneeskd.* **54**(II): 1686—90, 1910.
Westerman, C. W. J.: Behandeling van de peritonitis met de neuskatheter (Treatment of peritonitis with nasal catheter). *Ned. Tijdschr. Geneeskd.* **55**(I): 1956—7, 1911.
Van der Weyde, A. J.: Iets over steenssnijden en steensnijders (Something about lithotomy and lithotomists). *Ned. Tijdschr. Geneeskd.* **68**(II): 655—66, 1924.
Van der Weyde, A. J.: Eed voor een heelmeester in 1811 (Oath for a surgeon in 1811). *Ned. Tijdschr. Geneeskd.* **68**(II): 1258, 1924.
White [C. P.]: An account of a case in which the upper head of the os humeri was sawed off, a large portion of the bone afterwards exfoliated, and yet the entire motion of the limb was preserved. By Mr. White, surgeon, at Manchester. Communicated by Mr. Watson, F. R. S. *Philosoph. Trans.* **59**: 39—46, 1770.
Von Winniwarter, A.: *Beiträge zur Statistik der Carcinome* mit besondere Rücksicht auf die dauerende Heilbarkeit durch operative Behandlung. Stuttgart: F. Enke, 1878.
Wintgens, E.: *Johannes Monnikhoff en zijn legaat* (J. M. and his legacy). Thesis Leyden, 1879.
Withington, E. T.: *See* Hippocrates.
Wright, W. C.: *See* Lancisi.
Van Wy, G. J.: Bekroond antwoord op prijsvraag: 'Kunnen wij ons overtuigd houden, dat een waare kanker immer zonder de afzetting tot genezing is gebracht?'. (Can we be certain that a true cancer has ever been cured without amputation?). *Hand. Geneesk. Genootsch.* 'Servandis Civibus' **4**: 3—206, 1779.
Van Wyck, J.: *Waarneminge rakende eenen fungus* . . . waar vooraf gaan, briefswijze aanmerkingen op de voorreden van den Heere P. Vink . . . voor . . . Aanmerkingen op de chir. operatien van . . . Dionis (Observation relating to a fungus . . . preceded by remarks made in a letter to Mr. Vink . . . on . . . 'Aanmerkingen'). Rotterdam: H. Kentlink & J. Bosch, 1740.

Yperman, Jan: *De 'Cyrurgie' van meester Jan Yperman.* Ed. in Dutch by E. C. van Leersum after Mss in Brussels, Cambridge, Ghent and London. Leiden: A. W. Sijthoff, 1912.

Zaayer, J. H.: Overdruknarcose en experimentele slokdarmresectie (Insufflation anaesthesia and experimental oesophagus resection). *Ned. Tijdschr. Geneeskd.* **54**(II): 2295—7, 1910.
Zaayer, J. H.: Eenige gevallen van thorax-operatie uit de cliniek van prof. Korteweg (A few cases of thoracic operation from the clinic of professor K.). *Ned. Tijdschr. Geneeskd.* **57**(I): 1593—4, 1913.
Zaayer, J. H.: Heelkundige behandeling van bronchiectasen (Surgical treatment of bronchiectasis). *Ned. Tijdschr. Geneeskd.* **71**(II): 1724—37, 1927.

Zambon, J.-V.: Brugmans, voorloper van Semmelweis (B., precursor of S.). *Ned. Tijdschr. Geneeskd.* **127**: 1060—4, 1983.
Zimmerman, L. M., Veith, I.: *Great ideas in the history of surgery.* Baltimore: William & Wilkins, 1961.
Van Zuiden, D. S.: Op welke voorwaarden de hofschoenmaker van den Koning van Denemarken zijn breuk liet opereeren (On what terms the court shoemaker of the king of Denmark had his hernia operated upon). *Ned. Tijdschr. Geneeskd.* **62**(I): 1535, 1918.
Van der Zwaag, P.: *Wouter van Doeveren* (1730—1783). Thesis Free University Amsterdam, 1970.
Zwaveling, A., Hulsman, G.: Machiel Polano, laatste heelmeester van het oude tijdperk (M. P. last surgeon of the old era). *Ned. Tijdschr. Geneeskd.* **109**: 2091—5, 1965.

Index of Names

Numbers in italics refer to pages containing dates of birth and death

MIX
Papier aus verantwortungsvollen Quellen
Paper from responsible sources
FSC® C105338

If you have any concerns about our products,
you can contact us on
ProductSafety@springernature.com

In case Publisher is established outside the EU,
the EU authorized representative is:
Springer Nature Customer Service Center GmbH
Europaplatz 3, 69115 Heidelberg, Germany

Printed by Libri Plureos GmbH
in Hamburg, Germany